The Oxford Handbook
of Auditory Science
The Auditory Brain

The Oxford Handbook of Auditory Science
The Auditory Brain

VOLUME 2

Edited by

Adrian Rees
Institute of Neuroscience
Newcastle University
UK

and

Alan R. Palmer
MRC Institute of Hearing Research
Nottingham
UK

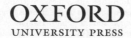

OXFORD
UNIVERSITY PRESS

OXFORD

UNIVERSITY PRESS

Great Clarendon Street, Oxford OX2 6DP

Oxford University Press is a department of the University of Oxford.
It furthers the University's objective of excellence in research, scholarship,
and education by publishing worldwide in

Oxford New York

Auckland Cape Town Dar es Salaam Hong Kong Karachi
Kuala Lumpur Madrid Melbourne Mexico City Nairobi
New Delhi Shanghai Taipei Toronto

With offices in

Argentina Austria Brazil Chile Czech Republic France Greece
Guatemala Hungary Italy Japan Poland Portugal Singapore
South Korea Switzerland Thailand Turkey Ukraine Vietnam

Oxford is a registered trade mark of Oxford University Press
in the UK and in certain other countries

Published in the United States
by Oxford University Press Inc., New York

British Library Cataloguing in Publication Data

Data available

Library of Congress Cataloging-in-Publication Data
Oxford handbook of auditory science : the auditory brain / edited by
Alan R. Palmer and Adrian Rees.
     p. ; cm.
  Includes bibliographical references and index.
  ISBN 978-0-19-923328-1 (pbk. : alk. paper) 1. Auditory
pathways–Physiology–Handbooks, manuals, etc. 2. Auditory
pathways–Diseases–Handbooks, manuals, etc. I. Palmer, A. R. (Alan R.)
II. Rees, Adrian. III. Title: Handbook of auditory science.
  [DNLM: 1. Auditory Pathways–physiology–Handbooks. 2. Auditory
Diseases, Central–physiopathology–Handbooks. 3. Evoked Potentials,
Auditory–physiology–Handbooks. WV 39 0985 2010]
  RF290.094 2010
  617.8–dc22   2009033182

Typeset in Minion by Glyph International, Bangalore, India
Printed in China
on acid-free paper through
Asia Pacific Offset

ISBN 978-0-19-923328-1

10 9 8 7 6 5 4 3 2 1

Series Preface

Auditory science has been, over the past three decades, one of the fastest growing areas of biomedical research. Worldwide there are now perhaps 10 000 researchers whose primary job is auditory research, and ten times that number working in allied, mainly clinical, hearing professions. This rapid growth is attributable to and, in turn, fuelled by several major developments in our understanding. While this Handbook focuses on fundamental research and underlying mechanisms, it does so from the perspective of understanding the impact of auditory science on the quality of our life. That impact has been realized through the explosive growth of digital technology and microelectronics, and delivered by devices as diverse as MP3 compression for music listening (based on models of perceptual coding) to the latest instruments for the management of hearing loss, including digital hearing aids and multichannel cochlear implants. The discovery of otoacoustic emissions (OAEs) – sounds produced by the cochlea – has enabled a step change both in our understanding of ear function and in the development of a clinical tool for deafness screening in newborn infants.

Fundamental research on the inner ear has shown that an elaborate system of sound-induced active processes, acting through the outer hair cells, serves to improve sensitivity, sharpen frequency tuning, dynamically modulate the mechanical response of the ear to sound, and create sound energy that passes back out of the ear. Each of these processes is also influenced by descending neural input to the hair cells. Most recently, the molecular machinery underlying these incredible phenomena has been explored and described in detail. The development, maintenance, and repair of the ear are also subjects of contemporary interest at the molecular level, as is the genetics of hearing disorders due to cochlear malfunctions. The auditory brain is responsible for sound (including speech) identification and localization. Through functional neuroimaging in humans, and the application of novel methods in animals, such as multichannel recordings of single unit activity, multiple cortical and subcortical areas necessarily involved in hearing and listening have now been identified and characterized. These areas occupy the superior (dorsal) temporal cortex, and extend into non-classical cortical regions, including the more rostral and ventral temporal lobe, the limbic system, and elsewhere in the frontal and parietal lobes. Understanding of subcortical processing has expanded through the use of molecular and cellular techniques *in vitro* and recordings in awake and behaving humans and animals *in vivo*. Increasingly, the widespread descending pathways are being shown to have profound functional importance, and to influence the coding of both simple and complex sounds. Recent studies of hearing (auditory perception) have shown how our perceptions relate to the underlying physiological mechanisms. For example, behavioural measures of peripheral auditory function have led to the development of sophisticated models of cochlear processing in humans. These models are having widespread influence in understanding both normal and pathological hearing. At the same time, there has been an increasing focus on auditory 'ecology', on complex sound perception in real (or virtual) environments. Traditional distinctions between spectral, temporal, and binaural processing have evolved into more functional concerns, including auditory scene analysis and auditory object perception.

Here, then, are the three major domains of auditory science – the ear, the brain, and hearing – and I am proud to present a corresponding three-volume Handbook. However, as the volume

editors and I started sifting through all the areas we wished to cover, a number of recent developments in our science became apparent that made us question the way in which we had decided to
partition the field. Spurred on by ever-increasing knowledge, the availability of enabling technology, and cultural shifts in attitudes towards 'relevance' and 'interdisciplinary' research, the three
domains have begun to blur into one. Several instances of this are hinted at above: a transition
from more segmented to more holistic approaches to audition; a shift in focus from more simple
to more complex and, hence, more realistic sounds; and a drilling down across traditional disci-
plinary boundaries from the phenomenological to the mechanistic and generic. Dynamic properties of hearing are becoming more prominent across all three domains, and beyond, as lifespan
development, adaptation, and learning receive increasing recognition. Reciprocal influences of
hearing on and from cognition (attention, memory, and emotion), action, and vision add to a
picture of a powerful, working, integrated sense that is arguably the most important we possess
for what makes us distinctly human – our social interaction with our world. Organizationally,
researchers at all levels (peripheral, central, and perceptual) now work increasingly together, with
many major and several new interdisciplinary centres of auditory science dotted across the
globe.

Our ambitious aim has been to deliver a working Handbook that would fill an unmet need for
a single reference work spanning all of auditory science. We wanted it to offer a basic background
for all those interested in the subject, from the curious undergraduate to the professional
researcher and clinician, while also capturing the excitement, and some of the detail, of the most
recent developments in this rapidly evolving discipline. Consequently, we set out with the conflicting aims of producing a comprehensive, even definitive work, but of completing it within the
minimum time possible. We optimistically targeted this at one year, recognizing that the finished
product would have a finite lifespan. In fact, the preparation of the chapters, from commissioning
to collection of the final versions of the final chapters, has taken about two years. Although
disappointing to us, Martin Baum, our very helpful and ever patient senior commissioning editor
at Oxford University Press, has tried to console us, suggesting that even this effort has been
something of a world record.

I knew at the outset of this project that its success would be completely dependent on the
recruitment of the right volume editors. I feel incredibly lucky and humbled to have retained the
services of four colleagues whose insight, experience, determination, interpersonal skills, and
sheer hard work have managed to get this Handbook together more quickly than some of my own
previous book chapters have taken to be read by the book's editors, and more professionally than
I had dreamed possible. Many, many thanks to all four – my dedication is to you.

David R. Moore
MRC Institute of Hearing Research
Nottingham
April 2009

Contents

Contributors

Richard A. Altschuler
Kresge Hearing Research Institute,
University of Michigan, Ann Arbor, USA

Jorge L. Armony
Douglas Mental Health University Institute,
McGill University, Montreal QC, Canada

Doris-Eva Bamiou
Neuro-otology Department,
National Hospital for Neurology and
Neurosurgery, Queen Square, London, UK

Daniel Bendor
Laboratory of Auditory Neurophysiology,
Department of Biomedical Engineering,
Johns Hopkins School of Medicine,
Baltimore, USA

Jos J. Eggermont
Department of Physiology and
Pharmacology, and
Department of Psychology,
University of Calgary,
Calgary AB, Canada

Yonatan I. Fishman
Department of Neurology,
Rose F. Kennedy Center,
Albert Einstein College of Medicine,
Bronx, NY, USA

Robert D. Frisina
Department of Otolaryngology,
University of Rochester Medical Center,
Rochester, NY, USA

Timothy D. Griffiths
Auditory Group
Institute of Neuroscience,
Newcastle University,
Newcastle upon Tyne, UK

Benedikt Grothe
Department Biology II,
Ludwig-Maximilians-Universität München,
Planegg-Martinsried, Germany

Troy A. Hackett
Department of Hearing and Speech Sciences,
Vanderbilt University School of Medicine,
Nashville, USA

Douglas E.H. Hartley
Department of Physiology, Anatomy and
Genetics, Sherrington Building,
University of Oxford, Oxford, UK

Jufang He
Department of Rehabilitation Sciences,
The Hong Kong Polytechnic University,
Hung Hom,
Kowloon, Hong Kong, China

Dexter R.F. Irvine
School of Psychology, Psychiatry and
Psychological Medicine,
Monash University, Australia
and
The Bionic Ear Institute,
East Melbourne, Australia

Andrew J. King
Department of Physiology, Anatomy and
Genetics, Sherrington Building,
University of Oxford, Oxford, UK

Achim Klug
Department of Physiology and Biophysics,
University of Colorado at Denver,
Aurora, USA

Shigeyuki Kuwada
Department of Neuroscience,
University of Connecticut Health Center,
Farmington, USA

Joseph E. LeDoux
Center for Neural Science,
New York University, New York, USA

Ruth Y. Litovsky
Department of Communicative Disorders,
University of Wisconsin, Waisman Center 521,
Madison, USA

Manuel S. Malmierca
Auditory Neurophysiology Unit,
Institute for Neuroscience of Castilla y León
Faculty of Medicine,
University of Salamanca,
Spain

Brian Malone
Coleman Memorial Laboratory,
Department of Otolaryngology and
Head and Neck Surgery,
University of California,
San Francisco, USA

Bradford J. May
Department of Otolaryngology-Head and
Neck Surgery,
Johns Hopkins University School of
Medicine, Baltimore, USA

David McAlpine
UCL Ear Institute,
332 Gray's Inn Road,
London, UK

Alan R. Palmer
MRC Institute of Hearing Research,
University Park,
Nottingham, UK

Adrian Rees
Auditory Group,
Institute of Neuroscience,
Newcastle University,
Newcastle upon Tyne, UK

Brett R. Schofield
Department of Anatomy and Neurobiology,
Northeastern Ohio Universities College of
Medicine,
Rootstown, USA

Christoph E. Schreiner
Coleman Memorial Laboratory,
Department of Otolaryngology and
Head and Neck Surgery,
University of California,
San Francisco, USA

Sophie K. Scott
Institute of Cognitive Neuroscience,
University College London,
London, UK

Robert V. Shannon
House Ear Institute,
Auditory Implant Research,
Los Angeles, USA

Susan E. Shore
Kresge Hearing Research Institute,
University of Michigan, Ann Arbor, USA

Donal G. Sinex
Department of Psychology,
Utah State University, Logan, USA

Mitchell Steinschneider
Department of Neurology,
Rose F. Kennedy Center,
Albert Einstein College of Medicine,
Bronx, USA

Xiaoqin Wang
Laboratory of Auditory Neurophysiology,
Department of Biomedical Engineering,
Johns Hopkins School of Medicine,
Baltimore, USA

Jason D. Warren
Dementia Research Centre,
Institute of Neurology,
National Hospital for Neurology and
Neurosurgery, Queen Square,
London, UK

Norman M. Weinberger
Center for the Neurobiology of
Learning and Memory,
Department of Neurobiology and Behavior
University of California Irvine,
Irvine, CA, USA

Tom C.T. Yin
Department of Physiology,
University of Wisconsin,
Madison, USA

Eric D. Young
Biomedical Engineering,
Johns Hopkins School of Medicine,
Baltimore, USA

Yanqin Yu
Department of Physiology,
Zhejiang University School of Medicine,
HangZhou, China

Chapter 1

Overview

Adrian Rees and Alan R. Palmer

The purpose of this volume is to introduce the reader to the fascinating complexity of what we have chosen to call the auditory brain: those neural centres and their connections that enable us to perceive and interpret sounds that have been transduced into neural activity by the cochlea.

Hearing, with its obvious link to language, is arguably the most important of all the senses in separating humans from other animals. The perception of sound underlies the enormous richness and complexity of our vocal communication, which, together with music, has been a primary driver of human intellectual and cultural development. However, long before we became creatures of the theatre or concert hall, hearing played an important part in our survival and evolution. Hearing alerted our ancestors to approaching predators, and signalled the presence of prey before it came in sight. Hearing not only allows us to detect the presence of such threats or opportunities, it also enables us to locate them; running in the direction of safety rather than into the jaws of the predator is an essential rule in winning the survival game! These vital advantages to humans and other animals that hearing provides makes stern demands on the system that is responsible for detecting and analysing the pressure waves that constitute sounds.

Vision, with a few exceptions, provides a limited view of an animal's surroundings, and this is particularly true of primates, carnivores, and other species that have sacrificed visual field for depth perception. Foveal vision enables the animal to select the object to view. Hearing, on the other hand, always samples the whole sound field; even by turning the head, or in some animals rotating the ears, towards a sound source it is not possible to exclude sounds originating from other sources and directions. Thus separating and distinguishing sound sources are essential processes for hearing, and particular challenges for the auditory brain.

Another important difference between hearing and other senses (e.g. vision and somatosensation) is in the spatial representation of objects. In vision, objects at different points in space stimulate topographically equivalent positions on the receptor array in the retina. In contrast, the spatial position of a sound source is not mapped onto the hair cell receptors arrayed along the basilar membrane in the inner ear. The displacement of the basilar membrane reflects the frequency and level of the components of a sound, so sound source location, for the most part, must be computed in the brain utilizing cues that are extracted from the spectral, temporal, and level differences at the ears that arise from sounds occupying different positions in space. Perhaps for this reason alone the organization of the auditory system with its many subthalamic nuclei linked by a bewildering pattern of connections is more complex than the equivalent pathways for other senses.

Sounds are waveforms defined by pressure fluctuations in the medium through which they propagate, and they are thus inherently time dependent. They are in constant flux, and auditory objects cannot in their entirety be frozen into a brief glimpse. This fundamental physical property of sounds has required the auditory brain to evolve the capacity to encode time-dependent information with an exquisite precision that exceeds that of any other sensory system. Viewed from a particular instant in time, all information-bearing elements of sounds, like syllables or words, have a history and a future, and virtually all sounds that have any biological significance are characterized by time-dependent changes in their parameters.

For all these reasons, the auditory brain can be rather intimidating for the new student. This is exacerbated by the fact that central auditory processing is usually given only superficial coverage by most neuroscience textbooks, and there are few resources between that level and the primary sources to help a reader who seeks a more detailed understanding of the field. Another potential difficulty for the newcomer is the diverse range of techniques that are harnessed to study the brain. These range from methods that address the structural and functional properties of single cells, like immunocytochemistry and single unit recording, to functional magnetic resonance imaging (fMRI), magnetoencephalography (MEG) and behaviour that provide a window on the function of the brain in its entirety. One of the challenges for neuroscience is to discover how these multiple levels of brain organization are interrelated and lead to perception.

Our aim here has been to bring together, in a single volume, an account of what is known about the brain mechanisms that underlie different facets of hearing; their anatomy and physiology, what changes occur during development and ageing, and the consequences when they malfunction. We have commissioned succinct, up-to-date accounts of the current state of knowledge, written by experts in their field. We hope these will not only serve as an introduction for those who are exploring auditory processing for the first time, but also provide a valuable resource for experienced auditory scientists who want to know more about a field outside their speciality. The book is intended to give an overview of the field, to identify the main concepts and controversies, and provide sufficient orientation to enable the reader to plunge with confidence into the primary literature.

Research monographs often tackle the auditory pathway on a hierarchical centre-by-centre basis, beginning at the auditory nerve and working chapter by chapter towards the cortex. This approach often reflects each author's focus of endeavour within the auditory pathway, and while useful to others studying the same brain area, it is less useful for the reader who wants to grasp the bigger picture. In contrast, each chapter in this volume explores its subject over the whole auditory pathway in an attempt to provide a more integrated account.

The organizing principle of the book is its arrangement into several themes that we believe define the field: how sounds are encoded for their identification and location; changes that occur in the auditory pathway throughout life; how sounds influence emotions, learning, and memory; and disorders of the auditory brain and its potential as a target for auditory prostheses.

Of course it is not possible to explore these functionally orientated themes without some scene setting that describes the anatomical substrate that underpins them. This is provided by Section 1 which outlines the anatomy of the auditory pathway and its synaptic organization, providing the contextual material on which the remainder of the book depends. Thus, Malmierca and Hackett (Chapter 2) describe the structural and functional organization of the ascending auditory pathway. They explain the location and cellular architecture of the auditory centres in the brainstem, thalamus, and cortex, together with the interconnecting pathways that carry the flow of information from the output of the cochlea to the cortex.

While this ascending, bottom-up pathway is clearly essential for sensation, it is also intuitively obvious, and increasingly apparent from experimental studies, that auditory perception relies extensively on past experience, attention, and emotional state analysed at higher levels of the pathway. The extensive, but often overlooked, network of descending, top-down connections whereby activity generated by these aspects of auditory processing can intercept and modify the upward flow of information is described by Schofield (Chapter 3).

In the final chapter in this section, Altschuler and Shore (Chapter 4) outline the roles of the many neurotransmitters and synaptic mechanisms that subserve the neuronal interactions in the auditory brain.

With this background in place, Section 2 addresses the theme of how sounds are encoded for their identification. Young (Chapter 5) tackles how spectrum and level, the most elemental properties of all sounds, are encoded. A significant part of this chapter discusses responses to pure tones, noise bursts, and other relatively simple stimuli. Such sounds have been invaluable probes for studying the auditory system, because the processing of sound begins with its analysis by frequency in the cochlea (see The Ear, Volume 1 of this Handbook). However, as is also apparent from Young's chapter, the auditory system is remarkably nonlinear, so that responses to simple sounds often fail to predict responses to more complex sounds.

The remaining chapters in this section develop this theme of complexity. In Chapter 6, Malone and Schreiner describe how sounds whose amplitudes fluctuate with time are encoded at different levels of the auditory pathway. This chapter emphasizes that temporal information in sounds resides not just in the rapid pressure fluctuations that determine the spectral content, or fine structure, of the waveform, but also in the slower variations of amplitude that shape the waveform's envelope.

Pitch is a quality that is so readily ascribed to many sounds, both simple and complex, that one might expect that pinpointing its manner of representation in the brain would be easy. Perhaps because so many facets of a stimulus can contribute to the pitch percept, understanding where and how it is encoded has proved elusive. Wang and Bendor (Chapter 7) reveal that neuronal recording and imaging techniques are now beginning to impact on this problem and provide evidence for brain areas specific for the analysis and representation of pitch.

The review of how different categories of stimuli are encoded is completed with two chapters that examine sounds that have the greatest biological significance; the sounds that animals generate themselves. In Chapter 8, Klug and Grothe focus on bats. These are particularly interesting species to study because they produce sounds not just for communication, but also for echolocating their prey. The auditory systems of these animals are beautifully adapted to these tasks, and thus provide a fascinating insight into how the auditory brain can become highly specialized, as well as revealing processing mechanisms of more general application.

Understanding how speech sounds are encoded and processed is of particular interest in understanding the human auditory system, and this is explored by Scott and Sinex (Chapter 9). Because it is unique to humans there are obvious limitations on the techniques we can apply to study the different brain centres involved. The advent of brain imaging in conscious humans has been a huge step forward for studying speech processing at the cortical level, but the technical limitations of such brain imaging techniques limit their usefulness for studying lower centres or for providing detailed neurophysiological mechanisms. Information about the responses of neurons to speech sounds currently is almost entirely limited to measurements made in animals and makes the assumption that the fundamental coding strategies in the mammalian auditory system are well conserved.

Sounds generated by people and animals are often characterized by the presence of many spectral components. In the real world, such sounds rarely occur in isolation, but in a cacophony of different, but similar sounds, as at the eponymous cocktail party. The challenge for the auditory brain is thus not just the recognition of isolated sounds, but also of segregation: components from a single source must be grouped together and segregated from those belonging to other sources. Given the overlap that often exists between frequency components originating from different sources, our capacity to form these auditory streams is remarkable, and far beyond the capability of any machine. Fishman and Steinschneider (Chapter 10) discuss how the brain might extract the cues upon which this process depends. It seems likely that we use top-down as well as bottom-up processing for this task. As discussed earlier, we know much less about the role of these descending influences in auditory processing, but the emerging story of this important aspect of the auditory brain is explored by He and Yu (Chapter 11).

Section 3 considers the second aspect of sound encoding, how sounds are located. Key to this process is that the ears are separated by the solid mass of the head and so sample the sound field differently. This arrangement leads to disparities in the timing and level of the sound waves between the ears, and Yin and Kuwada (Chapter 12) describe the neural circuits that can extract these cues to enable us to localize sounds in the horizontal plane. However, as May describes in Chapter 13, localizing sounds in the vertical plane relies on monaural mechanisms derived from cues generated by the interaction of the sound waves with the outer ear and the head. In Chapter 14, the final chapter in this section, Litovsky and McAlpine discuss how binaural mechanisms involved in locating sounds in space also make an important contribution to isolating single sound sources and segregating them from others.

Hearing, like most aspects of brain function, changes throughout life and these changes are examined in Section 4. It is easy to predict that development might play an important role in the auditory brain because the sensory cues that an animal receives will change as its head grows. In Chapter 15, Hartley and King discuss how the auditory brain matures during development and the impact that sensory experience during early life has on this process. Such plasticity in the auditory pathway was once believed only to occur during early development, but it is now recognized that plasticity also occurs in the adult animal. Irvine (Chapter 16) discusses how changing the input to the auditory brain, often as a consequence of an insult to the cochlea, can lead to a reorganization of neuronal connections and function. Much of the decline in hearing experienced with age is attributable to loss of function at the receptor level in the cochlea, but, as Frisina (Chapter 17) explains, processing in the auditory brain also declines during ageing because of changes in its intrinsic organization, as well as those induced by a reduced input.

Sounds are not just stimuli that we perceive; as anyone who has been reduced to tears by a piece of music can attest, they have a considerable capacity to influence our emotional and cognitive states. Some aspects of these processes are explored in Section 5. Weinberger (Chapter 18) discusses how the auditory cortex must be viewed as much more than just a sound analyser. Evidence shows that it is also a substrate of learning and memory, and thus directly influences the way sounds modify behaviour and cognitive state. Armony and LeDoux (Chapter 19) describe how the limbic system must be seen as an extension of the auditory brain, and they tease out the mechanisms whereby sounds contribute to our emotions.

The final section considers disorders of the auditory brain. While most hearing loss has its origin in pathological changes in the cochlea, subtle deficits in auditory processing arise from lesions in specific regions of the auditory pathway, or as a consequence of developmental or acquired disorders. In their survey of these conditions in Chapter 20, Griffiths *et al.* demonstrate that such cases can provide powerful insights into functional mechanisms of the auditory brain. The perception of phantom sounds known as tinnitus, an affliction bringing misery to many, is often associated with cochlear hearing loss. While sensorineural hearing loss is often a precipitating condition for tinnitus, recent research suggests that the origin of such phantom percepts lies in changes to the auditory brain, particularly the midbrain and cortex. How this condition manifests itself and the mechanisms that give rise to it are discussed by Eggermont (Chapter 21). In the past 25 years the astonishing success of cochlear implants has revolutionized the treatment of profound sensorineural deafness originating in the cochlea. In the final chapter (22) Shannon reports how this prosthetic technology can be taken a stage further by implanting electrodes directly into the brainstem or midbrain to provide benefit to those whose hearing loss results from bilateral loss of the auditory nerves.

While our intention is to represent as many different facets of the auditory brain as possible in one place, there are inevitably some gaps. For example, one area we have not been able to cover is the fascinating story that is emerging on multimodal interactions between the auditory brain and the other senses: perhaps these omissions can be included in a future edition.

We are immensely grateful to the authors who have contributed so much of their expertise and time to produce this volume. To produce a critical summary of a huge body of research within the confines of a short chapter is a difficult task, and we appreciate the generous spirit with which they accepted our editing to make them shorter still! We also wish to thank Martin Baum, our Editor at OUP, and his colleagues, for their help with the book's production. We hope the result is a wide ranging and accessible survey that also provides the researcher, hearing professional, or student with sufficient depth to gain a true insight into the organization and function of the auditory brain.

Section 1

Structural and functional organization of the auditory brain

Chapter 2

Structural organization of the ascending auditory pathway

Manuel S. Malmierca and Troy A. Hackett

The aim of this chapter is to highlight the structural organization of the ascending auditory system. We focus on the general plan of organization of the auditory system in mammals, since a major objective in hearing research is to understand the structure and function of the human auditory system, and to identify the causes of, and treatments for, hearing impairment.

The range of frequencies to which the ear responds varies between species. In the rat the frequency range is 0.25–70 kHz (reviewed in Malmierca, 2003), while it is about 2–70 kHz in the mouse, 0.2–45 in the guinea pig, and 0.125–60 in the cat. In humans the range is 0.02–20 kHz. The hearing of some animals, e.g., echolocating bats, is particularly tuned to certain frequencies of special importance to their behavior (reviewed in Fay and Popper, 1994) and they are considered to be 'auditory specialists' (Echteler *et al.*, 1994). The representation of frequency is a major organizing principle in the auditory system and thus the frequency range is an important influence on the anatomy of the structures in the auditory brain.

Sound waves are transmitted mechanically through the outer and middle ear to the sensory hair cells of the organ of Corti on the cochlear partition of the inner ear (see The Ear, Volume 1 of this Handbook). Auditory (cochlear) nerve fibers that synapse on the inner hair cells (IHCs) transmit information to the brainstem in the form of patterns of action potentials initiated in response to receptor potentials generated in the hair cells (Fig. 2.1). In the first relay center, i.e., the cochlear nucleus complex (CNC), the signals of the auditory nerve (AN) are shunted into a number of parallel ascending tracts, each with its own particular course and destination.

The ascending auditory tracts converge towards the auditory midbrain (Fig. 2.2); the inferior colliculus (IC) is an obligatory relay on the route to the auditory cortex. From the IC upwards, the auditory pathway can be divided into a 'core projection' where the tonotopic organization is very precise and a 'belt projection' where it is less defined (for review see Malmierca, 2003). In contrast to the single thalamic relay station between the periphery and cerebral cortex in the visual system, there is a minimum of three relays, several stages of convergence and divergence, and at least seven decussations that make the auditory system unique (Fig. 2.2).

2.1 The auditory nerve

The AN consists of two types of nerve fibers: *afferent* and *efferent* (for review see Slepecky, 1996). The afferent fibers transmit impulses to the CNC, while the efferent fibers convey impulses from the superior olivary complex to the organ of Corti (Fig. 2.1; Chapter 3).

There are two subtypes of afferent fibers (Fig. 2.1): the thick myelinated fibers arising from the bipolar type I spiral ganglion cells innervating the inner hair cells (IHCs), and the thin unmyelinated fibers arising from monopolar type II spiral ganglion cells innervating the outer hair cells (OHCs).

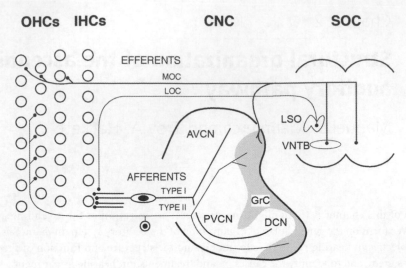

Fig. 2.1 Afferent and efferent innervation of the outer (OHC) and inner (IHC) hair cells in the cochlea. Afferent connections of type I and II auditory nerve fibers terminate among the anteroventral (AVCN), posteroventral (PVCN), and dorsal (DCN) cochlear nuclei. Efferent fibers of the olivocochlear bundle arise from the medial (MOC) and lateral (LOC) nuclei of the superior olivary complex (SOC) and terminate on OHCs and the afferent fibers that synapse on IHCs. (Modified and redrawn after Brown *et al.*, 1988.)

Studies in the cat have demonstrated that 90–95% of afferent AN fibres are type I fibers that contact only IHCs (Fig. 2.1). These are unbranched and each fiber terminates on a single IHC. Each IHC contacts about 20 different fibers (Spoendlin, 1972). The precise number of nerve fibers that synapse with each IHC varies, but seems to be larger in frequency regions that are functionally important. More recent studies have detailed the fine structure and organization of the innervation in several species (Warr, 1992).

The synapses between IHCs and afferent fibers are characterized at the presynaptic zone by the existence of a presynaptic bar surrounded by a number of synaptic vesicles (for review see Slepecky, 1996). The shape and size of these synaptic bars vary among the IHCs and it has been suggested that this change is due to the physiological characteristics of the postsynaptic fibers and the functional state of the IHCs (reviewed in Slepecky, 1996). In the cat, three types of type I fiber have been characterized based on morphological features that correlate with their spontaneous activity (low, medium, and high) and threshold sensitivity (Liberman *et al.*, 1990). Low threshold, high spontaneous rate fibers have large diameters and are located at the lateral side of the IHC, while high threshold, low spontaneous rate fibers are thinner and located on the medial side.

The unmyelinated type II fibers arise from small unipolar ganglion cells and constitute about 5% of all ganglion cells (Fig. 2.1). In contrast to type I, type II fibers are highly branched and a single fiber synapses onto 6–100 OHCs (Spoendlin, 1972) as they spiral down towards the base of the cochlea.

In addition to the afferent fibers, there are two systems of efferent fibers (Fig. 2.1): the lateral efferent system (LOC; lateral olivocochlear system) that innervates the IHCs and the medial efferent system (MOC; medial olivocochlear system) that innervates the OHCs (Warr, 1992). They make up the olivocochlear system which is the final part of the descending auditory pathway. This will be treated in detail by Schofield (see Chapter 3).

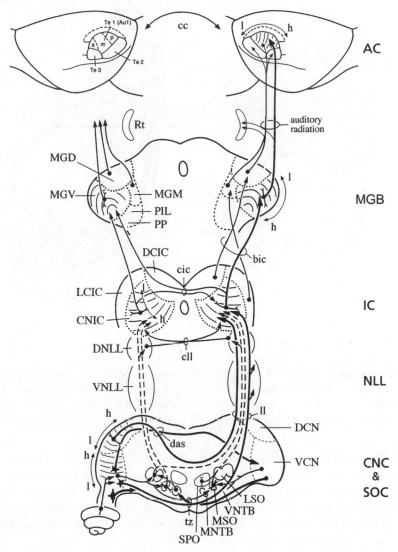

Fig. 2.2 Schematic diagram of the central auditory pathways in the rat associated with input from a single cochlea. Ascending and commissural projections between nuclei are indicated by *arrows* (*heavy lines*, strong connections; *dashed lines*, weaker connections). See List of Abbreviations for full names of structures. (Modified and redrawn after Brodal, 1981, AC is from Herbert *et al.*, 1991.)

2.2 The cochlear nuclear complex

The cochlear nuclear complex (CNC) (Fig. 2.3) is the site of termination of all AN fibers, and is thus the first relay center of the ascending auditory pathway (Cant and Benson, 2003). The axons of CNC projection neurons use three primary pathways to reach higher auditory structures: the dorsal, intermediate, and ventral acoustic striae (DAS, IAS, and VAS respectively; the VAS is also referred to as the trapezoid body (Fig. 2.4). The CNC receives descending projections from the auditory brainstem, midbrain and cortex as well as other non-auditory brain structures (for review see Malmierca, 2003).

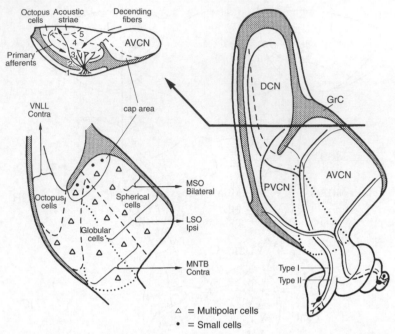

Fig. 2.3 Organization of the cochlear nucleus. *Right*, type I and II auditory nerve fiber inputs to the anteroventral and posteroventral nuclei (AVCN, PVCN) and dorsal nucleus (DCN). *Lower left*, distribution of neuronal types and associated projection to medial superior olive (MSO), lateral superior olive (LSO), and medial nucleus of the trapezoid body (MNTB). *Upper left* shows a cross section as indicated by the *arrow* indicating the connections of the dorsal cochlear nucleus pyramidal cells. (Redrawn after Osen, 1988.)

The CNC is situated laterally and superficially in the pons (Fig. 2.2). There are some interspecies variations in its location and spatial orientation, presumably secondary to differences in the shape of the brainstem. The CNC consists of a ventral cochlear nucleus (VCN) and a dorsal cochlear nucleus (DCN). The VCN is subdivided by the cochlear nerve root into an anteroventral (AVCN) and a posteroventral (PVCN) cochlear nucleus. The VCN is flattened mediolaterally. The DCN curves around the restiform body.

2.2.1 **Primary afferents**

The AN fibers terminate within the CNC in an orderly manner according to the sound frequencies to which they are tuned, giving rise to what is termed a tonotopic representation (Lorente de Nó, 1981). Each fiber bifurcates into an ascending branch which supplies the AVCN and a descending branch which supplies the PVCN and DCN (Figs 2.1 and 2.3). The anatomical distribution of the primary fibers forms the basis for the laminar tonotopic organization of the three subnuclei. This tonotopic organization has been demonstrated electrophysiologically, and also by c-*fos* immunocytochemistry (for review see Ryugo and Parks, 2003).

Myelinated type I and unmyelinated type II axons follow similar bifurcation patterns, but the total terminal area and mode of termination differ (Figs 2.1 and 2.3). Axon collaterals also arise from the main branches of the cochlear nerve all along their trajectory.

The mode of termination of the type I fibers and type II fibers has been described in detail (for review see Ryugo and Parks, 2003). Type I fibers supply all parts of the CNC except the superficial granule cell areas (Figs 2.1 and 2.3), and they have been found to have two basic types of terminals: large, axosomatic endings called 'endbulbs of Held' and small boutons. The endbulbs of Held arise mainly from the ascending branches, while small boutons arise from loosely ramifying collaterals of both ascending and descending branches.

The type II fibers innervate areas rich in granule cells and appear to supply the marginal shell of the VCN (Figs 2.1 and 2.3, and see below) (for review see Ryugo and Parks, 2003). It is not currently known whether type II fibers respond to sound stimulation.

2.2.2 The ventral cochlear nucleus

The VCN shows only minor interspecies variations (Fig. 2.3). Five main neuron types are recognized: spherical bushy, globular bushy, octopus, multipolar, and small cells (Osen, 1969; Brawer *et al.*, 1974; for discussion of analogies see Osen, 1969). The five main types may be collected into two groups with respect to dendritic patterns and main axonal targets. The first three types are segregated in distinct regions of the nucleus. The spherical bushy cells are found rostrally in the AVCN, the globular bushy cells lie centrally on both sides of the nerve root in the caudal AVCN and the rostral PVCN, and the octopus cells are found caudally in the PVCN. In contrast to the first three types, the multipolar and small cells are present throughout the VCN. The small cells are most abundant around the peripheral margins of the nucleus underneath the superficial granule cell layer. A large collection of small cells located dorsolaterally in a superficial location forms the *small cell cap* of the VCN (Osen, 1969). This is particularly conspicuous in the cat.

The *spherical bushy, globular bushy*, and *octopus neurons* (Figs 2.3 and 2.4) have non-tapering dendrites ending in bushy-like formations. They differ with regard to the number of root segments and the relative length of the stem dendrites and the terminal bush. In addition, each cell type receives different numbers of afferent cochlear fibers and projects to different targets. Both spherical and globular cells receive a small number of large axosomatic terminals, the bulbs of Held (for review see Ryugo and Parks, 2003), and have so-called primary-like responses (Fig. 2.4) to pure tone stimulation, similar to those of the AN fibers (Young *et al.*, 1988; Young and Davis, 2002). The spherical bushy cells (Fig. 2.4) project bilaterally to the medial superior olive and to the ipsilateral lateral superior olive (Cant and Benson, 2003). Like the somatic surface of the spherical bushy cells, that of the globular bushy cells is almost completely covered by synaptic terminals, and the fine structure of the terminals is very similar to that described for spherical cells, although they are not as large as the endbulbs that contact spherical bushy cells. The globular bushy cells (Fig. 2.4) project to the contralateral medial nucleus of the trapezoid body. The unique properties of both spherical and globular bushy cell membranes and their AN input make these cells capable of transmitting precise temporal information necessary for both high- and low-frequency sound localization (Young *et al.*, 1988; Young and Davis, 2002).

The *octopus cells* (Fig. 2.4) receive small boutons from collaterals arising from the descending branches of a number of primary fibers. They respond to a tone burst with a single spike and so are called onset units (Young *et al*, 1988; Young and Davis, 2002). They receive very few GABAergic and glycinergic inhibitory afferents, and they are the only VCN cells that do not receive inhibitory input from the DCN (Osen *et al.*, 1990). Their main projection is to the superior paraolivary nucleus on both sides, and to the contralateral ventral complex of the lateral lemniscus (for review see Cant and Benson, 2003). While their function is still unclear, it has been speculated that onset cells are involved in encoding short latency echoes, giving spatial depth to the sound. They are also capable of encoding the pitch period of periodic sounds like vowels in their temporal firing patterns (Oertel, 1999). While the globular and spherical bushy cell axons course ventrally in the trapezoid body, the octopus cell axons course dorsally above the restiform body in the intermediate acoustic stria.

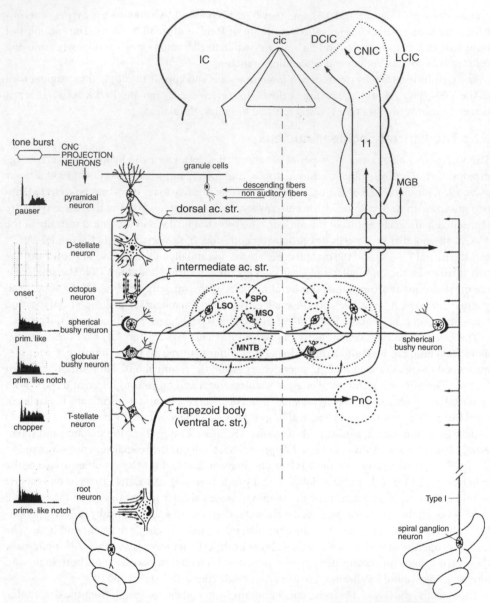

Fig. 2.4 Cell types and response profiles of neurons in the cochlear nucleus. For each type of neuron, a representative peristimulus time histogram (PSTH) is shown to its *left*. Major connections of each neuronal type are also illustrated. See List of Abbreviations for full names of structures. (Redrawn and modified from Moore and Osen, 1979.)

The *multipolar cells* (Figs 2.3 and 2.4) receive primary afferents by means of small boutons from many fibers, mainly on their moderately tapering and branched dendrites. There are two types of multipolar cell: I and II (Wickesberg and Oertel, 1988). Corresponding cell types, given other names, have also been described in the mouse and rat.

Multipolar type I cells (Fig. 2.4) correspond to the T-stellate cells described in the mouse and planar neurons in the rat. They have oriented dendritic arbors and project to the periolivary region of the superior olivary complex via the trapezoid body, and to the nuclei of the lateral lemniscus and the central nucleus of the IC through the lateral lemniscus (Adams, 1979; Cant and Benson, 2003; Malmierca *et al.*, 2005a). They also supply motoneurons of the middle ear muscles. Frequency-specific collaterals of these projecting axons are also given off to both the VCN and DCN (Lorente de Nó, 1981). The post-stimulus time histogram (PSTH) of these cells to pure tone stimuli show a regularly repeating, or 'chopper', firing pattern whose period is independent of the stimulus frequency. They may be specialized for conveying information about complex acoustic stimuli, including speech.

Multipolar type II cells (Fig. 2.4) correspond to the large D-stellate cells of the mouse and radiate cells in the rat. They have non-oriented dendritic arbors and project to the contralateral CNC, so they are also referred to as commissural neurons (Doucet and Ryugo, 1997). The axons give off widely dispersed collaterals to the ipsilateral VCN and DCN as they course through the dorsal acoustic stria (Smith and Rhode, 1989; Oertel *et al.*, 1990; Doucet and Ryugo, 1997). The D-stellate cells show glycine-like immunoreactivity (Osen *et al.*, 1990; Doucet *et al.*, 1999). Thus, they are the only known inhibitory projection neurons of the CNC. They respond to pure tone stimulation with an 'on-chop' pattern (two to three onset peaks followed by little or no sustained activity) (Fig. 2.3; Smith and Rhode, 1989; Arnott *et al.*, 2004) and often respond over a very large frequency range. A few published examples of type II multipolar cells with a slightly different form of PSTH (O_L, single onset peak followed by a pause and then a low level of sustained activity) have been reported, but it is not yet clear where these cells project and whether they constitute a separate subpopulation. It is unclear which features of these various forms of stellate cells cause them to display different PSTH patterns (chopper, on-chop, or O_L).

The *small cells* (Fig. 2.3) are abundant in the marginal shell of the VCN which is composed of the 'granule cell layer' and the subjacent 'cap area'. The granule cell layer is continuous over the exposed surface of the CNC and forms a lamina, partly separating the VCN and DCN (Mugnaini *et al.*, 1980a, b; for review see Cant and Benson, 2003). In the DCN, the granule cell layer is covered superficially by a molecular layer. The granule cell axons project as parallel fibers (Fig. 2.5) to the molecular layer (Mugnaini *et al.*, 1980a,b). The cap area is small in the rat, but it still distinguishable due to its large number of small cells, many of which show glycine- and/or GABA-like immunoreactivity (for review see Cant and Benson, 2003). The cap is supplied by both type I and type II fibers (Figs 2.1 and 2.3). In the cat, nearly all type I AN fibers that innervate the cap have low spontaneous rates in contrast to those terminating in the core (for review see Ryugo and Parks, 2003). The marginal shell also receives descending input, and its cells show a wide dynamic range (Ye *et al.*, 2000). Some of the cells in the marginal shell project to the IC (Adams, 1979; Malmierca *et al.*, 2005a), while others project to the MOC bilaterally, the LOC ipsilaterally (Ye *et al.*, 2000), and the medial geniculate body (MGB; Malmierca *et al.*, 2002). Very little information is available on the response features or the intrinsic membrane and synaptic features of those cells in the VCN classified as 'small', but these data suggest that the marginal shell (including the cap area) provides information about stimulus intensity as part of a feedback gain control system comprising the cochlea, cochlear nuclear complex, MOC, and OHCs (Ye *et al.*, 2000).

The CNC of some rodents contains a population of large cells scattered in the cochlear nerve root, between the main body of the VCN and the glial Schwann-cell border of the AN. These *cochlear root neurons* (Fig. 2.4) have dendrites oriented orthogonal to the AN fibers and receive small boutons from axon collaterals of AN fibers. The cochlear root neurons possess an exceptionally thick axon (5–7 µm) that projects mainly to the contralateral reticular pontine nucleus. These cells respond with a short latency and it has been suggested that these root neurons participate in the acoustic startle reflex (Sinex *et al.*, 2001).

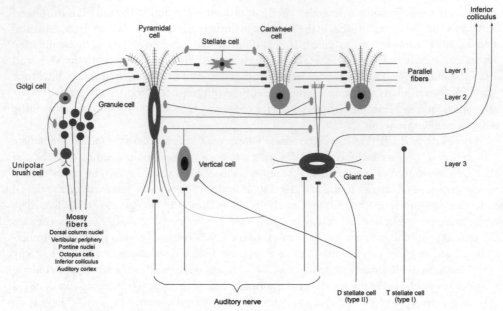

Fig. 2.5 Connection patterns of several types of neurons in the dorsal cochlear nucleus. Laminar and dendritic connection patterns are illustrated for each type of cell. (Redrawn after Oertel and Young, 2004.)

2.2.3 The dorsal cochlear nucleus

The DCN (Figs 2.3 and 2.5) shows large interspecies variations. It varies from being markedly laminated in rodents and carnivores, where it resembles the cerebellar cortex, to being non-laminated in humans and some bat species (Malmierca, 2003). It is virtually absent in some cetaceans. Each DCN cell type possesses unique anatomical, synaptic, and intrinsic membrane features that allow it to convert AN input into a response pattern characteristic of that cell type.

The three superficial layers of the DCN are related to the morphology of its principal fusiform (pyramidal) cells (Fig. 2.5). Pyramidal cell dendritic arbors are flattened perpendicular to the frequency gradient axis of the DCN (see, for example, Cant and Benson, 2003; Malmierca, 2003). The basal arbors of these pyramidal cells are flatter than the apical arbors. They are also supplied by primary afferents in a strictly tonotopic manner. The spiny apical dendritic arbors of pyramidal cells occupy layer 1, together with granule cell axons and several other types of interneurons (Fig. 2.5 and see below). Pyramidal cell bodies define layer 2 (Fig. 2.5), and their aspinous basal dendritic arbors delimit layer 3 (Fig. 2.5). The pyramidal cells are the main projection neurons of the DCN, supplying fibers to the contralateral IC via the DAS. In addition, some have a direct projection to the medial division of the medial geniculate body (Figs. 2.4 and 2.5; Malmierca *et al.*, 2002.). The deepest layer of the DCN contains two size categories of cells: the giant cells which project to the contralateral IC through the DAS and smaller glycinergic tuberuloventral interneurons.

Interneurons of the DCN may be divided into two systems: the tuberculoventral system, associated with the basal dendritic arbors of the pyramidal cells, and the granule cell system, associated with the apical dendritic arbors and cell bodies of pyramidal cells (Fig. 2.5).

The *tuberculoventral system* reciprocally interconnects the DCN and VCN. It contains both frequency-specific and diffuse projections (Cant and Benson, 2003; Malmierca, 2003). The frequency-specific projection from the DCN to the VCN originates from small interneurons, a subset of the glycinergic 'vertical cells' (Fig. 2.4). A separate set of vertical cells with only local collaterals contain both GABA and glycine, the relative amounts of which vary among species. They are located amongst the pyramidal cell basal dendrites in layer 3. The dendritic arbors of the vertical cells that project to the VCN are flattened and parallel to the pyramidal cell basal dendrites in the isofrequency planes. They receive primary afferents and project to the VCN, via the tuberculoventral tract, after giving off recurrent collaterals to the DCN which terminate on pyramidal cells (Oertel and Young, 2004). Thus, the vertical cells of the DCN provide tonotopically organized inhibition in both the DCN and VCN. The tonotopic, presumably excitatory projection from the VCN to the DCN is made up of the collaterals of type I multipolar or planar cells described above. The inhibitory projection from the VCN to DCN is composed of axons of the glycinergic commissural radiate or D-stellate cells. It has been speculated that off-characteristic frequency (CF) or wideband inhibition from tuberculoventral (vertical) cells might allow these cells to function as 'spectral contrast detectors' (Doucet et al., 1999). Some small cells of the marginal shell surrounding the AVCN also project to the DCN. They receive ascending inputs from type II AN fibers and descending cholinergic inputs (Ye et al., 2000). Thus, these cells may be important in the integration of neural activity in the ascending and descending systems. Finally, yet another type of neuron referred to as adendritic has been found to participate in the VCN to DCN projection.

The granule cell system includes the excitatory granule cells and unipolar brush cells as well as three types of inhibitory cells: the GABAergic Golgi and stellate cells and the glycinergic cartwheel cells (Fig. 2.5; Oertel and Young, 2004). The granule cells receive direct excitatory input from many sources, including the somatosensory system (Cant and Benson, 2003). Inhibitory input from these same sources also reaches the granule cells indirectly via the Golgi cells. The granule cells contribute parallel fibers to layer 1, where they form asymmetric contacts en passant with the dendritic spines of both pyramidal cells and cartwheel cells, and the smooth dendrites of the stellate cells. The unipolar brush cells may represent a source of feed-forward excitation to links along the mossy fibers (Oertel and Young, 2004). The stellate cells and cartwheel cells provide feed-forward inhibition to the pyramidal cells. Very little is known about the responses of cells in the granular cell system to auditory stimuli. Cartwheel cells show complex spikes (two or three action potentials riding on a depolarization) and weak responses to auditory stimuli that are difficult to classify.

Pyramidal and giant cell excitatory responses are more strongly influenced by their inhibitory inputs than are those of other projection neurons in the CNC, and have been classified as types III and IV (Oertel and Young, 2004). Much of the inhibition is thought to arise from two cell types, the DCN vertical cells and the glycinergic type II stellate cells in the VCN, described above. The vertical cells provide inhibition over a narrow frequency range while the on-chop, type II stellate cells generate inhibition over a wide frequency range. This inhibition also presumably accounts for the response patterns of these cells to pure tones, which have been classified as 'pauser' (onset response followed by a pause then a resumption of firing; see Fig. 2.4) and 'build-up' (a slow buildup of spike activity rather than an abrupt increase in firing). Behavioral studies in cats following surgical lesions of the DAS and IAS suggest that the DCN plays some role in directing attention to sound (see Chapter 13). The type IV units have been found to be sensitive to spectral notches created by the pinna that are important cues for localizing sounds particularly in the plane of elevation (see Chapter 13). DCN projection neurons receive and respond not only to auditory information, but also to somatosensory inputs from muscle proprioceptors in and around the pinna. Such evidence has led to speculation that the DCN output may be involved in coordinating pinna orientation with localization cues, and bilateral lesions of the DAS in cats result in reduced accuracy in head orientation responses to broad-band sounds, particularly in elevation.

2.2.4 Connections with higher centers

The ascending projections of the CNC (Fig. 2.4) have already been briefly discussed and will be considered in detail when the target nuclei are described. Here it suffices to point out that the projections are largely tonotopically organized, so that the isofrequency laminae of the CNC are connected with the corresponding isofrequency laminae of the higher centers.

The right and left CNC are interconnected by the fibers of presumed inhibitory (glycinergic) commissural neurons, as mentioned above (for review see Cant and Benson, 2003). The CNC also receives descending projections from the auditory cortex, the IC, the ventral complex of the lateral lemniscus, and the superior olivary complex (see Malmierca, 2003). A large proportion of the latter fibers may also be inhibitory, glycine, and/or GABA, being the transmitters. There are also excitatory descending fibers, e.g., collaterals of the cholinergic olivocochlear bundle (Osen *et al.*, 1984). These descending connections are reviewed in detail in Chapter 3.

2.3 The superior olivary complex

The superior olivary complex (SOC) comprises a number of closely grouped nuclei in the caudal pons (Fig. 2.6). In contrast to the CNC, the SOC shows considerable variation among species (Osen *et al.*, 1984). Three main nuclei are consistently identified: the lateral superior olive (LSO), medial superior olive (MSO), and medial nucleus of the trapezoid body (MNTB). These three nuclei are surrounded by diffuse cellular areas, collectively referred to as the periolivary region (PO) (Adams, 1983; Osen *et al.*, 1984; Schofield and Cant, 1991).

The architecture of the SOC structures varies across species (Fig. 2.6). The MSO is diminutive in the rat, while it is well developed in both the cat and humans. The LSO and MNTB are well developed in both the rat and cat, while they are quite small in humans. This may relate to differences between the animals' frequency range of hearing. The MSO responds mainly to low frequencies but also to a limited range of high frequencies, while the LSO responds to all tonal frequencies (for review see Malmierca, 2003). Both systems are important for directional hearing. The MSO is probably more important for localization of low-frequency sounds and analysis of interaural time differences, while the LSO and MNTB may code all frequencies and principally serve to detect interaural intensity differences.

2.3.1 The medial superior olive

The MSO is wedged between the LSO and the MNTB and appears as a transversely oriented row of 'principal cells' with dendrites extending in the medial and lateral directions. Two cell types populate the MSO: principal and non-principal cells. Principal cells are flattened multipolars, and extend rostrocaudally to form horizontal laminae (Smith, 1995). The MSO is tonotopically organized, with low-frequency tones represented dorsally and high-frequency tones ventrally, but most of the nucleus is devoted to low frequencies (Osen *et al.*, 1984).

The MSO receives direct and excitatory input from spherical bushy cells in the AVCN bilaterally (Fig. 2.4; for review see Malmierca, 2003). The MSO receives input from both sides, but the inputs remain segregated (Smith, 1995), such that the lateral dendrites receive inputs from the ipsilateral side, while the medial dendrites receive inputs from the contralateral side (Smith, 1995). This arrangement is reminiscent of the input configuration proposed in the Jeffress model for sound localization. The direct bilateral input suggests that the MSO neurons are ideally suited to measure interaural phase, or time, differences (Joris *et al.*, 1998).

The MSO has also been found to receive inhibitory inputs, primarily glycinergic, from the medial and lateral nuclei of the trapezoid body on the same side. The latter may also provide GABAergic inhibitory input (Smith, 1995).

SUPERIOR OLIVARY COMPLEX

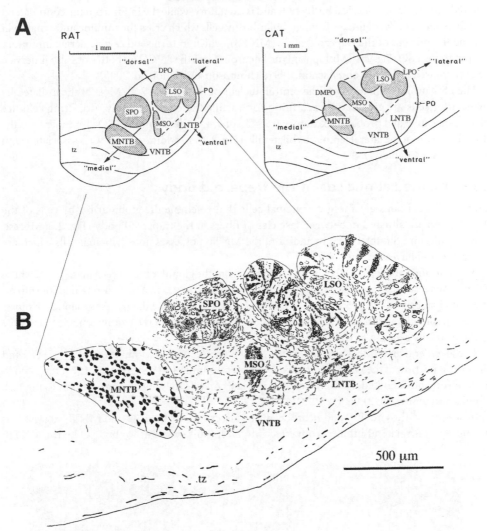

Fig. 2.6 Organization of the superior olivary complex (SOC). **A** Schematic diagram of the SOC in the rat and cat, showing relative locations of the major nuclei. See List of Abbreviations for full names of structures. (Redrawn from Osen *et al.*, 1984.) **B** Types of neurons and their distribution among nuclei of the SOC. (Redrawn after Friauf, 1993.)

The principal cells project to the IC and to the ipsilateral dorsal nucleus of the lateral lemniscus (Fig. 2.2), but the non-principal multipolar cells project elsewhere (for review see Helfert and Aschoff, 1997; Thompson and Schofield, 2000).

2.3.2 The lateral superior olive

The LSO forms an S-shaped row of flattened multipolar neurons, with dendrites oriented perpendicular to the long axis (Rietzel and Friauf, 1998). The LSO is tonotopically organized, with low frequencies represented laterally and high frequencies medially.

The LSO receives input that originates from the AVCN on both sides. The ipsilateral input is derived directly from spherical bushy cells and is excitatory, while the input from the contralateral AVCN is indirect. It originates from globular bushy cells which cross the midline and synapse in the medial nucleus of the trapezoid body (MNTB), which in turn sends a glycinergic inhibitory output to the LSO (Fig. 2.4). Multipolar type I neurons from the AVCN on both sides also innervate LSO (reviewed in Helfert and Aschoff, 1997; Thompson and Schofield, 2000).

The LSO projects bilaterally to the central nucleus of the IC (Fig. 2.2). Most of the ipsilaterally projecting cells are glycinergic, i.e., inhibitory, while the contralaterally projecting cells are glycine-negative and probably excitatory (see Chapter 4 for details). The LSO also innervates the dorsal nucleus of the lateral lemniscus bilaterally (Fig. 2.2). In addition, the LSO is associated with the LOC (see Chapter 3).

2.3.3 The medial nucleus of the trapezoid body

The MNTB contains glycinergic principal cells that resemble the globular bushy cells of the AVCN, and are situated in between fascicles of fibers in the trapezoid body (Fig. 2.6; Morest, 1968; Banks and Smith, 1992). In addition, the MNTB possesses non-principal cells which are elongated and have very few spines.

As mentioned above, the MNTB receives input from the globular bushy cells in the VCN whose thick axons terminate as large axosomatic calyces of Held (1893) in a one-to-one relationship on the principal cells of the MNTB (Fig. 2.4). These calyces constitute the largest synaptic terminals in the mammalian brain (Fig. 2.7A) and provide a fast and secure relay of information from the globular bushy cells to the LSO.

The glycinergic inhibitory neurons of the MNTB project widely within the ipsilateral SOC and the dorsal portion of the ventral complex of the lateral lemniscus (VLL; Adams, 1979; reviewed in Thompson and Schofield, 2000). Non-principal cells may be the source of projections to the VLL (Banks and Smith, 1992).

In summary, the circuitry and neurochemistry described for the LSO and MNTB suggest that excitatory contralateral input is converted into an inhibitory input to the LSO by the MNTB,

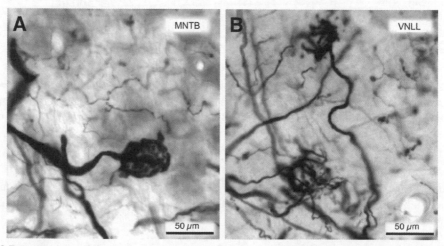

Fig. 2.7 Comparison of the endbulbs (calyces) of Held in the medial nucleus of the trapezoid body (MNTB) and ventral nucleus of the lateral lemniscus (VNLL). **A** Projections to the MNTB from the anterior ventral cochlear nucleus. **B** Projections to the VNLL from the posterior ventral cochlear nucleus. (Malmierca, unpublished data.)

which, combined with the excitatory ipsilateral input, allows the LSO to faithfully encode inter-aural intensity differences in the high-frequency range of audition (for review see Irvine, 1992).

2.3.4 The superior paraolivary nucleus

In rodents, there is a fourth distinct nucleus, the superior paraolivary nucleus (SPO), found in the dorsomedial part of the complex (Fig. 2.6; Osen *et al.*, 1984; Schofield and Cant, 1991; Schofield, 1995). It consists of GABAergic multipolar cells which are the largest in the SOC, and these receive inputs from octopus and multipolar cells in the contralateral VCN, from multipolar cells in the ipsilateral VCN, and a substantial glycinergic input from the MNTB on the same side. The SPO projects to the ipsilateral IC (Fig. 2.10; Schofield, 1995) and may represent a hyperdevelop-ment of the periolivary cells with a similar projection that are present in smaller numbers in other mammals (Adams, 1983). The physiological properties and functional role of this pathway are beginning to be disclosed: it may be involved in the analysis of temporal features of complex sounds (Dehmel *et al.*, 2002; Kulesza *et al.*, 2003).

2.3.5 Periolivary nuclei

The PO contains several distinct types of neurons with different projection patterns (Adams, 1983). Although there is some interspecies variation, the various cell types all appear to have specific locations within the superior olivary complex (Adams, 1983; Osen *et al.*, 1984).

The PO receives input from the VCN bilaterally, the lateral part from the ipsilateral side and the medial part from both sides (Fig. 2.4). These excitatory afferents arise mainly from multipolar type I neurons and possibly from octopus cells. Certain parts of the PO also receive input from the ipsilateral MNTB (probably inhibitory), ipsilateral IC (probably excitatory), and the dorsal nucleus of the lateral lemniscus (see Chapter 3).

PO cells project to the cochlea, the CNC, or the IC (Adams, 1983). The medial part of the PO participates in the MOC, which innervates the OHCs ipsi- and contralaterally, and is reciprocally connected with the CNC on both sides. The lateral part of PO is reciprocally connected with the ipsilateral CNC.

Of the cells projecting to the IC, cells situated medial to the MSO are connected to the ipsilateral IC, whereas those situated lateral to the MSO and ventral to the LSO project to the IC bilaterally (Adams, 1983; Osen *et al.*, 1984).

Special mention should be made of the ventral nucleus of the trapezoid body (VNTB) which is situated ventral to the MNTB. The VNTB is a heterogeneous group of cells situated strategically at the intersection of ascending projections from the CNC and descending projections from the IC (see Chapter 3). The VNTB receives major afferent projections from the globular bushy cells, octopus, and multipolar cells in the contralateral VCN (Friauf and Ostwald, 1988; Smith *et al.*, 1991; Thompson, 1998). The VNTB also receives projections from the multipolar cells in the ipsilateral PVCN (Thompson and Schofield, 2000) and the marginal shell of the AVCN from both sides (Ye *et al.*, 2000). Finally, the VNTB is the major target in the SOC for descending projections from the IC (see Chapter 3). Neuroanatomical and physiological evidence suggests that this descending projection may be involved in the activation of the olivocochlear neurons (Rajan, 1990).

2.4 The nuclei of the lateral lemniscus

Over the past decade, extraordinary progress has been made in understanding the anatomy and physiology of the nuclei of the lateral lemniscus (NLL). Although several cytoarchitectonic schemes were proposed for different species by different authors (for a detailed discussion see

Malmierca *et al.*, 1998, Malmierca, 2003), its subdivision into a dorsal nucleus (DNLL) and a ventral nucleus (VNLL; collectively referring to the cell groups ventral to the DNLL) is consistent with the presence of two distinct functional systems, a binaural *dorsal* system and a monaural *ventral* system (Covey and Casseday, 1991). Each system has its own unique connectional, neuro-chemical, and physiological properties (Covey and Casseday, 1991; Malmierca *et al.*, 1998).

2.4.1 The ventral complex of the lateral lemniscus: the monaural system

The VNLL consists of groups of neurons embedded within the lateral lemniscus (Fig. 2.2), located between the SOC and DNLL. It receives inputs mainly from the contralateral ear (Figs 2.2 and 2.7B), as opposed to the DNLL which receives inputs from both ears mostly through its connections with the superior olive. VNLL neurons exhibit a variety of shapes and sizes in Nissl stained sections. Most of them project to the ipsilateral IC in a laminar and tonotopic fashion, and it has been recently demonstrated that the VNLL is also organized in a laminar fashion, suggesting that it is tonotopically organized.

Based on the morphology of the dendritic arbors, two main types of VNLL neurons have been described: bushy and stellate cells. In slice preparations the bushy cells show an onset firing pattern and non-linear current–voltage relationship. In contrast, the stellate cells show a linear current–voltage relationship, but exhibit different firing patterns, which may be related to differences in the shape of the soma, and the branching pattern and orientation of their dendrites (Zhao and Wu, 2001). Similar firing patterns have been found in *in vivo* studies.

The *afferent projections* to the VNLL arise mainly from the contralateral VCN and ipsilateral MNTB. The majority of cells in the ventral part of the complex are glycine and/or GABA immunoreactive (see Chapter 4), although the incidence of colocalization of the two transmitters seems considerably higher than previously estimated. The VNLL neurons are suitable for encoding temporal events with high precision (Covey and Casseday, 1991).

2.4.2 The dorsal nucleus of the lateral lemniscus: the binaural system

The DNLL is a distinctive group of neurons embedded within the dorsal part of the lateral lemniscus (Fig. 2.2). In contrast to the VNLL, the DNLL receives input from both ears, and it projects to both ICs as well as to its counterpart on the opposite side through the commissure of Probst. The DNLL plays an important role in binaural processing, i.e., sound localization.

Several neuronal types have been described, depending on the species and the criteria used for cell classification. Regardless of the morphological type, all cells have similar membrane properties, with a sustained series of regular action potentials produced by the injection of positive current (Zhao and Wu, 2001).

Generally speaking, the DNLL receives collaterals from afferents that also innervate the IC (Fig. 2.10). Thus, DNLL receives contralateral inputs from the VCN and DNLL, ipsilateral input from the medial superior olive, superior paraolivary nucleus, and VLL, and bilateral inputs from the lateral superior olive. The DNLL projection to the IC is laminar and tonotopic and bilateral, with a predominant projection to the contralateral IC. Most DNLL cells are GABAergic and therefore have an inhibitory influence on IC (for review see Malmierca, 2003)

2.5 The inferior colliculus

The IC is the principal auditory nucleus in the midbrain and it is characterized by the convergence of inputs that previously diverge from lower auditory centers (Figs 2.2 and 2.4; Irvine, 1992; Casseday *et al.*, 2002; Malmierca, 2003; Loftus *et al.*, 2008). The IC consists of a central nucleus

(CNIC) surrounded by cortical regions (Figs 2.8 and 2.9). These collicular cortices include a dorsal cortex (DCIC) that covers the CNIC dorsally and caudally, a lateral cortex (LCIC) that covers it laterally, and a rostral cortex (RCIC) that covers it rostrally. However, the details of these subdivisions and the locations of the borders between them have been interpreted differently by different authors, and across species. A recent study by Loftus *et al.* (2008) has proposed a scheme that unifies these different views and has clarified the different cytoarchitectural schemes used by different authors.

The IC receives fibers from lower and higher auditory centers as well as from non-auditory structures. Neurons in the CNIC tend to be most strongly influenced by lower auditory centers, while neurons in the DCIC tend to be most strongly influenced by the descending pathways. Cells at the border between the the CNIC and DCIC may be influenced by a combination of ascending, descending, intrinsic, and commissural inputs.

The IC has ascending projections to the MGB and descending projections to the SOC and the CNC (Malmierca *et al.*, 1996; Peruzzi *et al.*, 1997; Oliver *et al.*, 1999; Cant and Benson 2007). In addition, the IC possesses well-developed intrinsic fiber systems and commissural connections that interconnect the two ICs (Saldaña and Merchán, 1992; Malmierca *et al.*, 1995, 2009a).

2.5.1 The central nucleus of the inferior colliculus

The CNIC is defined by the presence of 'fibrodendritic laminae', distinguishable in Golgi material as a parallel organization of afferent lemniscal fibers and neurons with flattened dendritic arbors,

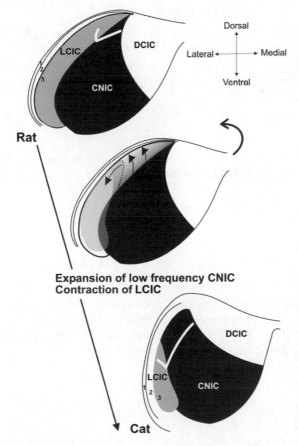

**Expansion of low frequency CNIC
Contraction of LCIC**

Rat

Cat

Fig. 2.8 Subdivisions of the inferior colliculus in the rat and cat. The low frequency representation in the central nucleus (CNIC) is expanded in cats and contracted in rats. The size of the lateral cortex (LCIC) is contracted in cats and expanded in rats. Dorsal cortex (DCIC). (From Loftus *et al.*, 2008.)

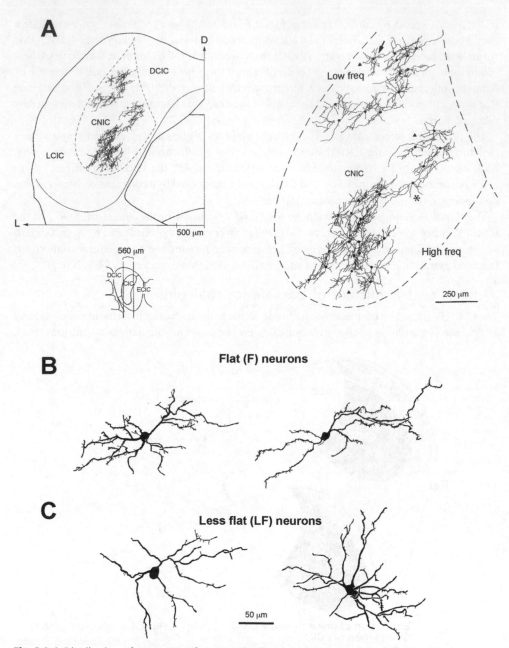

Fig. 2.9 A Distribution of two types of neurons in the central nucleus of the inferior colliculus (CNIC). **B** The dendritic arbors of flat neurons (F) are narrow (50 μm) and confined to laminae. **C** The arbors of less flat neurons (LF) are wider (100 μm) and segregated within intralaminar compartments. (Redrawn and modified from Malmierca *et al.*, 1993.)

usually called disk-shaped cells (Oliver and Morest, 1984; Faye-lund and Osen, 1985; Malmierca *et al.*, 1993). Stellate cells with non-oriented arbors also populate the IC. This characteristic laminar organization of the CNIC has been observed in all species studied and constitutes the structural basis for the tonotopic organization of the IC (Schreiner and Langner, 1997).

In the rat, Malmierca *et al.* (1993) defined two types of neuron: F (flat) and LF (less flat) (Fig. 2.9). These seem to correspond to the disk-shaped and stellate neurons described in the cat (Oliver and Morest, 1984). The F and LF neurons differ in several respects, including the thickness, branching pattern, and orientation of their dendritic arbor, and their location within the laminae. The dendritic arbor of the F neurons is about 50 μm thick and denser than that of the LF neurons. The F neurons are oriented strictly parallel to the ascending fibers and form laminae that are about 40–70 μm (one cell thick) (Faye-Lund and Osen, 1985). The laminae are separated by interlaminar compartments populated by the LF neurons. The dendritic arbors of the LF neurons are about 100 μm wide, and less dense than those of the F neurons. LF neuron arbors are roughly parallel to F neuron arbors (Malmierca *et al.*, 1993). In the rat, the interlaminar compartments are less distinct in the dorsomedial, low-frequency region than in the ventromedial, high-frequency region. It is likely that there are several types of F and LF cells with complex functional properties, as no correlation has been discovered between *in vitro* physiological response properties and the morphological classification of F and LF cells (Sivaramakrishnan and Oliver, 2001).

The CNIC receives *afferent (ascending) projections* (Fig. 2.10) that originate in the AVCN, PVCN, and DCN contralaterally, VLL and MSO ipsilaterally, and DNLL and LSO bilaterally (Malmierca 2003; Cant and Benson, 2006). Most experiments to study the afferent input to the IC have been performed in cats (for review see Malmierca, 2003). These show that the afferent fibers are tonotopically arranged and that many of the ascending systems show a 'banded' pattern of projections, with dense bands (about 200 μm thick) running parallel to the isofrequency fibrodendritic laminae. The terminal fields of the various ascending projections may also vary in their distribution along the main axis of the IC. For example, in the dorsal part of the CNIC, the axons from the DCN do not overlap with afferents from the LSO. The extent to which projections from different brainstem processing channels are, or are not, segregated in CNIC may be the basis for emergent functional properties in the CNIC (Kuwada *et al.*, 1997).

The CNIC projects to the ventral division of the MGB in a tonotopic manner, largely to the ipsilateral side, but also with a crossed component. The CNIC projections originate from both F and LF neurons (Peruzzi *et al.*, 1997; Oliver *et al.*, 1999). Although the majority of neurons that project from the CNIC to the MGB probably use glutamate as the neurotransmitter, there is a population of neurons in the IC that contain GABA and project to the MGB. The GABA-containing neurons in the IC provide short-latency, monosynaptic inputs to the thalamocortical projection neurons in the MGB (Peruzzi *et al.*, 1997). This is interesting because the *rat* MGB lacks GABAergic cells (Winer and Larue, 1988), and therefore this monosynaptic inhibitory input to the MGB may be important for the regulation of firing patterns in thalamocortical neurons in conjunction with the known GABAergic projection from the auditory part of the reticular thalamic nucleus.

IC neurons in the rat possess $GABA_A$, $GABA_B$, and glycine receptors (reviewed in Kelly and Caspary, 2005; see also Chapter 4) and about a quarter of the cells in the CNIC are GABAergic (Merchán *et al.*, 2005). Studies using microiontophoresis *in vivo* have demonstrated that both GABA and glycine inhibit IC neurons in several species (e.g., LeBeau *et al.*, 2001). IC neurons also possess NMDA and AMPA receptors, and microiontophoretic studies (see Chapter 4) have demonstrated that both AMPA and NMDA are involved in the maintenance of the response for the duration of the stimulus, while AMPA receptors also seem to be important at the response onset.

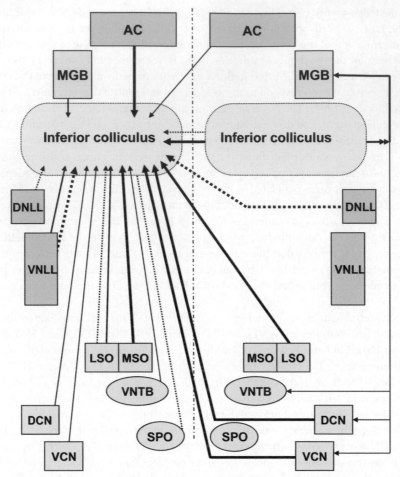

Fig. 2.10 Summary of major ascending and descending inputs to the inferior colliculus on one side of the brain from auditory nuclei in the brainstem, thalamus, and auditory cortex. Connection strength is denoted by the thickness of the *arrows*. *Continuous lines* represent excitatory connections while *dashed lines* do for inhibitory connections. See List of Abbreviations for full names of structures. (From Malmierca, 2004.)

Furthermore, both AMPA and NMDA receptors are involved in maintaining the firing of CNIC neurons to dynamically changing acoustic stimuli (reviewed in Kelly and Caspary, 2005).

Physiological studies have suggested that the laminae of the CNIC contain a highly organized representation of both spectral and temporal parameters (for review see Langner and Schreiner, 1988; Schreiner and Langner, 1988). Neurons in the IC show a variety of different frequency response areas that include both V-shaped and non-V-shaped (LeBeau *et al.*, 2001). Palombi and Caspary (1996) also studied binaural responses in the rat IC and classified them as suppression, summation, or mixed. Binaural suppression responses were more numerous at high frequencies and summation at low frequencies, as would be expected given the relative contribution of LSO and MSO across frequency. Nevertheless, iontophoretic application of GABA and glycine antagonists and intracellular recordings (Covey *et al.*, 1996; Kuwada *et al.*, 1997) have shown that neural inhibition contributes to the binaural response of neurons in the IC.

2.5.2 The dorsal cortex of the inferior colliculus

The DCIC covers the dorsomedial and caudal aspects of the CNIC (Figs 2.8 and 2.9). Three layers of the DCIC have been defined (Faye-Lund and Osen, 1985). The most superficial layer (layer 1) is a thin fibrocellular capsule that covers the entire exterior surface of the IC. It contains scattered, small, flattened neurons. Layer 2 is deeper and slightly thicker and consists of small and medium-sized, mostly multipolar neurons. Layer 3 contains small and medium-sized cells as well as large multipolar neurons near the border with the CNIC. Computer-assisted 3-D reconstructions of Golgi-impregnated neurons in the rat DCIC have demonstrated that the DCIC neurons as a group differ morphologically from the F neurons of the CNIC in several respects (Malmierca, 1993). A distinct feature of neurons in DCIC (and also LCIC) is the presence of nitric oxide. This has been revealed by means of NADPH-diaphorase staining for nitric oxide synthase in the rat and guinea pig. Nitric oxide is a neuromodulator that can interact with other systems such as NMDA. For this reason it has been implicated in long-term potentiation and neuronal plasticity, a phenomenon seen in the rat IC (Zhang and Wu, 2000).

As mentioned previously, some of the ascending input from lower auditory centers to the CNIC encroaches upon the DCIC, as do the intrinsic projections (Saldaña and Merchán, 1992; Malmierca *et al.*, 1995). The DCIC also receives input from the sagulum. In addition, it receives descending inputs bilaterally from the auditory cortex that originate largely from the primary auditory areas (see Chapter 3). The neocortical terminals in the DCIC form a banded pattern similar to that of the ascending projections to the CNIC. These neocortical terminals are tonotopically organized, with the isofrequency contours continuous with, and overlapping, those of the CNIC (see Chapter 3). The DCIC projects mainly to the dorsal division of the MGB (Cant and Benson, 2007).

2.5.3 The lateral cortex of the inferior colliculus

The LCIC (also termed in the literature the external cortex, or external nucleus) covers the CNIC laterally (Figs 2.8 and 2.9) and ventrally (Faye-Lund and Osen, 1985; Loftus *et al.*, 2008). Three layers are defined in the lateral part of the LCIC (Faye-Lund and Osen, 1985; Loftus *et al.*, 2008). Layer 1 is a continuation of the fibrodendritic capsule of the DCIC. Layer 2 is composed of small and medium-sized neurons which, in the LCIC, are partly aggregated in dense clusters in myelin-rich neuropil. These aggregates are rich in acetylcholinesterase and GABA. Layer 3 of the LCIC constitutes the largest part and appears to continue into the non-stratified rostral part (rostral cortex), that is topographically related to the fascicles of the commissural fibers. Although the functions of the LCIC are not known, it is likely that it plays an important role by providing auditory input to visual-motor areas that direct head and eye movements involved in gaze initiation. The LCIC may be a major source of binaural cues for gaze control in the superior colliculus (King *et al.*, 1998). In agreement with the multitude of inputs, neurons of the LCIC have been shown electrophysiologically to respond not only to auditory stimulation, but also to somatosensory input (Aitkin *et al.*, 1978). Thus, a second role of the LCIC could be in multisensory integration, distinct from the 'classical' auditory role of the central nucleus. The LCIC receives somatosensory input from the spinal cord, dorsal column nuclei, and spinal trigeminal nuclei in the cat (Zhou and Shore, 2006). Some neurons in the LCIC appear to have relatively large somatosensory receptive fields, in addition to auditory responses, which are broadly tuned with respect to frequency (Aitkin *et al.*, 1978). The multisensory integration in the LCIC mirrors similar types of function at the MGB of the belt or 'extralemniscal' auditory pathway. Finally, the LCIC may have a unique influence on the olivocochlear system. Recent studies show that electrical stimulation of LCIC has a broadly tuned effect on cochlear responses, in contrast to central nucleus stimulation which has sharply tuned effects (Ota *et al.*, 2004). Thus, the medial and lateral olivocochlear bundles may be differentially activated by the CNIC and LCIC, respectively.

2.5.4 The rostral cortex of the inferior colliculus

The neurons located rostral to the CNIC form the rostral cortex (RCIC). They include very large multipolar cells as well as small and medium-sized multipolar neurons, and thus differ from those of the CNIC and LCIC (Faye-Lund and Osen, 1985; Malmierca *et al.*, 1993).

The LCIC and RCIC, like the DCIC, receive input from the cerebral cortex, the ipsilateral MGB, and many non-auditory structures (for review see Malmierca, 2003). The LCIC and RCIC project to the dorsal and medial divisions of the MGB (Fig. 2.1). Thus, projections from the three subdivisions of the IC overlap, especially in the medial division. The functional role of the RCIC neurons is still unknown, although recent studies (Perez-Gonzalez *et al.*, 2005; Malmierca *et al.*, 2009b) have demonstrated that at least some neurons in this region and in other cortical regions of the IC may be specialized for detecting novel sounds.

2.5.5 Local intrinsic and commissural connections of the inferior colliculus

Fibers that form connections within the IC on one side are called local intrinsic fibers, while those that interconnect the two sides are termed commissural fibers (Fig. 2.10). Both types of fibers may represent collaterals of axons with projections to the thalamus or lower brainstem or, alternatively, they may be the sole projection of neurons whose connections are restricted to one or both ICs (for review see Malmierca, 2003). The intrinsic fibers form 'sheets' that are parallel to the isofrequency contours of the CNIC. The sheets extend into the DCIC, LCIC, and RCIC (Saldaña and Merchán, 1992; Malmierca *et al.*, 1995, 2009a). Recent studies show that the majority of these intrinsic and commissural projections may be excitatory, although about 25% of the commissural neurons are GABAergic (Hernandez *et al.*, 2006). Physiological evidence *in vivo* and *in vitro* (reviewed in Malmierca *et al.*, 2003, 2005b) shows that the commissural inputs may have either an excitatory or an inhibitory influence on the contralateral IC, and that they affect frequency response areas, binaural properties, and temporal firing patterns.

2.6 The medial geniculate body

The medial geniculate body (MGB) is a nuclear complex in the thalamus that mediates the last stage of subcortical auditory processing in the ascending pathway (Fig. 2.2). The structure is commonly divided into three major divisions: the ventral (MGV), dorsal (MGD), and medial or magnocellular (MGM), named to denote their relative locations within the complex (Fig. 2.11). Earlier descriptions of the structure recognized two divisions (see Jones, 2007), attesting to the difficulty in establishing subdivisions on the basis of architectonic features alone. Additional subdivisions are currently recognized in most species, usually representing smaller domains within each of the major subdivisions.

The connections of the MGB mainly include the IC and auditory cortex. For the most part, these connections are reciprocal, and vary such that each subdivision has a particular pattern of connections with other structures. The main source of ascending projections to the MGB is the IC (Fig. 2.10). Other inputs include the thalamic reticular nucleus and other auditory nuclei, including the SOC, NLL, and CNC. Ascending fibers enter the structure from the brachium of the IC and terminate among neurons in each subdivision. Connections with the auditory cortex pass through the posterior limb of the internal capsule.

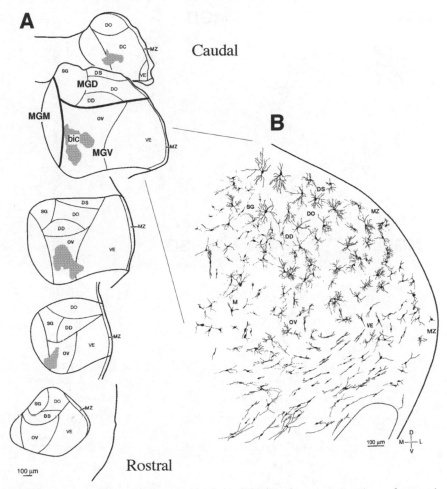

Fig. 2.11 Organization of the medial geniculate body (MGB) in the cat. **A** Drawings of coronal sections through the MGB, showing locations of nuclei and their subdivisions along the caudal–rostral axis. **B** Types of neurons located among nuclei of the MGB. bic brachium of the inferior colliculus; DC dorsal nucleus, caudal part; DD deep dorsal nucleus; DO dorsal nucleus; DS dorsal superficial nucleus; M medial division; MGD medial geniculate body, dorsal division; MGM medial geniculate body, medial division; MGV medial geniculate body, ventral division; MZ marginal zone; OV pars ovoidae of the ventral division; Sg suprageniculate nucleus; VE pars lateralis of the ventral division. (After Winer *et al.*, 1999.)

2.6.1 The ventral nucleus of the medial geniculate body

The principal cells of the MGV are the bi-tufted neurons, which have polarized dendritic fields extending from the poles of elongated soma. These neurons (Figs 2.11 and 2.12) are closely spaced and tend to be arranged in rows about 50–100 μm wide, with dendritic fields oriented from dorsolateral to ventromedial (Winer *et al.*, 1999). The fibrodendritic laminae correspond to the organized projection from the CNIC, within which precise tonotopic organization is preserved. The principal neurons are assumed to be glutamatergic, and most are immunoreactive for the calcium-binding protein parvalbumin (Jones, 2007). Except in rodents and bats, GABAergic interneurons are abundant in the MGV, accounting for at least a quarter of the population

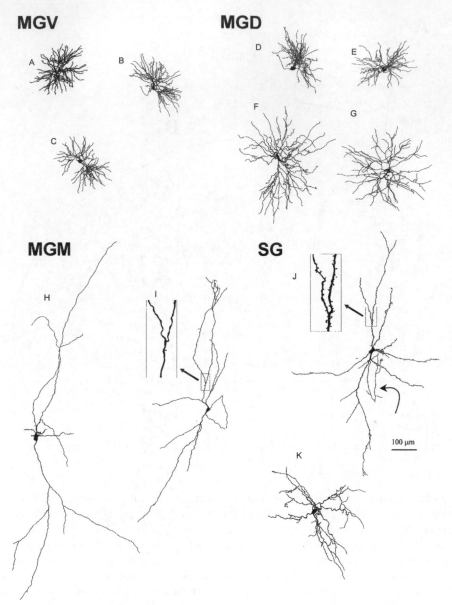

Fig. 2.12 Camera lucida drawings of neurons in the MGB of the rat. **A–C** Bi-tufted neurons in the MGV. **D–G** Bushy (**D** and **E**) and stellate (**F** and **G**) in the MGD. **H–I** Multipolar neurons in the MGM. (**J** and **K**). SG Stellate cells in the suprageniculate. (From Bartlett and Smith, 1999.)

(Winer and Larue, 1988). The principal neurons exhibit low threshold short-latency responses to tones and complex sounds. As noted for other nuclei in the ascending lemniscal pathway, these neurons are tuned to frequency and sensitive to both interaural time and intensity differences.

The main source of inputs to the MGV is the ipsilateral CNIC (Fig. 2.10), coupled with a weaker contralateral projection (Malmierca, 2003; Jones, 2007). Projections from the IC to the MGV appear to arise from both glutamatergic and GABAergic neurons (Bartlett and Smith,

1999). The MGV projection to the auditory cortex mainly terminates in layers III and IV of the primary (core) areas. The tonotopic organization of the projection is preserved in these areas.

2.6.2 The dorsal nucleus of the medial geniculate body

The MGD lies dorsal to the MGV, extending from the rostral to the caudal poles of the MGB (Fig. 2.11). The MGD is generally characterized by cell spacing, which is less dense than the MGV, and it lacks a laminar organization. In most species, at least two subdivisions are recognized on the basis of architectonic variations and connections (Burton and Jones, 1976; Winer, 1985). The most numerous in the MGD are radiate cells, which have radially symmetric dendritic fields with a simple branching pattern (Fig. 2.12). There is also a substantial number of tufted cells (Fig. 2.12). These have dendritic arbors that extend from each pole, and tend to be organized in thin sheets, especially dorsolaterally (Winer *et al.*, 1999). Compared to the MGV, parvalbumin density is reduced in the MGD, accompanied by a relative increase in the numbers of calbindin-positive cells (Jones, 2007). As in the MGV, GABAergic interneurons are abundant in the MGD in most species studied, accounting for a similar percentage of the population. Latencies in the MGD are typically longer than MGV, and the latency distribution is wider. Tonotopic organization is not apparent from recordings in any species and frequency tuning is generally broader (Jones, 2007).

The main sources of ascending auditory inputs to the MGD are the DCIC and LCIC (Malmierca, 2003; Jones, 2007). These inputs represent both glutamatergic and GABAergic neurons (Bartlett and Smith, 1999). The MGD mainly projects to the non-primary (belt) areas of the auditory cortex, within which tonotopy is weak or absent.

2.6.3 The medial nucleus of the medial geniculate body

The magnocellular, or medial, nucleus (MGM) borders the MGV and MGD medially (Fig. 2.11), extending from the rostral to the caudal poles of the MGB (Fig. 2.11). Although recognized as a single division, the MGM is rather heterogeneous with respect to cell types and connections. Dendritic configurations vary widely and there is no apparent laminar organization. In addition to the largest neurons, from which the MGM gets one of its names (magnocellular), at least four different types of cells have been identified (Winer and Morest, 1983). These neurons are further distinguished on the basis of distinctive projections to the auditory cortex. Calbindin reactive neurons project mainly to layers I and II of all auditory cortical areas, while projections to the middle layers represent both calbindin and parvalbumin neurons (Jones, 2007). GABAergic interneurons are present in similar proportions as the MGV and MGD (Malmierca, 2003). Consistent with various classes of neurons populating the MGM, response properties are highly variable. Some neurons are narrowly tuned to frequency and respond robustly at short latencies, similar to MGV neurons, while others are broadly tuned and have longer latencies.

Inputs to the MGM include both auditory and non-auditory sources. The main auditory inputs arise from the CNC and LCIC, as well as the CN, SOC, and VNLL (Malmierca *et al.*, 2002; Anderson *et al.*, 2006). Non-auditory inputs are not well defined, but include the deep layers of the superior colliculus and other nuclei that appear to drive responses to somatic, vestibular, visual, and nociceptive stimuli in some species (see Jones, 2007). In addition to the auditory cortex, the MGM also projects to the striatum and amygdala (Doron and Ledoux, 1999).

2.7 The auditory cortex

In the ascending auditory pathway, species differences are the most apparent in the auditory cortex (Fig. 2.13), where the number of areas identified ranges from 5 to 6 in mice and rats, 6 to 9 in cats and ferrets, 10 to 12 in primates, and over 30 in some studies of humans (Fig. 2.13). Species differences include the number of areas present, their relative position and arrangement, cell density, connections, and tonotopic organization. The tendency to identify more areas in larger brains may be a methodological artifact, in part, but it is likely that species differences will be reflected in the organization of the auditory cortex in other ways, as well.

A common theme is that a central primary region, or *core*, is surrounded by a variable number of secondary, or *belt*, areas (Fig. 2.13). In non-human primates, the core–belt scheme has been extended to include a third region, known as the *parabelt* (Kaas and Hackett, 2000).

2.7.1 The core region of the auditory cortex

Across species, the primary field (A1) and up to two other tonotopically organized areas may be considered part of the core region. Areas in the core are characterized by high cell density in a broad layer IV, dense myelination across laminae, and relatively high expression of several markers in the horizontal band involving layers III and IV, compared to secondary areas in the belt (e.g., cytochrome oxidase, acetylcholinesterase, parvalbumin) (Kaas and Hackett, 2000;

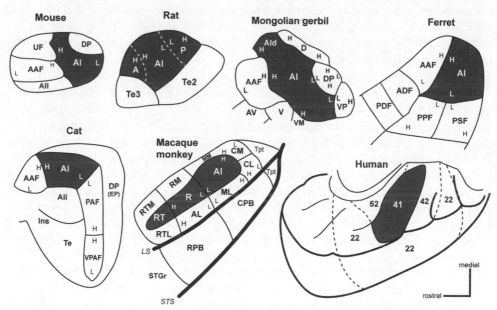

Fig. 2.13 Schematic drawings of the auditory cortex in several mammals. Primary (core) auditory areas are *shaded*. Belt areas are *unshaded*. Tonotopic gradients are indicated by H (high) and L (low) frequency. A Anterior area; A1 auditory area 1; AII auditory area 2; AAF anterior auditory field; ADF anterior dorsal field; AV anterior ventral area; CL caudolateral area; CM caudomedial area; D dorsal area; DC dorsocaudal area; DCB dorsocaudal belt area; DP dorsal posterior area; DRB dorsorostral belt area; PAF posterior auditory field; VPAF ventral posterior auditory field; Ins insula; MM middle medial area; P posterior area; PDF posterior dorsal field; R rostral area; RM rostromedial area; RT rostrotemporal area; RTL rostrotemporal lateral area; RTM rostrotemporal medial area; Te temporal area; V ventral area; VCB ventrocaudal belt area; VM ventral medial area; VRB ventrorostral belt area. *Numbers* denote Brodmann's areas. (Adapted from Bizley *et al.* (2005) (ferret); Brodmann (1909) (human); Budinger *et al.* (2000) (Mongolian gerbil); Kaas and Hackett (1998) (macaque monkey); Lee *et al.* (2004) (cat); Rutkowski *et al.* (2003) (rat); Stiebler *et al.* (1997) (mouse).)

Jones, 2003). At least eight different classes of pyramidal and non-pyramidal cells are distributed across the six layers of the auditory cortex (Fig. 2.14; Winer, 1992). Pyramidal cells tend to be glutamatergic and are concentrated in layers III and V. GABAergic cells are mainly non-pyramidal, and account for about one-fourth of the neurons in most layers, except layer I. Layer I has the fewest cells, where over 90% are small GABAergic neurons. Layer II contains both pyramidal and non-pyramidal neurons. The smaller cells are located superficially in layer II, while the larger pyramidal cells predominate near the border with layer III. About one-fourth of the non-pyramidal cells are GABAergic. Layer III is populated by several types of pyramidal and non-pyramidal cells of variable size. The largest pyramidal cells are deep in layer III (IIIb) at the border with layer IV. Their apical dendrites extend to layer I where they branch horizontally, while the basal dendrites spread widely within layers III and IV, contributing to the horizontal band involving layers IIIb and IV. Smaller pyramidal cells populate the more superficial parts of layer III. The non-pyramidal cells of layer III include tufted, stellate, and multipolar neurons of various sizes, and tend to be GABAergic. Layer IV receives a dense thalamocortical projection from the MGV. It is mainly populated by small tufted cells which have radially oriented somata and dendritic fields,

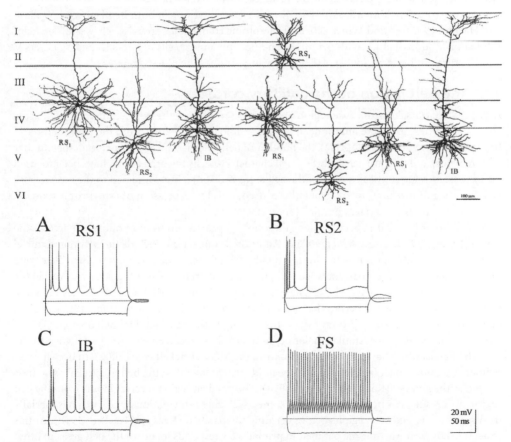

Fig. 2.14 Laminar distribution of neuron types and their response profiles in the auditory cortex of the rat. *Top*, spiny cells in layers II–VI. **A–D** Types of responses to square current pulses. **A** Regular spiking 1 (RS1), fast adaptation early in response. **B** Regular spiking 2 (RS2), adaptation throughout pulse. **C** Intrinsic bursting (IB), initial burst of spikes followed by regular spiking. **D** Fast spiking (FS), little or no adaptation. (Adapted from Hefti and Smith, 2000.)

and make mainly local projections. Layer V contains both pyramidal and non-pyramidal neurons. The somata of the conspicuous large pyramidal neurons located in layer Vb have apical dendrites that extend to layer I, with several branches along the way. The other pyramidal cells in layer V are smaller and more evenly distributed. GABAergic cells in layer V are mainly multipolar and bipolar varieties. Layer VI has perhaps the widest variety of cell types. These include several classes of pyramidal cells, along with multipolar, bipolar, and horizontal cells. Less than 20% of layer VI neurons are GABAergic (Winer, 1992).

The main source of ascending inputs to A1 and other core areas is the MGV (Winer, 1985; Jones, 2007; Lee and Winer, 2008a). The thalamocortical termination is concentrated in layers III and IV. The organization of these connections is topographic, reflecting tonotopic organization within the MGV, as well as the areas to which it projects. Additional inputs to the core include MGM, which projects broadly to all areas of the auditory cortex. Inputs from MGD are absent or minimal. The intracortical connections of the core mainly include other areas of the auditory cortex ipsilaterally, and sparse connections with areas beyond the auditory cortex. Tonotopically matched sites are more densely interconnected than non-matched sites (Lee and Winer, 2005), a feature that is likely to reflect an underlying organizational principle of the auditory cortex. Connections with the auditory cortex in the opposite hemisphere are concentrated in the homotopic (matching) area, and most strongly link identical best-frequency representations in both hemispheres (Wallace and Harper, 1997; Lee and Winer 2008b). Heterotopic connections are relatively weak. The main callosal projections include both pyramidal and non-pyramidal cells in layers III and V. Layers V and VI represent the main source of descending projections to the MGB and IC.

2.7.2 The belt region of the auditory cortex

Areas that lie outside of the core region are often referred to as the non-lemniscal or belt areas (Fig. 2.13). These areas are anatomically and physiologically distinct from the core fields, and from one another. In a given species, the number of belt fields is typically greater than the number of core fields, and they are generally less well characterized, as research efforts have been focused on the core. Architectonically, each of the belt areas is distinct, but compared to the core region, cell density and myelination are generally reduced, as is the expression of cytochrome oxidase, acetylcholinesterase, and parvalbumin (Jones, 2003).

Aside from inputs from the core, the main source of projections to most of the belt areas is the MGD (Jones, 2007; Lee and Winer, 2008a). Additional connections include the MGM and nuclei surrounding the MGB, such as the suprageniculate, limitans, posterior, and pulvinar. Belt areas tend to differ with respect to the balance of inputs from different thalamic nuclei. Area AAF in the cat is perhaps an extreme example, as it has strong inputs from the MGV and MGD (rostral pole). Coupled with response properties that are similar to neurons in A1 (Eggermont, 1998), AAF in cats could be considered a primary field. Interestingly, the caudomedial belt area (CM) (see Fig. 2.13) in monkeys has similar thalamic inputs to those received by AAF, in contrast to the other belt areas which have almost no input from the MGV (Hackett *et al.*, 2007). In non-human primates, an additional belt of areas has been identified lateral to the belt areas. This region is known as the *parabelt* (Kaas and Hackett, 1998). The parabelt region receives inputs from the belt region and MGD, but not the core; thus, some ascending information appears to pass serially through the core and belt regions before reaching the parabelt (Kaas and Hackett, 1998). At this time, it is not clear whether the parabelt in primates corresponds to any of the belt areas in other species, although the caudal posterior ectosylvian in cats has similar patterns of cortical and thalamic connections (Lee and Winer, 2008c).

In contrast to the core, areas in the belt and parabelt have widespread connections with areas outside the auditory cortex (Romanski *et al.*, 1999). In primates, several studies have noted that the organization of the belt and parabelt connections is topographic, such that caudal and rostral areas of the auditory cortex project to largely different areas of the temporal, frontal, and parietal lobes. This has been interpreted as evidence of functional segregation in the outputs of the auditory cortex to different parts of the cortex (Rauschecker and Tian, 2000).

2.8 Conclusions

The mammalian auditory system comprises a highly complex network of interconnected subcortical nuclei and cortical areas designed to extract, encode, and interpret acoustic signals in a dynamic auditory environment. A wide variety of neurons interconnected by multiple parallel pathways on both sides of the brain contribute to these computational tasks at all stages of processing. From these computations emerge information about the location and identity of auditory objects which is used to guide behavior. Precisely how the auditory system accomplishes these tasks is only partially understood, but sustained efforts to explore the structural and functional details of its organization are gradually filling in the gaps, as discussed throughout this volume.

List of abbreviations

AC	Auditory cortex
Ac str	Acoustic stria
AVCN	Anteroventral cochlear nucleus
bic	Brachium of the inferior colliculus
cc	Corpus callosum
cic	Commissure of the inferior colliculus
cll	Commissure of the lateral lemniscus
CNC	Cochlear nucleus complex
CNIC	Central nucleus of the inferior colliculus
das	Dorsal acoustic stria
DCIC	Inferior colliculus, dorsal cortex
DCN	Dorsal cochlear nucleus
DNLL	Dorsal nucleus of the lateral lemniscus
GrC	Granule cell layer
h	High frequency representation
IC	Inferior colliculus
l	Low frequency representation
LCIC	Lateral cortex of the inferior colliculus
ll	lateral lemniscus
MGB	Medial geniculate body
MGD	Medial geniculate body, dorsal nucleus
MGM	Medial geniculate body, medial nucleus
MGV	Medial geniculate body, ventral nucleus
LSO	Superior olivary complex, lateral nucleus
MNTB	Medial nucleus of the trapezoid body (SOC)
MSO	Superior olivary complex, medial nucleus
NLL	Nuclei of the lateral lemniscus
PIL	Posterior intralaminar nucleus
PO	Periolivary nuclei
PP	Peripeduncular nucleus
RCIC	Rostral cortex of the inferior colliculus

Rt	Reticular nucleus
SOC	Superior olivary complex
SPO	Superior periolivary nucleus
tz	Trapezoid body
VCN	Ventral cochlear nucleus
VNLL	Ventral nucleus of the lateral lemniscus
VNTB	Ventral nucleus of the trapezoid body (SOC)

References

Adams JC (1979) Ascending projections to the inferior colliculus. *J Comp Neurol* 183: 519–38.

Adams JC (1983) Cytology of periolivary cells and the organization of their projections in the cat. *J Comp Neurol* 215: 2752–89.

Aitkin LM, Dickhaus H, Schult W, Zimmermann M (1978) External nucleus of inferior colliculus, auditory and spinal somatosensory afferents and their interactions. *J Neurophysiol* 41: 837–47.

Anderson LA, Malmierca MS, Wallace MN, Palmer AR (2006) Evidence for a direct, short latency projection from the dorsal cochlear nucleus to the auditory thalamus in the guinea pig. *Eur J Neurosci* 24(2): 491–8.

Arnott RH, Wallace MN, Shackleton TM, Palmer AR (2004) Onset neurones in the anteroventral cochlear nucleus project to the dorsal cochlear nucleus. *J Assoc Res Otolaryngol* 5(2):153–70.

Banks MI, Smith PH (1992) Intracellular recordings from neurobiotin-labeled cells in brain slices of the rat medial nucleus of the trapezoid body. *J Neurosci* 12: 2819–37.

Bartlett EL, Smith PH (1999) Anatomic, intrinsic, and synaptic properties of dorsal and ventral division neurons in rat medial geniculate body. *J Neurophysiol* 81(5): 1999–2016.

Bizley JK, Nodal FR, Nelken I, King AJ (2005) Functional organization of ferret auditory cortex. *Cereb Cortex* 15: 1637–53.

Brawer JR, Morest DK, Kane EC (1974) The neuronal architecture of the cochlear nucleus of the cat. *J Comp Neurol* 155: 251–300.

Brodal A (1981) Neurological Anatomy In Relation to Clinical Medicine. Oxford University Press, Oxford.

Brodmann K (1909) Vergleichende lokalisationslehre der grosshirnrinde barth, Leipzig.

Brown MC, Liberman MC, Benson TE, Ryugo DK (1988) Brainstem branches from olivocochlear axons in cats and rodents. *J. Comp. Neurol.* 278, 591–603.

Budinger E, Heil P, Scheich H (2000) Functional organization of auditory cortex in the Mongolian gerbil (*Meriones unguiculatus*). IV. Connections with anatomically characterized subcortical structures. *Eur J Neurosci* 12: 2452–74.

Burton H, Jones EG (1976) The posterior thalamic region and its cortical projection in New World and Old World monkeys. *J Comp Neurol* 168(2): 249–301.

Cant NB, Benson CG (2003) Parallel auditory pathways: projection patterns of the different neuronal populations in the dorsal and ventral cochlear nuclei. *Brain Res Bull* 60: 457–74.

Cant NB, Benson CG (2006) Organization of the inferior colliculus of the gerbil (*Meriones unguiculatus*): differences in distribution of projections from the cochlear nuclei and the superior olivary complex. *J Comp Neurol* 495: 511–28.

Cant NB, Benson CG (2007) Multiple topographically organized projections connect the central nucleus of the inferior colliculus to the ventral division of the medial geniculate nucleus in the gerbil, *Meriones unguiculatus*. *J Comp Neurol* 503: 432–53.

Casseday JH, Fremouw T, Covey E (2002) The inferior colliculus, a hub for the central audiotory system. In: *Springer Handbook of Auditory Research* (eds Oertel D, Popper AN, Fay RR). Springer, New York.

Covey E, Casseday JH (1991) The monoaural nuclei of the lateral lemniscus in an echolocatin bat: parallel pathways for analyzing temporal features of sound. *J Neurosci* 11: 3456–70.

Covey E, Kauer JA, Casseday JH (1996) Whole-cell patch-clamp recording reveals subthreshold sound-evoked postsynaptic currents in the inferior colliculus of awake bats. *J Neurosci* **16**: 3009–18.

Dehmel S, Kopp-Scheinpflug C, Dörrscheidt GJ, Rübsamen R (2002) Electrophysiological characterization of the superior paraolivary nucleus in the Mongolian gerbil. *Hear Res* **172**: 18–36.

Doron NN, Ledoux JE (1999) Organization of projections to the lateral amygdala from auditory and visual areas of the thalamus in the rat. *J Comp Neurol* **412**(3): 383–409.

Doucet JR, Ryugo DK (1997) Projections from the ventral cochlear nucleus to the dorsal cochlear nucleus in rats. *J Comp Neurol* **385**: 245–64.

Doucet JR, Ross AT, Gillespie MB, Ryugo DK (1999) Glycine immunoreactivity of multipolar neurons in the ventral cochlear nucleus which project to the dorsal cochlear nucleus. *J Comp Neurol* **408**: 515–31.

Echteler SM, Fay RR, Popper AN (1994) Structure of the mammalian cochlea. In: *Comparative Hearing: Mammals* (eds Fay RR, Popper AN), pp. 134–71. Springer, Berlin.

Eggermont JJ (1998) Representation of spectral and temporal sound features in three cortical fields of the cat. Similarities outweigh differences. *J Neurophysiol* **80**(5): 2743–64.

Fay RR, Popper AN (1994) *Comparative Hearing in Mammals. Springer Handbook of Auditory Research.* Springer, New York.

Faye-Lund H, Osen KK (1985) Anatomic of the inferior colliculus in rat. *Anat Embryol* **175**: 35–52.

Friauf E (1993) Transient appearance of calbindin-D28k-positive neurons in the superior olivary complex of developing rats. *J. Comp. Neurol.* **334**, 59–74.

Friauf E, Ostwald J (1988) Divergent projections of physiologically characterized rat ventral cochlear nucleus neurons as shown by intra-axonal injection of horseradish peroxidase. *Exp Brain Res* **73**(2): 263–84.

Hackett TA, Smiley JF, Ulbert I, *et al.* (2007) Sources of somatosensory input to the caudal belt areas of auditory cortex. *Perception* **36**: 1419–30.

Hefti BJ, Smith PH (2000) Anatomy, physiology, and synaptic responses of rat layer V auditory cortical cells and effects of intracellular GABA(A) blockade. *J Neurophysiol* **83**(5): 2626–38.

Held H (1893) Die centralem Bahnen des Nervus acusticus bei der Katz. *Arch Anat Abtheil* **15**. 190–271.

Helfert RH, Aschoff A (1997) Superior olivary complex and nuclei of the lateral lemniscus. In: *Anatomical and Functional Aspects of the Cochlear Nucleus* (eds Ehret G, Romand R), pp. 193–257. Oxford Univerity Press, Oxford.

Herbert H, Aschoff A, Ostwald J (1991) Topography of projections from the auditory cortex to the inferior colliculus in the rat. *J. Comp. Neurol.* **304**, 103–122.

Hernández O, Rees A, Malmierca MS (2006) A GABAergic component in the commissure of the inferior colliculus in rat. *Neuroreport* **17**: 1611–14.

Irvine DRF (1992) Physiology of the auditory brainstem. In: *Springer Handbook of Auditory Pathway: Neurophysiology* (eds Popper AN, Fay RR), pp. 153–231. Springer, New York.

Jones EG (2003) Chemically defined parallel pathways in the monkey auditory system. *Ann N Y Acad Sci* **999**: 218–33.

Jones EG (2007) *The Thalamus*, 2nd edn, Vol II. Cambridge University Press, Cambridge, pp. 875–923.

Joris PX, Smith PH, Yin TCT (1998) Coincidence detection in the auditory system, 50 years after Jeffress. *Neuron* **21**: 1235–8.

Kaas JH, Hackett TA (1998) Subdivisions of auditory cortex and levels of processing in primates. *Audiol Neurootol* **3**(2–3): 73–85.

Kaas JH and Hackett TA (2000) Subdivisions of auditory cortex and processing streams in primates. *Proc Natl Acad Sci USA* **97**: 11793–9.

Kelly JB, Caspary DM (2005) Pharmachology of the inferior colliculus. In: *The Inferior Colliculus* (eds Winer JA, Schreiner C), pp. 248–81. Springer, New York.

King AJ, Jiang ZD, Moore DR (1998) Auditory brainstem projections to the ferret superior colliculus: anatomical contribution to the neural coding of sound azimuth. *J Comp Neurol* **390**: 342–65.

Kulesza RJ Jr, Spirou GA, Berrebi AS (2003) Physiological response properties of neurons in the superior paraolivary nucleus of the rat. *J Neurophysiol* **89**: 2299–312.

Kuwada S, Batra R, Yin TC, Oliver DL, Haberly L B, Stanford TR (1997) Intracellular recordings in response to monaural and binaural stimulation of neurons in the inferior colliculus of the cat. *J Neurosci* **17**: 7565–81.

Langner G, Schreiner CE (1988) Periodicity coding in the inferior colliculus of the cat. I. Neuronal mechanisms. *J Neurophysiol* **60**(6): 1799–822.

LeBeau FEN, Malmierca MS, Rees A (2001) Iontophoresis *in vivo* demonstrates a key role for GABA$_A$- and glycinergic inhibition in shaping frequency response areas in the inferior colliculus of guinea pig. *J Neurosci* **21**: 7303–312.

Lee CC, Winer JA (2005) Principles governing auditory cortex connections. *Cereb Cortex* **15**(11): 1804–814.

Lee CC, Winer JA (2008a) Connections of cat auditory cortex: I. Thalamocortical system. *J Comp Neurol* **507**(6): 1879–900.

Lee CC, Winer JA (2008b) Connections of cat auditory cortex: II. Commissural system. *J Comp Neurol* **507**(6): 1901–19.

Lee CC and Winer JA (2008c) Connections of cat auditory cortex: III. Corticocortical system. *J Comp Neurol* **507**(6): 1920–43.

Lee CC, Schreiner CE, Imaizumi K, Winer JA (2004) Tonotopic and heterotopic projection systems in physiologically defined auditory cortex. *Neuroscience* **128**: 871–87.

Liberman MC, Dodds LW, Pierce S (1990) Afferent and efferent innervation of the cat cochlea: quantitative analysis with light and electron microscopy. *J Comp Neurol* **301**: 443–60.

Loftus B, Malmierca MS, Oliver DL (2008) The cytoarchitecture of the inferior colliculus revisited: a common organization of the lateral cortex in rat and cat. *Neuroscience* **154**: 196–205.

Lorente de Nó R (1981) *The Primary Acoustic Nuclei*. Raven Press, New York.

Malmierca MS (2003) The structure and physiology of the rat auditory system: an overview. *Int Rev Neurobiol* **56**: 147–211.

Malmierca MS (2004) The inferior colliculus: A center for convergence of ascending and descending auditory information. *Neuroembry. Aging* **3**:215–229.

Malmierca MS, Blackstad TW, Osen KK, Karagülle T, Molowny RL (1993) The central nucleus of the inferior colliculus in rat. A Golgi and computer reconstruction study of neuronal and laminar structure. *J Comp Neurol* **333**: 1–27.

Malmierca MS, Rees A, LeBeau FEN, Bajaalie JG (1995) Laminar organization of frequency-defined local axons within and between the inferior colliculi of the guinea pig. *J Comp Neurol* **357**: 124–44.

Malmierca MS, LeBeau FEN, Rees A (1996) The topographical organization of descending projections from the central nucleus of the inferior colliculus in guinea pig. *Hear Res* **93**: 167–80.

Malmierca MS, Leergard TB, Bajo VM, Bjaalie JG (1998) Anatomic evidence of a 3-D mosaic pattern of tonotopic organization in the ventral complex of the lateral lemniscus in cat. *J Neurosci* **19**: 10603–18.

Malmierca MS, Merchán M, Henkel CK, Oliver DL (2002) Direct projections from the dorsal cochlear nucleus to the auditory thalamus in rat. *J Neurosci* **22**: 10891–7.

Malmierca MS, Hernández O, Falconi A, Lopez-Poveda EA, Merchán MA, Rees A (2003) The commissure of the inferior colliculus shapes frequency response areas in rat: an *in vivo* study using reversible blockade with microinjection of kynurenic acid. *Exp Brain Res* **153**: 522–9.

Malmierca MS, Saint Marie RL, Merchan MA, Oliver DL (2005a) Laminar inputs from dorsal cochlear nucleus and ventral cochlear nucleus to the central nucleus of the inferior colliculus: two patterns of convergence. *Neuroscience* **136**: 883–94.

Malmierca MS, Hernández O, Rees A (2005b) Intercollicular commissural projections modulate neuronal responses in the inferior colliculus. *Eur J Neurosci* **21**: 2701–10.

Malmierca MS, Hernández O, Antunes FM, Rees A (2009a) Divergent and point-to-point connections in the commissural pathway between the inferior colliculi. *J. Comp. Neurol.* **514**: 226–239.

Malmierca MS, Cristaudo S, Pérez-González D, Covey E (2009b) Stimulus-specific adaptation in the inferior colliculus of the anesthetized rat. *J Neurosci* **29**: 5483–93.

Merchán M, Aguilar LA, Lopez-Poveda EA, Malmierca MS (2005) The inferior colliculus of the rat: quantitative immunocytochemical study of GABA and glycine. *Neuroscience* **136**: 907–25.

Moore JK, Osen KK (1979) The cochlear nuclei in man. *Am J Anat* **154**: 393–418.

Morest DK (1968) The collateral system of the medial nucleus of the trapezoid body of the cat, its neuronal architecture and relation to the olivo-cochlear bundle. *Brain Res* **9**: 288–311.

Mugnaini E, Osen KK, Dahl A-L, Friedrich V L Jr, Korte G (1980a) Fine structure of granule cells and related interneurons (termed Golgi cells) in the cochlear nuclear complex of cat, rat and mouse. *J Neurocytol* **9**: 537–70.

Mugnaini E, Warr WB, Osen KK (1980b) Distribution and light microscopic features of granule cells in the cochlear nuclei of cat, rat, and mouse. *J Comp Neurol* **191**: 581–606.

Oertel D (1999) The role of timing in the brain stem auditory nuclei of vertebrates. *Annu Rev Physiol* **61**: 497–519.

Oertel D, Young ED (2004) What's a cerebellar circuit doing in the auditory system? *Trend Neurosci* **27**: 104–10.

Oertel D, Wu SH, Garb MW, Dizack, C (1990) Morphology and physiology of cells in slice preparations of the posteroventral cochlear nucleus of mice. *J Comp Neurol* **295**: 136–54.

Oliver DL, Morest DK (1984) The central nucleus of the inferior colliculus in the cat. *J Comp Neurol* **222**: 237–64.

Oliver DL, Ostapoff EM, Beckius GE (1999) Direct innervation of identified tectothalamic neurons in the inferior colliculus by axons from the cochlear nucleus. *Neuroscience* **93**: 643–58.

Osen KK (1969) Cytoarchitectureof the cochlear nuclei in the cat. *J Comp Neurol* **136**: 453–83.

Osen KK (1988) Anatomy of the mammalian cochlear nuclei, A review. In: *Auditory Pathway, Structure and Function* Auditory Pathway, Structure and Function (J. Syka and R. B. Masterton Eds.), pp. 65–75, Plenum Press, New York.

Osen KK, Mugnaini E, Dahl AL, Christiansen AH (1984) Histochemical localization of acetylcholinesterase in the cochlear and superior olivary nuclei. A reappraisal with emphasis on the cochlear granule cell system. *Arch Ital Biol* **122**: 169–212.

Osen KK, Ottersen OP, Størm-Mathisen J (1990) Colocalization of glycine-like and GABA-like inmunoreactivities, a semiquantitative study of individual neurons in the dorsal cochlear nucleus of cat. In: *Glycine Neurotransmission* (eds Ottersen OP, Størm-Mathissen J), pp. 417–51. Wilcy, Chichester.

Ota Y, Oliver DL, Dolan DF (2004) Frequency-specific effects on cochlear responses during activation of the inferior colliculus in the guinea pig. *J Neurophysiol* **91**: 2185–93.

Palombi PS and Caspary DM (1996) Responses of young and aged Fischer 344 rat inferior colliculus neurons to binaural tonal stimuli. *Hear Res* **100**: 59–67.

Perez-Gonzalez D, Malmierca MS, Covey E (2005) Novelty detector neurons in the mammalian auditory midbrain. *Eur J Neurosci* **22**(11): 2879–85.

Peruzzi D, Bartlett E, Smith PH, Oliver DL (1997) A monosynaptic GABAergic input from the inferior colliculus to the medial geniculate body in rat. *J Neurosci* **17**: 3766–77.

Rajan R (1990) Electrical stimulation of the inferior colliculus at low rates protects the cochlea from auditory desensitization. *Brain Res* **506**: 192–204.

Rauschecker JP and Tian B (2000) Mechanisms and streams for processing of "what" and "where" in auditory cortex. *Proc Natl Acad Sci USA* **97**(22): 11800–6.

Rietzel HJ, Friauf E (1998) Neuron types in the rat lateral superior olive and developmental changes in the complexity of their dendritic arbors. *J Comp Neurol* **390**: 20–40.

Romanski LM, Tian B, Fritz J, Mishkin M, Goldman-Rakic PS, Rauschecker JP (1999) Dual streams of auditory afferents target multiple domains in the primate prefrontal cortex. *Nat Neurosci* **2**(12): 1131–6.

Rutkowski RG, Miasnikov AA, Weinberger NM (2003) Characterisation of multiple physiological fields within the anatomical core of rat auditory cortex. *Hear Res* 181: 116–30.

Ryugo DK, Parks TN (2003) Primary innervation of the avian and mammalian cochlear nucleus. *Brain Res Bull* 60: 435–56.

Saldaña E, Merchán MA (1992) Intrinsic and commissural connections of the rat inferior colliculus. *J Comp Neurol* 319: 417–37.

Schofield BR (1995) Projections from the cochlear nucleus to the superior paraolivary nucleus in guinea pigs. *J Comp Neurol* 360: 135–49.

Schofield BR, Cant NB (1991) Organization of the superior olivary complex in the guinea pig. I. Cytoarchitecture, cytochrome oxidase histochemistry, and dendritic morphology. *J Comp Neurol* 314: 645–70.

Schreiner CE, Langner G (1988) Coding of temporal patterns in the central auditory nervous system. In: *Auditory Function* (eds. Edelman GM, Gall WE, Cowan WM), pp. 337–40. Wiley, New York.

Schreiner CE, Langner G (1997) Laminar fine structure of frequency organization in auditory midbrain. *Nature* 388: 383–6.

Sinex DG, López DE, Warr WB (2001) Electrophysiological responses of cochlear root neurons. *Hear Res* 370: 1–11.

Sivaramakrishnan S, Oliver DL (2001) Distinct K^+ currents result in physiologically distinct cell types in the inferior colliculus of the rat. *J Neurosci* 21: 2861–77.

Slepecky NB (1996) Structure of the mammalian cochlea. In: *The Cochlea. Springer Handbook of Auditory Research* (eds Dallos P, Popper AN, Fay RR), pp. 44–129. Springer, New York.

Smith PH (1995) Structural and functional differences distinguish principal from nonprincipal cells in the guinea pig MSO slice. *J Neurophysiol* 73: 1653–67.

Smith PH, Rhode WS (1989) Structural and functional properties distinguish two types of multipolar cells in the ventral cochlear nucleus. *J Comp Neurol* 282: 595–616.

Smith PH, Joris PX, Carney LH, Yin TCT (1991) Projections of physiologically characterized globular bushy cell axons from the cochlear nucleus of the cat. *J Comp Neurol* 304: 387–407.

Spoendlin H (1972) Innervation densities of the cochlea. *Acta Otolaryngol* 73: 235–48.

Stiebler I, Neulist R, Fichtel I, Ehret G (1997) The auditory cortex of the house mouse: left-right differences, tonotopic organization and quantitative analysis of frequency representation. *J. Comp. Physiol A: Sensory, Neural, and Behavioral Physiology* 181: 559–571.

Thompson AM (1998) Heterogeneous projections of the cat posteroventral cochlear nucleus. *J Comp Neurol* 390: 439–53.

Thompson AM, Schofield BR (2000) Afferent projections of the superior olivary complex. *Micr Res Tech* 51: 330–54.

Wallace MN, Harper MS (1997) Callosal connections of the ferret primary auditory cortex. *Exp Brain Res* 116(2): 367–74.

Warr WB (1992) Organization of olivocochlear efferent systems in mammals. In: *The Mammalian Auditory Pathway, Neuroanatomy* (eds Webster DB, Popper AN, Fay RR), pp. 410–48. Springer, Berlin.

Wickesberg RE, Oertel D (1988) Tonotopic projection from the dorsal to the anteroventral cochlear nucleus of mice. *J Comp Neurol* 268: 389–99.

Winer JA (1985) The medial geniculate body of the cat. *Adv Anat Embryol Cell Biol* 86: 1–97.Winer JA (1992) The functional architecture of the medial geniculate body and the primary auditory cortex. In: *The Mammlian Auditory Pathway. Neuroanatomy* (eds Webster DB, Popper AN, Fay RR), pp. 222–409. Springer, New York.

Winer JA, Larue DT (1988) Anatomy of glutamic acid decarboxylase immunoreactive neurons and axons in the rat medial geniculate body. *J Comp Neurol* 278(1): 47–68.

Winer JA, Morest DK (1983) The medial division of the medial geniculate body of the cat: implications for thalamic organization. *J Neurosci* 3(12): 2629–51.

Winer JA, Kelly JB, Larue DT (1999) Neural architecture of the rat medial geniculate body. *Hear Res* 130: 19–41.

Ye Y, Machado DG, Kim DO (2000) Projection of the marginal shell of the anteroventral cochlear nucleus to olivocochlear neurons in the cat. *J Comp Neurol* 420: 127–38.

Young ED, Davis KA (2002) Circuitry and function of the dorsal cochlear nucleus. In: *Springer Handbook of Auditory Research. Volume 15: Integrative Functions in the Mammalian Auditory Pathway* (eds Oertel D, Fay RR, Popper AN), pp. 160–206. Springer, New York.

Young ED, Shofner WP, White JA, Robert JM, Voigt HF (1988) Response properties of cochlear nucleus neurons in relationship to physiological mechanisms. In: *Auditory Function. Neurobiological Bases of Hearing* (eds Edelman GM, Gall WE, Cowan WM), pp. 277–312. Wiley, New York.

Zhang Y, Wu SH (2000) Long-term potentiation in the inferior colliculus studied in rat brain slice. *Hear Res* 147: 92–103.

Zhao M, Wu SH (2001) Morphology and physiology of neurons in the ventral nucleus of the lateral lemniscus in rat brain slices. *J Comp Neurol* 433: 255–71.

Zhou J, Shore S (2006) Convergence of spinal trigeminal and cochlear nucleus projections in the inferior colliculus of the guinea pig. *J Comp Neurol* 495: 100–112.

Chapter 3

Structural organization of the descending auditory pathway

Brett R. Schofield

3.1 Introduction

The descending auditory system extends from the cerebral cortex to the cochlea. The circuitry suggests a variety of functions. A prominent theme has been feedback, whereby a higher level alters neuronal processing at lower levels and thus modifies the information transmitted in the ascending pathways. Such a role might not only control what information reaches consciousness, for example, but also improve the system's ability to extract salient information. Other descending projections may have protective roles such as minimizing damage due to loud sounds. The past decade has seen a resurgence of interest in the descending pathways. One area of advancement is associated with the olivocochlear system; the advances include insights into cellular and molecular aspects of the system, physiological effects on the cochlea, and the central circuitry that converges onto olivocochlear cells. A second area of advancement is the discovery that auditory cortex has more extensive subcortical projections than previously believed. It was well established that auditory cortex projects directly to the thalamus and inferior colliculus (IC); the new findings reveal significant projections to subcollicular centers such as the cochlear nucleus (CN) and nuclei in the superior olivary complex (SOC) and lateral lemniscus (LL). These findings raise many questions about the brainstem circuits that are under direct influence of cortical projections.

This chapter reviews descending projections that arise at each level of the auditory system. For reasons of space, we focus on pathways that both originate and terminate within the main ascending auditory pathways; we do not consider descending projections to other targets, such as the striatum (which may involve audio-motor coordination), the periaqueductal gray (e.g., for vocalization), or cranial nerve nuclei (e.g., for middle ear reflexes). Feedback 'loops', such as those formed by connections between the cortex and thalamus, continue to be important conceptual tools for understanding the descending systems. Interestingly, early workers considered the possibility of cognitive roles of descending systems, allowing for attentional effects as far 'down' as the cochlea (see discussion in Huffman and Henson, 1990). These views incorporated the concept of descending chains or multisynaptic pathways that provide the anatomical substrate for higher order effects to be exerted all the way to the cochlea. This review presents evidence for both loops and descending chains. The discussion begins with the olivocochlear system and progresses to successively higher levels of the auditory pathway.

3.2 The olivocochlear system

The SOC is a source of descending projections to the cochlea and the CN. The connections to the cochlea form the olivocochlear system. The SOC comprises medial and lateral superior olivary nuclei (MSO and LSO, respectively), often considered the principal nuclei, and cell groups surrounding the principal nuclei that are collectively termed the periolivary nuclei. Some of these cell groups form well-circumscribed nuclei whereas others are less well defined. The nuclei and the nomenclature vary across species and studies (for comparisons see Schofield and Cant, 1991; Schwartz, 1992; Helfert and Aschoff, 1997). For the present account, we will refer to the nuclei as identified in Fig. 3.1A.

Rasmussen (1946, 1960) identified the olivocochlear system and described two parts: an uncrossed projection and a crossed projection (Fig. 3.1B). The crossed and uncrossed axons collect in the dorsal brainstem to form the olivocochlear bundle (OCB) on each side. Along their course, many OCB axons give collaterals to various brainstem nuclei. The OCB axons leave the brain with the vestibular nerve, cross over to the auditory nerve via the vestibulocochlear anastomosis, and then continue to the cochlea to terminate in the organ of Corti.

Within the brainstem, the axons of crossed fibers travel close to the floor of the IV ventricle, which allows investigators to stimulate or cut the crossed fibers selectively. This technical issue makes the crossed axons accessible and distinguishable from uncrossed axons, allowing a great deal of data to be collected on both the crossed and uncrossed projections and reinforcing the distinction between crossed and uncrossed systems. Subsequent work by Warr and colleagues (e.g., Warr and Guinan, 1979) led to a major new perspective on the organization of OC projections: medial and lateral olivocochlear systems (MOC and LOC, respectively). As discussed below, the 'uncrossed' projection contains prominent MOC and LOC components, whereas the 'crossed' projection is dominated by the MOC system. The utility of the MOC and LOC terminology is that it appears to reflect substantial functional distinctions within the olivocochlear system. The MOC and LOC systems differ with regard to a wide range of characteristics, including location and morphology of the cells of origin, the neurotransmitters released by their axons, and the patterns of termination in the cochlea and brainstem.

OC cells have been characterized in many species. The cells of origin are scattered within the SOC (Fig. 3.1B). The medial and lateral systems are named according to the location of their cell bodies relative to a line drawn through the MSO (Fig. 3.1B).

3.2.1 The MOC system

In most species studied, the MOC cells are concentrated in the ventral nucleus of the trapezoid body (VNTB). They extend rostrally as far as the ventral nucleus of the lateral lemniscus, and may even invade it. Their cell bodies and myelinated axons are larger on average than those of most LOC cells, whose axons are mostly unmyelinated. About two-thirds of the MOC cells project to the contralateral cochlea. Most of the remaining cells project to the ipsilateral cochlea, and a few (1–5%) send branching axons to innervate the cochleae on both sides (Robertson et al., 1987).

In the cochlea, the MOC axons terminate on the outer hair cells (Fig. 3.1C). The projections are tonotopically organized, although not all parts of the cochlea are innervated with equal density by MOC axons (Guinan, 1996). Individual MOC cells respond to a narrow range of frequencies, allowing for frequency-specific effects of MOC projections on cochlear function (Guinan, 1996). The MOC axons release acetylcholine onto the outer hair cells. Activation of this system reduces the gain of the cochlear amplifier. It has been suggested that one function of the MOC system is to reduce masking and improve the ability of the system to respond to signals in a noisy environment (reviewed by Guinan, 1996).

Many MOC axons provide collaterals to the CN and to the vestibular nuclei (VN) (Fig. 3.1B; Brown, 1993). In the CN, the axons terminate in close relation to the granule cell area (grca) surrounding the VCN. Electron microscopic studies have identified the targets as stellate cells of

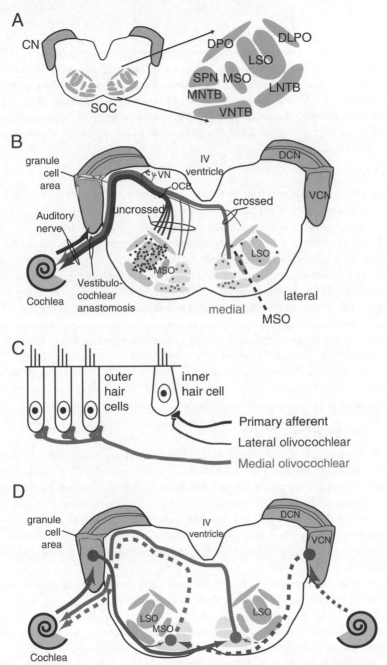

Fig. 3.1 Organization of superior olivary complex (SOC) and olivocochlear projections. **A** Schematic cross section through the brainstem in guinea pig showing location of the SOC (*blue*) and its component nuclei (*inset*). The cochlear nucleus (CN) is also shown for reference (*gray*). **B** The origins and axonal course of medial (*green*) and lateral (*red*) olivocochlear axons projecting to a single cochlea. Cells of origin are shown by *green* and *red dots*. OCB Olivocochlear bundle. **C** The terminations of medial olivocochlear axons (*green*) on outer hair cells and lateral olivocochlear axons (*red*) on sensory endings (primary afferents) associated with inner hair cells in the cochlea. **D** Projections from the cochlear nucleus (*blue*) to medial olivocochlear cells (*green*) that project to the left cochlea. *Solid lines* show the main pathway by which input to the left ear could affect the left cochlea; *dashed lines* show the main pathway by which input to the right ear could affect the left cochlea. DLPO Dorsolateral periolivary nucleus.

the VCN, whose dendrites extend into the granule cell area (Benson and Brown, 1990). These collateral projections have been proposed to 'compensate' for MOC effects on the cochlea (Benson and Brown, 1990). In this scenario, the MOC projections to the cochlea reduce cochlear output, while collaterals to the CN 'inform' a population of CN cells about the gain adjustment to allow these cells to accurately encode sound intensity. This idea of a 'feedback gain control system' has been expanded, with increasingly detailed characterization of cochlear and CN circuit components (for review see Ye *et al.*, 2000).

Inputs to MOC cells

MOC cells receive bilateral inputs from the VCN and descending inputs from the inferior colliculus and auditory cortex (described below). They also receive presumed modulatory inputs that use serotonin (from cells in the raphe nuclei), noradrenalin (from cells in the locus ceruleus), or substance P (source unknown) as neurotransmitters (reviewed in Thompson and Schofield, 2000). The majority of MOC cells are binaural, i.e., they can be influenced by stimulation of either ear (Guinan, 1996). Nonetheless, input from one ear (usually the contralateral) is often dominant. Consequently, MOC cells are usually activated best by stimulation of the contralateral ear (see Fig. 3.1D). This means that MOC cells with crossed axons could provide feedback to the ear that best drives them (solid lines in Fig. 3.1D). In contrast, MOC cells that have *uncrossed* axons could provide a pathway for stimulation of one ear to affect the opposite ear (dashed lines in Fig. 3.1D). Stimulation of the inferior colliculus also has been used to activate the OC system, presumably through the descending projections to MOC cells. Activation of MOC cells by auditory cortex, either directly or via a synapse in the colliculus, has been invoked to explain the effects of 'higher level' functions, such as attention, on function of the cochlea.

3.2.2 **The LOC system**

The LOC cells are scattered in and around the LSO and usually outnumber MOC cells (Fig. 3.1B). The cells are smaller on average than MOC cells. The majority (85–95%) project ipsilaterally to the cochlea. The axons are unmyelinated and thinner than MOC axons. In the cochlea, LOC axons terminate primarily on auditory nerve fibers that innervate the inner hair cells (Fig. 3.1C). The LOC axons also show uneven innervation along the length of the cochlea (see Guinan, 1996). The large ipsilateral projection is slightly reduced for low frequencies, whereas the small contralateral projection is biased toward low frequencies. The projections appear to be organized tonotopically.

In comparison to MOC cells, the LOC cells are more heterogeneous, and may comprise subsets. Vetter *et al.* (1991) distinguished 'intrinsic' LOC neurons that reside within the body of the LSO and 'shell' LOC cells that surround the LSO in rats. Not all species have OC neurons within the LSO; it is unclear whether functions served by 'intrinsic' LOC cells, such as those in rats, are absent in other species or are served by other ('non-intrinsic') LOC cells.

One area of variation among LOC cells is the presence of collaterals to brainstem nuclei. Some reports suggest a lack of collaterals, whereas others indicate collaterals to the CN and to the vestibular nuclei (Fig. 3.1B). Intrinsic LOC cells may lack collaterals whereas many shell LOC cells have collaterals to the CN (Horvath *et al.*, 2000). A second source of axonal variation is the pattern of termination in the cochlea: some LOC cells appear to terminate on *outer* rather than inner hair cells. The termination patterns may vary across species.

LOC cells are also heterogeneous with respect to neurotransmitters (Eybalin, 1993). Acetylcholine is released by most or all LOC cells. Numerous other neurotransmitters, including gamma aminobutyric acid (GABA), calcitonin gene-related peptide (CGRP), dopamine, enkephalin, and dynorphin, have been described as co-localizing with acetylcholine in LOC cells. In some species there may be subsets of LOC cells that release GABA or dopamine and not acetylcholine (Vetter *et al.*, 1991; Darrow *et al.*, 2006).

The questions surrounding LOC cells extend to their response properties. Inputs to LOC cells likely include the ipsilateral CN as well as noradrenergic and serotoninergic nuclei of the brainstem. However, the thin, unmyelinated LOC axons are difficult to record from and harder to stimulate than MOC axons. Guinan (1996) suggested that most of the data available on the effects of the OC system are in general likely attributable to the MOC system. Recent studies, using indirect means to isolate LOC effects, suggest that we may soon gain a more informed view of LOC function (e.g., Le Prell *et al.*, 2005; Darrow *et al.*, 2007).

3.2.3 Functions of the OC system

As described above, the OC system may play an important role in setting cochlear gain. This function alone has important implications for the interrelated issues of intensity encoding, dynamic range, masking, and hearing in noisy environments. Guinan (1996) elaborates on these and other functions such as selective attention and protection of the cochlea from damage resulting from intense sounds.

3.3 Origins and targets of central descending pathways

This section describes briefly the descending projections from the major subdivisions of the auditory pathways to lower auditory centers. We describe the cells of origin and the patterns of axonal termination. An important issue for subsequent discussion is the identity of the cells that are contacted by the descending axons. In particular, we would like to know the projections of the target cells in order to characterize the circuitry. The target cells are sometimes inferred from experiments with single anterograde tracers, and occasionally examined with electron microscopy. The latter technique allows for definitive identification of synapses, but rarely identifies the projections of the target cells. In a small number of cases, the latter issue has been addressed with multi-labeling light microscopy, in which one tracer is used to label the descending pathway and one or more additional tracers are used to label the pathways that may be contacted by the descending projection.

3.3.1 Superior olivary complex: projections to the cochlear nucleus

The SOC projects bilaterally to the CN. The cells of origin are scattered throughout the periolivary nuclei. The details vary across species, but in general the ipsilateral projections are more numerous and originate from more widely spread nuclei than the contralateral projections (Fig. 3.2). The projecting cells use a variety of neurotransmitters; the SOC is the main source of GABAergic, glycinergic, and cholinergic inputs to the CN, and a minor source of glutamatergic inputs (Helfert and Aschoff, 1997).

Olivary projections terminate throughout the CN (Schwartz, 1992; Helfert and Aschoff, 1997). Details of projections from individual nuclei are limited, but the evidence suggests that different nuclei can have different patterns of termination within the CN and that at least some of the projections are organized tonotopically (e.g., Warr and Beck, 1996).

Targets identified by projections

The CN has a variety of cell types that give rise to distinct ascending pathways (see Chapter 2). Consequently, it is of great interest to identify the cell types contacted by specific olivary inputs. The widespread olivary projections to the CN suggest that many CN cell types are directly contacted by olivary axons. However, there are only a few examples in which specific olivary cell types

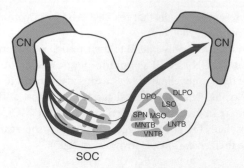

Fig. 3.2 Projections (*red arrows*) from the left superior olivary complex (SOC) to the cochlear nuclei (CN) on each side. In this and subsequent figures, *blue shading* shows the target areas of the projections and *pink shading* shows the location(s) of the cells of origin. In this figure, the thickness of the *arrows* shows the relative size of each projection (as measured by the number of cells of origin); *absence of arrows associated with a pink nucleus* (e.g., left LSO) indicates that there are very few cells of origin in that nucleus. The *arrows* do not indicate the actual course of axons through the brainstem.

have been associated with input to specific CN cells. Benson and Brown (1990) identified multipolar cells in the VCN as targets of MOC collaterals in the CN; the heterogeneity of the multipolar population means that the projections of these particular multipolar cells are unknown. Schofield (1994) identified projections from medial nucleus of the trapezoid body (MNTB) principal cells to globular bushy cells and multipolar cells in the ipsilateral VCN. Again, the projections of the multipolar cells are unknown, but those of globular bushy cells are well characterized; they project to the ipsilateral lateral nucleus of the trapezoid body (LNTB) and to the contralateral MNTB. The circuitry suggests a role in analysis of binaural disparities important for sound localization (see discussion in Schofield, 1994). Further speculation on the functions of olivo-CN projections awaits more detailed information associating olivary cell types with projections to specific CN cell types.

3.3.2 **Inferior colliculus**

The IC can be divided into several subdivisions, some of which may be species specific (Oliver, 2005). We identify a central nucleus (ICc), external cortex (ICx), and dorsal cortex (ICd) because this general scheme facilitates discussion across species. The IC projects to numerous targets, including the nuclei of the lateral lemniscus, the superior olivary complex, and the cochlear nucleus (Fig. 3.3A). The following description is based primarily on detailed studies in rats and guinea pigs (Caicedo and Herbert, 1993; Malmierca *et al.*, 1996).

Collicular projections to the nuclei of the lateral lemniscus and adjacent areas

The IC projects in a frequency-specific pattern to the ipsilateral dorsal nucleus of lateral lemniscus (DNLL) (see Caicedo and Herbert, 1993). Additional projections, with no apparent topography, end in the ipsilateral sagulum (Sag) horizontal cell group (h) (between the dorsal and intermediate nuclei of the lateral lemniscus (INLL)) and in regions medial to the ventral nucleus of the lateral lemniscus (VNLL) (the paralemniscal zone, pl). Sparse projections to the INLL and VNLL are sometimes described[1]. The ICc contributes to most or all of these projections, and is the sole

---

[1] More substantial projections to VNLL are sometimes described; these are difficult to distinguish from projections to the SOC (see Caicedo and Herbert, 1993).

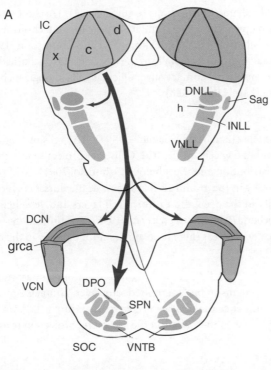

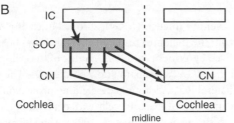

Fig. 3.3 Descending projections from the inferior colliculus (IC). **A** Projections (*red arrows*) from the left IC to brainstem targets. Conventions as in Fig. 3.2. **B** Pathways (*red arrows*) that appear to be contacted directly by axons descending from cells in the left IC (*black arrow*).

source of the topographic projections to the DNLL. The ICx projects to the sagulum and horizontal cell group, and the ICd projects primarily to the sagulum.

Collicular projections to the SOC

IC projections to the SOC are almost exclusively ipsilateral (reviewed by Thompson and Schofield, 2000). The cells of origin occur throughout the IC; in general, they are most numerous in the ICc and ICx, although the relative contribution from different subdivisions varies across species.

The targets of projections from the ICc and the ICx are similar. The majority of terminals are in the ipsilateral VNTB, with additional terminals in the superior paraolivary nucleus (SPN) and the dorsal periolivary nucleus (DPO). There is a small contralateral projection, primarily to the VNTB (Thompson and Schofield, 2000). Projections from the ICc to the ipsilateral VNTB are topographic according to frequency. Topography is not apparent in ICc projections to other SOC nuclei, or in the projections from the ICx.

Targets identified by projections As a group, the periolivary nuclei project to numerous places including the IC, CN, and cochlea. While the cells that project to these targets are intermingled, those that project to the IC form a population largely distinct from those that project to the cochlea or CN (i.e., few cells send collateral projections to these targets) (Aschoff and Ostwald, 1988; Schofield, 2002). Descending projections from the IC appear to contact olivary cells that project ipsilaterally or contralaterally to the cochlea (Thompson and Thompson, 1993; Vetter *et al.*, 1993) or ipsilaterally, contralaterally, or bilaterally to the CN (Fig. 3.3B; Schofield and Cant, 1999). It appears that collicular axons do *not* contact olivocollicular cells, though such a negative finding is difficult to demonstrate (Faye-Lund, 1988).

Collicular projections to the CN

The IC projects bilaterally to the CN (reviewed by Saldaña, 1993). The cells of origin are most numerous in the ICc and ICx, with a few cells in the ICd. Cells that project to the ipsilateral or contralateral CN are similar in distribution and morphology (Schofield, 2001).

The IC axons terminate bilaterally in the granule cell area and in the dorsal cochlear nucleus (DCN), where they end primarily in the deep and fusiform cell layers and, less densely, in the molecular layer (Caicedo and Herbert, 1993; Malmierca *et al.*, 1996). The projections to the DCN appear to be organized tonotopically, whereas there is no apparent topography in the projections to the granule cell area.

Targets identified by projections It is usually assumed that IC projections contact fusiform cells in the DCN; whether this is true remains to be determined. However, contacts onto other cell types in DCN would also likely influence the fusiform cells through intrinsic connections, so ultimately it is likely that IC projections to the CN affect the ascending projection from the DCN to the IC.

3.3.3 **Thalamus**

The medial geniculate body comprises a ventral nucleus (MGv), a dorsal nucleus (MGd), and a medial nucleus (MGm). A projection from the thalamus to the ipsilateral IC has been described in cats, gerbils, monkeys, and rats (reviewed by Winer *et al.*, 2002). Some of the cells of origin are located in the MGm and, in gerbils, in the MGd (Kuwabara and Zook, 2000). The descending axons of these cells terminate in the ipsilateral ICx. Additional descending projections arise from intralaminar thalamic nuclei. A prominent group of thalamic cells with descending projections is located in the subparafascicular nucleus (SPF; Fig. 3.4; Yasui *et al.*, 1992). The SPF receives inputs from the IC, regions surrounding the MG, and the auditory cortex, as well as somatosensory inputs from the spinal cord. Outputs of the SPF include non-auditory (e.g., hypothalamus, spinal cord) as well as auditory targets. The latter include ascending projections to auditory cortex as well as bilateral descending projections to the IC, the superior paraolivary nucleus of the SOC, and the CN (Fig. 3.4).

3.3.4 **Auditory cortex**

The auditory cortex (AC) projects directly to a range of targets (Fig. 3.5A). The projections to the MG and IC are by far the largest. Projections to targets below the IC were noted in a few early studies, but were not really appreciated until the landmark study by Feliciano *et al.* (1995). The 'new' targets include the cochlear nuclei, nuclei in and around the superior olivary complex, and regions adjacent to the nuclei of the lateral lemniscus.

Cortical projections to the thalamus

Projections to the auditory thalamus originate from all areas of AC and terminate in all subdivisions of the MG as well as numerous nuclei nearby (reviewed by Rouiller and Welker, 2000; Smith and Spirou, 2002; Winer, 2005). In general, each cortical area projects to multiple thalamic nuclei.

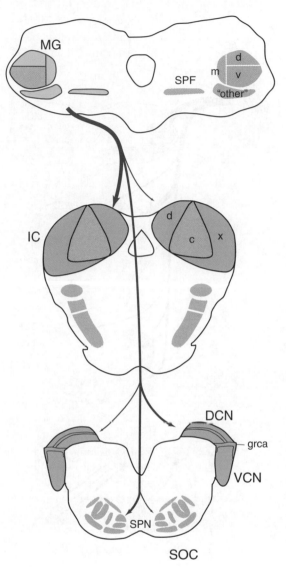

Fig. 3.4 Descending projections from the thalamus. MG Medial geniculate and its medial (m), dorsal (d), and ventral (v) divisions. SPF Subparafascicular nucleus of the thalamus; 'other' refers to a collection of various thalamic nuclei (see text for discussion). Conventions as in Fig. 3.2.

Almost all the areas project to the MGm, with additional, denser projections to MGv or MGd. Comparisons across species are complicated by the variable organization (and terminology) for thalamic and cortical areas. Nonetheless, one can identify common patterns.

Corticothalamic projections form parallel descending pathways that reflect the organization of the ascending pathways. Three systems can be distinguished: a tonotopic (or lemniscal) system, a diffuse (or non-tonotopic) system, and a polysensory system. This level of organization can also be extended to the cortico-collicular projections, and will be discussed below.

In general, the corticothalamic projections are topographic. Those from tonotopically organized cortical areas connect cortical and thalamic regions of similar frequency representation, presumably allowing for frequency-specific interactions. The significance of topography in projections from the non-tonotopically organized areas is unclear.

The majority of corticothalamic projections originate from pyramidal cells in cortical layer VI; these projections typically terminate in the thalamus as thin axons with small boutons. The boutons

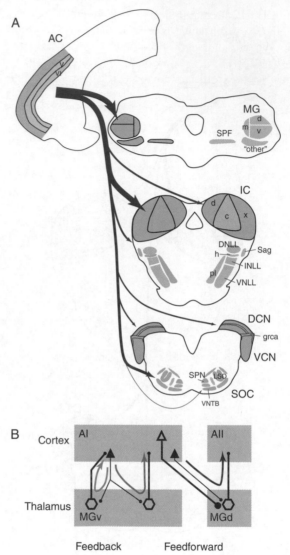

Fig. 3.5 Descending projections from the auditory cortex (AC). **A** Projections (*red arrows*) from the left AC to thalamic and brainstem auditory nuclei. Conventions as in Fig. 3.2. **B** Examples of cortico-thalamo-cortical circuits. *Gray boxes* represent cortical and thalamic areas. Projections from AI originate from layer VI cells (*solid triangles*) and layer V cells (*open triangle*). Some projections to MGv contact thalamocortical cells that project back to the same cortical column, forming a feedback circuit (*blue arrow*). Other projections contact cells in MGv that project back to a different part of A1; these projections (*green arrow*) form a 'local feedforward system'. Finally, projections from A1 go to MGd, where they contact thalamocortical cells that project to a different cortical area (AII). This pathway (*red arrow*) forms a 'distant feedforward' system. Additional circuits (e.g., involving MGm) exist, but are not shown.

contain round synaptic vesicles and form asymmetric synapses, consistent with excitatory physiologic effects (Bartlett *et al.*, 2000). Their targets include thalamocortical cells, interneurons and cells in the nearby thalamic reticular nucleus (the latter cells are GABAergic and project into the MG). These types of projections occur in all the auditory thalamic nuclei. A smaller number of projections originate from cortical layer V pyramidal cells; these projections typically comprise thicker axons and larger boutons. These axons originate in multiple cortical areas and terminate in restricted regions of the MG (especially the MGd), where they contact thalamocortical cells. These axons also contain round vesicles and form asymmetric synapses, consistent with excitatory effects.

A prominent feature of the corticothalamic projection is reciprocity, whereby a cortical region projects to the part of the thalamus from which it receives input. These connections could allow for a feedback function, which is often considered the primary role of corticothalamic projections. Reciprocity, and feedback, may occur at the level of a single cortical column and the corresponding group of thalamic cells that project to that column (Rouiller and Welker, 2000; Fig. 3.5B, blue arrow). Other corticothalamic axons terminate in a non-reciprocal fashion. These connections could allow for a 'feedforward' effect, whereby information from a cortical region could be sent to other parts of cortex (in the same or other cortical areas) via the thalamus. A 'local feedforward' circuit involves corticothalamic axons that contact thalamocortical cells that project to other columns in the same cortical area (Fig. 3.5B, green arrow). 'Distant feedforward' circuits involve corticothalamic axons that contact thalamocortical cells that project to different cortical areas (Fig. 3.5B, red arrow).

Feedback and feedforward ideas can be viewed within a broader framework of cortico-thalamo-cortical relationships that relate the pathways to axon morphology and physiological effects on thalamic cells. Sherman and Guillery (1996) describe drivers and modulators of thalamic cells, and although their work has focused on the visual and somatosensory thalamus, it may also apply to the auditory thalamus (Smith and Spirou, 2002). In so-called first-order thalamic nuclei, such as the MGv, corticothalamic inputs converge with ascending inputs on thalamic cells. The ascending inputs drive the thalamic cells whereas the cortical inputs play a modulatory role. In 'higher order' thalamic nuclei, such as the MGd, the 'driver' inputs are the large axons and terminals that originate from cortical layer V cells. Smaller axons, from cortical layer VI, are 'modulators'. The higher order thalamic nuclei also receive ascending inputs (e.g., from the IC), and it is unclear how these inputs interact with the cortical drivers. The higher order nuclei are seen as playing a role in a corticothalamic feedforward system, in which large layer V axons contact thalamic cells that relay information to another cortical area. An appealing aspect of these ideas is their apparent applicability across numerous species and systems (Rouiller and Welker, 2000). Nonetheless, exceptions exist, and other forms of processing may occur in the thalamus (see, e.g., Smith et al., 2007).

Cortical projections to the IC

Projections to the IC originate bilaterally in multiple AC areas (reviewed by Winer et al., 2002). The extent to which different areas project to the IC varies across species; in general, there are heavy projections from the core primary areas, while projections from the non-primary areas are more variable.

The cells of origin are located primarily in cortical layer V. This includes a large population that projects ipsilaterally to the IC and a smaller population that projects contralaterally (or bilater-ally) to the IC. Morphologically, these cells are pyramidal cells, probably of several varieties (Winer and Prieto, 2001; Bajo and Moore, 2005). Additional cells of origin are located in layer VI; these project to the ipsilateral IC. The layer VI cells are probably also pyramidal cells, but their morphology has not been described in detail.

The corticocollicular axons are distributed ipsilaterally to all IC subdivisions and contralaterally to the ICd and, in some species, to the ICx. The ipsilateral projections are denser than the contral-ateral ones. On the ipsilateral side, the terminations are much denser in the ICd and ICx than in the ICc. In fact, the projection to the ICc has been controversial; it is described as dense in rats (Saldaña et al., 1996) and less so in monkeys (Fitzpatrick and Imig, 1978), cats (Winer et al., 1998), gerbils (Budinger et al., 2000; Bajo and Moore, 2005), ferrets (Bajo et al., 2007), and guinea pigs (Peterson and Schofield, 2007).

Projections from tonotopic cortical areas are topographic. Both anatomical (Bajo et al., 2007) and physiological (Lim and Anderson, 2007) studies have demonstrated a tonotopic projection to ICc. Numerous studies have demonstrated frequency-specific effects on ICc cells (reviewed by Suga and Ma, 2003), though it is not clear whether these are due to direct AC projections to the ICc.

Projections to the ICd and ICx terminate in diffuse clouds or in more focused patches. An individual cortical area can project to multiple regions of the IC, and multiple cortical areas can project to a single part of the IC. The significance of this divergence and convergence has not been identified (Winer, 2005).

Further organization is seen in the projections to the ICd. The ICd is layered, and the projections from different AC areas terminate with distinct patterns in these layers. Different authors identify three or four layers in the ICd, but the key issue here is layer I vs deeper layers. AC areas that are tonotopically organized (e.g., A1) project to all ICd layers but terminate most heavily in the deeper layers (Winer *et al.*, 1998). Non-tonotopically organized AC areas can also project to multiple ICd layers, but usually project most heavily to layer I.

The boutons of cortical axons are small compared to lemniscal inputs to the IC (Jones and Rockel (1973) described these terminals in the 'dorsomedial' part of the central nucleus, an area corresponding to the ICd in the terminology used here). These terminals contain round vesicles and form asymmetric synapses with dendritic spines and, occasionally, dendritic shafts.

Functional roles of the corticocollicular and corticothalamic systems The corticothalamic and corticocollicular projections can be viewed together as forming several parallel systems (Fig. 3.6; Rouiller, 1997). The 'tonotopic' system involves the tonotopically organized cortical fields, the MGv and the ICc. This descending pathway parallels the 'lemniscal' ascending pathways. The 'diffuse' (or 'non-tonotopic') descending system involves non-tonotopic cortical fields (e.g., AII), the ICd, and the MGd. The 'polysensory' (or 'multimodal') system is associated with many cortical areas (including those associated with the tonotopic and diffuse systems) and with the ICx and MGm, both of which receive direct somatosensory inputs. It is presumed that these different systems serve distinct functions. The polysensory system is so named primarily because of somatosensory inputs to both the ICx and the MGm. The diffuse system 'originates' from the ICd, which is dominated by inputs from auditory cortex. This fact, along with a behavioral study following lesions of the ICd in cats (Jane *et al.*, 1965), has led to the suggestion that the diffuse system is involved in auditory attention. The tonotopic system is the largest and, as its name implies, is well suited for analysis according to frequency. Obviously, this covers a broad area; much remains to be learned about the functional roles of these three systems.

Targets identified by projections AC axons potentially could contact IC cells that project to any number of targets, including the MG, SOC, or CN. The IC cells that project to these targets are

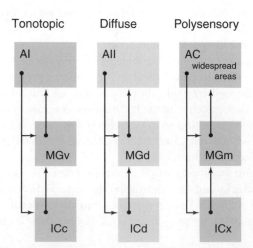

Fig. 3.6 Components of three different systems that interconnect the cortex, thalamus and midbrain areas. See text for discussion.

intermingled, but those that project to the MG form a population distinct from those that project to the CN or the SOC (Schofield, 2000; Coomes and Schofield, 2004c). Cortical axons appear to contact cells in the ipsilateral IC that project ipsilaterally or contralaterally to the MG (Fig. 3.7A; Mitani et al., 1983; Peterson and Schofield, 2007). Cortical axons also contact cells in ipsilateral IC that project to the ipsilateral SOC or to either CN as well as cells in the contralateral IC that project to either CN (Fig. 3.7A; Schofield and Coomes, 2006).

Cortical projections to the NLL and adjacent areas

AC projections to the region of the lemniscal nuclei have been described in greatest detail in rats (Feliciano et al., 1995) and gerbils (Budinger et al., 2000). In rats, terminals of cortical axons occur in areas surrounding the main nuclei of the lateral lemniscus: in a paralemniscal area medial to the VNLL, in the 'horizontal cell group' between the INLL and DNLL, and in the sagulum. The projections are ipsilateral and originate in area Te1[2] (Feliciano et al., 1995). In gerbils, terminations occur in the DNLL and adjacent areas, including the cuneiform nucleus. These projections arise from cells in the anterior auditory field (but not from A1) and from non-primary areas (Budinger et al., 2000). The laminar identity and morphology of the cells of origin have not been identified in either species.

Cortical projections to the SOC

Projections to the SOC originate from cells in cortical layer V (Doucet et al., 2002). The cells of origin are spread across multiple cortical areas, including primary and non-primary areas in the rat (Doucet et al., 2002); guinea pig (Coomes and Schofield, 2004b), and gerbil (Budinger et al., 2000).

In rats, cortical axons from Te1 terminate ipsilaterally in the LSO and VNTB and along the dorsal margin of the SOC. A much smaller number of terminations occur in a similar pattern on the contralateral side. The projections in guinea pigs appear more robust, with terminations occurring in most SOC nuclei, excepting only the MSO. Again, the contralateral terminations are similar in pattern but much less dense. Details of cortico-olivary terminations in gerbils have not been determined, but the main target appears to be the VNTB (Budinger et al., 2000).

Targets identified by projections Cortical projections to the SOC appear to contact olivary cells that project to a number of targets (Fig. 3.7B). Cortical projections to the ipsilateral SOC contact MOC cells that project to the opposite cochlea (Mulders and Robertson, 2000) as well as SOC cells that project ipsilaterally, contralaterally or bilaterally to the CN (Schofield and Coomes, 2006), or ipsilaterally or contralaterally to the IC (Peterson and Schofield, 2007). Cortical projections to the *contralateral* SOC contact cells that project to the ipsilateral CN or ipsilateral or contralateral IC (Schofield and Coomes, 2006; Peterson and Schofield, 2007).

Cortical projections to the CN

Cortical projections to the CN originate from Te1 in rats (Weedman and Ryugo, 1996a), A1 in mice (Meltzer and Ryugo, 2006), and A1 and other cortical fields in guinea pigs (Jacomme et al., 2003; Schofield and Coomes, 2005b; Schofield et al., 2006). The cells of origin are layer V pyramidal cells.

---

[2] Te1 (temporal area 1) is defined cytoarchitectonically (Zilles, 1985) and was initially considered equivalent to primary auditory cortex. Subsequent study indicates that Te1 contains multiple auditory areas; it may be equivalent to the group of areas commonly referred to as 'core' AC areas (e.g., primary auditory cortex and the anterior auditory field of cats or the dorsocaudal field of guinea pigs; see Rutkowski et al., 2003 for discussion).

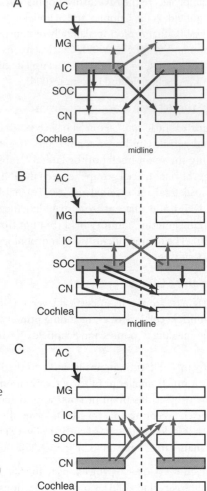

Fig. 3.7 Ascending pathways (*blue arrows*) and descending pathways (*red arrows*) originating at different levels that appear to be contacted directly by corticofugal axons (*black arrows*) descending from the left AC. The locations of the cells contacted by the descending projections are shown by *gray shading*. **A** Pathways that originate in the IC. **B** Pathways that originate in the SOC. **C** Pathways that originate in the CN.

The AC projects bilaterally to the CN. The patterns of termination are similar on the two sides. In rats, most terminals are in the granule cell area. The boutons contain round synaptic vesicles and form asymmetric junctions, typical of excitatory synapses (Weedman and Ryugo, 1996b). In mice, additional terminals are scattered in DCN. In guinea pigs, the heaviest terminations are in the granule cell area, small cell cap, and fusiform cell layer of the DCN, with additional terminals in other DCN layers and throughout much of the VCN.

Targets identified by projections Electron microscopy has demonstrated that granule cell dendrites are major targets of cortical axons (Weedman and Ryugo, 1996b; Meltzer and Ryugo, 2006). Granule cell axons are confined to the CN, indicating cortical inputs to intrinsic CN circuits, but the presence of cortical boutons outside the granule cell areas suggests that they have additional targets. Evidence from light microscopy suggests that cortical terminals contact CN cells that project ipsilaterally, contralaterally, or bilaterally to the IC (Schofield and Coomes, 2005a; Fig. 3.7C). The targeted cells include fusiform cells and giant cells in the DCN and multipolar cells in the VCN.

3.4 Collateral projections in descending pathways

Collateral projections, whereby axons branch to innervate multiple nuclei, are prominent in some but not all descending pathways. The possible functions of branched projections are numerous, and include coordinating activity at multiple sites or adjusting sensitivity or gain in the pathway. The alternative to collaterals is for projections to arise from different cell types or different populations of a single cell type. Projections originating from different cell types could allow for specialized processing; e.g., bushy cells and multipolar cells in the ventral cochlear nucleus (VCN) each receive auditory nerve input, but process that input in different ways and project to different targets. Projections originating from different populations, even of a single cell type, could allow for differential processing if the two populations receive different inputs. Again, the consequence would be that different information is sent to the targets. The presence of collateral projections from olivocochlear cells to other brainstem nuclei has been discussed above. Below we discuss collaterals in several additional descending pathways.

3.4.1 Olivary projections to the CN

As described above, all the periolivary nuclei project to the ipsilateral CN, and many project to the contralateral CN. Cells that send collateral projections to the CN on both sides are distributed across many of the periolivary nuclei, but the majority of such cells are located in the VNTB (Schofield and Cant, 1999). Interestingly, VNTB cells that project bilaterally to the CN appear to be targets of descending projections from both the IC and the AC (Schofield and Cant, 1999; Schofield and Coomes, 2006).

3.4.2 Corticofugal projections

Given the list of cortical targets, one could imagine many opportunities for collateral projections. Wong and Kelly (1981) were the first to look for collateral projections from auditory cortex. They found that different populations of cells project to the thalamus and the IC. Doucet et al. (2002, 2003) studied projections to the IC, SOC, and CN and concluded that the most common pattern of projection is for a pyramidal cell to project to a single brainstem target. In guinea pigs, the projection from AC to the contralateral IC is about 10% the size of that to the ipsilateral IC (as measured by number of cells of origin). About 6% of the corticocollicular cells in layer V project to both ICs (Fig. 3.8). This is a small percentage of the overall population, but represents a very large percentage of the contralateral projection (average 46%; maximum observed 81%) (Coomes et al., 2005). The authors conclude that a large number of cells project to one target – the ipsilateral IC – and that a significant second population projects bilaterally. There are also AC cells that project to the ipsilateral IC and to one or the other CN (Coomes and Schofield, 2004a). Fewer cortical cells project to the CN than to the IC, so cells with these collateral projections are relatively few. Nonetheless, such cells form a large percentage of the population that projects to the CN. In addition, a small number of cells send collaterals to three targets: left and right IC and one CN. It was concluded that projections from layer V form two general patterns: (1) projections to a single target and (2) projections to multiple targets. Most layer V cells show the single-target pattern. The minority of cells with divergent (collateral) projections may be in a position to exert broader effects; certainly they are likely to serve a different function than cells with single projection targets.

3.4.3 Other descending projections

There is little evidence for collaterals in descending projections from the IC. The IC projections to the ipsilateral and contralateral CN arise from different cell groups (Schofield, 2002).

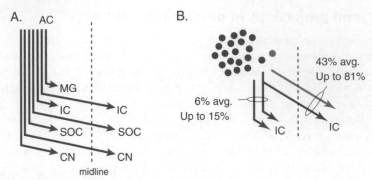

Fig. 3.8 Patterns of collateral projections from auditory cortex (AC). In this figure (unlike previous figures), *branching arrows* indicate branching axons. **A** *Independent arrows* indicate that many of the projections to different subcortical targets originate from different populations of cortical cells. **B** Cortical projections to the inferior colliculus (IC). The collateral branching pattern is shown with quantitative data from guinea pigs (Coomes *et al.*, 2005). The relative proportions of cells of origin are shown as *circles*. *Purple* indicates cells that send collateral projections to both sides; *red* and *blue* indicate cells that project to one side or the other. The *numbers* refer to average and maximum values for collateral projections to the indicated side; e.g., '*purple*' cells made up 43% on average, and up to 81%, of the cells that project to the contralateral IC ('*blue*' plus '*purple*' populations). The '*purple*' population made up 6% on average (up to 15%) of the population that projected to the ipsilateral IC ('*purple*' plus '*red*').

Whether colliculo-olivary cells have collaterals (e.g., to the CN) is more difficult to assess. The possibility of collaterals in descending projections from the thalamus has not been addressed.

3.5 Functional roles of central descending projections

The descending systems have been characterized as forming feedback loops or descending chains (Huffman and Henson, 1990; Spangler and Warr, 1991). Loops include descending projections to cells that project to higher centers. Figure 3.9A summarizes the ascending auditory pathways that appear to be contacted directly by cortical axons. Projections from a single side of cortex appear to reach ascending pathways on both sides of the brain, and include pathways that extend all the way from the CN to the cortex. In addition to obvious loops (e.g., AC-MG-AC), there are pathways by which the cortex on one side can apparently affect the ascending pathways to the *opposite* cortex (e.g., via AC projections to contralateral IC). These circuits are reminiscent of the feedforward circuits attributed to some cortico-thalamo-cortical circuits, discussed above.

Descending chains involve descending projections that terminate on cells that project to lower levels, forming multisynaptic descending pathways. Figure 3.9B summarizes the descending pathways that appear to be contacted by cortical axons. From the earliest research on descending pathways, it was assumed that multi-neuronal chains extended from cortex to the cochlea (the shortest route based on anatomy known at the time was from AC to IC to SOC to cochlea). Recent research supports some of the implied links, but also demonstrates additional possibilities, such as the direct cortical projections to olivocochlear cells.

Clearly, recent evidence supports the idea of loops and chains in the descending pathways. However, these concepts seem inadequate to capture the full expanse of descending systems, which can now be appreciated as a complex array of multiple, often parallel, descending pathways. The concept of feedforward effects, discussed above, applies to a descending pathway that affects information that ascends to some region *other* than the source of the descending projections. The patterns of convergence and divergence provide additional functional implications.

Divergence is prominent and would appear to allow auditory cortex to exert influence over virtually all levels of the central auditory pathways. Could divergent projections act to suppress or enhance transmission through a particular ascending pathway? For example, could cortical projections influence a cell in the IC as well as cells in the CN or SOC that provide that IC cell with its main ascending inputs?

The multiplicity of descending pathways also leads to convergence. Ultimately, convergence is meaningful only at the cellular level (i.e., inputs that innervate the same nucleus do not actually converge unless they innervate the same *cells*). Nonetheless, convergence of multiple descending pathways on a single area, e.g., the CN, emphasizes the possibility of multiple functions. An important step is to relate specific inputs (i.e., cell types) with their cellular targets. In the CN, perhaps the best understood example is the collateral projection from MOC cells to cells in the VCN, whereby the MOC collaterals could allow a small subset of CN cells to continue to encode the actual sound intensity (discussed in Section 3.2.1). A second pathway to the CN characterized by cell types is the projection from principal cells of the MNTB to the CN (Schofield, 1994). Both the MNTB principal cells and one of their CN targets, globular bushy cells, are considered to play a role in the analysis of interaural disparities that are important for sound localization. The anatomy of this circuit suggests that it may enhance the processing of interaural disparities by SOC cells (see discussion in Schofield, 1994).

Less is known about other descending projections to the CN. Figure 3.10 summarizes the termination patterns of the descending projections. The first point is that not all sources of projections terminate throughout the CN. Different CN cell types have different distributions within the CN and different patterns of projections outside the CN. It follows that different CN cell types, and thus different circuits, will receive different combinations of descending inputs. Second, given that cells at different levels of the auditory system have different response characteristics, it is likely that they will have different effects in the CN. This possibility is extended by a third factor, which is that the descending pathways use a variety of neurotransmitters. The cortical inputs

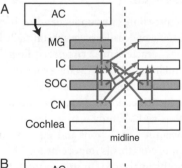

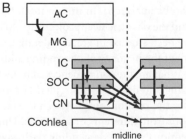

Fig. 3.9 Subcortical pathways that have been identified as receiving direct inputs from auditory cortex. The pathways are drawn from the perspective of projections originating from left auditory cortex (*black arrows*). **A** Ascending pathways (*blue*). **B** Descending pathways (*red*).

Fig. 3.10 Schematic illustrating descending pathways to the cochlear nucleus (CN). *Arrows* indicate the sources of projections: *Blue* – auditory cortex (AC); *orange*: subparafascicular nucleus of the thalamus (SPF); *green* – inferior colliculus (IC); *red* – superior olivary complex (SOC). The general pattern of terminations is indicated by color in the enlarged views of the CN; *darker shading* indicates denser projections. scc Small cell cap.

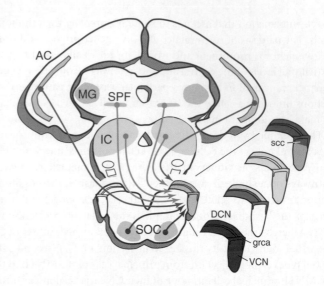

presumably use glutamate, whereas the olivary inputs probably use acetylcholine, GABA, glycine, and glutamate (and perhaps others). The transmitters associated with thalamic and collicular projections to the CN are unknown.

Convergence occurs in regions above the CN as well. Descending projections from the AC and IC converge in the SOC and appear to contact olivocochlear and olivo-CN cells. Do these inputs actually converge on the same cells? For example, does an individual olivocochlear cell receive inputs from both AC and IC, or do some olivocochlear cells receive AC inputs and other olivocochlear cells receive IC inputs? The IC is also a target of converging projections, including massive projections from multiple AC areas and smaller projections from the thalamus. Little is known about the underlying circuitry of either of these projections.

3.6 **Issues for future research**

The incomplete picture of the circuitry limits our understanding of the functions of the descending system. Studies over the last couple of decades have substantially increased our understanding of connections between areas, but characterizing a *circuit* requires that one identify (1) synaptic connections between a pathway and its targets and (2) the projections of those post-synaptic cells. In some instances, direct synaptic connections can be identified physiologically, but more often this issue requires ultrastructural identification of synapses with the electron microscope (EM). In many instances, the labor-intensive EM study is preceded by light microscopic studies that provide suggestive evidence for synaptic connections and, equally importantly, provide guidance for where synaptic contacts might occur (this is important for EM studies, which are limited in the size of tissue samples that can be analyzed). In this context, the cortical projections to the thalamus and cochlear nucleus and the olivocochlear projections (to the cochlea and, via collaterals, to the cochlear nucleus) have been studied in greatest detail. Considerable work remains to characterize the synaptic circuitry of the majority of descending auditory pathways.

Many other questions remain. What are the consequences of branching axons? Do single axons branch to innervate both ascending and descending circuits? For axons that innervate multiple targets (say, IC and CN), what are the relationships between the targeted circuits? What are the functions of descending projections from different cortical areas? Under what conditions (acoustic stimuli; behavioral state; attention) are the descending pathways active? A few studies have looked at the role of attention or behavioral state on early auditory processing (e.g., Ryan and Miller, 1977), but little is known about the underlying circuits.

This chapter has focused narrowly on projections from auditory regions to lower auditory circuits. A broader perspective would include descending projections from 'non-auditory' nuclei, such as the amygdala or basal ganglia (for a review of these broader descending systems see Winer, 2005). There is also a need to examine descending projections to lower circuits that extend beyond the ascending auditory pathways, such as circuits involved in orientation, vocalization, and middle ear reflexes. Finally, numerous modulatory systems (e.g., noradrenergic, serotoninergic) have been identified as inputs to olivocochlear cells. It seems likely that similar inputs affect many, perhaps all, descending pathways, but almost nothing is known about this aspect of the descending system.

Acknowledgments

The work described here that was done in the author's laboratory was supported by NIH DC04391 and DC05277. Special thanks to Susan Motts for comments on an early draft and Debbie Heeter for assistance with the figures.

References

Aschoff A, Ostwald J (1988) Distribution of cochlear efferents and olivo-cochlear neurons in the brainstem of rat and guinea pig. *Exp Brain Res* 71: 241–51.

Bajo VM, Moore DR (2005) Descending projections from the auditory cortex to the inferior colliculus in the gerbil, *Meriones unguiculatus. J Comp Neurol* 486: 101–16.

Bajo VM, Nodal FR, Bizley JK, Moore DR, King AJ (2007) The ferret auditory cortex: descending projections to the inferior colliculus. *Cereb Cortex* 17: 475–91.

Bartlett EL, Stark JM, Guillery RW, Smith PH. (2000) Comparison of the fine structure of cortical and collicular terminals in the rat medial geniculate. *Neuroscience* 100: 811–28.

Benson TE, Brown MC (1990) Synapses formed by olivocochlear axon branches in the mouse cochlear nucleus. *J Comp Neurol* 295: 52–70.

Brown MC (1993) Fiber pathways and branching patterns of biocytin-labeled olivocochlear neurons in the mouse brainstem. *J Comp Neurol* 337: 600–613.

Budinger E, Heil P, Scheich H (2000) Functional organization of auditory cortex in the Mongolian gerbil (*Meriones unguiculatus*). IV. Connections with anatomically characterized subcortical structures. *Eur J Neurosci* 12: 2452–74.

Caicedo A, Herbert H (1993) Topography of descending projections from the inferior colliculus to auditory brainstem nuclei in the rat. *J Comp Neurol* 328: 377–92.

Coomes DL, Schofield BR (2004a) Projections from individual cortical cells to multiple targets in the auditory brainstem in guinea pigs. *Assoc Res Otolaryngol Abstr* 27: 120.

Coomes DL, Schofield BR (2004b) Projections from the auditory cortex to the superior olivary complex in guinea pigs. *Eur J Neurosci* 19: 2188–200.

Coomes DL, Schofield BR (2004c) Separate projections from the inferior colliculus to the cochlear nucleus and thalamus in guinea pigs. *Hear Res* 191: 67–78.

Coomes DL, Schofield RM, Schofield BR (2005) Unilateral and bilateral projections from cortical cells to the inferior colliculus in guinea pigs. *Brain Res* 10426: 62–72.

Darrow KN, Simons EJ, Dodds L, Liberman MC (2006) Dopaminergic innervation of the mouse inner ear: evidence for a separate cytochemical group of cochlear efferent fibers. *J Comp Neurol* 498: 403–414.

Darrow KN, Maison SF, Liberman MC (2007) Selective removal of lateral olivocochlear efferents increases vulnerability to acute acoustic injury. *J Neurophysiol* 97: 1775–85.

Doucet JR, Rose L, Ryugo DK (2002) The cellular origin of corticofugal projections to the superior olivary complex in the rat. *Brain Res* **925**: 28–41.

Doucet JR, Molavi DL, Ryugo DK (2003) The source of corticocollicular and corticobulbar projections in area Te1 of the rat. *Exp Brain Res* **153**: 61–6.

Eybalin M (1993) Neurotransmitters and neuromodulators of the mammalian cochlea. *Physiol Rev* **73**: 309–73.

Faye-Lund H (1988) Inferior colliculus and related descending pathways in rat. *Ups J Med Sci* **93**: 1–17.

Feliciano M, Saldaña E, Mugnaini E (1995) Direct projections from the rat primary auditory neocortex to nucleus sagulum, paralemniscal regions, superior olivary complex and cochlear nuclei. *Audit Neurosci* **1**: 287–308.

Fitzpatrick KA, Imig TJ (1978) Projections of auditory cortex upon the thalamus and midbrain in the owl monkey. *J Comp Neurol* **177**: 537–555.

Guinan JJ Jr (1996) Physiology of olivocochlear efferents. In: *The Cochlea*, vol. 8 (eds Dallos P, *et al.*), pp. 435–502. Springer, New York.

Helfert RH, Aschoff A (1997) Superior olivary complex and nuclei of the lateral lemniscus. In: *The Central Auditory System* (eds Ehret G, Romand R), pp. 193–258. Oxford University Press, New York.

Horvath M, Kraus KS, Illing RB (2000) Olivocochlear neurons sending axon collaterals into the ventral cochlear nucleus of the rat. *J Comp Neurol* **422**: 95–105.

Huffman RF, Henson OW Jr (1990) The descending auditory pathway and acousticomotor systems: connections with the inferior colliculus. *Brain Res Rev* **15**: 295–323.

Jacomme AV, Nodal FR, Bajo VM, *et al.* (2003) The projection from auditory cortex to cochlear nucleus in guinea pigs: an in vivo anatomical and in vitro electrophysiological study. *Exp Brain Res* **153**: 467–76.

Jane JA, Masterton RB, Diamond IT (1965) The function of the tectum for attention to auditory stimuli in the cat. *J Comp Neurol* **125**: 165–91.

Jones EG, Rockel AJ (1973) Observations on complex vesicles, neurofilamentous hyperplasia and increased electron density during terminal degeneration in the inferior colliculus. *J Comp Neurol* **147**: 93–118.

Kuwabara N, Zook JM (2000) Geniculo-collicular descending projections in the gerbil. *Brain Res* **878**: 79–87.

Le Prell CG, Halsey K, Hughes LF, Dolan DF, Bledsoe SC Jr (2005) Disruption of lateral olivocochlear neurons via a dopaminergic neurotoxin depresses sound-evoked auditory nerve activity. *J Assoc Res Otolaryngol* **6**: 48–62.

Lim HH, Anderson DJ (2007) Antidromic activation reveals tonotopically organized projections from primary auditory cortex to the central nucleus of the inferior colliculus in guinea pig. *J Neurophysiol* **97**: 1413–27.

Malmierca MS, Beau FENL, Rees A (1996) The topographical organization of descending projections from the central nucleus of the inferior colliculus in guinea pig. *Hear Res* **93**: 167–80.

Meltzer NE, Ryugo DK (2006) Projections from auditory cortex to cochlear nucleus: a comparative analysis of rat and mouse. *Anat Rec A Discov Mol Cell Evol Biol* **288**: 397–408.

Mitani A, Shimokouchi M, Nomura S (1983) Effects of stimulation of the primary auditory cortex upon colliculogeniculate neurons in the inferior colliculus of the cat. *Neurosci Lett* **42**: 185–89.

Mulders WH, Robertson D (2000) Evidence for direct cortical innervation of medial olivocochlear neurones in rats. *Hear Res* **144**: 65–72.

Oliver DL (2005) Neuronal organization in the inferior colliculus. In: *The Inferior Colliculus* (eds Winer JA, Schreiner CE), pp. 69–114. Springer, New York.

Peterson DC, Schofield BR (2007) Projections from auditory cortex contact ascending pathways that originate in the superior olive and inferior colliculus. *Hear Res* **232**: 67–77.

Rasmussen GL (1946) The olivary peduncle and other fiber projections of the superior olivary complex. *J Comp Neurol* **14**: 141–219.

Rasmussen GL (1960) Efferent fibers of the cochlear nerve and cochlear nucleus. In: *Neural Mechanisms of the Auditory and Vestibular Systems* (eds Rasmussen GL, Windle WF), pp. 105–15. Charles C. Thomas, Springfield, Illinois.

Robertson D, Cole KS, Corbett K (1987) Quantitative estimate of bilaterally projecting medial olivocochlear neurones in the guinea pig brainstem. *Hear Res* **27**: 177–81.

Rouiller EM (1997) Functional organization of the auditory pathways. In: *The Central Auditory System* (eds Ehret G, Romand R), pp. 3–96. Oxford University Press, New York.

Rouiller EM, Welker E (2000) A comparative analysis of the morphology of corticothalamic projections in mammals. *Brain Res Bull* **53**: 727–41.

Rutkowski RG, Miasnikov AA, Weinberger NM (2003) Characterisation of multiple physiological fields within the anatomical core of rat auditory cortex. *Hear Res* **181**: 116–30.

Ryan A, Miller J (1977) Effects of behavioral performance on single-unit firing patterns in inferior colliculus of the rhesus monkey. *J Neurophysiol* **40**: 943–56.

Saldaña E (1993) Descending projections from the inferior colliculus to the cochlear nuclei in mammals. In: *The Mammalian Cochlear Nuclei: Organization and Function* (ed. Merchan MA), pp. 153–65. Plenum Press, New York.

Saldaña E, Feliciano M, Mugnaini E (1996) Distribution of descending projections from primary auditory neocortex to inferior colliculus mimics the topography of intracollicular projections. *J Comp Neurol* **371**: 15–40.

Schofield BR (1994) Projections to the cochlear nuclei from principal cells in the medial nucleus of the trapezoid body in guinea pigs. *J Comp Neurol* **344**: 83–100.

Schofield BR (2000) Distinct origins of ascending and descending projections from the inferior colliculus in guinea pigs. *Assoc Res Otolaryngol Abst* **23**: 35.

Schofield BR (2001) Origins of projections from the inferior colliculus to the cochlear nucleus in guinea pigs. *J Comp Neurol* **429**: 206–20.

Schofield BR (2002) Ascending and descending projections from the superior olivary complex in guinea pigs: different cells project to the cochlear nucleus and the inferior colliculus. *J Comp Neurol* **453**: 217–25.

Schofield BR, Cant NB (1991) Organization of the periolivary nuclei in pigmented guinea pigs: distribution of cells that send axon collaterals to the inferior colliculus, the cochlear nucleus, or both. *Assoc Res Otolaryngol Abst* **14**: 19.

Schofield BR, Cant NB (1999) Descending auditory pathways: projections from the inferior colliculus contact superior olivary cells that project bilaterally to the cochlear nuclei. *J Comp Neurol* **409**: 210–23.

Schofield BR, Coomes DL (2005a) Projections from auditory cortex contact cells in the cochlear nucleus that project to the inferior colliculus. *Hear Res* **206**: 3–11.

Schofield BR, Coomes DL (2005b) Auditory cortical projections to the cochlear nucleus in guinea pigs. *Hear Res* **199**: 89–102.

Schofield BR, Coomes DL (2006) Pathways from auditory cortex to the cochlear nucleus in guinea pigs. *Hear Res* **216–217**: 81–9.

Schofield BR, Coomes DL, Schofield RM (2006) Cells in auditory cortex that project to the cochlear nucleus in guinea pigs. *J Assoc Res Otolaryngol* **7**: 95–109.

Schwartz IR (1992) The superior olivary complex and lateral lemniscal nuclei. In: *The Mammalian Auditory Pathway: Neuroanatomy* (eds Webster DB, *et al.*), pp. 117–67. Springer, New York.

Sherman SM, Guillery RW (1996) Functional organization of thalamocortical relays. *J Neurophysiol* **76**: 1367–95.

Smith PH, Spirou GA (2002) From the cochlea to the cortex and back. In: *Integrative Functions in the Mammalian Auditory Pathway* (eds Oertel D, *et al.*), vol. 15, pp. 6–71. Springer, New York.

Smith PH, Bartlett EL, Kowalkowski A (2007) Cortical and collicular inputs to cells in the rat paralaminar thalamic nuclei adjacent to the medial geniculate body. *J Neurophysiol* **98**: 681–695.

Spangler KM, Warr WB (1991) The descending auditory system. In: *Neurobiology of Hearing: The Central Auditory System* (eds Altschuler RA, *et al.*), pp. 27–45. Raven Press, New York.

Suga N, Ma X (2003) Multiparametric corticofugal modulation and plasticity in the auditory system. *Nat Rev Neurosci* **4**: 783–94.

Thompson AM, Schofield BR (2000) Afferents of the superior olivary complex. *Microsc Res Tech* **51**: 330–54.

Thompson AM, Thompson GC (1993) Relationship of descending inferior colliculus projections to olivocochlear neurons. *J Comp Neurol* **335**: 402–12.

Vetter DE, Adams JC, Mugnaini E (1991) Chemically distinct rat olivocochlear neurons. *Synapse* **7**: 21–43.

Vetter DE, Saldaña E, Mugnaini E (1993) Input from the inferior colliculus to medial olivocochlear neurons in the rat: a double label study with PHA-L and cholera toxin. *Hear Res* **70**: 73–86.

Warr WB, Beck JE (1996) Multiple projections from the ventral nucleus of the trapezoid body in the rat. *Hear Res* **93**: 83–101.

Warr WB, Guinan JJ Jr (1979) Efferent innervation of the organ of Corti: two separate systems. *Brain Res* **173**: 152–5.

Weedman DL, Ryugo DK (1996a) Pyramidal cells in primary auditory cortex project to cochlear nucleus in rat. *Brain Res* **706**: 97–102.

Weedman DL, Ryugo DK (1996b) Projections from auditory cortex to the cochlear nucleus in rats: synapses on granule cell dendrites. *J Comp Neurol* **371**: 311–24.

Winer JA (2005) Decoding the auditory corticofugal systems. *Hear Res* **207**: 1–9.

Winer JA, Prieto JJ (2001) Layer V in cat primary auditory cortex (AI): cellular architecture and identification of projection neurons. *J Comp Neurol* **434**: 379–412.

Winer JA, Chernock ML, Larue DT, Cheung S (2002) Descending projections to the inferior colliculus from the posterior thalamus and the auditory cortex in rat, cat, and monkey. *Hear Res* **168**: 181–95.

Winer JA, Larue DT, Diehl JJ, Hefti BJ (1998) Auditory cortical projections to the cat inferior colliculus. *J Comp Neurol* **400**: 147–74.

Wong D, Kelly JP (1981) Differentially projecting cells in individual layers of the auditory cortex: a double-labeling study. *Brain Res* **230**: 362–6.

Yasui Y, Nakano K, Mizuno N (1992) Descending projections from the subparafascicular thalamic nucleus to the lower brain stem in the rat. *Exp Brain Res* **90**: 508–18.

Ye Y, Machado DG, Kim DO (2000) Projection of the marginal shell of the anteroventral cochlear nucleus to olivocochlear neurons in the cat. *J Comp Neurol* **420**: 127–38.

Zilles K (1985) *The Cortex of the Rat*. Springer, Berlin.

Chapter 4

Central auditory neurotransmitters

Richard A. Altschuler and Susan E. Shore

This chapter reviews neurotransmitters and receptors in the auditory pathway. We first discuss the major transmitter classes (the excitatory and inhibitory amino acids) in the core ascending auditory pathway and describe the characteristics of their receptors. This is followed by a more detailed examination of neurotransmission in auditory nuclei at different stages in the pathway. Finally, we briefly review neurotransmission in the descending pathways. References for the cell types and their connections in the ascending and descending pathways are given in Chapters 2, 3 and will only be provided in this chapter in the context of neurotransmitters and receptors.

4.1 Overview of the core ascending pathway

We will use the 'core' nomenclature (see Chapter 2) to refer to the exclusively auditory, tonotopically organized nuclei of the auditory pathway. Neurons in the core auditory pathway exhibit some of the highest firing rates of the central nervous system. Many of its synapses mediate rapid excitation of the postsynaptic neuron, followed by fast recovery that permits rapid responses. This allows a frequency rate-code to be established, maintained, and transmitted along the ascending auditory neuraxis. This is accomplished by the use of the excitatory amino acid glutamate, acting on ionotropic glutamate receptors composed of specific subunits around a cationic channel (for review see Parks, 2000).

4.2 Excitatory amino acids

There are three types of ionotropic glutamate receptors: alpha-amino-3-hydroxy-5-methyl-4-isoxazolepropionate (AMPA), N-methyl-D-aspartate (NMDA), and kainate receptors as well as metabotropic glutamate receptors (mGLURs). In the auditory pathways the immediate action of glutamate is achieved through the binding of glutamate to the AMPA receptor, while binding to the NMDA receptor modulates the response. Both the AMPA and NMDA receptors are composed of several subunits, each with unique placements in the active zone of the synapse, which determine their specific response characteristics.

4.2.1 AMPA receptors

There are four major subunits for the AMPA glutamate receptor: GLUR1, 2, 3, and 4 (also called GLURA, B, C, and D) (e.g. Hollmann and Heinemann, 1994). The mRNAs for GLUR1–4 subunits have two alternative splicings and their translation results in production of alternative isoforms termed 'flip' and 'flop'. Use of the 'flop' splice variant generally provides a more rapid desensitization (about fourfold quicker) than use of 'flip' variants. The GLUR2 subunit in AMPA receptors influences Ca^{2+} permeability. With high GLUR2 placement Ca^{2+} permeability is lower and AMPA receptors gate more slowly, particularly when the flip version is used, while lower GLUR2 placement provides for higher permeability, resulting in a high Ca^{2+} ion flow.

AMPA receptors of many auditory neurons have higher permeability to divalent cations than most other central nervous system AMPA receptors, leading to rapid desensitization and deactivation (for review see Trussell, 1997). This is accomplished through a relatively 'auditory specific' configuration of AMPA receptor subunits. These 'auditory specific' AMPA receptors express high GLUR4 (flop) and very low GLUR2. The AMPA receptors at 'auditory specific' synapses may also contain GLUR3. The GLUR3/GLUR4 configuration of subunits in flop versions provides AMPA receptors with rapidly gated channels and low calcium permeability, providing a rapid response, desensitization, and recovery, allowing for high fidelity and preservation of timing.

This 'auditory specific' configuration of the AMPA receptor is found in most synapses of the binaural pathway in the auditory brain stem (Schmid et al., 2001) including those apposing end-bulb terminals of the auditory nerve on spherical and globular bushy cells in the ventral cochlear nucleus (VCN) (Wang et al., 1998). Similar receptor configurations are found apposing the connections from VCN to principal cells of the medial and lateral superior olivary nuclei (MSO, LSO), the superior peraolivary nucleus (SPN), and octopus cells of the VCN. Other examples include the end-bulb synapses between globular bushy cells and the principal cells of the medial nucleus of the trapezoid body (MNTB) (Geiger et al., 1995) and LSO connections to the dorsal nucleus of the lateral lemniscus (DNLL). The 'auditory specific' AMPA receptor composition is also found in many synapses in the monaural auditory ascending pathway, including auditory nerve connections to the basal dendrites of fusiform cells. In contrast, these types of receptors are not found on the inferior colliculus (IC) neurons receiving direct monaural inputs from T-multipolar stellate cells, fusiform, and giant cells, which often form synapses with receptors containing high levels of the GLUR2 flip subunit (Schmid et al., 2001).

4.2.2 NMDA receptors

Glutamate also binds to NMDA receptors that are present at glutamatergic synapses in the ascending auditory pathways. NMDA receptors can modulate neuronal activity, influence long-term potentiation, and impart neural plasticity, as evidenced in the reorganization of fields in the primary auditory cortex after deafness (e.g. Ji et al., 2005) and changes in the auditory space map in the IC in birds (Feldman et al., 1996). In the MNTB, Forsythe and Barnes-Davies (1993) found that NMDA receptors were more involved in slow excitatory postsynaptic currents (EPSCs), while fast EPSCs of MNTB principal neurons were primarily mediated by AMPA receptors. Like the AMPA receptor, the NMDA receptor has different subunits: the NMDAR1 subunit with eight splice variants and the NMDAR2 subunit with four types (A–D) form heteromeric complexes (e.g. Monyer et al., 1992). Alternatively spliced exons in the NMDAR1 subunit encode a sequence in the N-terminal domain (termed the N1 cassette) and adjacent sequences in the C-terminal domain (termed the C1 and C2 cassettes) (e.g. Hollmann and Heinemann, 1994). The presence of the N1 cassette allows for larger current flow at the receptor channel (Hollmann and Heinemann, 1994). The presence or absence of the C1 and C2 cassettes influences intracellular phosphorylation in downstream pathways. There is a diversity in NMDAR1 receptor expression in the auditory brain stem (for review see Sato et al., 2000) that could give differences in responses under the conditions in which NMDA receptors play a role (e.g. plasticity or high levels of activity).

4.2.3 Metabotropic glutamate receptors

Metabotropic glutamate receptors (mGLURs) are coupled to G-proteins and have a slower, longer-lasting action than the ionotropic NMDA and AMPA receptors. In the dorsal cochlear nucleus (DCN) mGLURs reduce parallel fiber-evoked excitation (Molitor and Manis, 1997), while mGLURs can influence (increase or decrease) the gain of auditory nerve-driven activity in the VCN (Sanes et al., 1998).

4.3 Inhibitory amino acids

Most inhibition in the ascending auditory pathway is accomplished by synapses using the inhibitory amino acids gamma amino butryic acid (GABA) and glycine, which, like the excitatory amino acid glutamate, act on ionotropic receptors that provide rapid responses. There is a rostral-to-caudal gradient in the number of GABA and glycinergic synapses in the central auditory system: glycine terminals are more abundant in medullary and pontine auditory brain stem nuclei, while GABA terminals are more abundant in midbrain, thalamus, and cortical auditory regions. Co-localization of glycine with GABA is common in the lower auditory brain stem and less common elsewhere.

4.3.1 GABA receptors

GABA acts on ionotropic GABA-A receptors as well as metabotropic GABA-B receptors. GABA-A receptors are composed of different combinations of alpha, beta, gamma, and delta subunits that combine to form a ligand-gated chloride channel. There are different sub-types of each subunit as well as splice variants for several sub-types. Most GABA-A receptors in the core lemniscal ascending auditory pathway use beta 3 and gamma 2L subunits, with diversity generated by the incorporation of different alpha subunits in the composition of the receptors (Campos et al., 2001). The alpha 1 and 5 subunits provide faster kinetics than the alpha 3 subunit. There does not appear to be an 'auditory' GABA-A receptor configuration to match the rapid kinetics of the auditory AMPA receptor, although there are many GABAergic endings on neurons in the auditory pathways. In the superior olivary complex (SOC) and lateral lemniscus (LL) there is high expression of the alpha 3 subunit in addition to, or instead of, alpha 1 and alpha 5 (Campos et al., 2001). In the IC, larger cells show the highest expression of the alpha 1 subunit (Shiraishi et al., 2001).

4.3.2 Glycine receptors

Glycine receptors are composed of different combinations of alpha and beta subunits that combine to form a ligand-gated chloride channel. Glycine receptors composed of alpha 1, alpha 3, and beta subunits are found along most of the ascending auditory pathways (for reviews see Friauf et al., 1997; Sato et al., 2000). Alpha 1 subunit expression is lower in the medial geniculate body (MGB) and the primary auditory cortex than in the auditory brain stem (Friauf et al., 1997), perhaps reflecting the paucity of glycinergic terminals in these higher centers. Similarly, the SOC nuclei, such as the LSO and MSO, which receive numerous glycinergic inputs have high alpha 1 expression, while SOC nuclei receiving less glycinergic input, such as the MNTB and VNTB, have lower alpha 1 and higher alpha 3 subunit expression (Sato et al., 2000), resulting in a less sensitive receptor configuration.

4.4 Divisions of the ascending auditory pathway

4.4.1 Ventral cochlear nucleus inputs

The neurotransmitter components of inputs to the ventral cochlear nucleus are summarized in Fig. 4.1. Type I auditory nerve fibers are excited by glutamatergic input from hair cells and in turn use glutamate as their neurotransmitter. Type I auditory nerve fibers terminate on all the major classes of VCN projection neurons, except for the shell region, while type II auditory nerve fibers have their major endings in the shell regions surrounding the magnocellular regions of the CN. The neurotransmitter of type II auditory nerve terminals has not yet been established, but there are indications that it is not glutamate (Zhou et al., 2007). There are four major cell types in the

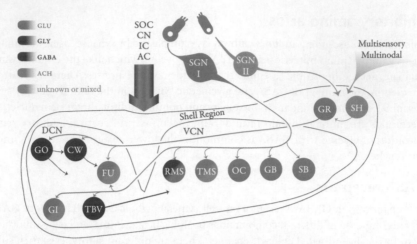

Fig. 4.1 The transmitter composition of the inputs to the cochlear nucleus. DCN Dorsal cochlear nucleus, VCN ventral cochlear nucleus. Glutamate (GLU) (*green*) is an excitatory amino acid found in type I spiral ganglion neurons (SGN I) projecting to VCN and DCN, as well as granule cells in the shell region projecting to DCN and in spherical bushy cells (SB), globular bushy cells (GB), and octopus cells (OC) in the VCN. Glutamate is co-contained with other transmitters in T-multipolar stellate (TMS) and radiate multipolar stellate cells (RMS) in the VCN and fusiform (FU) and giant (GI) cells in the DCN. Glycine (*purple*) is found in radiate multipolar stellate cells (RMS) in the VCN and cartwheel (CW) and tuberculoventral (TBV) cells in the DCN. Golgi cells (GO) and cartwheel cells co-contain GABA (*red*) and glycine (*purple*). The transmitter of type II spiral ganglion neurons (SGN II) is not known (*blue*). There are multiple transmitters in the inputs from the superior olivary complex (SOC), contralateral cochlear nucleus (CN), inferior colliculus (IC), and auditory cortex (AC), including acetylcholine (ACH) (*orange*). *Blue* reflects an unknown transmitter or presence of multiple transmitters within neurons.

magnocellular region of the VCN: spherical bushy cells, globular bushy cells, octopus cells, and stellate multipolar cells (for reviews see Cant and Benson, 2003; Chapter 2). Stellate multipolar cells are a heterogeneous class that includes T-stellate multipolar projection neurons (type 1) of the core ascending auditory pathway (Cant and Benson, 2003; Chapter 2) as well as radiate-commissural and radiate multipolar cells (type 2), which project to the contra- and ipsilateral CN, respectively (Shore *et al.*, 1992; Doucet and Ryugo, 2006).

Glutamate

The termination pattern for glutamatergic terminals on spherical and globular bushy cells is atypical for neurons in the central nervous system. While most neurons typically receive glutamatergic terminals on their dendrites and inhibitory amino acid terminals on their somata, the auditory nerve ends on the somata of spherical and globular bushy cells, with large end-bulbs covering much of the somata of spherical bushy cells. Auditory nerve endings on T-stellate multipolar and octopus cells are more typical and terminate primarily on dendrites. However, radiate multipolar stellate cells (also called D-stellate), like bushy cells, receive many auditory nerve terminals on their somata (Doucet and Ryugo, 2006). Typical of glutamatergic neurons, the auditory nerve terminals contain large, round vesicles and make asymmetrical synaptic contacts (Altschuler *et al.*, 1981; Hackney *et al.*, 1996). The receptors apposing auditory nerve synapses with bushy and octopus cells are AMPA glutamate receptors (for reviews see Parks, 2000; Petralia *et al.*, 2000) with GluR3 and GluR4 subunits in the flop splice form (Hunter *et al.*, 1993; Wang *et al.*, 1998).

As mentioned above, this subunit composition allows for rapid gating of channels, rapid densensitization, and rapid deactivation with low calcium permeability. Stellate multipolar cells receive smaller auditory nerve terminals (Hackney *et al.*, 1996) and are more diverse in their AMPA receptor configurations, reflecting the heterogeneity in this cell class (Hunter *et al.*, 1993; Wang *et al.*, 1998; Parks, 2000; Petralia *et al.*, 2000; Schmid *et al.*, 2001).

Inhibitory amino acids

Numerous inhibitory amino acid inputs to the VCN that originate in the SOC contain GABA, or glycine, or co-contain GABA and glycine (Ostapoff *et al.*, 1997). Glycine is most common in the ipsilateral projections from lateral and ventral nuclei of the trapezoid body (LNTB and VNTB) and GABA is most common in projections from the contralateral VNTB (Ostapoff *et al.*, 1997). Radiate multipolar cells are glycinergic and project to the contralateral CN and the DCN (Wenthold, 1987; Babalian *et al.*, 2002; Doucet and Ryugo, 2006).

GABA receptors

Numerous terminals containing glycine or containing both GABA and glycine contact spherical and globular bushy cells, although these cells also receive some contacts from terminals containing only GABA (Kolston *et al.*, 1992; Juiz *et al.*, 1996). The low number of GABA-only terminals is reflected in the relatively low GABA-A binding in the VCN compared to the DCN (Juiz *et al.*, 1989, 1994). The GABA-A receptors for spherical and globular bushy cells have alpha 1, 3, and 5 subunits, octopus cells have alpha 1 units while stellate multipolar cells have alpha 1 and 3 subunits (Campos *et al.*, 2001). There is also considerable GABA-B binding and immunolocalization throughout the CN, where it is found to be greatest in the DCN (Juiz *et al.*, 1994; Lujan *et al.*, 2004).

Glycine receptors

Glycine receptors are found on most VCN neurons (Wenthold *et al.*, 1988; Sato *et al.*, 2000) accompanied by high levels of glycine binding (Sanes *et al.*, 1987). Both alpha 1 and alpha 2 subunits of the glycine receptor are expressed in bushy, multipolar, and octopus cells in VCN. However, the alpha 1 subunit is more strongly expressed on spherical and globular bushy cells as well as on stellate multipolar cells that receive glycinergic input from tuberculoventral cells of the DCN. Alpha 3 is highly expressed on octopus cells (Sato *et al.*, 2000) that do not receive tuberculoventral input.

4.4.2 Ventral cochlear nucleus outputs

The neurotransmitter components of the projections from the VCN are summarized in Fig. 4.2. The targets of specific VCN projection neurons are described in Chapter 2 and have been reviewed by Cant and Benson (2003) and will not be discussed in detail in this section. Like the auditory nerve, the ascending projections from the VCN to the superior olivary complex, nuclei of the lateral lemniscus, and the inferior colliculus are largely glutamatergic (Suneja *et al.*, 1995; Alibardi 1998, 2003). There are also sub-types of stellate multipolar cells sending commissural projections that are both glycinergic and possibly also glutamatergic, crossing to the contralateral CN as well as projecting to the ipsilateral DCN (Wenthold, 1987; Babalian *et al.*, 2002; Zhou and Shore, 2006). Serotonin is found in cell bodies of a small population of VCN projection neurons (Thompson and Lauder, 2005).

4.4.3 Dorsal cochlear nucleus inputs

Glutamate

The neurotransmitter components of inputs to the DCN are summarized in Fig. 4.1. While all VCN projection neurons receive glutamatergic excitation from the auditory nerve, this is not the

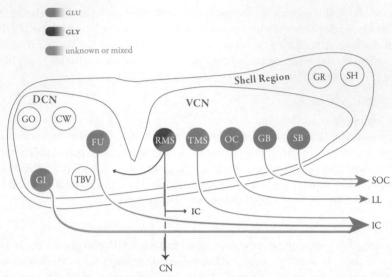

Fig. 4.2 The neurotransmitter composition of the output from the cochlear nucleus. Glutamate (GLU) (*green*) is used by projections from spherical bushy cells (SB), globular bushy cells (GB), and octopus cells (OC) in the ventral cochlear nucleus (VCN) that project to the superior olivary complex (SOC) and the lateral lemniscal nuclei (LL). Glutamate is also used by some T-multipolar stellate cells (TMS) projecting to the inferior colliculus (IC) and radiate multipolar stellate cells (RMS), both of which occur in the VCN. It is also used by some, but not necessarily all, fusiform (FU) and giant (GI) cells in the dorsal cochlear nucleus (DCN) projecting to the inferior colliculus (IC). Glycine (GLY) (*purple*) is used by many radiate multipolar stellate cells (RMS) of the VCN that project to the DCN and the contralateral cochlear nucleus (CN).

case for all neurons in the DCN. Here, the auditory nerve makes direct glutamatergic synapses on the basal dendrites of fusiform cells, giant cells, and tuberculoventral cells, while the parallel fiber axons of granule cells in the CN shell region provide the glutamatergic excitation to cartwheel cells, Golgi cells, stellate cells, and the apical dendrites of fusiform cells (Osen *et al.*, 1995; Rubio and Juiz, 2004). The synaptic connections onto the fusiform cell are therefore complex and have provided a valuable model system for the study of multiple glutamatergic inputs and their modulation by inhibitory inputs. While both auditory nerve and parallel fibers make glutamatergic synapses on fusiform cells, the composition of AMPA receptors apposing their terminals is quite different. Rubio and Wenthold (1999) found that the GluR4 AMPA subunit is placed in the AMPA receptors at synapses in the basal dendrites of fusiform cells, while there is little placement of the GLUR2 subunit into the AMPA receptors in this location. Thus these receptors have the 'auditory specific' AMPA receptor configuration that is typical for synapses that receive glutamatergic input from the auditory nerve. On the other hand, there is high GLUR2 and no placement of GLUR4 in the AMPA receptor subunits found in the apical dendritic synapses that receive input from glutamatergic parallel fiber axons of granule cells in the shell region (for reviews see Parks, 2000; Petralia *et al.*, 2000). This configuration is also seen in parallel fiber synapses on cartwheel cells. Gardner *et al.* (2001) reported that the latter synapses had AMPA receptors with slower gating, consistent with higher levels of GluR2 and flip isoforms. Fusiform cells with parallel fiber and auditory nerve inputs apposed by receptors with different compositions had intermediate kinetic properties compared to the rapid gating found in VCN neurons.

Bilak *et al.* (1996) reported that while NMDAR1 was expressed in most neuronal types, granule cells in the DCN had little, if any, expression, unlike their heavily labeled counterparts in the small cell shell and the cerebellum. The metabotropic mGluR1 alpha subunit has a wide distribution in DCN, particularly in the dendritic spines of cartwheel cells and in dendrites of unipolar brush cells. mGluR2 expression is high in Golgi cells as well as unipolar brush cells (Wright *et al.*, 1996; Petralia *et al.*, 2000). Molitor and Manis (1997) reported that expression of the mGLUR receptor, which induced depression of activation in the DCN, was greatest at parallel fiber synapses.

GABA and glycine

Fusiform cells receive many GABA, glycine, and GABA/Gly terminals, while tuberculoventral and cartwheel cells receive only GABA and glycine terminals. Glycine and GABA/Gly terminals are both apposed by glycine receptors (Rubio and Juiz, 2004). Many, but not all, cartwheel cells label for glycine (e.g. Wenthold *et al.*, 1987; Gates *et al.*, 1996). These provide inhibitory input to fusiform cells that modulates the excitation mediated by granule cells and auditory nerve fibers (Golding and Oertel, 1996). GABAergic input from intrinsic neurons of the molecular layer as well as from the SOC provide additional inhibitory inputs to fusiform cells (Golding and Oertel, 1996). The GABA-A receptors of cartwheel, Golgi, fusiform, and giant cells are mostly composed of the alpha 3, beta 3, and gamma 2L subunits (Campos *et al.*, 2001). Metabotropic GABA-B receptors are found both pre- and post-synaptically. GABA-B1 immunostaining is observed in the molecular and fusiform cell layers in both pre- and post-synaptic locations that are often associated with glutamatergic input, particularly on the dendritic spines of fusiform cells that receive parallel fiber terminals from granule cells (Lujan *et al.*, 2004).

4.4.4 Dorsal cochlear nucleus outputs

The neurotransmitter components in the ascending projections of DCN neurons are summarized in Fig. 4.2. Fusiform cells give rise to the major ascending projection of the DCN, ending predominantly in the contralateral IC with smaller projections to the ipsilateral IC and nuclei of the lateral lemniscus (see Cant and Benson, 2003; Chapter 2). The smaller population of giant cells in the deep layer of the DCN receives glutamatergic input from the auditory nerve, but also receives inhibitory amino acid terminals. Giant cells send their axons along with those of fusiform cells into the dorsal acoustic striae to terminate in the IC and lateral lemniscal nuclei (for reviews see Cant and Benson, 2003; Chapter 2).

Some, but not all, fusiform cells immunostain for glutamate, but not for GABA or glycine (Alibardi, 1999). Similarly, some giant cells also immunostain for glutamate, and some immunostain for glycine (Kolston *et al.*, 1992). Interestingly, Oliver (1985) reported that while some terminals from fusiform and giant cells onto IC neurons contained large round vesicles consistent with glutamate as a transmitter, other terminals contained small round vesicles, the shape of which were more consistent with acetylcholine as the neurotransmitter. There may therefore be diversity in the transmitters of the projection from the DCN to the IC which requires further study. This may be an exception to the otherwise largely glutamatergic projection from the CN into the ascending core auditory pathway.

4.4.5 The shell region of the cochlear nucleus

Auditory input to the shell region of the CN is largely from type II spiral ganglion neurons onto dendrites of shell neurons as well as onto synaptic nests (Hurd *et al.*, 1999; Ryugo *et al.*, 2003; Benson and Brown, 2006), although there is some input from type I neurons as well. The shell region of the cochlear nucleus contains Golgi cells as well as several additional neuronal types (Hutson and Morest, 1996; Hurd *et al.*, 1999; Ryugo *et al.*, 2003). This is an area that integrates auditory and non-auditory inputs and there are many different neurotransmitters from multiple sources, including neuropeptides, biogenic amines, and amino acid transmitters (for reviews see

Ryugo *et al.*, 2003; Shore and Zhou, 2006). The non-auditory input includes glutamatergic mossy fibers and *en passant* endings from the trigeminal and cuneate nuclei of the somatosensory system that end on granule cells and shell neurons (Ryugo *et al.*, 2003; Shore and Zhou, 2006). The non-auditory input is higher in shell regions than in the VCN or DCN (Ryugo *et al.*, 2003; Shore and Zhou, 2006). Granule cells are themselves glutamatergic (Oliver *et al.*, 1983; Altschuler *et al.*, 1984; Godfrey *et al.*, 1988) and give rise to the parallel fiber input to the DCN. Many of the shell neurons are glycinergic and/or GABAergic (Kolston *et al.*, 1992), while unipolar brush neurons are glutamatergic (Kalinichenko and Okhotin, 2005). Glutamate concentrations are high in regions containing granule cell bodies as well as in regions where their axons terminate (Godfrey *et al.*, 1988, 2000). While auditory nerve terminals are associated with vesicular glutamate transporter 1, the non-auditory (including somatosensory) glutamatergic inputs, highest in the shell region, are more associated with vesicular glutamate transporter 2 (Zhou *et al.*, 2007).

The metabotropic glutamate receptor mGluR1 alpha is enriched in unipolar brush cells (Wright *et al.*, 1996). In addition to glutamatergic input, granule cells receive an unknown source of inhibitory amino acid input and have alpha 1 and alpha 6, beta 3, and gamma 2L subunits in their GABA-A receptors (Campos *et al.*, 2001), comparable to the granule cells of the cerebellum, and different from all other neurons in the ascending auditory pathway.

Acetylcholine (ACh)

Cholinergic neurons contribute a major input to both the ventral and dorsal divisions of the cochlear nucleus. Much of the cholinergic input to the CN is from collaterals of the olivocochlear sytem projection to the cochlea; however, some VNTB neurons may send cholinergic projections that go only to the CN (Godfrey *et al.*, 1988, 2000; Fujino and Oertel, 2001). Cholinergic inputs act on nicotinic and muscarinic receptors of CN neurons with predominantly excitatory postsynaptic effects (Fujino and Oertel, 2001). Studies showing the formation of new cholinergic synapses (Meidinger *et al.*, 2006), changes in muscarinic acetylcholine receptor binding in the CN following peripheral auditory lesions (Jin and Godfrey, 2006), and changes in sensitivity to acetylcholine following acoustic trauma (Chang *et al.*, 2002) implicate cholinergic synapses in neural plasticity of the auditory system.

Biogenic amines

Noradrenergic (norepinephrine) input to all divisions of the CN originates in the locus coeruleus (Kromer and Moore, 1980). There is also serotonergic input to the CN from the raphe nuclei (Thompson and Thompson, 2001), with highest density in the molecular layer of the DCN and shell regions, and lowest density in magnocellular areas of the VCN. Dopamine is associated with the lateral olivocochlear efferents (see section 4.4.14) which may send collateral branches to the CN.

Neuropeptides

Several neuropeptide transmitters are localized or co-localized in non-primary inputs to the VCN, DCN, and shell regions of the CN. These include enkephalin, neurotensin, substance P, cholecystokinin (CCK), and neuropeptide Y. The distributions of calcitonin gene-related peptide (CGRP) and neuropeptide Y terminals are higher in the shell regions than the magnocellular regions.

Non-traditional neurotransmitters/neuromodulators: endocannabinoids and nitric oxide

There is evidence that the non-traditional neurotransmitters/neuromodulators endocannabinoids and nitric oxide play a role in the ascending auditory pathways. Endocannabinoids modulate glutamate release in the DCN (Tzounopoulus *et al.*, 2007) and are strongly implicated in the mechanisms underlying plasticity that depend on spike timing. Nitric oxide is used as a neuro-transmitter in some neurons in the CN and in several regions of the superior olivary complex, including the MNTB, LSO, SPN, VNTB, and MSO (Fessenden *et al.*, 1999; Schaeffer *et al.*, 2003) and is assumed to play a neuromodulatory role as well as regulating blood flow.

4.4.6 The superior olivary complex and lemnsical nuclei (SOC-LL)

Several major nuclei in the core ascending auditory pathway are located in the brain stem between the CN and IC in the superior olive and the lateral lemniscus (SOC-LL). These nuclei play an important role in processing ascending signals for binaural interaction. Some nuclei are involved in circuitry within the SOC-LL, such as the MNTB which receives largely excitatory glutamatergic input from the CN and transforms this into largely inhibitory (glycinergic) inputs ('sign-switch') to many other SOC-LL nuclei. The LNTB also provides inhibitory projections within the SOC-LL, often using both GABA and glycine. Most SOC-LL nuclei project to the IC, with glutamatergic projections from the MSO and LSO, GABAergic projections from the DNLL, VNLL, and SPN, and glycinergic projections from the LSO and VNLL (Fig. 4.4). SOC neurons also give rise to descending projections, including olivocochlear projections (e.g. LSO, VNTB), which will be discussed in a later section and are reviewed in Chapter 3. The neurotransmitter components of inputs from the 'core' ascending auditory pathway into nuclei of the SOC-LL are summarized in Fig. 4.3, while Fig. 4.4 summarizes the neurotransmitter components of the brainstem projections to the IC.

Glutamate

Principal cells in all major SOC and LL nuclei receive direct excitatory glutamatergic inputs from the ipsi- and/or contralateral CN, and LL receives excitatory glutamatergic input from the LSO. The AMPA receptor composition in these regions has not been extensively examined, but where it has been assessed, it largely follows the auditory AMPA receptor pattern, i.e. with high levels of GLUR3 and 4 and low levels of GLUR2 components. There are also many glycinergic and GABAergic synapses on SOC and LL neurons that originate largely in other SOC and LL regions, or are intrinsic to each nucleus.

Glycine

The neurons of the MNTB provide large, glycinergic inputs to the lateral and medial superior olivary nuclei (LSO, MSO), superior paraolivary nucleus (SPN), and LNTB. The MNTB itself and the ventral nucleus of the trapezoid body (VNTB) receive smaller glycinergic connections from other MNTB neurons. The alpha 1 subunit of the glycine receptor is highly expressed in neurons that receive many glycinergic terminals (e.g. LSO) and has lower expression in regions receiving less glycinergic input, such as the MNTB and VNTB, where alpha 3 subunit expression is higher (Sato *et al.*, 2000).

GABA

The GABAergic and GABA/Gly terminals found on many SOC neurons largely originate in the LNTB and VNTB, and can thus be considered intrinsic to the SOC (Adams and Mugnaini, 1984, 1990). On the other hand, the IC receives many GABAergic projections from the VNLL and DNLL. The GABAergic neurons of the DNLL also send a major projection to the contralateral DNLL. Descending GABAergic inputs from the IC terminate in both the LL and SOC nuclei where GABA-A receptors composed of the alpha 3, beta 3, and gamma 2L subunits predominate (Campos *et al.*, 2001).

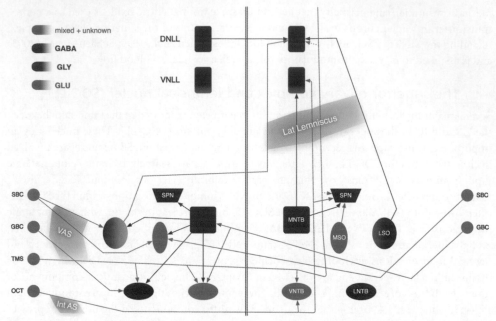

Fig. 4.3 The neurotransmitter composition of ascending inputs to the superior olivary complex and lateral lemniscal nuclei. There is an excitatory amino acid (glutamate – GLU (*green*) projection from spherical bushy cells (SB), globular bushy cells (GB), and octopus cells (OC) and T-multipolar stellate cells via the ventral acoustic stria (VAS) and intermediate acoustic stria (Int AS). The medial superior olive (MSO) and the lateral superior olive (LSO) also provide glutamatergic (*green*) projections. The medial nucleus of trapezoid body (MNTN) provides a glycinergic (GLY) (*purple*) projection. The dorsal and ventral nuclei of the lateral lemniscus (DNLL, VNLL) receive inputs via the lateral lemniscus (Lat Lemniscus) and the DNLL receives a commissural GABAergic (GABA) (*red*) input from the contralateral DNLL. Outputs from the lateral and ventral nuclei of the trapezoid body (LNTB, VNTB), the superior paraolivary nucleus (SPN), and the VNLL are not shown, though their transmitter composition is color coded.

LSO

LSO principal neurons receive a major inhibitory glycinergic projection from neurons in the MNTB (Bledsoe *et al.*, 1990) and a major excitatory glutamatergic projection from the ipsilateral CN. These LSO neurons compute interaural intensity differences for localizing sounds by comparing the strength of the excitatory input from spherical bushy cells of the ipsilateral CN with the inhibitory glycinergic input from ipsilateral neurons in MNTB, which in turn is driven by the CN on the opposite side. The glutamatergic projection from the CN contacts auditory type AMPA receptors composed of GluR3 and 4 flop subunits (Schmid *et al.*, 2001) to give rapid kinetics. The glycinergic projection from MNTB contacts glycine receptors that have high expression of the alpha 1 rather than the alpha 3 subunit (Sato *et al.*, 2000), so giving rapid kinetics to the inhibition that matches the excitation. NMDA receptors may play a role in binaural processing by modulating contralateral inhibitory glycinergic input (Wu and Kelly, 1992). LSO neurons send a crossed, excitatory, glutamatergic projection to the contralateral DNLL and IC and an uncrossed, ipsilateral, inhibitory, glycingergic projection to the ipsilateral DNLL and IC (Saint Marie *et al.*, 1989b; Glendenning *et al.*, 1991).

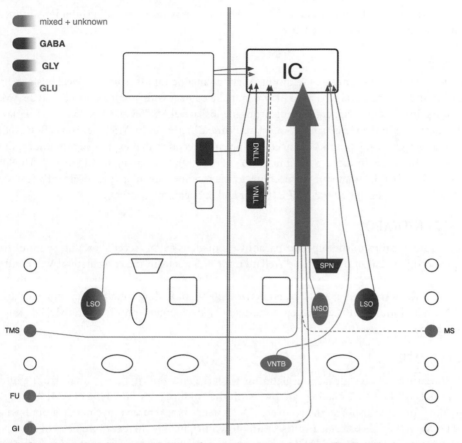

Fig. 4.4 The neurotransmitter composition of ascending inputs to the inferior colliculus (IC). There is glutamatergic (GLU) (*green*) excitatory amino acid input from stellate multipolar cells (TMS, MS), from some fusiform (FU) and giant cells (GI), from the medial superior olive (MSO), and from some of the neurons in the lateral superior olive (LSO) and ventral nucleus of the lateral lemniscus (VNLL) as well as from the contralateral IC. There is GABAergic (GABA) (*red*) input from the superior paraolivary nucleus (SPN), the dorsal nucleus of the lateral lemniscus (DNLL), and some neurons in the VNLL and contralateral IC. There is glycinergic input (GLY) (*purple*) from some neurons in the LSO and VNLL. The ventral nucleus of the lateral lemniscus (VNTB) has neurons using multiple transmitters (*blue*) including glutamate, GABA, glycine, and acetylcholine. Some of these neurons project to the IC.

4.4.7 **MNTB**

Principal neurons of the MNTB receive major glutamatergic input from globular bushy cells in the VCN via end-bulb terminals. The receptors opposing the end-bulbs are the 'auditory specific' type of AMPA receptor (as described previously) specialized for rapid neurotransmission (Forsythe and Barnes-Davies, 1993, Geiger *et al.*, 1995). The principal neurons also receive GABAergic and glycinergic innervation (Adams and Mugnaini, 1990; Awatramani *et al.*, 2004) from intrinsic collaterals (glycine) and from LNTB (GABA and glycine), which likely disinhibit and thus modify the relay function of the MNTB during sound localization.

MNTB neurons do not provide an ascending core projection to the IC, but have an important function in glycinergic inhibitory modulation of the ascending signal, not only for the LSO, but also for most other SOC nuclei and the VNLL. They also provide a descending inhibitory influence to the cochlear nucleus (see Chapter 3).

4.4.8 **MSO**

The neurons in MSO compare the timing of glutamatergic inputs from spherical bushy cells in the ipsi- and contralateral CN, both of which make contact with 'auditory specific'-type AMPA receptors. Inhibitory, glycinergic inputs from the ipsilateral MNTB and VNTB may also play an important role in the processing of interaural time differences by MSO neurons (Brand *et al.*, 2002). These glycinergic inputs connect with glycine receptors that express high numbers of the alpha 1 rather than the alpha 3 subunit (Sato *et al.*, 2000), thus giving rapid kinetics. The MSO sends excitatory (glutamatergic) projections to the inferior colliculus (predominantly ipsilateral to it) as well as to the ipsilateral DNLL (Oliver and Schneiderman, 1989).

4.4.9 **SPN/DMPO**

GABAergic neurons in the superior paraolivary nucleus (SPN) receive excitatory input from glutamatergic axons of octopus and stellate multipolar cells in the contralateral VCN and the MSO (e.g. Kulesza *et al.*, 2003; Chapter 2). The GABAergic neurons, in turn, project to the ipsilateral IC (Kelly *et al.*, 1998; Saldaña and Berrebi, 2000), providing an inhibitory influence driven by CN excitation. The SPN also receives modulatory glycinergic inputs from the MNTB (Kulesza *et al.*, 2003).

4.4.10 **LNTB**

LNTB neurons receive glutamatergic input via large end-bulb-type terminals from globular bushy cells of the VCN, making synapses with the 'auditory specific' type of AMPA receptor, providing for rapid response and recovery. LNTB neurons also receive glycinergic input from the MNTB as well as GABAergic inputs of unknown origin. The main subnucleus of the LNTB contains both glycinergic and GABAergic neurons as well as neurons co-containing both GABA and glycine, while in contrast the posteroventral subnucleus is composed almost exclusively of glycinergic neurons. LNTB neurons function as interneurons for processing within the SOC, and also project to the CN (Shore *et al.*, 1991).

4.4.11 **VNTB**

The VNTB is the major, and, in some species the only, source of descending medial olivocochlear efferents (MOC) to the cochlea. It receives ascending glutamatergic input from the CN and descending input from the inferior colliculus, primarily onto the MOC neurons. The VNTB also receives a direct descending input from the auditory cortex, primarily onto the VNTB neurons that project to the ipsilateral IC or the cochlea. In addition, the VNTB sends major projections to the CN, particularly the molecular layer of contralateral DCN, and the contralateral LSO, and smaller projections to the LL. Acetylcholine is found in a large number of VNTB neurons (Sherriff and Henderson, 1994; Yao and Godfrey, 1998), but there are also many inhibitory GABAergic and glycinergic neurons throughout the VNTB (Ostapoff *et al.*, 1997). The cholinergic neurons project to multiple regions including the CN, cochlea, and cochlear root neurons (Sherriff and Henderson, 1994; Gomez-Nieto *et al.*, 2007). Their influence is predominantly excitatory in the CN and where they inhibit outer hair cell motility in the cochlea. The GABAergic and glycinergic projections of the VNTB can inhibit other SOC and LL nuclei, and also project to the contralateral CN (Ostapoff *et al.*, 1997). VNTB neurons giving rise to descending projections are innervated by glutamatergic, cholinergic, and GABA/glycinergic terminals, many with dense core vesicles suggesting co-containment of neuropeptides and/or biogenic amines (Benson and Brown, 2006). The transmitter or transmitters of the ascending projection from the VNTB that terminates in the inferior colliculus have not been identified but could be acetylcholine, since that is the predominant neurotransmitter type in VNTB neurons.

4.4.12 VNLL

The VNLL is part of the monaural pathway to the IC. Principal cells of the VNLL receive excitatory glutamatergic input from the contralateral VCN, largely from octopus cells (Alibardi, 2003). There is also a major inhibitory glycinergic input to VNLL that originates in the ipsilateral MNTB (Glendenning *et al.*, 1981) and acts on glycine receptors on VNLL principal cells that express the alpha 1 subunit. Two-thirds of VNLL cells are either GABAergic or glyinergic, with many co-containing both GABA and glycine (Riquelme *et al.*, 2001). These neurons provide a large inhibitory projection to the ipsilateral IC, with perhaps a small projection directly to the auditory thalamus (medial geniculate nucleus).

4.4.13 DNLL

The DNLL is a binaural nucleus because in addition to excitatory glutamatergic inputs from the ipsilateral CN, there is also an excitatory glutamatergic input from the contralateral LSO and the ipsilateral MSO. An inhibitory glycinergic projection arises in the ipsilateral LSO and an inhibitory GABAergic projection comes from the contralateral DNLL (Glendenning *et al.*, 1981; Pollak, 1997). As in the VNLL, GABAergic terminals in the DNLL neurons contact GABA-A receptors that express the alpha 1 subunit in addition to beta 3 and gamma 2L subunits (Campos *et al.*, 2001). While there are both excitatory and inhibitory DNLL neurons, the majority are GABAergic (Adams and Mugnaini, 1984), and project to the central nuclei of both ICs, producing long-lasting inhibition that may be important for functions such as echo suppression (Pecka *et al.*, 2007).

4.4.14 SOC-LL 1

Biogenic amines

Noradrenergic input, largely from locus coeruleus, provides an excitatory influence onto lateral olivocochlear neurons (LOCs) of the lateral superior olive and MOC neurons of the VNTB (Mulders and Robertson, 2005) as well as less dense input to principal neurons across all SOC nuclei (Mulders and Robertson, 2005).

Dopaminergic neurons in the LSO, the periolivary shell region surrounding the LSO, and in the LNTB project to the organ of Corti as LOC neurons (Mulders and Robertson, 2004; Niu *et al.*, 2004). Dopaminergic neurons are also found in MNTB (Reuss *et al.*, 1999), VNLL, and DNLL (Wynne and Robertson, 1996; Tong *et al.*, 2005).

Serotonergic innervation varies among species, with a periolivary distribution in some and in others additional innervation of principal cells in LSO and MSO (Thompson and Hurley, 2004). Serotonergic and adrenergic terminals are also found on neurons in the SOC and IC that project to the CN (Behrens *et al.*, 2002).

Neuropeptides

Neuropeptide neurotransmitters or neuromodulators are found in SOC neurons that project to the cochlea and CN (see section 4.5.3). Neuropeptides can also influence SOC neurons: enkephalin and neurotensin input to the MSO and MNTB might arise from periolivary cells. Enkephalin containing inputs to VNTB, SPN, and LSO have been identified together with CCK and somatostatin input onto principal cells of the VNTB and MNTB. Substance P input is found in shell regions of the SOC which may arise from multimodal inputs. There are also CGRP positive neurons in the LSO that have both ascending and descending projections (Reuss *et al.*, 1999).

4.4.15 The inferior colliculus – central regions

The neurotransmitter components of ascending inputs to the inferior colliculus from the CN and SOC-LL neurons are summarized in Fig. 4.4. The central nucleus of the IC (ICC) is most involved in the core ascending auditory pathway. Cant and Benson (2003) divided the central nucleus into two divisions based on different ascending input patterns. Zone 1 receives the bulk of its input from the contralateral CN (predominantly glutamatergic from T-stellate multipolar cells of the VCN and some of the fusiform and giant cells of the DCN), the ipsilateral MSO (predominantly glutamatergic), and both ipsilateral (glutamatergic) and contralateral (glycinergic) LSO. Zone 2 receives the bulk of its input from the contralateral CN (predominantly glutamatergic) and bilaterally from the lateral lemniscus (predominantly GABAergic). There is also a large commissural input from the other IC, which has both glutamargic (Saint Marie, 1996) and GABAergic components, with the glutamatergic component making up the large majority (approximately 80%) (Hernández *et al.*, 2006). Glutamatergic and GABAergic neurons of the central nucleus of the IC then project predominantly to neurons in the ventral division of the medial geniculate nucleus, continuing the core ascending auditory pathway. Approximately 25% of neurons in the central nucleus of the IC are GABAergic (Merchán *et al.*, 2005).

Glutamate and glutamate receptors

There is monaural, excitatory glutamatergic input from the CN and binaural, excitatory glutamatergic input from the LSO and MSO to the IC. In contrast to CN and SOC neurons of the binaural pathway, most neurons in the central nucleus of the IC express high levels of GluR2 flip (Schmid *et al.*, 2001), resulting in many glutamatergic synapses with Ca^{2+} impermeable AMPA receptors and therefore slower kinetics than the 'auditory specific' AMPA synapses seen in lower brain stem regions.

Inhibitory amino acids and their receptors

The largest GABAergic input to the ICC is from the VNLL, with additional ascending GABAergic inputs from the SPN and DNLL and the contralateral IC. Application of GABA to IC neurons results in inhibition of spontaneous rates and acoustically evoked firing rates, whereas blocking GABA-A receptors increases the discharge rates of many IC neurons (e.g. Caspary *et al.*, 2002) and broadens frequency tuning (Zhang *et al.*, 1999). On the other hand, blocking GABA-B receptors can increase discharge rates (Ma *et al.*, 2002). GABA-A receptors in large ICC cells used more alpha 1 and gamma 2L subunits, while small cells used more alpha 2 and gamma 2S subunits (Shiraishi *et al.*, 2001), suggesting that cell classes in the central nucleus of the IC may differ in their response to GABA. With aging there is an increase in the alpha 2 and gamma 1 subunits across ICC neurons, leading to a more sensitive receptor configuration (Caspary *et al.*, 1999). There are many GABAergic neurons in all divisions of the IC. Approximately 25% of those in the central nucleus are GABAergic (Merchán *et al.*, 2005) and many contribute inhibitory input to the medial geniculate body (MGB). As mentioned earlier, glycine is less prevalent in the more rostral auditory nuclei, and thus there are few glycine positive neurons in the IC and it receives less glycinergic than GABAergic input. The largest glycinergic input to the IC is from the ipsilateral LSO (Saint Marie *et al.*, 1989b; Glendenning *et al.*, 1991, 1992), although some glycinergic inputs also originate in VNLL.

Biogenic amines

Serotonergic inputs, originating in the Raphe nuclei, terminate primarily on those IC neurons that project to the CN and can alter firing rates of these neurons (Hurley and Pollak, 2005). Noradrenergic input to the IC originates in the locus coeruleus, while dopaminergic input of unknown origin has been demonstrated to the central nucleus as well as to the lateral and dorsal cortex (Tong *et al.*, 2005).

4.4.16 Belt/shell regions

Glutamate

The regions surrounding the central nucleus of the inferior colliculus (IC), including the dorsal cortex and lateral (external) cortex, constitute part of the paralemniscal, non-classical 'belt' auditory pathways that incorporate multi-modal pathways. These shell regions receive a large glutamatergic input likely from multiple auditory and non-auditory sources. A major source of input to the lateral cortex originates from somatosensory nuclei (for review see Shore, 2008), some of which is glutamatergic.

GABA

The shell/belt regions of the IC, including the dorsal cortex and lateral (external) cortex, contain many GABAergic neurons, which are organized into focal patches or clusters of 'neurochemical modules' (Chernock *et al.*, 2004) that may be involved in direction-dependent sharpening of tuning.

Acetylcholine

While few cholinergic terminals are located in the central nucleus, they are abundant in shell regions. Most of the cholinergic input to these regions appears to originate in non-auditory regions and terminates in the lateral (external) and dorsal cortices, which are involved in multi-modal/multisensory integration (Jain and Shore, 2006; Shore, 2008). Post-synaptically, there is evidence of numerous alpha 7 nicotinic acetylcholine receptors (nAChR), especially in the external nucleus when compared to the central nucleus and lower regions of the auditory brain stem. The alpha 7 nAChR is predominantly localized on somata or proximal dendrites (Happe and Morley, 2004).

4.4.17 Medial geniculate body (MGB)

Amino acid transmitters

The ventral division of the MGB is most involved in the core ascending auditory pathway and receives the majority of its ascending input from the ipsilateral ICC. While the projection from ICC to the MGB is primarily glutamatergic, there is also an important GABAergic component (10–30% of the axons) of this projection (for reviews see Winer.*et al.*, 2005; Winer and Lee, 2007), as well as a small, direct GABAergic projection from DNLL (Peruzzi *et al.*, 1997).

Many of the neurons in the MGB are GABA immunopositive (Huang *et al.*, 1999), averaging 33% of the neurons in the ventral division, 26% in the dorsal division, and 18% in the medial division in the cat and primate, where most of these are small interneurons, rather than projection neurons.

Acetylcholine

Almost all thalamocortical projection neurons in the MGB are excited by acetylcholine acting at muscarinic and/or nicotinic acetylcholine receptors, although some neurons are inhibited by acetylcholine (Tebecis, 1972). The source of cholinergic input to the MGB is not from the classicial lemniscal auditory ascending pathway, however, and therefore is most likely from non-auditory regions.

Projections

The MGB influences the auditory cortex through projections terminating directly in the auditory cortex and through indirect projections that connect to other regions that in turn project to the auditory cortex (Winer and Lee, 2007). The direct connection to the auditory cortex is predominantly glutamatergic, projecting from the ventral division of the MGB to the primary auditory cortex, A1. The medial and dorsal divisions of the MGB are belt/paralemniscal and send their direct projections predominantly to secondary and association areas of the auditory cortex. The indirect connections from the MGB to the auditory cortical areas are through projections from the MGB to the amygdale and limbic cortical regions, in turn influencing the bidirectional limbic–auditory cortex interaction (Shinonaga et al., 1994) as well as projections to thalamic reticular nuclei (Crabtree, 1998). The medial and dorsal divisions of the MGB are also involved in circuits for multisensory integration as well as for auditory learning and conditioning (for review see Weinberger, 1998 and Chapter 18).

4.4.18 The auditory cortex

Amino acid transmitters

The organization of the primary auditory cortex including its inputs and outputs has been recently reviewed (Winer and Lee, 2007). As in other regions of the cerebral cortex, the pyramidal output projection neurons are predominantly glutamatergic while the multipolar interneurons with intrinsic connections are predominantly GABAergic. These interneurons are found in all layers of primary auditory cortex, but are highest in layer 1 (for reviews see Prieto et al., 1994a,b; Winer et al., 2005; Winer and Lee, 2007). The percentage of neurons in primary auditory cortex that are GABAergic is approximately 25%, slightly higher than in other neocortical regions (Prieto et al., 1994a). There is also a small population of auditory cortical neurons that are cholinergic (Kamke et al., 2005).

The thalamocortical input to the primary auditory cortex from the core auditory ascending pathway is largely glutamatergic and arises primarily from the ipsilateral ventral division of the MGB. Neurons in primary auditory cortex also receive glutamatergic input from other cortical areas, both ipsi- and contralateral as well as from the collaterals of its own pyramidal neurons. Indeed, geniculo-cortical excitation provides only about one third of the input onto A1 pyramidal neurons, mostly to the layer IV neurons, with the bulk of cortico-cortical inputs onto apical dendrites of pyramidal neurons in the supragranular layers. There are also many GABA terminals on auditory cortical neurons. These are found across all layers, with highest density in layer Ia, intermediate density in layers Ib–IVb, and lowest density in layers V and VI (Preito et al., 1994a). The source of these terminals is most often the local GABA interneurons, but others are from extrinsic sources such as basal forebrain. Wang et al. (2000, 2002) found that GABA acts on GABA-A receptors to modulate the intensity and frequency response ranges of neurons in the primary auditory cortex, an effect that is enhanced by the activation of GABA-B receptors.

Acetylcholine

There are also many cholinergic terminals on neurons in the primary auditory cortex, mostly originating from basal forebrain regions, including ipsilateral putamen, globus pallidus, and internal capsule, as well as more medial nuclei of the basal forebrain (Kamke et al., 2005). This cholinergic input to the auditory cortex from nucleus basalis is involved in plasticity in the primary auditory cortex and tonotopic reorganization (Kilgard and Merzenich, 1998; Ji and Suga, 2003). The cholinergic input can act on muscarinic (Ji and Suga, 2003) and/or nicotinic (Metherate and Hsieh, 2003) receptors. Reorganization can still occur after removal of cholinergic input (Kilgard, 2005), which suggests that it plays more of a role in modulation than in the induction of plastic changes. The glutamatergic input from MGB, IC, and other cortical neurons can induce reorganization through its action on NMDA receptors (e.g. Ji *et al.*, 2005) and the action of cholinergic input onto nicotinic receptors can influence glutamate release (Metherate and Hsieh, 2003).

Biogenic amines

Auditory cortical neurons also receive input from neurons using biogenic amines as transmitter (Descarries *et al.*, 1975) with serotonergic input from Raphe nuclei as well as noradrenergic input from the locus coreleus, which may also contribute to plasticity.

4.5 Descending auditory pathways

4.5.1 Auditory cortex

The pyramidal neurons of layers V and VI provide a largely glutamatergic output from the auditory cortex that forms a corticofugal feedback loop to the MGB as well as a less direct feedback loop to colliculo-geniculate neurons in the IC. In addition to these connections to MGB and IC there are projections from the auditory cortex to the ipsilateral VNTB and SPN, as well as to the contralateral SOC neurons that project to the IC (Chapter 3). A direct projection from primary auditory cortex also terminates in the shell region of the CN (Weedman and Ryugo, 1996).

4.5.2 IC

The central nucleus of the IC sends a large, predominantly glutamatergic, projection to the ipsilateral DNLL and VNLL, MOC neurons of the VNTB, and rostral periolivary nuclei (Vetter *et al.*, 1993; Chapter 2). ICC neurons also send a descending projection to the ipsilateral DCN (Shore *et al.*, 1991; Chapter 2). Neurotransmitters for these descending projections have not been definitively established, but, based on ultrastructural examination, they appear to be both glutamatergic and GABAergic.

4.5.3 SOC

The SOC gives rise to five descending projections: (1) MOC efferents, (2) LOC efferents, (3) shell olivocochlear efferents, (4) CN-projection neurons, and (5) SOC connections to cochlear root neurons.

Medial olivocochlear projections (MOCs)

Medial olivocochlear efferents (MOCs) originate in the VNTB (and SPN in some species) and project to outer hair cells in the cochlea. Acetylcholine is their major transmitter, often co-colocalized with CGRP (Eybalin, 1993). There is also a small GABAergic sub-population of MOC neurons in the VNTB (Fex and Altschuler, 1984). The MOC efferents give off collaterals to both divisions of the CN before they exit from the brain stem. Kraus and Illing (2004) report that cholinergic projections of MOC neurons to the CN show plasticity following unilateral deafness. The MOC and non-MOC cholinergic inputs from SOC to CN have also been implicated in tinnitus-associated firing rate changes (Chang *et al.*, 2002). Based on the ultrastructure of their terminals and vesicle shapes, MOC neurons in VNTB receive a major glutamatergic input as well as an inhibitory amino acid and cholinergic input (Benson and Brown, 2006). These authors suggest that stellate multipolar cells are one source of the glutamatergic terminals, providing for a 'reflex' response driven by the auditory nerve and providing rapid feedback to outer hair cells via the projections of MOC neurons. Descending glutamatergic inputs from the IC may be another source of excitatory input to MOC neurons; these are not considered part of the MOC reflex pathway.

Lateral olivocochlear projections (LOCs)

Lateral olivocochlear efferents (LOC) originate within or around the LSO and project to the cochlea after giving off collaterals to the CN. In the cochlea they terminate on the peripheral processes of type I auditory nerve fibers. While acetylcholine was the first neurotransmitter localized to the LOC (for reviews see Eyablin, 1993; Raphael and Altschuler, 2003), many additional neurotransmitters are often co-contained in LOC neurons. These include enkephalin, dynorphin, dopamine, and CGRP. A separate population of LOC neurons contains GABA (for reviews see Eyablin, 1993; Raphael and Altschuler, 2003). Shell olivocochlear efferents (ShOC) constitute a subdivision of the LOC system that originates in periolivary neurons around the LSO and project to the cochlea where they terminate on auditory nerve peripheral processes (Brown, 1987; Vetter and Mugnaini, 1992; Warr *et al.*, 1997). They use acetylcholine (Vetter and Mugnaini, 1992) and/or dopamine (Niu and Canlon, 2002; Niu *et al.*, 2004) as transmitters and may co-contain other neurotransmitters, as do other LOC neurons.

4.5.4 **SOC–CN connections**

The VCN and DCN both receive GABAergic and glycinergic input from the ipsilateral lateral nucleus of the trapezoid body, while the DCN receives GABAergic input from DMPO/SPN (Shore *et al.*, 1991). There is also a glycinergic projection to the CN from the MNTB (Schofield, 1994). There is a major bilateral cholinergic projection originating in non-MOC neurons of theVNTB to both VCN and DCN (Vetter *et al.*, 1993).

4.5.5 **SOC to cochlear root neurons**

Cochlear root neurons are found in the auditory nerve and modiolus of the cochlea in many, but not all, species, where they provide a more direct pathway for the acoustic startle reflex. They receive descending cholinergic input from the VNTB (Gómez-Nieto *et al.*, 2007).

4.6 **Conclusions**

This chapter has emphasized the importance of both the inhibitory and excitatory amino acids as major determinants of information transfer along the core ascending auditory pathways. These amino acid transmitters, along with specialized receptors, allow for the rapid responses necessary for processing auditory information. The balance of synaptic strength between these inhibitory and excitatory influences plays a key role in the actions of individual neurons in normal neurotransmission, and changes in the balance of these influences are involved in processes such as 'active listening'. Pathological imbalances in synaptic strength can occur after peripheral end organ damage, noise overstimulation, or during aging and can lead to tinnitus, hyperacusis, and other central auditory processing disorders.

Other neurotransmitters also play key roles in modulating information processing in the ascending auditory pathways, often through the belt, but also within the core component. Their inputs combine with those using amino acid transmitters to play a key role in multisensory and multimodal integration as well as learning and conditioning. Both the amino acid transmitters and multiple other transmitters also play key roles in the descending auditory pathways and associated processing.

Acknowledgements

We would like to thank Ben Yates for expertly preparing the figures and Mabel Render for her expert secretarial assistance.

References

Adams JC, Mugnaini E (1984) Dorsal nucleus of the lateral lemniscus: a nucleus of GABAergic projection neurons. *Brain Res Bull* **13**(4): 585–90.

Adams JC, Mugnaini E (1990) Immunocytochemical evidence for inhibitory and disinhibitory circuits in the superior olive. *Hear Res* **49**(1–3): 281–98.

Alibardi L (1998) Ultrastructural and immunocytochemical characterization of neurons in the rat ventral cochlear nucleus projecting to the inferior colliculus. *Ann Anat* **180**(5): 415–26.

Alibardi L (1999) Fine structure, synaptology and immunocytochemistry of large neurons in the rat dorsal cochlear nucleus connected to the inferior colliculus. *J Hirnforsch* **39**(4): 429–39.

Alibardi L (2003) Ultrastructure and immunocytochemical characteristics of cells in the octopus cell area of the rat cochlear nucleus: comparison with multipolar cells. *Ann Anat* **185**(1): 21–33.

Altschuler RA, Neises GR, Harmison GG, Wenthold RJ, Fex J (1981) Immunocytochemical localization of aspartate aminotransferase immunoreactivity in cochlear nucleus of the guinea pig. *Proc Natl Acad Sci USA* **78**(10): 6553–7.

Altschuler RA, Wenthold RJ, Schwartz AM, *et al.* (1984) Immunocytochemical localization of glutaminase-like immunoreactivity in the auditory nerve. *Brain Res* **291**(1): 173–8.

Awatramani GB, Turecek R, Trussell LO (2004) Inhibitory control at a synaptic relay. *J Neurosci* **24**(11): 2643–7.

Babalian AL, Jacomme AV, Doucet JR, Ryugo DK, Rouiller EM (2002) Comissural glycinergic inhibition of bushy and stellate cells in the anteroventral cochlear nucleus. *Neuroreport* **13**(4): 555–8.

Behrens EG, Schofield BR, Thompson AM (2002) Aminergic projections to cochlear nucleus via descending auditory pathways. *Brain Res* **955**(1–2): 34–44.

Benson TE, Brown MC (2006) Ultrastructure of synaptic input to medial olivocochlear neurons. *J Comp Neurol* **499**(2): 244–57.

Bilak MM, Bilak SR, Morest DK (1996) Differential expression of N-methyl-D-aspartate receptor in the cochlear nucleus of the mouse. *Neuroscience* **75**(4): 1075–97.

Bledsoe SC Jr, Snead CR, Helfert RH, Prasad V, Wenthold RJ, Altschuler RA (1990) Immunocytochemical and lesion studies support the hypothesis that the projection from the medial nucleus of the trapezoid body to the lateral superior olive is glycinergic. *Brain Res* **517**(1–2): 189–94.

Brand A, Behrend O, Marquardt T, McAlpine D, Grothe B. (2002) Precise inhibition is essential for microsecond interaural time difference coding. *Nature* **417**(6888): 543–7.

Brown MC (1987) Morphology of labeled efferent fibers in the guinea pig cochlea. *J Comp Neurol* **260**(4): 605–18.

Campos ML, de Cabo C, Wisden W, Juiz M, Merlo D (2001) Expression of GABA(A) receptor subunits in rat brainstem auditory pathways: cochlear nuclei, superior olivary complex and nucleus of the lateral lemniscus. *Neuroscience* **102**(3): 625–38.

Cant NB, Benson CG (2003) Parallel auditory pathways: projection patterns of the different neuronal populations in the dorsal and ventral cochlear nuclei. *Brain Res Bull* **60**(5–6): 457–74.

Caspary DM, Holder TM, Hughes LF, Milbrandt JC, McKernan RM, Naritoku DK (1999) Age-related changes in GABA(A) receptor subunit composition and function in rat auditory system. *Neuroscience* **93**(1): 307–12.

Caspary DM, Palombi PS, Hughes LF (2002) GABAergic inputs shape responses to amplitude modulated stimuli in the inferior colliculus. *Hear Res* **168**(1–2): 163–73.

Chang H, Chen K, Kaltenbach JA, Zhang J, Godfrey DA (2002) Effects of acoustic trauma on dorsal cochlear nucleus neuron activity in slices. *Hear Res* **164**(1–2): 59–68.

Chernock ML, Larue DT, Winer JA (2004) A periodic network of neurochemical modules in the inferior colliculus. *Hear Res* **188**(1–2): 12–20.

Crabtree JW (1998), Organization in the auditory sector of the cat's thalamic reticular nucleus, *J Comp Neurol* **390**: 167–82.

Descarries L, Beaudet A, Watkins KC (1975) Serotonin nerve terminals in adult rat neocortex. *Brain Res* **100**(3): 563–88.

Doucet JR, Ryugo DK (2006) Structural and functional classes of multipolar cells in the ventral cochlear nucleus. *Anat Rec A Discov Mol Cell Evol Biol* **288**: 331–44.

Eybalin M (1993) Neurotransmitters and neuromodulators of the mammalian cochlea. *Physiol Rev* **73**(2): 309–73.

Feldman DE, Brainard MS, Knudsen EI (1996) Newly learned auditory responses mediated by NMDA receptors in the owl inferior colliculus. *Science* **271**(5248): 525–8.

Fessenden JD, Altschuler RA, Seasholtz AF, Schacht J (1999) Nitric oxide/cyclic guanosine monophosphate pathway in the peripheral and central auditory system of the rat. *J Comp Neurol* **404**(1): 52–63.

Fex J, Altschuler RA (1984) Glutamic acid decarboxylase immunoreactivity of olivocochlear neurons in the organ of Corti of guinea pig and rat. *Hear Res* **15**(2): 123–31.

Forsythe ID, Barnes-Davies M (1993) The binaural auditory pathway: membrane currents limiting multiple action potential generation in the rat medial nucleus of the trapezoid body. *Proc Biol Sci* **251**(1331): 143–50.

Friauf E, Hammerschmidt B, Kirsch J (1997) Development of adult-type inhibitory glycine receptors in the central auditory system of rats. *J Comp Neurol* **385**(1): 117–134.

Fujino K, Oertel D (2001) Cholinergic modulation of stellate cells in the mammalian ventral cochlear nucleus. *J Neurosci* **21**(18): 7372–83.

Gardner SM, Trussell LO, Oertel D (2001) Correlation of AMPA receptor subunit composition with synaptic input in the mammalian cochlear nuclei. *J Neurosc* **21**(18): 7428–37.

Gates TS, Weedman DL, Pongstaporn T, Ryugo DK (1996) Immunocytochemical localization of glycine in a subset of cartwheel cells of the dorsal cochlear nucleus in rats. *Hear Res* **96**(1–2): 157–66.

Geiger JR, Melcher T, Koh DS, *et al.* (1995) Relative abundance of subunit mRNAs determines gating and Ca^{2+} permeability of AMPA receptors in principal neurons and interneurons in rat CNS. *Neuron* **5**(1): 193–204.

Glendenning KK, Brunso-Bechtold JK, Thompson GC, Masterton RB (1981) Ascending auditory afferents to the nuclei of the lateral lemniscus. *J Comp Neurol* **197**(4): 673–703.

Glendenning KK, Masterton RB, Baker BN, Wenthold RJ (1991) Acoustic chiasm. III: Nature, distribution, and sources of afferents to the lateral superior olive in the cat. *J Comp Neurol* **310**(3): 377–400.

Glendenning KK, Baker BN, Hutson KA, Masterton RB (1992) Acoustic chiasm V: Inhibition and excitation in the ipsilateral and contralateral projections of LSO. *J Comp Neurol* **319**(1): 100–122.

Godfrey DA, Parli JA, Dunn JD, Ross CD (1988) Neurotransmitter microchemistry of the cochlear nucleus and superior olivary complex. In: *Auditory Pathway* (eds Syka J, Masterton RB), pp. 107–121. Kluwer, Dordrecht.

Godfrey DA, Farms WB, Godfrey TG, Mikesell NL, Liu J (2000) Amino acid concentrations in rat cochlear nucleus and superior olive. *Hear Res* **150**(1–2): 189–205.

Golding NL, Oertel D (1996) Context-dependent synaptic action of glycinergic and GABAergic inputs in the dorsal cochlear nucleus. *J Neurosci* **16**(7): 2208–19.

Gómez-Nieto R, Rubio ME, López DE (2007) Cholinergic input from the ventral nucleus of the trapezoid body to cochlear root neurons in rats. *J Comp Neurol* **506**(3): 452–68.

Hackney CM, Osen KK, Ottersen OP, Storm-Mathisen J, Manjaly G (1996) Immunocytochemical evidence that glutamate is a neurotransmitter in the cochlear nerve: a quantitative study in the guinea-pig anteroventral cochlear nucleus. *Eur J Neurosci* 8(1): 79–91.

Happe HK, Morley BJ (2004) Distribution and postnatal development of alpha 7 nicotinic acetylcholine receptors in the rodent lower auditory brainstem. *Brain Res Dev* 153(1): 29–37.

Hernández O, Rees A, Malmierca MS (2006) A GABAergic component in the commissure of the inferior colliculus in rat. *Neuroreport* 17(15): 1611–14.

Hollmann M, Heinemann SF (1994) Cloned glutamate receptors. *Annu Rev Neurosci* 17; 31–108.

Huang CL, Larue DT, Winer JA. (1999) GABAergic organization of the cat medial geniculate body. *J Comp Neurol*.415(3): 368–92.

Hunter C, Petralia RS, Vu T, Wenthold RJ (1993) Expression of AMPA-selective glutamate receptor subunits in morphologically defined neurons of the mammalian cochlear nucleus. *J Neurosci* 13(5):1932–46.

Hurd LB, Hutson, KA, Morest DK (1999) Cochlear nerve projections to the small cell shell of the cochlear nucleus: the neuroanatomy of extremely thin sensory axons. *Synapse* 33(2): 83–117.

Hurley LM, Pollak GD (2005) Serotonin shifts first-spike latencies of inferior colliculus neurons. *J Neurosc* 25(34): 7876–86.

Hutson KA, Morest DK (1996) Fine structure of the cell clusters in the cochlear nerve root: stellate, granule, and mitt cells offer insights into the synaptic organization of local circuit neurons. *J Comp Neurol* 371(3): 397–414.

Jain R, Shore SE (2006) External inferior colliculus integrates trigeminal and acoustic information: unit responses to trigeminal nucleus and acoustic stimulation in the guinea pig. *Neurosci Lett* 395: 71–5.

Ji W, Suga N (2003) Development of reorganization of the auditory cortex caused by fear conditioning: effect of atropine. *J Neurophysiol* 90(3): 1904–1909.

Ji W, Suga N, Gao E (2005) Effects of agonists and antagonists of NMDA and ACh receptors on plasticity of bat auditory system elicited by fear conditioning. *J Neurophysiol* 94(2): 1199–211.

Jin YM, Godfrey DA (2006) Effects of cochlear ablation on muscarinic acetylcholine receptor binding in the rat cochlear nucleus. *J Neurosci Res* 83(1): 157–66.

Juiz JM, Helfert RH, Wenthold RJ, De Blas AL, Altschuler RA (1989) Immunocytochemical localization of the GABAA/benzodiazepine receptor in the guinea pig cochlear nucleus: evidence for receptor localization heterogeneity. *Brain Res* 504: 173–9.

Juiz JM, Albin RL, Helfert RH, Altschuler RA (1994) Distribution of GABAA and GABAB binding sites in the cochlear nucleus of the guinea pig. *Brain Res* 639: 193–201.

Juiz JM, Helfert RH, Bonneau JM, Wenthold RJ, Altschuler RA (1996) Three classes of inhibitory amino acid terminals in the cochlear nucleus of the guinea pig. *J Comp Neurol* 373(1): 11–26.

Kalinichenko SG, Okhotin VE (2005) Unipolar brush cells – a new type of excitatory interneuron in the cerebellar cortex and cochlear nuclei of the brainstem. *Neurosci Behav Physiol* 35(1): 21–36.

Kamke MR, Brown M, Irvine DR (2005) Origin and immunolesioning of cholinergic basal forebrain innervation of cat primary auditory cortex. *Hear Res* 206(1–2): 89–106.

Kelly JB, Liscum A, van Adel B, Ito M (1998) Projections from the superior olive and lateral lemniscus to tonotopic regions of the rat's inferior colliculus. *Hear Res*.116(1–2): 43–54.

Kilgard MP (2005) Cortical map reorganization without cholinergic modulation. *Neuron* 48: 529–30.

Kilgard MP, Merzenich MM (1998) Cortical map reorganization enabled by nucleus basalis activity. *Science* 279: 1714–18.

Kolston J, Osen KK, Hackney CM, Ottersen OP, Storm-Mathisen J (1992) An atlas of glycine- and GABA-like immunoreactivity and colocalization in the cochlear nuclear complex of the guinea pig. *Anat Embryol (Berl)* 186(5): 443–65.

Kraus KS, Illing RB (2004) Superior olivary contributions to auditory system plasticity: medial but not lateral olivocochlear neurons are the source of cochleotomy-induced GAP-43 expression in the ventral cochlear nucleus. *J Comp Neurol* 475(3): 374–9.

Kromer LF, Moore RY (1980) Norepinephrine innervation of the cochlear nuclei by locus coeruleus neurons in the rat. *Anat Embryol* **8**(2): 227–44.

Kulesza RJ, Spirou GA, Berribe AS (2003) Physiological response properties of neurons in the superior paraolivary nucleus of the rat. *J Neurophysiol* **89**(4): 2299–312.

Lujan R, Shigemoto R, Kulik A, Juiz JM (2004) Localization of the GABAB receptor 1a/b subunit relative to glutamatergic synapses in the dorsal cochlear nucleus of the rat. *J Comp Neurol* **475**(1): 36–46.

Ma CL, Kelly JB, Wu SH (2002) Presynaptic modulation of GABAergic inhibition by GABA(B) receptors in the rat's inferior colliculus. *Neuroscience* **114**(1): 207–15.

Meidinger MA, Hildebrandt-Schoenfeld H, Illing RB (2006) Cochlear damage induces GAP-43 expression in cholinergic synapses of the cochlear nucleus in the adult rat: a light and electron microscopic study. *Eur J Neurosci* **23**(12): 3187–99.

Merchán M, Aguilar LA, Lopez-Poveda EA, Malmierca MS (2005) The inferior colliculus of the rat: quantitative immunocytochemical study of GABA and glycine. *Neuroscience* **136**(3): 907–925.

Metherate R, Hsieh CY (2003) Regulation of glutamate synapses by nicotinic acetylcholine receptors in auditory cortex. *Neurobiol Learn Memory* **80**(3): 285–90.

Molitor SC, Manis PB (1997) Evidence for functional metabotropic glutamate receptors in the dorsal cochlear nucleus. *J Neurophysiol* **77**(4): 1889–905.

Monyer H, Sprengel R, Schoepter R, *et al.* (1992) Heteromeric NMDA-receptor; molecular and functional distinction of subtypes. *Science* **256**: 1217–21.

Mulders WH, Robertson D (2004) Dopaminergic olivocochlear neurons originate in the high frequency region of the lateral superior olive of guinea pigs. *Hear Res* **187**(1–2): 122–30.

Mulders WH, Robertson D (2005) Diverse responses of single auditory afferent fibres to electrical stimulation of the inferior colliculus in guinea-pig. *Exp Brain Res* **160**: 235–44.

Niu X, Canlon B (2002) Activation of tyrosine hydroxylase in the lateral efferent terminals by sound conditioning. *Hear Res* **174**(1–2): 124–32.

Niu X, Bogdanovic N, Canlon B (2004) The distribution and the modulation of tyrosine hydroxylase immunoreactivity in the lateral olivocochlear system of the guinea-pig. *Neuroscience* **125**(3): 725–33.

Oliver DL, Potashner SJ, Jones DR, Morest DK (1983) Selective labeling of spiral ganglion and granule cells with D-aspartate in the auditory system of cat and guinea pig *J Neurosci* **3**: 455–72.

Oliver DL (1985) Quantitative analyses of axonal endings in the central nucleus of the inferior colliculus and distribution of 3H-labeling after injections in the dorsal cochlear nucleus. *J Comp Neurol* **237**(3): 343–59.

Oliver DL, Schneiderman A (1989) An EM study of the dorsal nucleus of the lateral lemniscus: inhibitory, commissural, synaptic connections between ascending auditory pathways. *J Neurosci* **9**(3): 967–82.

Osen KK, Storm-Mathisen J, Ottersen OP, Dihle B (1995) Glutamate is concentrated in and released from parallel fiber terminals in the dorsal cochlear nucleus: a quantitative immunocytochemical analysis in guinea pig. *J Comp Neurol* **357**(3): 482–500.

Ostapoff EM, Benson CG, Saint Marie RL (1997) GABA- and glycine-immunoreactive projections from the superior olivary complex to the cochlear nucleus in guinea pig. *J Comp Neurol* 381(4): 500–512.

Parks TN (2000) The AMPA receptors of auditory neurons. *Hear Res* **147**(1–2): 77–91.

Pecka M, Zahn TP, Saunier-Rebori B, *et al.* (2007) Inhibiting the inhibition: a neuronal network for sound localization in reverberant environments. *J Neurosci* **27**(7): 1782–90.

Peruzzi D, Sivaramakrishnan S, Oliver DL (1997) A monosynaptic GABAergic input from the inferior colliculus to the medial geniculate body in rat. *J Neurosci* **17**: 3766–77.

Petralia RS, Rubio ME, Wang YX, Wenthold RJ (2000) Differential distribution of glutamate receptors in the cochlear nuclei. *Hear Res* **147**(1–2): 59–69.

Pollak GD (1997) Roles of GABAergic inhibition for the binaural processing of multiple sound sources in the inferior colliculus. *Ann Otol Rhinol Laryngol Suppl* **168**: 44–54.

Prieto JJ, Peterson BA, Winer JA (1994a) Morphology and spatial distribution of GABAergic neurons in cat primary auditory cortex (AI). *J Comp Neurol* **344**(3): 349–58.

Prieto JJ, Peterson BA, Winer JA (1994b) Laminar distribution and neuronal targets of GABAergic axon terminals in cat primary auditory cortex (AI). *J Comp Neurol* **344**(3): 383–402.

Raphael Y, Altschuler RA (2003) Structure and innervation of the cochlea. *Brain Res Bull* **60**: 397–422.

Reuss S, Disque-Kaiser U, De Liz S, Ruffer M, Riemann R (1999) Immunfluorescence study of neuropeptides in identified neurons of the rat auditory superior olivary complex. *Cell Tissue Res* **297**(1): 13–21.

Riquelme R, Saldaña E, Osen KK, Ottersen OP, Merchán MA (2001) Colocalization of GABA and glycine in the ventral nucleus of the lateral lemniscus in rat: an in situ hybridization and semiquantitative immunocytochemical study. *J Comp Neurol* **432**(4): 409–424.

Rubio ME, Juiz JM (2004) Differential distribution of synaptic endings containing glutamate, glycine, and GABA in the rat dorsal cochlear nucleus. *J Comp Neurol* **477**(3): 253–72.

Rubio ME, Wenthold RJ (1999) Differential distribution of intracellular glutamate receptors in dendrites. *J Neurosci* **19**(13): 5549–62.

Ryugo DK, Haenggeli CA, Doucet JR (2003) Multimodal inputs to the granule cell domain of the cochlear nucleus. *Exp Brain Res* **153**(4): 477–85.

Saint Marie RL (1996) Glutamatergic connections of the auditory midbrain: selective uptake and axonal transport of D-[3H]aspartate. *J Comp Neurol* **373**(2): 255–70.

Saint Marie RL, Morest DK, Brandon CJ (1989a) The form and distribution of GABAergic synapses on the principal cell types of the ventral cochlear nucleus of the cat. *Hear Res* **42**(1): 97–112.

Saint Marie RL, Ostapoff EM, Morest DK, Wenthold RJ (1989b) Glycine-immunoreactive projection of the cat lateral superior olive: possible role in midbrain ear dominance. *J Comp Neurol* **279**(3): 382–96.

Saldaña E, Berrebi AS (2000) Anisotropic organization of the rat superior paraolivary nucleus. *Anat Embryol (Berl)* **202**(4): 265–79.

Sanes DH, Geary WA, Wooten GF, Rubel EW (1987) Quantitative distribution of the glycine receptor in the auditory brain stem of the gerbil. *J Neurosci* **17**(11): 3793–80.

Sanes DH, McGee J, Walsh EJ (1998) Metabotropic glutamate receptor activation modulates sound level processing in the cochlear nucleus. *J Neurophysiol* **80**(1): 209–217.

Sato K, Shiraishi S, Nakagawa H, Kuriyama H, Altschuler RA (2000) Diversity and plasticity in amino acid receptor subunits in the rat auditory brain stem. *Hear Res* **147**(1–2): 137–44.

Schaeffer DF, Reuss MH, Riemann R, Reuss S (2003) A nitrergic projection from the superior olivary complex to the inferior colliculus of the rat. *Hear Res* **183**(1–2): 67–72.

Schmid S, Guthmann A, Ruppersberg JP, Herbert H (2001) Expression of AMPA receptor subunit flip/flop splice variants in the rat auditory brainstem and inferior colliculus. *J Comp Neurol* **430**(2): 160–67.

Schofield BR (1994) Projections to the cochlear nuclei from principal cells in the medial nucleus of the trapezoid body in guinea pigs. *J Comp Neurol* **344**(1): 83–100.

Sherriff FE, Henderson Z (1994) Cholinergic neurons in the ventral trapezoid nucleus project to the cochlear nuclei in the rat. *Neuroscience* **58**(3): 627–33.

Shinonaga Y, Takada M, Mizuno N (1994) Direct projections from the non-laminated divisions of the medial geniculate nucleus to the temporal polar cortex and amygdala in the cat, *J. Comp Neurol* **340**: 405–426.

Shiraishi S, Shiraishi Y, Oliver DL, Altschuler RA (2001) Expression of GABA(A) receptor subunits in the rat central nucleus of the inferior colliculus. *Mol Brain Res* **96**(1–2): 122–32.

Shore SE (2008) Auditory–somatosensory interactions. In: *Encyclopedia of Neuroscience* (ed. L. Squire). Academic Press, New York.

Shore SE, Zhou J (2006) Somatosensory influence on the cochlear nucleus and beyond. *Hear Res* **216–217**: 90–99.

Shore SE, Helfert RH, Bledsoe SC Jr, Altschuler RA, Godfrey DA (1991) Descending projections to the dorsal and ventral divisions of the cochlear nucleus in guinea pig. *Hear Res* 52(1): 255–68.

Shore SE, Godfrey DA, Helfert RH, Altschuler RA, Bledsoe SC Jr (1992) Connections between the cochlear nuclei in guinea pig. *Hear Res* 62(1): 16–26.

Suneja SK, Benson CG, Gross J, Potashner SJ (1995) Evidence for glutamatergic projections from the cochlear nucleus to the superior olive and the ventral nucleus of the lateral lemniscus. *J Neurochem* 64(1): 161–71.

Tebecis AK (1972) Cholinergic and non-cholinergic transmission in the medial geniculate nucleus of the cat. *J Physiol* 226(1): 153–72.

Thompson AM, Hurley LM (2004) Dense serotonergic innervation of principal nuclei of the superior olivary complex in mouse. *Neurosci Lett* 356: 179–82.

Thompson AM, Lauder JM (2005) Postnatal expression of the serotonin transporter in auditory brainstem neurons. *Dev Neurosci* 27(1): 1–12.

Thompson AM, Thompson GC (2001) Serotonin projection patterns to the cochlear nucleus. *Brain Res* 907(1–2): 195–207.

Tong L, Altschuler RA, Holt AG (2005) Tyrosine hydroxylase in the rat auditory midbrain: distribution and changes following deafness. *Hear Res* 206: 28–41.

Trussell LO (1997) Cellular mechanisms for preservation of timing in central auditory pathways. *Curr Opin Neurobiol* 7(4): 487–92.

Tzounopoulos T, Rubio ME, Keen JE, Trussell LO (2007) Coactivation of pre- and postsynaptic signaling mechanisms determines cell-specific spike-timing-dependent plasticity. *Neuron* 54(2): 291–301.

Vetter DE, Mugnaini E (1992) Distribution and dendritic features of three groups of rat olivocochlear neurons. *Anat Embryol* 185: 1–16.

Vetter DE, Saldaña E, Mugnaini E (1993) Input from the inferior colliculus to medial olivocochlear neurons in the rat: a double label study with PHA-L and cholera toxin. *Hear Res* 70(2): 173–86.

Wang J, Caspary D, Salvi RJ (2000) GABA-A antagonist causes dramatic expansion of tuning in primary auditory cortex. *Neuroreport* 11(5): 1137–40.

Wang J, McFadden SL, Caspary D, Salvi R (2002) Gamma-aminobutyric acid circuits shape response properties of auditory cortex neurons. *Brain Res* 944(1–2): 219–31.

Wang YX, Wenthold RJ, Ottersen OP, Petralia RS (1998) Endbulb synapses in the anteroventral cochlear nucleus express a specific subset of AMPA-type glutamate receptor subunits. *J Neurosci* 18(3): 1148–56.

Warr WB, Boche JB, Neely ST (1997) Efferent innervation of the inner hair cell region: origins and terminations of two lateral olivocochlear systems. *Hear Res* 108(1–2): 89–111.

Weedman DL, Ryugo, DK (1996) Projections from auditory cortex to the cochlear nucleus in rats: synapses on granule cell dendrites. *J Comp Neurol* 371: 311–24.

Weinberger NM (1998) Physiological memory in primary auditory cortex: characteristics and mechanisms. *Neurobiol Learn Mem* 70(1–2): 226–51.

Wenthold RJ (1987) Evidence for a glycinergic pathway connecting the two cochlear nuclei: an immunocytochemical and retrograde transport study. *Brain Res* 415(1): 183–7.

Wenthold RJ, Huie D, Altschuler RA, Reeks KA (1987) Glycine immunoreactivity localized in the cochlear nucleus and superior olivary complex. *Neuroscience* 22(3): 897–912.

Wenthold RJ, Parakkal MH, Oberdorfer MD, Altschuler RA (1988) Glycine receptor immunoreactivity in the ventral cochlear nucleus of the guinea pig. *J Comp Neurol* 276(3): 423–35.

Winer JA, Lee CC (2007) The distributed auditory cortex. *Hear Res* 229(1–2): 3–13.

Winer JA, Miller LM, Lee CC, Schreiner CE (2005) Auditory thalamocortical transformation: structure and function. *Trends Neurosci* 28(5): 255–63.

Wright DD, Blackstone CD, Huganir RL, Ryugo DK (1996) Immunocytochemical localization of the mGluR1 alpha metabotropic glutamate receptor in the dorsal cochlear nucleus. *J Comp Neurol* 364(4): 729–45.

Wynne B, Robertson D (1996) Localization of dopamine-beta-hydroxylase-like immunoreactivity in the superior olivary complex of the rat. *Audiol Neurotol* **1**(1): 54–64.

Wu SH, Kelly JB (1992) Synaptic pharmacology of the superior olivary complex studied in mouse brain slice. *J Neurosci* **12**(8): 3084–97.

Yao W, Godfrey DA (1998) Immunohistochemical evaluation of cholinergic neurons in the rat superior olivary complex. *Microscopy Res Technique* **41**(3): 270–83.

Zhang H, Xu J, Feng AS (1999) Effects of GABA-mediated inhibition on direction-dependent frequency tuning in the frog inferior colliculus. *J Comp Physiol* **184**(1): 85–98.

Zhou J, Shore S (2006) Convergence of spinal trigeminal and cochlear nucleus projections in the inferior colliculus of the guinea pig. *J Comp Neurol* **495**(1): 100–112.

Zhou J, Nannapaneni N, Shore S (2007) Vesicular glutamate transporters 1 and 2 are differentially associated with auditory nerve and spinal trigeminal inputs to the cochlear nucleus. *J Comp Neurol* **500**(4): 777–87.

Section 2

Information coding in the auditory brain: sound identification

Chapter 5

Level and spectrum

Eric D. Young

5.1 Introduction

The representation of sounds by the auditory system varies in its nature at different levels of the system. In the auditory nerve (AN) and cochlear nucleus (CN), the representation is a direct spectrotemporal one, meaning an isomorphic representation of the physical characteristics of the stimulus itself. In this representation, each neuron's activity provides information about the time-varying energy in a narrow frequency band of the stimulus. A complete representation of the stimulus is provided by a population code, made up of neurons sensitive to the whole range of frequencies (Pfeiffer and Kim, 1975; Sachs and Young, 1979). In the AN and CN, there are two representations, one for each ear.

At more central parts of the auditory system, the activity from the two ears is merged so that the representation contains information about binaural disparities (interaural time and intensity differences) along with the spectrotemporal description of the stimuli. This synthesis occurs in the inferior colliculus (IC) (Winer and Schreiner, 2005). Finally, in cortex, one observes the initial steps in the analysis of the auditory scene and the auditory objects that make it up (Nelken, 2004).

This chapter provides a review of the evidence for the summary statements in the preceding paragraphs, concentrating on two aspects of the neural representation: first, the representation of stimulus spectrum, i.e. of the frequency content of sounds; and second, the encoding of sound intensity or sound level. Of course a complete discussion of auditory neural representations necessarily includes the temporal aspects of the signal and the information encoded in signal onsets, offsets, and temporal modulations (e.g. Rosen, 1992; Joris *et al.*, 2004). However, temporal aspects of auditory signal processing are considered elsewhere in this volume and even the subject of spectral processing is larger than can be discussed in one chapter. A recent book (Malmierca and Irvine, 2005) contains more detailed and comprehensive reviews of many aspects of spectral processing.

5.2 Auditory filters and the representation of frequency

The basic organization of the auditory representation of sound is established in the cochlea. For this chapter, what is most important about cochlear physiology is the frequency decomposition of sound performed by the basilar membrane (BM) through its tuning properties. Each point on the BM is maximally responsive to a particular frequency, its best frequency (BF), with less sensitivity to adjacent frequencies. Thus each point on the BM is a *bandpass filter* tuned to a different frequency, where the word filter means a device that is selective by responding only to a limited range of frequencies (for a readable introduction to frequency analysis see Hartmann, 1997).

5.2.1 Tuning curves

The frequency tuning of the BM (Robles and Ruggero, 2001) can be observed indirectly by studying the tuning of AN fibers. Figure 5.1A shows typical threshold tuning curves of a number of AN fibers from the cat ear. The tuning curves were constructed by presenting short tone bursts of various frequencies (abscissa) and, for each frequency, increasing the sound level until the fiber began to respond (the threshold, ordinate). The BF of the fiber is the frequency at which it has the lowest threshold; presumably this corresponds to the BF of the point on the BM innervated by the fiber. Figure 5.1A shows data from cat AN fibers with BFs ranging from 0.6 to 7 kHz (only a portion of the cat's full range of 0.1–60 kHz). The tuning curves are all approximately V-shaped near their BFs, consistent with a bandpass filter. The filter analogy is a good one, in that an AN fiber can often be accurately modeled as a bandpass filter followed by a model that produces action potentials with the usual properties of refractoriness and adaptation (e.g. de Boer and de Jongh, 1978; Deng and Geisler, 1987; Zhang and Carney, 2005).

There is a direct method of computing the best bandpass filter to model each AN fiber from responses to broadband noise (e.g. Lewis *et al.*, 2002). In this method, the spike-train produced by the fiber in response to the noise is obtained in an experiment; the acoustic signal immediately preceding each action potential is averaged across the spike train. The result is the so-called reverse-correlation or revcor function. The Fourier transform of the revcor is very similar to the fiber's tuning curve and is the frequency-dependent gain of the desired bandpass filter. The fact that filtering is roughly the same for tones and noise is an important result, because it strengthens the bandpass filter interpretation of the tuning curves of AN fibers. The two are not necessarily the same for nonlinear neurons in more central parts of the auditory system, discussed later.

5.2.2 Perceptual auditory filters

The perception of sound by human observers can also be analyzed based on the idea of a parallel bank of bandpass filters. Many perceptual phenomena can be explained as reflecting the operation of an auditory filterbank as the first step in sound processing (reviewed by Moore, 2004). Perceptual auditory filters are usually derived for human observers from masking experiments. The filters in Fig. 5.1B were computed by asking observers to detect a tone that is masked by a preceding noise signal consisting of two bands of noise, one at frequencies below the tone and the other at higher frequencies (Oxenham and Shera, 2003). In such an experiment, the noise is a more effective masker, making it harder to hear the tone, as the frequencies included in the noise come closer to the tone frequency. The filter is derived as the function of frequency that best explains the masking data based on the assumption that the listener has available only the signal at the output of one filter centered on the tone frequency. The noise masks the tone to the extent that the noise contains energy within the passband of that filter. The results in Fig. 5.1B show filters centered at 1, 2, 4, 6, and 8 kHz; they are plotted as filter gains (i.e. output signal amplitude divided by input signal amplitude as a function of frequency) and can be compared to the tuning curves in Fig. 5.1A by inverting them. Clearly the perceptual filters are similar in shape to the tuning curves; it is generally believed that perceptual filters reflect the tuning of the cochlea.

5.2.3 The frequency map on the BM

The frequencies to which successive points on the BM are tuned are laid out roughly logarithmically along its length. The mapping of frequency into place or position along the membrane is shown for the cat cochlea in Fig. 5.1C (Liberman, 1982). This figure shows results obtained by recording from single AN fibers, determining their BFs, and then filling them with a dye. The dye allowed the filled fibers to be followed to their origin on the BM (i.e. to the inner hair cell innervated) so the position

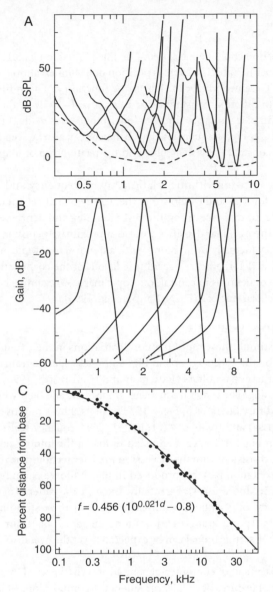

Fig. 5.1 Frequency selectivity of the auditory system. **A** Tuning curves of 11 AN fibers from a cat ear (Miller *et al.*, 1997). Each curve is a plot of threshold versus tone frequency for one fiber, constructed by increasing the sound level of a tone until the fiber gave a criterion increase in discharge rate at each frequency (1 spike in 50 ms). *Dashed line* shows the minimum thresholds in the most sensitive cats. The frequency at which the lowest threshold is observed in a particular fiber is its BF. **B** Auditory filters derived from masking experiments in human observers for probe tone frequencies of 1, 2, 4, 6, and 8 kHz (Oxenham and Shera, 2003). Each *curve* shows the gain function of a bandpass filter centered on the probe frequency that would produce the masking data observed in an experiment in which the probe tone is masked by bands of noise. **C** The tonotopic organization of the cat cochlea plotted as the BF of a fiber (*abscissa*) versus the position on the BM at which the fiber contacts a hair cell (*ordinate*) (Liberman, 1982). The line is a fit to the data points, from 52 AN fibers whose BFs and innervation points were measured. The formula of the line is given in the form developed by Greenwood (1961). *f* is the BF of a fiber in kiloHertz and *d* is the place innervated, as a fraction of distance from base to apex. Notice that the ordinate scale is reversed from the original. (Redrawn from the sources quoted.)

of each fiber's termination could be measured. The line plotted in Fig. 5.1B is a mathematical fit to the data showing fiber BF (abscissa) versus position of BM innervation (ordinate); the formula of the line is shown (Greenwood, 1961). This same function has been fit to the BM tuning of several mammals, with different constants. For BFs above 1–3 kHz in the cat, the relationship between frequency and place is approximately logarithmic, as is evident from the straight-line appearance of Fig. 5.1C at high frequencies. This behavior can also be seen from the formula; for high frequencies, the constant 0.8 is negligible and the relationship of frequency and distance is $d \approx 47 \log_{10}(f/0.456)$.

Two aspects of the near-logarithmic relationship of frequency and BM place are worth mentioning. First, anatomical studies show that the density of hair cells and AN fibers is roughly constant as a function of distance along the BM (Keithley and Schreiber, 1987); as a result, Fig. 5.1C implies that these cellular densities are also approximately constant in equal logarithmic increments of frequency (actually BF). Second, with a uniform tonotopic projection of AN fibers into higher auditory nuclei, the near-logarithmic layout of the cochlea translates into a near-logarithmic allocation of neurons in central tonotopic maps. An example is provided by the map of BF in the dorsal cochlear nucleus (DCN; Spirou et al., 1993).

5.2.4 Cochlear spectrograms

Real-world auditory stimuli show rapid temporal variations in their frequency content. Three examples are shown by the spectrograms in Fig. 5.2. These spectrograms were produced by a parallel bank of linear bandpass filters (Patterson and Holdsworth, 1996) that was designed to model cochlear processing. The center frequencies of the filters and their widths are modeled after human perceptual auditory filters, as in Fig. 5.1B. The plots show stimulus energy as a color scale on axes of time (abscissa) and frequency (ordinate). The frequency scales on the ordinates are near-logarithmic as in Fig. 5.1C, except adjusted to match the human ear. The energy (color) scales are logarithmic, consistent with the discussion in a later section. The resulting spectrograms are a model for the 'excitation pattern' produced in the auditory system by a complex stimulus (Pfeiffer and Kim, 1975; Moore, 2004). Essentially, these are the patterns of excitation that would be produced in the array of peripheral auditory neurons by these stimuli. In fact, they are not quite correct because the spectrogram is a linear model and does not capture nonlinear properties of the cochlea. Nonetheless, this model can be expected to get the overall excitation pattern about right.

The first signal is a segment of computer-generated speech, the word 'basketball', which serves to illustrate a number of features of cochlear frequency decomposition. At low frequencies, there are prominent horizontal bars of high energy (red) that represent low-order harmonics of the voice signal, which is approximately periodic. The first bar is the fundamental frequency of the voice (at 0.1–0.13 kHz). The second, third, and fourth harmonics are also visible. The harmonics are not seen at higher frequencies (above about 1 kHz) because the filters become wide enough that each filter contains more than one harmonic within its bandwidth, so the harmonics are not resolved. Instead, the pattern of energy peaks produced by the formant resonances of the vocal tract dominates at higher frequencies; the trajectory of the first four formants are shown by the white lines (these are the formants used in the computer synthesis). The first (lowest frequency) formant is mixed with the voice harmonics (0.3–0.7 kHz), but the higher formants correspond clearly to energy peaks in the spectrogram except during silences (the deep blue regions).

The temporal fluctuations of the voicing of the stimulus are clearly seen as vertical striations in the spectrogram. These are most clear during the vowels, where they correspond to the puffs of air released by the glottis and thus represent the periodicity of the voiced portions of the stimulus. They are clearest at high frequencies where multiple harmonics interact within each filter.

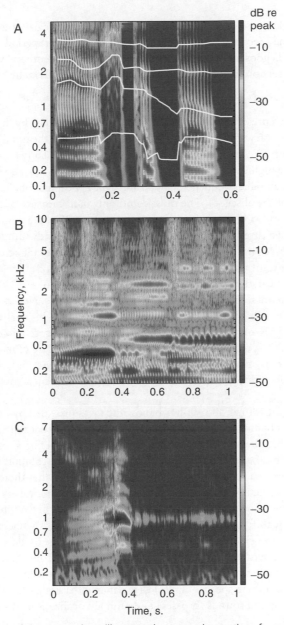

Fig. 5.2 Spectrograms of three sounds to illustrate the approximate time-frequency distribution of energy in the cochlea. The spectrogram shows the energy in the stimulus on a decibel color scale, according to the calibration bar at *right*. The spectrograms were produced by passing the signal through a parallel gammatone filterbank of 100 or 200 filters with their center frequencies and bandwidths set to model human auditory filters (using the program provided by Slaney, 1993). Each horizontal line in the spectrograms is the envelope of one filter output, computed from its analytic signal, and measured in decibels relative to the peak envelope value. **A** Spectrogram of the word 'basketball' computer synthesized to match the same word spoken by a male voice (provided courtesy of R. McGowan of Sensimetrics Corp.). *White lines* show the trajectories of the first four formant frequencies in the synthesis. **B** Spectrogram of a short segment of music consisting of a string and percussion instrument. **C** The 'honk' of a Canada goose, courtesy of Tony Phillips (http://www.math.sunysb.edu/~tony/birds/ geese.html).

The second example is a segment of music in which the harmonic patterns associated with the notes are plain and the spectra are reasonably stable in time for short periods. The third example is a 'honk' of a Canada goose. This sound is mainly defined by its temporal variation, beginning with a short periodic section (before ~0.35 s) and terminating in a dramatic broadband transient.

5.2.5 Bandwidths of cochlear filters

The properties of the representations in Fig. 5.2 are largely determined by the bandwidths of the filters and the way they vary with frequency. Note that the widths of the tuning curves in Fig. 5.1A vary substantially with BF. The lowest BF tuning curve (with BF 0.5 kHz) has a bandwidth of 0.35 kHz, whereas the highest BF tuning curve (with BF 7 kHz) has a bandwidth of 1.2 kHz (the bandwidth gets wider at higher frequencies, opposite to the appearance of Fig. 5.1A because of the logarithmic scaling of the abscissa). The most commonly used measure of tuning-curve bandwidth is the relative bandwidth or Q_{10}, equal to the ratio of the BF of the tuning curve to its width (in Hertz) 10 dB above threshold. If tuning curves had a fixed bandwidth on logarithmic axes (a constant tuning curve shape in Fig. 5.1A), the Q_{10} would be constant across frequency; if the bandwidths were constant on linear axes (a fixed number of Hertz), then Q_{10} would increase linearly with BF. In the cat, the Q_{10} values increase from ~1.5 at low BFs (0.3 kHz) to ~8–10 above 10 kHz (Fig. 5.3A), neither constant on linear nor logarithmic axes. Nevertheless, the tuning is sharper, relative to BF, at high BFs. The same behavior is observed in other mammalian species (e.g. humans in Fig. 5.1B and the gerbil; Schmiedt, 1989). An interpretation of the variation in tuning curve bandwidth is that it compensates for the low-pass nature of many natural acoustic stimuli, such as speech. By making bandwidths wider at higher frequencies, the average stimulus energy passing through auditory filters could be made roughly constant across different frequency bands.

An important insight into auditory filter bandwidths was provided by Lewicki (2002), who derived optimum filter banks for representing different ensembles of natural sounds. The assumption used in deriving the filters was that the signals carried by the AN fibers connected to different points on the BM should be statistically independent. Such a representation is desirable because it requires fewer neurons to represent the stimulus, in the sense that there is no redundancy among the neurons' responses, and because it leads to certain theoretical efficiencies in learning and pattern recognition. The resulting filters were bandpass filters like AN tuning curves. Their bandwidths changed with frequency in a way similar to that of real AN fibers (Fig. 5.3B), except that the exact bandwidth behavior depended on the sound ensemble used to derive the filters. In Fig. 5.3B, the different symbols show filter bandwidths derived from three sound ensembles, identified next to the curves. The lines show regression fits to the cat AN data in Fig. 5.3A. The ensemble consisting of human speech (circles) gave bandwidths similar to the cat tuning curves, whereas the environmental sounds (crosses) and animal vocalizations (pluses) gave wider or narrower filters.

The slopes of the Q_{10} values in Fig. 5.3B do not correspond to the constant-energy hypothesis described above. Instead they are best understood in terms of the temporal characteristics of the modulation envelopes of the stimuli. The animal vocalizations consisted of relatively long sine-wave-like stimuli that were best matched by filters of roughly constant (narrow) bandwidth, giving large Q_{10} values that increased rapidly, and close to linearly, with BF. The environmental sounds contained brief transient components that were best represented by filters with short time envelopes, and therefore broad frequency responses, and low Q_{10}. The impulse responses of the filters derived from speech matched ones derived for AN fibers using reverse correlation (Carney and Yin, 1988; Smith and Lewicki, 2006); in particular, both sets of filters showed temporal asymmetries characteristic of the tuning of AN fibers.

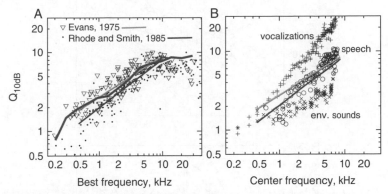

Fig. 5.3 A Relative bandwidths of tuning curves (Q_{10}s) of AN fibers from three data sets, two identified in the legend and the third from unpublished data of T. Ji and E.D. Young (*blue*). The lines are fits to those data (i.e. to logQ_{10} versus log *BF*). **B** Q_{10}s of the filters derived theoretically as described in the text by Lewicki (2002) for three different sound datasets: *crosses* are from environmental sounds, *circles* are from speech, and *pluses* are from animal and bird vocalizations. The lines are the same as in A. (Modified from Lewicki, 2002.)

It is not clear what sets the actual bandwidths of cochlear tuning in human or animal ears. The computational results in Fig. 5.3B suggest that an evolutionary optimization of bandwidths might lead to different results depending on the acoustic environment and the nature of the important signals within it. In this regard, there is recent evidence that humans and old-world monkeys have cochlear filtering with bandwidths as much as half as wide as common laboratory animals (Shera *et al.*, 2002; Joris *et al.*, 2006; but see Ruggero and Temchin, 2005).

5.3 The representation of sound level: compression

5.3.1 Basilar membrane velocity

In both physiological and psychophysical studies, the sound pressure of the stimulus is typically specified on a logarithmic scale, in terms of decibels relative to some appropriate reference level, such as 20 µPa (dB SPL). This is done for convenience, to deal with the wide dynamic range of hearing (100 dB or more), but it also may be close to the way the auditory system represents sound. As with frequency, the basic scaling of sound pressure is set by the properties of BM transduction. The velocity of BM motion in response to a stimulus increases as a power function of sound pressure, as $(const)P^n$, where the exponent n varies with frequency and sometimes also with sound level; examples are shown for one position on the BM in Fig. 5.4A (Ruggero *et al.*, 1997). In this log-log plot, the slope of the line is the exponent in the power-law relationship between sound intensity and BM velocity. For frequencies near the BF of the BM point (9–12 kHz in this case), the growth has an exponent near 1 at low (near-threshold) sound levels and an exponent of 0.2–0.3 at higher levels (Robles and Ruggero, 2001). For frequencies away from BF (3, 6, and 16 kHz), the slope is close to 1, meaning linear BM response growth.

The portion of the near-BF data with a slope less than 1 is *compressive*, meaning the stimulus intensity is being compressed by BM transduction (Rhode, 1984). Compression is a result of the amplification of BM motion by outer hair cells, which is large at low sound levels and progressively smaller as the sound level increases, yielding the low slope at higher sound levels. Compression is important for a variety of perceptual aspects of hearing (Oxenham and Bacon, 2003). The most obvious one is that the dynamic range of the physical signal (more than five

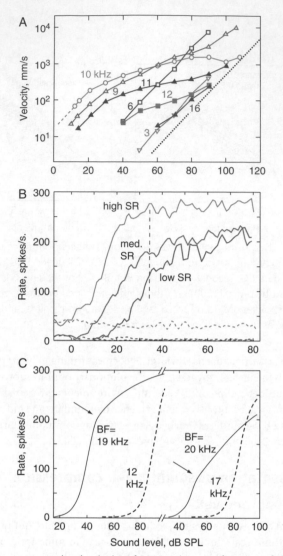

Fig. 5.4 A The root mean square (rms) velocity of BM motion as a function of the sound pressure level for a tone presented to the ear. Data are reproduced from the 10-kHz place on the chinchilla BM (Ruggero *et al.*, 1997). The frequency of the tone is given by the parameter next to each plot, colored to correspond to the data for that frequency. Note that velocity and sound pressure are both measured on logarithmic axes, so that the power law relationship discussed in the text becomes a straight line: log(*velocity*) = (*const*) + *n* log *P* = (*const*) + *n*.d*B*/20, where *dB* is the sound level in decibels. The *heavy dotted line at right* shows linear growth of BM velocity (i.e. *n*=1). 10 kHz is the BF because the largest BM velocity occurs in response to 10 kHz at low sound levels (0–40 dB), despite the fact that larger velocities occur at high levels at other frequencies. The curve for 10 kHz is extrapolated at low sound levels (*dashed line at left*), assuming a linear response. This extrapolation is based on the behavior of data from other ears. **B** Discharge rate versus sound level for cat AN fibers; data are responses to 200 ms BF tone bursts for three fibers from the same cat with BFs between 5.36 and 6.18 kHz. *Solid lines* show rates in response to the tone bursts at sound levels in 1-dB steps across a 100-dB range; *dashed lines* show rates of spontaneous activity preceding each tone burst. The fibers are examples of so-called low (*blue*), medium (*orange*), and high (*green*) spontaneous-rate fibers. **C** Smoothed rate versus level functions for two AN fibers from the guinea pig ear; rates are shown for BF tones (*solid lines*) and for tones at a frequency below BF (*dashed*). *Arrows* show the levels at which compression is assumed to set in. (A redrawn from Ruggero *et al.*, 1997; C redrawn from Yates *et al.*, 1990.)

orders of magnitude, 100 dB) is compressed down to only one or two orders in the BM vibration, i.e. at the input of the hair cells and neurons. This compression is essential because the neural elements have much smaller dynamic ranges; the hair cells and AN fibers can only change their responses over a limited range of BM vibrations. For AN fibers, this range is about, 20–30 dB (Sachs and Abbas, 1976; Palmer and Evans, 1982; Yates *et al.*, 1990).

5.3.2 **AN fiber discharge rates**

AN fibers signal the sound level of the stimulus by changing their discharge rates; as sound level (and BM motion) increases, fibers increase their discharge rates (see Fig. 5.4B). The rate functions in Fig. 5.4B are representative of three classes of AN fibers identified in cats (Liberman, 1978). The fibers with the lowest thresholds usually have substantial spontaneous activity, meaning ongoing spiking in the absence of a stimulus (~40 spikes/s in this case for the 'high SR' example). Rate functions of these fibers have a steep dynamic portion (between 0 and ~30 dB SPL here) with a relatively constant rate at higher sound levels, called *rate saturation* (ignoring the irregularities in these rate functions, which reflect the randomness of AN discharge). High SR fibers respond to sound levels low enough to be on the linear portion of the BM input/output function (the dashed portion at the left side of the 10-kHz plot in Fig. 5.4A). Thus the high SR rate functions represent the input/output relationship of a neuron in the absence of compression. The fiber goes from spontaneous rate to saturation over an ~30-dB range of sound pressures. Because the slope of the BM input/output function is 1 at low sound levels (Fig. 5.4A), this 30-dB range of sound levels corresponds to a 30-dB (1.5 decade) range of basilar membrane velocities. Thus an ANF can encode a 1–2 decade range of BM velocities.

Medium and low spontaneous-rate fibers have higher thresholds and apparently wider dynamic ranges on the sound level axis. Often, as in the examples shown in Fig. 5.4B, there is a break (i.e. a sharp decrease) in the slope of these rate functions at about the sound level (the vertical dashed line) where the BM slope should change from linear to compressive (Sachs and Abbas, 1976; Yates *et al.*, 1990). Thus the medium and low SR fibers sample both the linear (at low sound levels) and the compressive (at higher sound levels) portion of the BM response. To the extent that the compressive range is included, their discharge rates change over a wider range of sound levels.

Two kinds of experiments demonstrate the effects of the frequency-dependent compression shown in Fig. 5.4A. In both, it is assumed that BM response grows linearly with sound level for frequencies well below BF, but in a compressive fashion at BF. In a neurophysiological experiment, plots of discharge rate versus sound level are steeper for tone frequencies below BF than for tones at BF (Fig. 5.4C; Yates *et al.*, 1990). Of course, this is only so at sound levels high enough to produce compressive responses at BF (at levels above the arrows in Fig. 5.4C). The dashed lines have slopes corresponding to linear growth of BM response, because they are responses to tones at frequencies below BF. The ratio of the slopes of the low-frequency and the compressive portion of the BF rate functions gives a measure of compression. This measure turns out to be very close to that expected from BM measurements.

The second evidence comes from a psychophysical two-tone masking experiment which measured the intensity of a low-frequency masker required to just mask a probe tone. It is assumed that the listener uses fibers with BFs at the probe frequency to detect the probe. The fibers' response to the low-frequency masker should grow linearly with sound pressure, while the response to the probe should be compressed. Thus the masker level at masked threshold should grow more slowly than the level of the probe. The ratio of the two growth rates should be the compression ratio (Oxenham and Plack, 1997). In this experiment also, the inferred compression is roughly the same as that measured with direct observation of the BM.

5.3.3 Loudness and intensity discrimination

In principle, it should be possible to derive the properties of perceptual loudness of auditory stimuli from the response growth functions shown in Fig. 5.4. In fact, the growth of loudness is predictable from the growth of BM velocity at BF, i.e. loudness grows in a way that resembles the 9–12 kHz data in Fig. 5.4A (Schlauch et al., 1998). Despite this correspondence, it has been difficult to account for loudness growth based on the responses of AN fibers. Assuming that perceptual loudness is proportional to the integrated discharge rate across some population of AN fibers yields a loudness model that differs in several details from perceptual loudness, both in normal ears (Relkin and Doucet, 1997) and in ears damaged by acoustic trauma (Heinz et al., 2005). In both cases the results suggest that some properties of loudness are attributable to aspects of response growth in central neurons (Syka, 2002).

There has been more success in accounting for perceptual intensity discrimination on the basis of AN responses (reviewed by Colburn et al., 2003), i.e. accounting for a person's ability to detect changes in the intensity of a stimulus. From Figs 5.1A and 5.4B, it is clear that a change in sound level will produce an increase in discharge rate in fibers responding to the sound (at least in those that are not saturated) and also a spread of activity along the BM, corresponding to the widening of tuning curves at higher sound levels. The limit on performance in the intensity-discrimination task is the randomness of the neural response, which has the effect of adding neural 'noise' to the representation of sound level. Analyses using statistical decision theory have shown that the changes in the discharge rate of AN fibers are more than sufficient to support the performance of human observers in basic intensity discrimination tests, although to account for all the features of intensity discrimination it may be necessary for the brain to take advantage of features of the neural discharge other than rate, specifically the temporal patterns of spike trains (Colburn et al., 2003).

5.4 Rate is locally proportional to log stimulus intensity

The choice of the logarithmic (decibel) measure of acoustic stimulus intensity is not arbitrary. On theoretical grounds, the best choice for an auditory intensity measure would be one that approximates the basilar membrane response (Fig. 5.4A). However, this signal is complex: it varies with frequency and position along the basilar membrane (Cooper and Rhode, 1995; Ruggero et al., 1997) and is probably different for tones versus complex stimuli due to nonlinear interactions within stimuli (Ruggero et al., 1992; Cooper and Rhode, 1997; Rhode, 2007). Thus a direct BM amplitude measure is not feasible; a logarithmic measure of intensity is a reasonable approximation, however, for the reasons given below.

The neural representation of intensity should be somehow matched to the intensities that are encountered in a natural environment, so the distribution of intensities in natural sounds is a potentially useful source of information. This intensity analysis has been done by collecting ensembles of several classes of sounds, including human speech, music, animal vocalization, and environmental (but not biological) sounds (Attias and Schreiner, 1997; Escabi et al., 2003). The sound ensembles were decomposed into frequency bands using bandpass filters whose frequency spacing and width resemble cochlear filters (similar to Fig. 5.2) and the magnitude of the temporal envelope at the output of partially overlapping filters was sampled. Figure 5.5 shows distributions of these magnitudes, for all frequency bands, plotted on a linear amplitude scale (left) and on a logarithmic scale (right). Results are shown for two ensembles, but the results are similar for all the ensembles analyzed.

The bandpassed stimulus amplitudes vary over a wide range of intensities, approximately ±50 dB in the logarithmic plots. When plotted on a linear scale, the low intensity side of the distribution (below the mode) is hardly visible because, on a linear scale, these values fit in a small

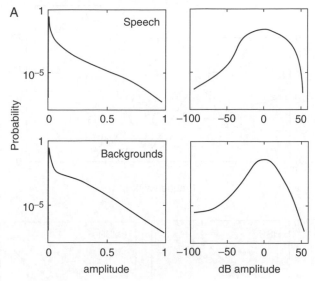

Fig. 5.5 Distributions of sound intensity sampled from an ensemble of speech and a second ensemble of background sounds. The sounds were analyzed as described in the text, producing samples of the amplitude of the sound after decomposing it with a cochlear-like parallel filterbank. In the *left two plots*, sound amplitude is plotted in linear units on the *abscissa* (normalized by the maximum amplitude) and in the *right* as decibels, i.e. 20 $\log_{10}$ of the linear amplitudes. In the *right plots*, the mean amplitude is subtracted so that the *abscissa* shows amplitudes in decibels relative to the mean value. (Redrawn from Escabi *et al.*, 2003.)

number of bins that are obscured by the ordinate. In the logarithmic plot, however, it is clear that there is a wide range of both quiet and loud portions of the stimuli. In particular, there are large tails on the low-intensity side. There is no reason to think that the quiet parts of the stimuli are less important than the loud parts. In fact information is likely to be conveyed by both peaks and valleys of sound intensity (e.g. by the stop, quiet, periods in speech as well as by the formant peaks). In this sense, the logarithmic stimulus intensity measure seems to provide a more complete description of natural stimuli than a linear measure.

The argument of the previous paragraph is supported by the properties of neurons in the AN and ventral cochlear nucleus (VCN). In a variety of situations, these peripheral neurons give rate changes to complex stimuli that are approximately linear functions of decibel stimulus level (e.g. May and Huang, 1997). An example is shown by the analysis of responses to a speech-like stimulus shown in Fig. 5.6 (May *et al.*, 1997). The stimulus is a steady vowel with the spectrum shown by the green line in Fig. 5.6A. Seven stimulus features are marked: the first three formants *F1–F3* and the four troughs at surrounding frequencies (*T0–T3*). By changing the sampling rate of the D/A converter used to generate the sound, the frequency content of the stimulus can be shifted along the log frequency axis, as shown in the inset of Fig. 5.6A. For each neuron, the sampling rate was set to align particular features of the stimulus with the BF of each neuron studied; in the inset, F1, *T1*, and F2 are aligned.

In Fig. 5.6B, the average discharge rates across four populations of AN fibers and CN neurons are plotted as a function of the feature level, i.e. the absolute level in dB SPL of the stimulus feature aligned with BF. Data are shown for AN fibers, where the straight line approximation is fit to all seven features, in the top two plots and for CN neurons from two populations, which were studied only with *F1*, *T1*, and *F2* aligned with BF, in the bottom two. Each line color and symbol

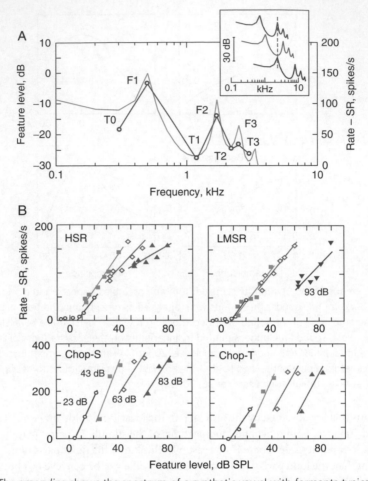

Fig. 5.6 A The *green line* shows the spectrum of a synthetic vowel with formants typical of /eh/ as in 'met' (on the *left ordinate*). The signal is periodic, so the spectrum has energy only at harmonics of 100 Hz. The formants *F1–F3* and the troughs between the formants *T0–T3* are marked. The *inset* shows the spectra of the same signal at three different A/D sampling rates, chosen to align the first formant *F1* (*brown*), the trough *T1* (*orange*), and the second formant *F2* (*green*) with a BF of 2.2 kHz (*dashed line*). *Blue lines in the main plot* show the driven discharge rates (rate minus spontaneous rate, *right-hand ordinate*) of an AN fiber with this BF in response to the vowel presented at seven different sampling rates, chosen to place each feature at BF. The *ordinates* of the two plots are scaled and aligned arbitrarily to emphasize that rate follows spectrum level at BF. **B** Mean discharge rates of four populations of neurons plotted against the sound level of the vowel feature at the neuron's BF. The stimuli were presented at five different overall stimulus levels (23–93 dB SPL) identified by different *colors* and *symbols*. The overall stimulus level corresponds to 0 dB on the ordinate in A, so the F1 feature is always 2 dB below the overall level, the F2 level is 10 dB below, etc. Rates were computed from responses to 0.4-s presentations of the stimulus and averaged across neurons regardless of BF. The *top two plots* are from AN fibers with high spontaneous rates (*HSR* at *left*) and low and medium spontaneous rates (*LMSR* at *right*). The *bottom two plots* are from two populations of so-called chopper neurons in the VCN (for a description see Blackburn and Sachs, 1989). The AN fibers were studied with all seven features aligned on BF, whereas the choppers were studied with only F1, T1, and F2 aligned on BF. (Redrawn from May *et al.*, 1997.)

type shows results for one overall stimulus sound level (ranging from 23 to 93 dB SPL). Consider first the AN data for the high (*HSR*) and low+medium (*LMSR*) populations. There is an approximately linear relationship of rate and dB sound level and the relationship holds for both high and low sound levels, over about a 40-dB range for each overall stimulus level. It is important that the linear relationship applies for stimulus alignments that place at BF a component that is louder than the average level of the stimulus (the formant peaks) as well as for alignments that place a component at BF that is softer than the average level (the troughs). This linearity supports the view expressed above that both loud and quiet parts of the stimulus should be encoded. The remaining data in the bottom row of Fig. 5.6 show similar results for two populations of so-called chopper neurons in the VCN. Chopper neurons seem to be specialized for encoding spectral shapes (Blackburn and Sachs, 1990; Yu and Young, 2000).

Of course, rate is proportional to log stimulus intensity over a limited range. At low and high sound levels, the neuron's rate saturates (see Fig. 5.6B) by the decrease in slope at the highest level (83 dB) or by the saturation at spontaneous rate.

A final argument for a logarithmic measure of stimulus level is provided by papers in which models of the input/output processing in neurons were constructed using either a linear or logarithmic measure of stimulus level (Escabi *et al.*, 2003; Gill *et al.*, 2006). The model is discussed in a later section; it postulates a linear relationship between the stimulus, described in a way similar to the spectrograms in Fig. 5.2, and the neuron's rate. However, the stimulus amplitude was specified in several ways, including linearly as sound pressure or nonlinearly as log sound pressure or as the amplitude of the signal passing through a nonlinear cochlear model. In both studies, the model does better if the logarithm of stimulus amplitude is used than if just the amplitude is used. In one case, the neurons' response rates and information rates were higher with log stimulus amplitudes (Escabi *et al.*, 2003); in the other the ability of the model to predict responses in a validation test is better (Gill *et al.*, 2006). The best performance in the second study occurred when a nonlinear cochlear model was used, perhaps because of the amplitude compression built into the model.

5.5 What is the representation of stimulus spectrum?

Figure 5.2 suggests that the representation of stimulus spectrum should be spectrotemporal in that the frequency content of a stimulus changes with time; thus the neural representation must characterize both the distribution of energy along the frequency axis and the time variations. A simple approach to analyzing the neural representation of sounds is to assume that it is a time-varying sequence of spectral representations, where the spectral representations are encoded as the strength of neural activity as a function of BF. Spectrotemporal representations of time-varying auditory stimuli have been reconstructed, mainly in peripheral neurons (e.g. Delgutte, 1980; Miller and Sachs, 1983; Sinex and Geisler, 1984), but also in central nuclei (e.g. Delgutte *et al.*, 1998; Wong and Schreiner, 2003; Mesgarani *et al.*, 2008).

5.5.1 Spectrotemporal representation of speech

Figure 5.7A shows an example of a spectrotemporal representation in the form of the instantaneous discharge rates of a population of AN fibers responding to the first 40 ms of the syllable /da/ (Miller and Sachs, 1983; Shamma, 1985b). The plot is on axes of time and BF and each point in this two-dimensional array is the probability of spiking in AN fibers, computed by averaging the discharge rates of fibers of similar BFs (grouped into 1/64 decade logarithmic BF bins and 1/16 ms time bins). Note that the BF axis runs from low frequencies at the top to high frequencies at the bottom. The formant frequencies, i.e. the frequencies at which there are peaks of energy, vary over

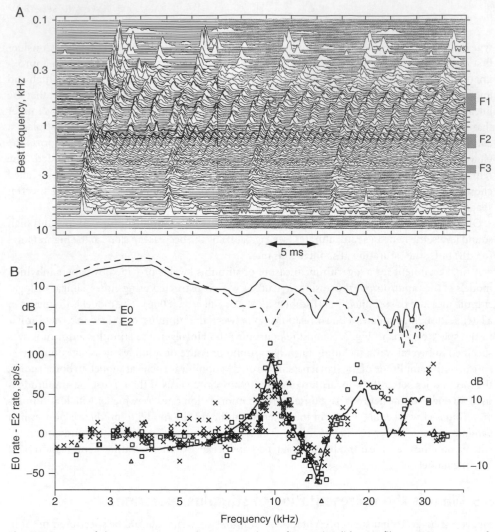

Fig. 5.7 Aspects of the spectrotemporal representations of two stimuli by AN fibers. **A** Responses of a population of 275 fibers from an anesthetized cat to the first 50 ms of the syllable /da/ (data from Miller and Sachs, 1983, analyzed by Shamma, 1985a, b). The plot shows instantaneous rate versus time (*abscissa*) and BF (*ordinate*) for AN fibers averaged in logarithmic groups according to BF. The *gray bars at right* show the range of the first three formant frequencies during the stimulus; the formants changed linearly over the time period to model the formant transition of the /d/; F1 increased (0.5–0.7 kHz), and F2 and F3 decreased (1.6–1.2 and 2.8–2.4 kHz). The break in the plot was caused by stitching together two pictures from the original presentation of these data. **B** A rate profile for the difference in responses of a population of 354 fibers from four cats. The spectra of the two noise stimuli are shown at the *top* of the figure. The spectral shapes, called *E0* and *E2*, are head-related transfer functions for the cat ear from two directions in space. The stimuli were broad-band noise filtered to have these spectra; they were presented at ~20 dB spectrum level. The rate plot below shows the rates of individual AN fibers (data points) in response to a 200-ms presentation of *E0* minus the rate of the same fibers in response to 200 ms of *E2*. The *heavy line* in the plot below is the decibel difference between the two stimulus spectra, arbitrarily scaled to make the peak to peak values match. The rate scale is on the *left ordinate* and the decibel scale is on the *right ordinate*. The zero points (0 rate difference and 0 dB difference) are aligned. The *symbols* indicate the spontaneous rate classification (as in Fig. 5.4B) of the fibers; low SR – *squares*; medium SR – *triangles*; high SR – *crosses*. (**A** redrawn from Shamma, 1985a; **B** redrawn from Rice *et al.*, 1995.)

the duration shown here, as described in the figure caption; the shaded bars at right show the ranges of the first three formants.

The plot in Fig. 5.7A shows the population response as it is conveyed to the brain in the AN. The time delays due to propagation of the stimulus down the BM are shown by the delays of the responses at low BFs relative to high BFs. Note that the fibers are phase-locked to the stimulus. The temporal pattern of fibers' responses can be seen by reading across the plot from left to right at a fixed BF. The pattern is near-periodic, repeating along the time axis; the frequency of the repeat varies with BF. Phase-locking allows one to immediately see which of the many frequency components of the stimulus is driving the response in any particular neuron. As has been shown many times for speech-like stimuli (Young and Sachs, 1979; Delgutte and Kiang, 1984a; Sinex and Geisler, 1984; Palmer *et al.*, 1986), fibers tend to phase-lock to the formant frequency nearest their BF; this occurs because the formants are the largest amplitude components of the stimulus, but cochlear nonlinearities emphasize this pattern. Responses to the formants suppress responses to smaller stimulus components. Thus there is a broad band of locking to F1 for BFs between 0.4 and 1 kHz in Fig. 5.7A, recognizable as a pattern that repeats at ~2 ms. At higher BFs, bands of fibers locked to F2 (between 1 and 2 kHz) and F3 (near 2.5 kHz) can be seen as patterns periodic at higher frequencies. Finally, at the lowest and highest BFs, fibers are locked to the fundamental frequency of the stimulus (120 Hz).

5.5.2 Decoding the spectrotemporal representation

It is useful to discuss how the pattern of neural activity shown in Fig. 5.7A could be decoded to provide information about the stimulus. The first way is a direct time-domain decoding of the phase-locking by circuits sensitive to the period of the responses. For example, a CN neuron could respond when its AN fiber inputs were phase-locked to a frequency near its BF. In principle, such a mechanism provides a powerful and robust code for spectral shape (the averaged localized synchronized rate or ALSR (e.g. Young and Sachs, 1979; Sachs *et al.*, 1983; Delgutte, 1984; Palmer, 1990). By counting only responses phase locked to frequencies near a fiber's BF, the ALSR ignores the spread of excitation from a strong stimulus component at another frequency (evident in Fig. 5.7A by the wide band of phase-locking to F1). The phase-locking measure clearly shows the formants of a speech sound and provides a stable representation at high sound levels and in the presence of background noise. A problem with the phase-locking measure is that little evidence for it has been found in central auditory circuits and it is not clear how it could be implemented with neural hardware at frequencies up to several kiloHertz (but see Loeb *et al.*, 1983).

A second possible coding scheme takes advantage of the coherence of phase-locking across a range of BFs (Shamma, 1985b; Carney, 1994; Heinz *et al.*, 2001), shown by the approximately vertical alignment of response peaks in Fig. 5.7A. For each formant, fibers of different but nearby BFs tend to respond synchronously. Moreover, there are sharp transitions in the coherent spiking where the responses shift from one formant to the next, for example the phase-locking shifts from F1 to F2 at BFs near 1 kHz in the figure. The synchrony is also modified at low BFs (<0.7 kHz, at the top of the figure) by the delays in the propagation of sound on the BM, but this is a gradual effect, quite different from the abrupt and complete desynchronization between the formants. The second coding scheme could use monaural synchrony detection (Deng and Geisler, 1987; Carney, 1990) in CN neurons to make them sensitive to the cross-BF coherence shown in Fig. 5.7A. Thus CN neurons would respond strongly when their AN inputs fired synchronously across BF, as for a range of BFs responding to a formant, and weakly at the transitions from one dominant pattern of phase-locking (formant) to the next. Another computational possibility would be a lateral inhibitory network (Shamma, 1985a) to accomplish the calculation. Versions of such a system have been shown to be useful for auditory coding in various tasks (Carney *et al.*, 2002;

Colburn *et al.*, 2003) and evidence for cross-BF synchrony sensitivity has been found in the responses of neurons in VCN (Carney, 1990).

The third possible encoding scheme is the simplest, to measure the discharge rate across BF, called a rate-place code (Sachs and Young, 1979; Delgutte and Kiang, 1984b). From Fig. 5.6, it is clear that a neuron's discharge rate provides information about the amount of energy in the stimulus at frequencies near the neuron's BF. Thus a plot of rate versus BF should resemble the spectrum of the stimulus. Figure 5.7B shows an example of such a population rate representation (Rice *et al.*, 1995). In this case the representation is for the difference in responses to two stimuli; the difference is shown because it is clearer than the representation of either stimulus alone. The spectra of the stimuli are shown at the top of the figure; these are broadband noises filtered with two cat head-related transfer functions, called *E0* and *E2*. These spectra have peaks and valleys that are produced by the acoustics of the head and external ear (Musicant *et al.*, 1990). In the experiment, the two noises were presented separately and the rates of a population of AN fibers measured in response to both noises. The plot below shows the differences in the discharge rates plotted against BF, on the same frequency axis as the spectra. Each data point shows the rate difference for one fiber. The heavy line shows the dB difference between the stimuli, scaled arbitrarily so that the peak to peak values of the dB difference and rate difference plots match approximately. Note that the rate-place profile gives an accurate estimate of the spectral differences between the stimuli, except at low BFs and some high BFs. Although a rate representation is straightforward in terms of neural mechanisms, it is not robust at high sound levels and in the presence of background sounds. In either case, the quality of the rate representation decreases (Sachs and Young, 1979; Delgutte and Kiang, 1984a, c). At high sound levels, the discharge rates reach their maximum, or saturating level (as in Fig. 5.4B), and the sensitivity to differences in amplitude across the spectrum is lost. This can be seen for the HSR fiber in Fig. 5.6B as a decrease in the slope of the lines at high sound levels. With background noise, the responses to the noise mask responses to the stimulus at low signal to noise ratios, so that the distinguishing features of the stimulus responses are lost.

5.5.3 Spectral representations in the central nervous system

Population representations like those in Fig. 5.7 have been reconstructed for neurons in the subcortical central auditory system in a few cases. These central representations differ from the representation in the AN in two ways: first, the central rate representation in the VCN is more robust, meaning that the features in the spectral representation are more stable as sound level increases (Blackburn and Sachs, 1990) and in the presence of background noise (May *et al.*, 1996). Second, there is a tendency for the representations to become more dynamic, i.e. to emphasize the time variations in the stimulus, as the recording site moves centrally (e.g. in the IC) (Delgutte *et al.*, 1998). However the basic principles of the spectrotemporal population representation, as currently described, do not differ fundamentally from those described in Fig. 5.7. By contrast, the representation of spectra in auditory cortex appears to go beyond a simple spectrotemporal population code, as is discussed in a later section.

5.6 Mechanisms of spectral processing in auditory neurons

The discussion in previous sections treats neurons as if each one represents the energy in the stimulus at the neuron's BF. For AN fibers this is a good approximation because of their narrow and simple tuning. However, the receptive fields of auditory neurons become more complex and diverse in central parts of the auditory system (e.g. Spirou and Young, 1991; Sutter and Schreiner, 1991; Ramachandran *et al.*, 1999). Most obviously, the excitatory tuning curves of AN fibers are augmented by one or more inhibitory regions, so that the idea of representing the frequency selectivity of auditory neurons by a bandpass filter is insufficient. Thus more complex models of auditory receptive fields are needed. There is a large literature dealing with this problem. The following is a selective discussion that does not attempt to review the entire literature.

5.6.1 Response maps: V and I responses

The most common method for determining the receptive field maps of auditory neurons is to record systematically the responses to tones of various frequencies and sound levels. Figure 5.8A–C shows plots of discharge rate versus frequency across a range of sound levels, so-called response maps, for neurons in the cat IC (Ramachandran *et al.*, 1999). These three response maps are representative of three classes of response commonly seen in neurons at all levels of the auditory system, especially in unanesthetized preparations (reviewed by Davis, 2005; Sutter, 2005). These examples from the IC are for responses to tones in the contralateral ear, usually the dominant ear in the IC. Ipsilateral response maps were also determined; they are often different from contralateral maps and are described below.

The type V neuron in Fig. 5.8A shows a V-shaped excitatory area reminiscent of AN tuning curves. These neurons have little or no apparent inhibitory input in that they give only excitatory responses to tones (increases in discharge rate from spontaneous rate). In the cat IC, the ipsilateral ear gives a similar V-shaped excitatory tuning curve. Usually, IC neurons excited by both ears are sensitive to interaural time difference (reviewed by Palmer and Kuwada, 2005), as are type V neurons in IC.

The type I neuron in Fig. 5.8B also has a V-shaped excitatory area with significant inhibitory areas at lower and/or higher frequencies. In the cat IC, type I neurons have purely inhibitory V-shaped response maps from the ipsilateral ear (Davis *et al.*, 1999). Such excitatory-inhibitory neurons encode differences in interaural sound level (e.g. Semple and Kitzes, 1987; Irvine and Gago, 1990). Type I response maps are commonly observed at all levels of the auditory system, beginning with monaural neurons in the CN. Evidence from iontophoresis of inhibitory neurotransmitter antagonists (strychnine or bicuculline) suggests that the inhibitory inputs to neurons with type I response maps have a single V-shaped tuning that is centered at or near BF, but with a wider bandwidth than the excitatory inputs; thus the apparent inhibitory 'sidebands' are actually only the visible part of a broadly tuned inhibitory input (Yang *et al.*, 1992; Palombi and Caspary, 1996; LeBeau *et al.*, 2001). In IC, several inhibitory circuits involving convergence of excitatory and inhibitory inputs have been identified that probably contribute to type I responses (Pollak *et al.*, 2003).

5.6.2 O responses and level tuning

Type O neurons (Fig. 5.8C) have an inhibitory area that includes BF. Excitatory areas are seen at low sound levels near BF and often in other places, such as high levels at low frequencies and along the edge of the inhibitory areas just above BF (the arrow in this example). Similar response maps are seen in the DCN (so-called type IV neurons) (Young and Davis, 2002). In fact, the type O neurons in IC seem to be related to DCN type IV neurons, in that many type O neurons stop responding when the output tract of the DCN is blocked with lidocaine (Davis, 2002), although some O responses are created by inhibitory synapses in the IC (LeBeau *et al.*, 2001). Similar response maps are observed in auditory cortex, in neurons with 'closed' response maps having an island of excitation with inhibition or no response at lower and higher sound levels (Sutter and Schreiner, 1991; Sadagopan and Wang, 2008). Whether the neurons in cortex are related to the brainstem type O neurons is not known, but they often have properties that differ in the details from brainstem type O neurons.

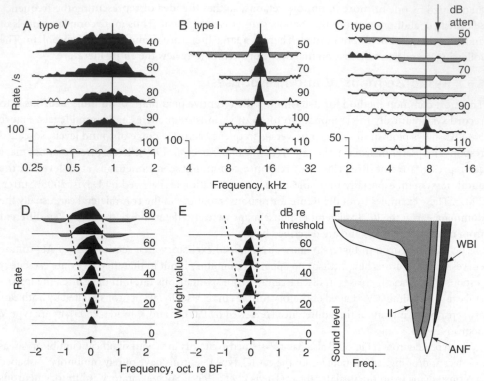

Fig. 5.8 Examples of receptive fields of auditory neurons, taken from the IC. **A–C** Response maps of three neuron types in IC for stimulation of the contralateral ear. The map consists of plots of discharge rate versus frequency at several sound levels; sound level is given as decibel attenuation at *right*. 0 dB is approximately 100 dB SPL. Rate plots at different sound levels are shifted vertically to avoid overlap; the rate scale at *lower left* applies to all plots in a map. The spontaneous rate for each plot is given by the *horizontal line*. Excitatory areas (rate increases above spontaneous) are colored *black*; inhibitory areas (rate decreases below spontaneous) are *gray*. The *vertical line* is the BF. **D** Model tone response map typical of most neuron types in CN and type I neurons in IC. **E** Response map for the same model neuron made up of first-order weight functions, computed as described in the text. Each weight function was computed from test stimuli at a different sound level, given at *right* on the plot. The *dashed lines* on **D** and **E** are identical and are drawn to bracket the excitatory area in **D**. **F** Model of type IV response maps in DCN which shows the tuning curves of one excitatory (ANF) and two inhibitory (II and WBI) neurons that converge on DCN principal cells (for a full explanation see Young and Davis, 2002). The excitatory and inhibitory areas of type IV response maps result if type II neurons make the strongest synapse, followed by AN fibers and finally WBI neurons. (**A–C** from Ramachandran *et al.*, 1999.)

In the case of DCN, type IV responses are recorded from the principal cells of the nucleus. Response maps similar to the one in Fig. 5.8C have been shown to be generated in DCN by over-lapping excitatory and inhibitory inputs, with tuning curves aligned as in Fig. 5.8F (reviewed in Young and Davis, 2002). The excitatory input (unfilled tuning curve marked 'ANF') is from AN fibers or perhaps collaterals of VCN neurons; the two inhibitory inputs (shaded) are from interneurons in the CN; they have the property of responding to narrowband stimuli like tones (the so-called type II neuron) and to broadband stimuli like noise (the so-called wide-band inhibitor, WBI). Computational models based on this circuit do a good job of reproducing type IV response characteristics (e.g. Hancock and Voigt, 1999).

In cortex, neurons with characteristics like type O have the additional property that their thresholds range widely so that they form a representation of sound intensity (Pfingst and O'Connor, 1981; Suga and Manabe, 1982; Sadagopan and Wang, 2008). Thus each neuron gives excitatory responses to BF tones over a narrow range of sound levels (20–30 dB), but that excitatory area may be at any sound level. Each neuron is 'tuned' for sound level as well as frequency. This differs from CN and IC in that all type O neurons in those nuclei have low thresholds, near the threshold for hearing. Thus the population of type O neurons in cortex forms a map in which both frequency and sound level are encoded (Sadagopan and Wang, 2008). This is an example of an elaborated sound representation in auditory cortex, i.e. one that adds an additional axis (in this case sound level) to the usual tonotopic, or frequency, axis.

5.6.3 Auditory receptive fields derived from broadband stimuli, the STRF

Tuning curves and response maps do not give an explicit model from which neural responses can be predicted; thus it is hard to know whether a response map, for example, is a complete and accurate representation of the spectral processing by a neuron. An extension of the idea of a tuning curve can be used for this purpose. The goal is to predict the discharge rate $r(t)$ of the neuron from the frequency content of the stimulus $S(f,t)$. S is a measure of the energy in the stimulus at frequency f and time t and is thus a representation like those shown in Fig. 5.2. It is commonly assumed that the discharge rate is linearly proportional to a weighted version of S. The weights are a function $g(f,t)$, called the STRF. The weights vary with frequency f, thus capturing the neuron's tuning, that is the neuron's tendency to respond more strongly at some frequencies than others. The time variable t is a necessary part of g because there are delays in the neural processing, so that the time variation of g shows how the neuron weights the stimulus components at different times. The neuron's response is then the convolution of g and S as in the equation below:

$$r(t) = \sum_f \sum_x g(f,x) S(f,t-x) \tag{5.1}$$

Essentially, the rate at time t is given by a linear weighting of the stimulus at times $t–x$ preceding t. The STRF model sums over time lags x and frequencies f to produce its estimate of the response. The STRF can be computed from properly chosen broadband test stimuli (e.g. noise or some natural stimulus) in a number of ways, described elsewhere (Klein *et al.*, 2000; Theunissen *et al.*, 2001; Lewis *et al.*, 2002). In this model, S is usually measured linearly, i.e. as stimulus power; however, as discussed in a previous section, the model actually works better if S is measured logarithmically, as the logarithm of stimulus power.

Insights gained from the STRF are discussed in a later section. Before discussing the STRF, it is useful to consider a simplified model in which the time axis is not included in the model. This simplification allows spectral processing to be studied separately; it is justified because g is usually separable into a time and a frequency component (i.e. $g(f,t) = g_1(f) g_2(t)$), at least for neurons in the IC and lower levels of the auditory system (Depireux *et al.*, 2001; Qiu *et al.*, 2003). For the simplified model, the goal is to compute the average discharge rate r over some time window (say the duration of a 200-ms stimulus) from the average spectrum $S(f)$ of the stimulus over the same time window (Yu and Young, 2000; Young and Calhoun, 2005). Given this assumption, it is clear that this model should only be applied to neurons that give tonic responses for which the average rate is an appropriate measure (Young *et al.*, 2005). In this model,

$$r = r_0 + \sum_j w_j S(f_j) + \cdots, \tag{5.2}$$

meaning that the rate is a sum of a constant r_0 plus the stimulus spectrum S weighted by the weights w_j, which take the place of the STRF in Eqn. 5.1. The weights have a simple interpretation; they are the slopes of the lines in plots like Fig. 5.6B and as such represent the 'gain' of the neuron for energy in the stimulus at frequencies f_j. If f_j is excitatory (inhibitory), the weight is positive (negative). The difference between the analysis of Fig. 5.6B and Eqn. 5.2 is that Eqn. 5.2 explicitly considers the weights at different frequencies and sums across their effects; in Fig. 5.6B, it was assumed that the neurons could be approximated as responding to only one frequency, the BF.

5.6.4 Weight functions versus tone response maps: level tolerance

The weights w_j are computed from broadband noise-like stimuli (Young and Calhoun, 2005), in a way similar to the STRF. Thus a plot of w_j versus f_j gives a measure of a neuron's tuning for broadband stimuli. A series of such plots computed for stimuli of different sound levels forms a weight-function response map (Fig. 5.8E). The weights are positive (black fill) at frequencies that are excitatory and negative (gray fill) at frequencies that are inhibitory. Note that the weights vary with sound level. This behavior is shown also in Fig. 5.6B where the slopes of the lines vary with sound level, especially for AN fibers, as the neuron goes from threshold to saturation.

For comparison, the tone response map of the same neuron is shown in Fig. 5.8D. These two maps are models typical of type I neurons in VCN and IC. This example illustrates that the weight functions are more level tolerant than the tone response map, meaning that they change less as sound level increases. To aid the comparison, identical dashed lines are drawn on Figs 5.8D and E; these lines were chosen to just bracket the excitatory part of the response map in Fig. 5.8D and have been repeated in Fig. 5.8E. Clearly the tone response map widens with sound level, whereas the weight-function response map does not, except near threshold. The property of level tolerance changes markedly in the first few levels of the auditory system. In the AN, both types of response map widen with sound level and there is no level tolerance (Evans, 1972; Liberman, 1978; Young and Calhoun, 2005). In VCN and IC, tone maps usually widen with sound level (Bourk, 1976; Ramachandran *et al.*, 1999), but weight-function response maps do not (Yu, 2003). In cortex, neurons with level-tolerant tone response maps (or tuning curves) are common (Sadagopan and Wang, 2008); in cats, such neurons are more common in the ventral part of the cortex (Schreiner and Sutter, 1992). Thus level tolerance seems to be established in a continuous process throughout the auditory system.

The level tolerance observed for weight-function tuning in CN and IC is probably a consequence of using broadband stimuli to compute the weights. Presumably, for broadband stimuli, the gain for off-BF responses is reduced by inhibition or suppression by the stronger stimulus components near BF. Of course, such suppression does not occur in a tone response map, where only one frequency is present at a time. The inhibition or suppression could be partially from cochlear suppression (so-called two-tone suppression), but the involvement of central inhibitory circuits is suggested because AN tuning is not level tolerant for either tones or noise.

5.6.5 Linear and nonlinear responses

The ellipsis in Eqn. 5.2 is a statement that this equation is an approximation. Neurons are nonlinear, meaning that the assumption that rate can be represented as a sum across frequency of weights times stimulus energy (and time in Eqn. 5.1) is an approximation which often is not accurate. As an example of what is meant by nonlinear, consider the responses of a neuron to the sum of two tones. For a linear interaction, the response to the two tones together is a sum of their responses presented separately; Eqns 5.1 and 5.2 predict exactly that interaction. However, in many cases the interaction is multiplicative, an example of which would be a neuron that gives no response to one tone but responds well to the second and then gives no response when both tones are presented together. The usual interpretation of that neuron is that the first tone inhibits the second. Another example is a coincidence neuron that responds to neither tone, but responds strongly when they are presented together. Responses like these two examples usually require additional terms in either Eqn. 5.1 or 5.2.

Either model can be tested by comparing its predictions to the rates generated by the real neuron in response to a battery of stimuli. The test is most rigorous when the test stimuli are different from the stimuli used to generate the model. The weight-function model works well for neurons in VCN and type I neurons in IC, especially if a second-order term is added to provide a mild nonlinear model (Yu and Young, 2000; Yu, 2003). By contrast, neurons in DCN and type O neurons in IC are more nonlinear and are usually poorly fit by this model. The STRF model has mainly been tested for neurons in the IC and cortex where neurons are more nonlinear (e.g. Eggermont *et al.*, 1983; Theunissen *et al.*, 2000; Escabi and Schreiner, 2002; Machens *et al.*, 2004). Some progress has been made in improving the performance of the STRF model, but that work is beyond the scope of this chapter (e.g. Sharpee *et al.*, 2004; Bandyopadhyay *et al.*, 2007; Gill *et al.*, 2008).

Nonlinearity signals the presence of important signal-processing properties in neurons and thus is an important problem for studies of spectral processing. For example, neurons become more nonlinear as they become more selective (Escabi and Schreiner, 2002). The best-studied nonlinear neurons in the auditory system are those in the cortex of songbirds, which may be selective for songs over other stimuli or even selective for one song over other very similar ones (e.g. Margoliash, 1986; Doupe and Konishi, 1991; Grace *et al.*, 2003; Cousillas *et al.*, 2005). This behavior is not predictable from linear models of neurons like the STRF (Theunissen *et al.*, 2000). Such stimulus selectivity seems to be necessary for specialized tasks, like the learning and control of complex behaviors. In that sense, much of the study of high-level processing in the auditory system reduces to ways of studying nonlinear neurons. Presently there are no general methods for this task.

5.7 **The STRF model: rate and scale**

Examples of STRFs for neurons in the IC are shown in Fig. 5.9A–F (Escabi and Read, 2005). These are the kernels $g(f,t)$ from Eqn. 5.1 plotted on time (abscissa) and frequency (ordinate) axes, with the magnitude of g indicated by a color scale from maximum (excitation; red) to minimum (inhibition; blue). The light blue color is zero. The time axis should be interpreted as time before spikes, so a particular pixel in an STRF shows the effect of energy at that frequency on the probability of spiking a certain time later, the time delay being the displacement along the abscissa. Each STRF applies only at one sound level, and STRFs usually change with sound level (Lesica and Grothe, 2008).

Analysis of STRFs has led to a biological interpretation of the cortical representation of natural stimuli in terms of modulation spectra, i.e. in terms of the modulation of the amplitude of the stimulus in time or frequency (Chi *et al.*, 1999; Singh and Theunissen, 2003). The examples shown in Fig. 5.9 differ in their sensitivity to modulation, either modulation of the stimulus energy in time, called 'rate', or modulation of the shape of the spectrum along the frequency axis, called 'scale' (Kowalski *et al.*, 1996; Calhoun and Schreiner, 1998). To illustrate the meaning of scale, note that neuron C would be strongly excited by broad spectral peaks extending over ~2 octaves (low scale) whereas neuron B has a rapidly varying weighting along the frequency axis and would respond best to narrow spectral peaks (high scale). Neuron A is in between. Similar comments apply in the time domain: neuron A weights events broadly across tens of milliseconds (low rate), whereas neurons E and F are matched to stimuli with rapid temporal modulations (high rate). Neurons in both IC and cortex are tuned to the modulations of stimulus spectrum along the frequency and time axes and each neuron usually has a particular best rate and best scale (reviewed by Chi *et al.*, 2005; Escabi and Read, 2005).

Tuning to rate and scale can be demonstrated by performing a 2-D Fourier transform of the STRF. The result expresses the neuron's response as a function of rate (the transformed temporal modulation rate in Hertz) and scale (the transformed spectral modulation in cycles/octave). Figure 5.9G shows the best rate and scale for neurons in the cat IC, determined as the maxima along the rate and scale axes of the 2-D Fourier transform of the STRF; the red letters identify the data points for the STRFs shown in Figs. 5.9A–F. The plot shows a tradeoff of best rate and best scale; high scale neurons respond to low rates and vice-versa (Qiu *et al.*, 2003). Such a tradeoff is

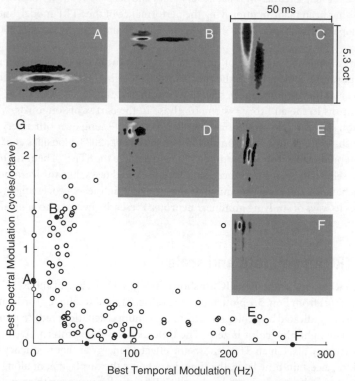

Fig. 5.9 A–F Examples of the STRFs of neurons in the IC of anesthetized cats. These two-dimensional plots show the values of the STRF kernel function *g(f,t)* in Eqn. 5.2 as a *color scale* against axes of time (*abscissa*) and frequency (*ordinate*). Time zero is at the *left* of each plot; the logarithmic frequency axis varies, but always has a range of 5.3 oct. as indicated. The *color axis* runs from *dark blue* (most negative) to *red* (most positive) and is zero at *light blue*. **G** Scatter plot of the best rate (*abscissa*) and scale (*ordinate*) for neurons in IC. The *red letters* mark the data points for the six examples. (Modified from Escabi and Read, 2005, with permission.)

seen in IC, but not in cortex, where a scatter plot like Fig. 5.9G would show a uniform distribution of data (Miller *et al.*, 2002; Mesgarani *et al.*, 2008). Note, however, that best rates in cortex are much lower than in IC, meaning that the high-rate sensitivity (>100 Hz) in the lower tail in Fig. 5.9G may simply be lost in synaptic processing between IC and cortex.

It can be argued that the usefulness of features such as best rate and best scale is limited in models of auditory processing, given that the STRF does not do well in predicting responses of nonlinear neurons to arbitrary stimuli. However, it is often found that the failures of low-order auditory models like the weight function or STRF are of a quantitative rather than a qualitative nature (Nelken *et al.*, 1997; Machens *et al.*, 2004; Reiss *et al.*, 2007). That is, the linear model gets the response roughly correct in shape, just not in amplitude. Thus the STRF model may give a useful measure of neural properties such as best rate and best scale, even though it does not predict actual discharge rates accurately.

5.8 Cortical representation of sounds

5.8.1 Rate and scale representation of speech

The neural representation was described above as a spectrotemporal representation of stimulus energy. However, it seems likely that sounds are analyzed in cortex in terms of additional features. In this section, the representation is described in terms of rate and scale (Chi *et al.*, 2005). Rate and scale were not arbitrarily chosen for this analysis, because cortical neurons are selective for rate and scale, as for the IC neurons in Fig. 5.9. Moreover rate and scale are a complete representation in the sense that the original stimulus can be reconstructed from a representation in terms of rate and scale as a function of frequency.

Figure 5.10 shows population representations of ten speech sounds; the data were obtained in the cortex of awake ferrets (Mesgarani *et al.*, 2008). Each column shows data from one phoneme (speech sound), for four vowels and six consonants, labelled at the top. The sounds were presented in a large number of sentences and responses were averaged across multiple repetitions of each phoneme in different contexts. The speech spectrograms (see Fig. 5.3) of the sounds are shown in the top row of the figure. Responses of cortical neurons to the phonemes are shown in the second row of the figure on the same time axis and on an ordinate showing BF. Thus the plots in the second row are like Fig. 5.7A except that the color scale shows the average rates of the neurons across several repetitions of the phoneme in different contexts. Consistent with other work (Bar-Yosef *et al.*, 2002; Wong and Schreiner, 2003; Engineer *et al.*, 2008), there is not a close resemblance of the spectrograms of the stimuli in the top row and the tonotopic representations in the second row; examples of poor resemblance are provided by the responses to /ɛ/, /i/, /f/, and /v/ where the regions of high discharge rate do not correspond well to the regions of high energy in the stimulus. The third and fourth rows show the same neural data, except now the neurons are grouped on the ordinate according to their best scale (third row) or best rate (fourth row). There was no relationship between BF and best scale or rate, so there is a complete reordering of neurons on the ordinates among the second, third, and fourth rows.

In some cases, the neurons seem to respond to the different speech sounds in ways that correspond to their scale and rate sensitivities. For example the vowels /ɛ/ and /e/ stimulate low scale neurons because these vowels have broad-band frequency content; the remaining two vowels have narrower bandwidth and thus evoke responses at high scale. The orderly nature of the rate and scale responses suggests that the cortical representation of speech sounds could be organized in terms of these features as well as BF. Because BF, best rate, and best scale are not correlated, one can think of the cortex as providing a three-dimensional representation of the spectra of complex sounds.

5.8.2 The nature of the cortical representation

The example in Fig. 5.10 suggests that the auditory cortex could be organized to represent multiple features of stimulus spectra in overlapping and interleaved maps. The rate and scale representation is merely one possibility which is suggested by the STRF data from cortical neurons. Sound level has previously been discussed as an additional dimension of the cortical representation.

There are several features of cortical responses to sound which complicate the problem of specifying the cortical representation (Nelken, 2004). First, cortical neurons are often selective for sounds that are behaviorally important for the animal. Neurons may respond specifically to a species' own vocalizations, for example, in a way not predicted by the sound's physical properties and not matched by neurons from another species responding to the same sounds (e.g. Wang and Kadia, 2001; Grace *et al.*, 2003; Cousillas *et al.*, 2005; Schnupp *et al.*, 2006). Moreover, regions of cortex may be organized according to computationally derived features important for analyzing sounds, as for sonar ranging in the bat (Suga, 1990) or pitch (Bendor and Wang, 2005).

Second, as mentioned above, cortical neurons may respond to sounds in ways that express high levels of nonlinearity. An example is combination sensitivity in which the neuron requires the

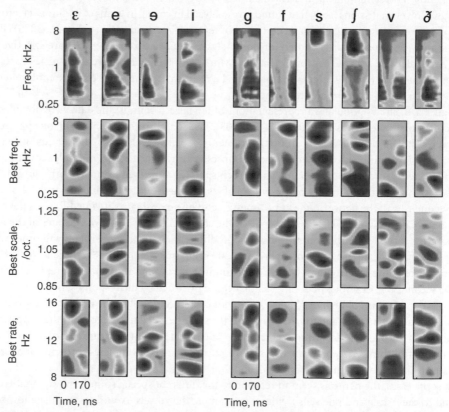

Fig. 5.10 Responses of a population of 90 cortical neurons to ten phonemes presented in various sentence contexts. The average spectrograms of the phonemes are shown on the *top row*. The population rate responses are shown in the *next three rows* on axes of time (*abscissa*) and BF (*ordinate, second row*), best scale (*ordinate, third row*), and best rate (*ordinate, fourth row*). BF, best scale, and best rate are the values of each parameter to which the neuron gives the largest response in a STRF. (Redrawn from Mesgarani *et al.*, 2008, with permission.)

presence of two different sounds (e.g. different frequencies or different harmonics) in order to respond (reviewed by Kanwal and Rauschecker, 2007). Another example is that responses to a complex scene consisting of a mixture of sounds may not be dominated by the most intense components of the sound, even if they have the highest sound level within the response map of the neuron (Bar-Yosef *et al.*, 2002).

Third, the receptive field of a cortical neuron may not be a fixed property. Rather, it can vary according to the immediate history of stimulation or the presence of a behavioral task that focuses attention on a particular frequency range (Fritz *et al.*, 2003; Weinberger, 2007). Also, cortical neurons can alter the receptive fields of subcortical neurons via descending connections (Suga, 2008). A third example is the phenomenon of oddball responses, in which the response of a neuron to a particular stimulus depends on its probability of occurring: common sounds evoke weaker responses than rare sounds (Ulanovsky *et al.*, 2003).

These examples suggest that it is not possible to specify *the* cortical representation of a sound. Instead the cortex seems to be analyzing sounds according to the objects that they represent or the behavioral implications of the sounds for the animal.

5.9 **Conclusions**

The neural representation of complex sounds in the peripheral auditory system is like the physical representation of the sounds shown in Fig. 5.2. There is a near-logarithmic allotment of neurons to different BF bands (Fig. 5.1), so that the frequency axis of the representation is near-logarithmic. The bandwidths of the filters vary with frequency in a way that may optimize the representation according to the stimulus ensemble (Fig. 5.3). The amplitude representation also seems to be logarithmic, in that the discharge rates of peripheral neurons are proportional to the decibel stimulus level over some range (Fig. 5.6).

The response properties of peripheral auditory neurons are strongly dependent on stimulus level, for example the widths of response maps (Fig. 5.8). Stabilizing the stimulus representation across sound level occurs in CN and continues in more central nuclei, as reflected in level-tolerant tuning (Fig. 5.8D, E). Finally, in cortex there is a specific representation of stimulus level, in the form of level-tuned neurons.

Two important topics related to stimulus level that were not covered because of lack of space are intensity adaptation and contrast sensitivity. The former means the adjustment of the dynamic range of a neuron (the range of sound levels over which its rate changes as stimulus level changes) in the presence of background sounds (e.g. Rees and Palmer, 1988; Dean *et al.*, 2005). Contrast sensitivity means the adaptation of neurons to stimulus contrast, which can be measured as the variance in stimulus level, either through time or across frequency (Barbour and Wang, 2003; Kvale and Schreiner, 2004; Nagel and Doupe, 2006; Reiss *et al.*, 2007). Both effects serve to stabilize the neural representation as stimulus intensity parameters change.

Ultimately the neural representation of a sound is the unique pattern of activity that it induces in the population of auditory neurons. It is easy to understand this representation in peripheral parts of the system where it is an isomorphic representation of the spectrotemporal features of the sound, modified in a limited way by peripheral nonlinearities such as suppression and adaptation. It is more difficult to describe the representation in cortex for the reasons discussed above. Most important, the isomorphic spectrotemporal representation seems to be augmented in cortex by a complex, and unknown, battery of other represented features, illustrated by the sound-level and rate/scale representations discussed. Although it is easy to show that a battery of stimuli are discriminable or identifiable from the responses of populations of cortical neurons through learning algorithms (Schnupp *et al.*, 2006; Engineer *et al.*, 2008; Mesgarani *et al.*, 2008), this approach does not produce an understanding of the nature of the representation itself. The nature of cortical representations is a central question for continuing research on the auditory system.

Acknowledgements

Preparation of this manuscript was supported by NIDCD grant DC00115. Comments on the manuscript by Paul Nelson, Alan Palmer, and Adrian Rees helped in its preparation.

References

Attias H, Schreiner CE (1997) Temporal low-order statistics of natural sounds. *Adv Neural Info Proc Sys* 9.

Bandyopadhyay S, Reiss LA, Young ED (2007) Receptive field for dorsal cochlear nucleus neurons at multiple sound levels. *J Neurophysiol* 98: 3505–15.

Bar-Yosef O, Rotman Y, Nelken I (2002) Responses of neurons in cat primary auditory cortex to bird chirps: effects of temporal and spectral context. *J Neurosci* 22: 8619–32.

Barbour DL, Wang X (2003) Contrast tuning in auditory cortex. *Science* 299: 1073–5.

Bendor D, Wang X (2005) The neuronal representation of pitch in primate auditory cortex. *Nature* 436: 1161–5.

Blackburn CC, Sachs MB (1989) Classification of unit types in the anteroventral cochlear nucleus: PST histograms and regularity analysis. *J Neurophysiol* 62: 1303–29.

Blackburn CC, Sachs MB (1990) The representation of the steady-state vowel sound /ε/ in the discharge patterns of cat anteroventral cochlear nucleus neurons. *J Neurophysiol* 63: 1191–212.

Bourk TR (1976) *Electrical Responses of Neural Units in the Anteroventral Cochlear Nucleus of the Cat*. Thesis, Massachusetts Institute of Technology, Cambridge.

Calhoun BM, Schreiner CE (1998) Spectral envelope coding in cat primary auditory cortex: linear and non-linear effects of stimulus characteristics. *Eur J Neurosci* 10: 926–40.

Carney LH (1990) Sensitivities of cells in anteroventral cochlear nucleus of cat to spatiotemporal discharge patterns across primary afferents. *J Neurophysiol* 64: 437–56.

Carney LH (1994) Spatiotemporal encoding of sound level: models for normal encoding and recruitment of loudness. *Hear Res* 76: 31–44.

Carney LH, Yin TCT (1988) Temporal coding of resonances by low-frequency auditory nerve fibers: single-fiber responses and a population model. *J Neurophysiol* 60: 1653–77.

Carney LH, Heinz MG, Evilsizer ME, Gilkey RH, Colburn HS (2002) Auditory phase opponency: a temporal model for masked detection at low frequencies. *Acustica-Acta Acustica* 88: 334–47.

Chi T, Gao Y, Guyton MC, Ru P, Shamma S (1999) Spectro-temporal modulation transfer functions and speech intelligibility. *J Acoust Soc Am* 106: 2719–32.

Chi T, Ru P, Shamma SA (2005) Multiresolution spectrotemporal analysis of complex sounds. *J Acoust Soc Am* 118: 887–906.

Colburn HS, Carney LH, Heinz MG (2003) Quantifying the information in auditory-nerve responses for level discrimination. *J Assoc Res Otolaryngol* 4: 294–311.

Cooper NP, Rhode WS (1995) Nonlinear mechanics at the apex of the guinea-pig cochlea. *Hear Res* 82: 225–43.

Cooper NP, Rhode WS (1997) Mechanical responses to two-tone distortion products in the apical and basal turns of the mammalian cochlea. *J Neurophysiol* 78: 261–70.

Cousillas H, Leppelsack HJ, Leppelsack E, Richard JP, Mathelier M, Hausberger M (2005) Functional organization of the forebrain auditory centres of the European starling: a study based on natural sounds. *Hear Res* 207: 10–21.

Davis KA (2002) Evidence of a functionally segregated pathway from dorsal cochlear nucleus to inferior colliculus. *J Neurophysiol* 87: 1824–35.

Davis KA (2005) Spectral processing in the inferior colliculus. In: Auditory Spectral Processing (eds Malmierca MS, Irvine DRF), pp 169–205. Elsevier, Amsterdam.

Davis KA, Ramachandran R, May BJ (1999) Single-unit responses in the inferior colliculus of decerebrate cats II. Sensitivity to interaural level differences. *J Neurophysiol* 82: 164–75.

de Boer E, de Jongh HR (1978) On cochlear encoding: potentialities and limitations of the reverse-correlation technique. *J Acoust Soc Am* 63: 115–35.

Dean I, Harper NS, McAlpine D (2005) Neural population coding of sound level adapts to stimulus statistics. *Nat Neurosci* 8: 1684–9.

Delgutte B (1980) Representation of speech-like sounds in the discharge patterns of auditory-nerve fibers. *J Acoust Soc Am* 68: 843–57.

Delgutte B (1984) Speech coding in the auditory nerve: II. Processing schemes for vowel-like sounds. *J Acoust Soc Am* 75: 879–86.

Delgutte B, Kiang NYS (1984a) Speech coding in the auditory nerve. I. Vowel-like sounds. *J Acoust Soc Am* 75: 866–78.

Delgutte B, Kiang NYS (1984b) Speech coding in the auditory nerve. III. Voiceless fricative consonants. *J Acoust Soc Am* 75: 887–96.

Delgutte B, Kiang NYS (1984c) Speech coding in the auditory nerve. V. Vowels in background noise. *J Acoust Soc Am* 75: 908–18.

Delgutte B, Hammond BM, Cariani PA (1998) Neural coding of the temporal envelope of speech: relation to modulation transfer functions. In: Psychophysical and Physiological Advances in Hearing (eds Palmer AR, et al.), pp 595–603. Whurr, London.

Deng L, Geisler CD (1987) A composite auditory model for processing speech sounds. *J Acoust Soc Am* 82: 2001–12.

Depireux DA, Simon JZ, Klein DJ, Shamma SA (2001) Spectro-temporal response field characterization with dynamic ripples in ferret primary auditory cortex. *J Neurophysiol* 85: 1220–34.

Doupe AJ, Konishi M (1991) Song-selective auditory circuits in the vocal control system of the zebra finch. *PNAS* 88: 11339–43.

Eggermont JJ, Aertsen AMHJ, Johannesma PIM (1983) Prediction of the responses of auditory neurons in the midbrain of the grass frog based on the spectro-temporal receptive field. *Hear Res* 10: 191–202.

Engineer CT, Perez CA, Chen YH, *et al.* (2008) Cortical activity patterns predict speech discrimination ability. *Nat Neurosci* 11: 603–8.

Escabi MA, Read HL (2005) Neural mechanisms for spectral analysis in the auditory midbrain, thalamus, and cortex. *Int Rev Neurobiol* 70: 207–52.

Escabi MA, Schreiner CE (2002) Nonlinear spectrotemporal sound analysis by neurons in the auditory midbrain. *J Neurosci* 22: 4114–31.

Escabi MA, Miller LM, Read HL, Schreiner CE (2003) Naturalistic auditory contrast improves spectrotemporal coding in the cat inferior colliculus. *J Neurosci* 23: 11489–504.

Evans EF (1972) The frequency response and other properties of single fibres in the guinea-pig cochlear nerve. *J Physiol* 226: 263–87.

Evans EF (1975) The sharpening of cochlear frequency selectivity in the normal and abnormal cochlea. *Audiology* 14: 419–42.

Fritz J, Shamma S, Elhilali M, Klein D (2003) Rapid task-related plasticity of spectrotemporal receptive fields in primary auditory cortex. *Nat Neurosci* 6: 1216–23.

Gill P, Zhang J, Woolley SMN, Fremouw T, Theunissen FE (2006) Sound representation methods for spectro-temporal receptive field estimation. *J Comput Neurosci* 21: 5–20.

Gill P, Woolley S, Fremouw T, Theunissen FE (2008) What's that sound? Auditory area CLM encodes stimulus surprise, not intensity or intensity changes. *J Neurophysiol* 99: 2809–20.

Greenwood DD (1961) Critical bandwidth and the frequency coordinates of the basilar membrane. *J Acoust Soc Am* 33: 1344–56.

Grace JA, Amin N, Singh NC, Theunissen FE (2003) Selectivity for conspecific song in the zebra finch auditory forebrain. *J Neurophysiol* **89**: 472–87.

Hancock KE, Voigt HF (1999) Wideband inhibition of dorsal cochlear nucleus type IV units in cat: a computational model. *Ann Biomed Eng* **27**: 73–87.

Hartmann WM (1997) *Signals, Sound, and Sensation.* AIP Press, Woodbury, New York.

Heinz MG, Colburn HS, Carney LH (2001) Rate and timing cues associated with the cochlear amplifier: level discrimination based on monaural cross-frequency coincidence detection. *J Acoust Soc Am* **110**: 2065–84.

Heinz MG, Issa JB, Young ED (2005) Auditory-nerve rate responses are inconsistent with common hypotheses for the neural correlates of loudness recruitment. *J Assoc Res Otolaryngol* **6**: 91–105.

Irvine DRF, Gago G (1990) Binaural interaction in high-frequency neurons in inferior colliculus of the cat: effects of variations in sound pressure level on sensitivity to interaural intensity differences. *J Neurophysiol* **63**: 570–91.

Joris PX, Schreiner CE, Rees A (2004) Neural processing of amplitude-modulated sounds. *Physiol Rev* **84**: 541–77.

Joris PX, Ramirez CL, McLaughlin M, van der Heijden M (2006) Spectral and temporal properties of the auditory nerve in old-world monkeys. *Abstr ARO Midwinter Res Mtg* **29**: 302.

Kanwal JS, Rauschecker JP (2007) Auditory cortex of bats and primates: managing species-specific calls for social communication. *Front Biosci* **12**: 4621–40.

Keithley EM, Schreiber RC (1987) Frequency map of the spiral ganglion in the cat. *J Acoust Soc Am* **81**: 1036–42.

Klein DJ, Depireux DA, Simon JZ, Shamma SA (2000) Robust spectrotemporal reverse correlation for the auditory system: Optimizing stimulus design. *J Comput Neurosci* **9**: 85–111.

Kowalski N, Depireux DA, Shamma SA (1996) Analysis of dynamic spectra in ferret primary auditory cortex. II. Prediction of unit responses to arbitrary dynamic spectra. *J Neurophysiol* **76**: 3524–34.

Kvale MN, Schreiner CE (2004) Short-term adaptation of auditory receptive fields to dynamic stimuli. *J Neurophysiol* **91**: 604–12.

LeBeau FEN, Malmierca MS, Rees A (2001) Iontophoresis In vivo demonstrates a key role for GABAA and glycinergic inhibition in shaping frequency response areas in the inferior colliculus of guinea pig. *J Neurosci* **21**: 7303–12.

Lesica NA, Grothe B (2008) Dynamic spectrotemporal feature selectivity in the auditory midbrain. *J Neurosci* **28**: 5412–21.

Lewicki MS (2002) Efficient coding of natural sounds. *Nat Neurosci* **5**: 356–63.

Lewis ER, Henry KR, Yamada WM (2002) Tuning and timing in the gerbil ear: Wiener-kernel analysis. *Hear Res* **174**: 206–21.

Liberman MC (1978) Auditory-nerve response from cats raised in a low-noise chamber. *J Acoust Soc Am* **63**: 442–55.

Liberman MC (1982) The cochlear frequency map for the cat: labeling auditory-nerve fibers of known characteristic frequency. *J Acoust Soc Am* **72**: 1441–9.

Loeb GE, White MW, Merzenich MM (1983) Spatial cross-correlation. *Biol Cybern* **47**: 149–63.

Machens CK, Wehr MS, Zador AM (2004) Linearity of cortical receptive fields measured with natural sounds. *J Neurosci* **24**: 1089–100.

Malmierca MS, Irvine DRF (2005) *Auditory Spectral Processing* (also Int Rev Neurobiol, vol. 70). Elsevier, Amsterdam.

Margoliash D (1986) Preference for autogenous song by auditory neurons in a song system nucleus of the white-crowned sparrow. *J Neurosci* **6**: 1643–61.

May BJ, Huang AY (1997) Spectral cues for sound localization in cats: a model for discharge rate representations in the auditory nerve. *J Acoust Soc Am* **101**: 2705–19.

May BJ, Huang A, LePrell G, Hienz RD (1996) Vowel formant frequency discrimination in cats: comparison of auditory nerve representations and psychophysical thresholds. *Aud Neurosci* 3: 135–62.

May BJ, LePrell GS, Hienz RD, Sachs MB (1997) Speech representation in the auditory nerve and ventral cochlear nucleus. In: Acoustical Signal Processing in the Central Auditory System (ed. Syka J), pp 413–29. Plenum Press, New York.

Mesgarani N, David SV, Fritz JB, Shamma S (2008) Phoneme representation and classification in primary auditory cortex. *J Acoust Soc Am* 123: 899–909.

Miller LM, Escabi MA, Read HL, Schreiner CE (2002) Spectrotemporal receptive fields in the lemniscal auditory thalamus and cortex. *J Neurophysiol* 87: 516–27.

Miller MI, Sachs MB (1983) Representation of stop consonants in the discharge patterns of auditory-nerve fibers. *J Acoust Soc Am* 74: 502–17.

Miller RL, Schilling JR, Franck KR, Young ED (1997) Effects of acoustic trauma on the representation of the vowel / / in cat auditory nerve fibers. *J Acoust Soc Am* 101: 3602–16.

Moore BCJ (2004) *An Introduction to the Psychology of Hearing*. Elsevier, Amsterdam.

Musicant AD, Chan JCK, Hind JE (1990) Direction-dependent spectral properties of cat external ear: new data and cross-species comparisons. *J Acoust Soc Am* 87: 757–81.

Nagel KI, Doupe AJ (2006) Temporal processing and adaptation in the songbird auditory forebrain. *Neuron* 51: 845–59.

Nelken I (2004) Processing of complex stimuli and natural scenes in the auditory cortex. *Curr Opin Neurobiol* 14: 474–80.

Nelken I, Kim PJ, Young ED (1997) Linear and non-linear spectral integration in type IV neurons of the dorsal cochlear nucleus: II. Predicting responses using non linear methods. *J Neurophysiol* 78: 800–11.

Oxenham AJ, Bacon SP (2003) Cochlear compression: perceptual measures and implications for normal and impaired hearing. *Ear Hear* 24: 352–66.

Oxenham AJ, Plack CJ (1997) A behavioral measure of basilar-membrane nonlinearity in listeners with normal and impaired hearing. *J Acoust Soc Am* 101: 3666–75.

Oxenham AJ, Shera CA (2003) Estimates of human cochlear tuning at low levels using forward and simultaneous masking. *J Assoc Res Otolaryngol* 4: 541–54.

Palmer AR (1990) The representation of the spectra and fundamental frequencies of steady-state single- and double-vowel sounds in the temporal discharge patterns of guinea pig cochlear-nerve fibers. *J Acoust Soc Am* 88: 1412–26.

Palmer AR, Evans EF (1982) Intensity coding in the auditory periphery of the cat: responses of cochlear nerve and cochlear nucleus neurons to signals in the presence of bandstop masking noise. *Hear Res* 7: 305–23.

Palmer AR, Kuwada S (2005) Binaural and spatial coding in the inferior colliculus. In: The Inferior Colliculus (eds Winer JA, Schreiner CE), pp 377–410. Springer, New York.

Palmer AR, Winter IM, Darwin CJ (1986) The representation of steady-state vowel sounds in the temporal discharge patterns of the guinea pig cochlear nerve and primary-like cochlear nucleus neurons. *J Acoust Soc Am* 79: 100–13.

Palombi PS, Caspary DM (1996) GABA inputs control discharge rate primarily within frequency receptive fields of inferior colliculus neurons. *J Neurophysiol* 75: 2211–19.

Patterson RD, Holdsworth J (1996) Neural activity patterns and auditory images. *Adv Speech Hear Lang Proc* 3B: 547–63.

Pfeiffer RR, Kim DO (1975) Cochlear nerve fiber responses: distribution along the cochlear partition. *J Acoust Soc Am* 58: 867–9.

Pfingst BE, O'Connor TA (1981) Characteristics of neurons in auditory cortex of monkeys performing a simple auditory task. *J Neurophysiol* 45: 16–34.

Pollak GD, Burger RM, Klug A (2003) Dissecting the circuitry of the auditory system. *Trend Neurosci* 26: 33–9.

Qiu A, Schreiner CE, Escabi MA (2003) Gabor analysis of auditory midbrain receptive fields: spectro-temporal and binaural composition. *J Neurophysiol* **90**: 456–76.

Ramachandran R, Davis KA, May BJ (1999) Single-unit responses in the inferior colliculus of decerebrate cats I. Classification based on frequency response maps. *J Neurophysiol* **82**: 152–63.

Rees A, Palmer AR (1988) Rate-intensity functions and their modification by broadband noise for neurons in the guinea pig inferior colliculus. *J Acoust Soc Am* **83**: 1488–98.

Reiss LA, Bandyopadhyay S, Young ED (2007) Effects of stimulus spectral contrast on receptive fields of dorsal cochlear nucleus neurons. *J Neurophysiol* **98**: 2133–43.

Relkin EM, Doucet JR (1997) Is loudness simply proportional to the auditory nerve spike count?. *J Acoust Soc Am* **101**: 2735–40.

Rhode WS (1984) Cochlear mechanics. *Annu Rev Physiol* **46**: 231–46.

Rhode WS (2007) Mutual suppression in the 6 kHz region of sensitive chinchilla cochlea. *J Acoust Soc Am* **121**: 2805–18.

Rhode WS, Smith PH (1985) Characteristics of tone-pip response patterns in relationship to spontaneous rate in cat auditory nerve fibers. *Hear Res* **18**: 159–68.

Rice JJ, Young ED, Spirou GA (1995) Auditory-nerve encoding of pinna-based spectral cues: rate representation of high-frequency stimuli. *J Acoust Soc Am* **97**: 1764–76.

Robles L, Ruggero MA (2001) Mechanics of the mammalian cochlea. *Physiol Rev* **81**: 1305–52.

Rosen S (1992) Temporal information in speech: acoustic, auditory and linguistic aspects. *Phil Trans R Soc Lond B* **336**: 367–73.

Ruggero MA, Temchin AN (2005) Unexceptional sharpness of frequency tuning in the human cochlea. *PNAS* **102**: 18614–19.

Ruggero MA, Rich NC, Recio A, Narayan SS (1997) Basilar-membrane responses to tones at the base of the chinchilla cochlea. *J Acoust Soc Am* **101**: 2151–63.

Ruggero MA, Robles L, Rich NC, Recio A (1992) Basilar membrane responses to two-tone and broadband stimuli. *Phil Trans R Soc Lond B* **336**: 307–15.

Sachs MB, Abbas PJ (1976) Phenomenological model for two tone suppression. *J Acoust Soc Am* **60**: 1157–63.

Sachs MB, Young ED (1979) Encoding of steady-state vowels in the auditory nerve: representation in terms of discharge rate. *J Acoust Soc Am* **66**: 470–9.

Sachs MB, Voigt HF, Young ED (1983) Auditory nerve representation of vowels in background noise. *J Neurophysiol* **50**: 27–45.

Sadagopan S, Wang X (2008) Level invariant representation of sounds by populations of neuron in primary auditory cortex. *J Neurosci* **28**: 3415–26.

Schlauch RS, DiGiovanni JJ, Ries DT (1998) Basilar membrane nonlinearity and loudness. *J Acoust Soc Am* **103**: 2010–20.

Schmiedt RA (1989) Spontaneous rates, thresholds and tuning of auditory-nerve fibers in the gerbil: comparisons to cat data. *Hear Res* **42**: 23–35.

Schnupp JW, Hall TM, Kokelaar RF, Ahmed B (2006) Plasticity of temporal pattern codes for vocalization stimuli in primary auditory cortex. *J Neurosci* **26**: 4785–95.

Schreiner CE, Sutter ML (1992) Topography of excitatory bandwidth in cat primary auditory cortex: single-neuron versus multiple-neuron recordings. *J Neurophysiol* **68**: 1487–502.

Semple MN, Kitzes LM (1987) Binaural processing of sound pressure level in the inferior colliculus. *J Neurophysiol* **57**: 1130–47.

Shamma SA (1985a) Speech processing in the auditory system. II: Lateral inhibition and the central processing of speech evoked activity in the auditory nerve. *J Acoust Soc Am* **78**: 1622–32.

Shamma SA (1985b) Speech processing in the auditory system. I: The representation of speech sounds in the responses of the auditory nerve. *J Acoust Soc Am* **78**: 1612–21.

Sharpee T, Rust NC, Bialek W (2004) Analyzing neural responses to natural signals: maximally informative dimensions. *Neural Comput* **16**: 223–50.

Shera CA, Guinan JJ, Oxenham AJ (2002) Revised estimates of human cochlear tuning from otoacoustic and behavioral measurements. *PNAS* **99**: 3318–23.

Sinex DG, Geisler CD (1984) Comparison of the responses of auditory nerve fibers to consonant-vowel syllables with predictions from linear models. *J Acoust Soc Am* **76**: 116–21.

Singh NC, Theunissen FE (2003) Modulation spectra of natural sounds and ethological theories of auditory processing. *J Acoust Soc Am* **114**: 3394–411.

Slaney M (1993) *An Efficient Implementation of the Patterson-Holdsworth Auditory Filter Bank.* Apple Computer Technical Report #35. Apple Computer Inc, Cupertino, California.

Smith EC, Lewicki MS (2006) Efficient auditory coding. *Nature* **439**: 978–82.

Spirou GA, Young ED (1991) Organization of dorsal cochlear nucleus type IV unit response maps and their relationship to activation by bandlimited noise. *J Neurophysiol* **65**: 1750–68.

Spirou GA, May BJ, Wright DD, Ryugo DK (1993) Frequency organization of the dorsal cochlear nucleus in cats. *J Comp Neurol* **329**: 36–52.

Suga N (1990) Cortical computational maps for auditory imaging. *Neural Networks* **3**: 3–21.

Suga N (2008) Role of corticofugal feedback in hearing. *J Comp Physiol A* **194**: 169–83.

Suga N, Manabe T (1982) Neural basis of amplitude-spectrum representation in auditory cortex of the mustached bat. *J Neurophysiol* **47**: 225–5.

Sutter ML (2005) Spectral processing in the auditory cortex. In: Auditory Spectral Processing (eds Malmierca MS, Irvine DRF), pp 253–98. Elsevier, Amsterdam.

Sutter ML, Schreiner CE (1991) Physiology and topography of neurons with multipeaked tuning curves in cat primary auditory cortex. *J Neurophysiol* **65**: 1207–26.

Syka J (2002) Plastic changes in the central auditory system after hearing loss, restoration of function, and during learning. *Physiol Rev* **82**: 601–36.

Theunissen FE, Sen K, Doupe AJ (2000) Spectral-temporal receptive fields of nonlinear auditory neurons obtained using natural sounds. *J Neurosci* **20**: 2315–31.

Theunissen FE, David SV, Singh NC, Hsu A, Vinje WE, Gallant JL (2001) Estimating spatio-temporal receptive fields of auditory and visual neurons from their responses to natural stimuli. *Network Comput Neural Syst* **12**: 289–316.

Ulanovsky N, Las L, Nelken I (2003) Processing of low-probability sounds by cortical neurons. *Nat Neurosci* **6**: 391–8.

Wang X, Kadia SC (2001) Differential representation of species-specific primate vocalizations in the auditory cortices of marmoset and cat. *J Neurophysiol* **86**: 2616–20.

Weinberger NM (2007) Associative representational plasticity in the auditory cortex: a synthesis of two disciplines. *Learn Mem* **14**: 1–16.

Winer JA, Schreiner CE (2005) *The Inferior Colliculus.* Springer, New York.

Wong SW, Schreiner CE (2003) Representation of CV-sounds in cat primary auditory cortex: intensity dependence. *Speech Comm* **41**: 93–106.

Yang L, Pollak GD, Resler C (1992) GABAergic circuits sharpen tuning curves and modify response properties in the mustache bat inferior colliculus. *J Neurophysiol* **68**: 1760–74.

Yates GK, Winter IM, Robertson D (1990) Basilar membrane nonlinearity determines auditory nerve rate-intensity functions and cochlear dynamic range. *Hear Res* **45**: 203–20.

Young ED, Calhoun BM (2005) Nonlinear modeling of auditory-nerve rate responses to wideband stimuli. *J Neurophysiol* **94**: 4441–54.

Young ED, Davis KA (2002) Circuitry and function of the dorsal cochlear nucleus. In: Integrative Functions in the Mammalian Auditory Pathway (eds Oertel D, et al.), pp 160–206. Springer, New York.

Young ED, Sachs MB (1979) Representation of steady-state vowels in the temporal aspects of the discharge patterns of populations of auditory-nerve fibers. *J Acoust Soc Am* **66**: 1381–403.

Young ED, Yu JJ, Reiss LA (2005) Non-linearities and the representation of auditory spectra. *Int Rev Neurobiol* 70: 135–68.

Yu JJ (2003) *Spectral Information Encoding in the Cochlear Nucleus and Inferior Colliculus: A Study Based on the Random Spectral Shape Method*. Thesis, Johns Hopkins, Baltimore.

Yu JJ, Young ED (2000) Linear and nonlinear pathways of spectral information transmission in the cochlear nucleus. *PNAS* 97: 11780–6.

Zhang X, Carney LH (2005) Response properties of an integrate-and-fire model that receives subthreshold inputs. *Neur Comput* 17: 2571–601.

Chapter 6

Time-varying sounds: amplitude envelope modulations

Brian Malone and Christoph E. Schreiner

6.1 Introduction

Auditory signals are necessarily extended in time, which implies that all auditory processing can be construed as a form of temporal coding. In the case of an unmodulated 'pure' tone, however, the only temporal variation in the signal occurs at onset and offset. Of course, a pure tone consists of sinusoidal variations in pressure at the tone frequency, but the parameters defining the tone, such as its frequency and amplitude, are constant while it endures. Time-varying sounds, by contrast, exhibit fluctuations in amplitude or frequency. Nearly all naturally occurring, ecologically relevant sounds exhibit ongoing changes in their temporal structure, and answers to fundamental perceptual and informational questions regarding incoming sounds, such as 'who or what or where' require the accurate discrimination of such changes.

When discussing fluctuations in frequency and amplitude, it is useful to distinguish between the fine structure and the envelope of a temporal waveform. The fine structure is more closely associated with the spectral content of the signal, and refers to relatively fast pressure variations, typically exceeding several hundred Hertz (Hz). Superimposed on the fine structure are relatively slow changes in the overall signal magnitude (Fig. 6.1A). These changes define the envelope of the signal (for a mathematical treatment of the envelope, see Hartmann, 1997). For pure tones, the fine structure is a sinusoidal variation in pressure, and the envelope is said to be flat. By combining the fine structure of one sound with the envelope of a different sound to form 'auditory chimeras,' researchers have demonstrated that envelope cues dominate speech recognition, and fine structure dominates pitch perception and sound localization (Smith *et al.*, 2002).

In this chapter, we focus on one class of experimental stimuli that involves relatively simple modulations of the envelope: sinusoidal modulations of amplitude. We stress that these stimuli cannot capture the full complexity of auditory temporal processing, which has also been studied with a range of informative paradigms (e.g., forward masking, gap detection, and duration discrimination). The coding of time-varying sounds is really a subset of the broader issue of how context, impacts the processing of acoustic signals. There is abundant evidence that the auditory system is sensitive to the context in which a particular sound occurs (Sanes *et al.*, 1998; Galazyuk *et al.*, 2000; Malone and Semple, 2001; Malone *et al.* 2002; Ulanovsky *et al.*, 2004). All enduring sounds, in a sense, provide their own context because the features of the sound in the past bear on how it will be processed in the present due to activity-dependent biophysical mechanisms throughout the auditory pathway. The encoding of time-varying signals is thus necessarily complex because these mechanisms, as well as passive filtering mechanisms operating in cells and synapses, have their own time constants, and these too inform the neural representation of the stimulus as it passes through the system.

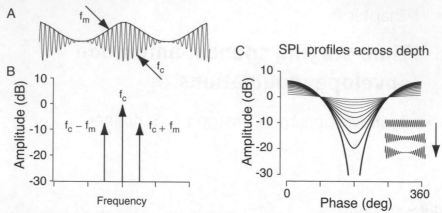

Fig. 6.1 Introduction to sinusoidal amplitude modulation. **A** Fluctuations in sound pressure that constitute a SAM stimulus. These rapid changes are referred to as the fine structure of the carrier signal (f_c). Overlaid on the outline of this stimulus is the envelope of the modulating stimulus (f_m), which in this case occurs at a much lower frequency ($f_m \ll f_c$). **B** Representation of a SAM stimulus in the spectral domain shows that the stimulus contains power at three frequencies: the carrier, f_c, and two sidebands, $f_c \pm f_m$. The relative height of the sidebands is determined by the modulation depth, m, such that a fully (100%) modulated stimulus has sidebands at –6 dB relative to the carrier. **C** Representations of SAM stimuli for a range of modulation depths with respect to an axis defined in decibels of sound pressure level (dB SPL) relative to an unmodulated pure tone. As the modulation depth increases, the asymmetry between the cyclical increases and decreases in the 'instantaneous' amplitude of SAM signals grows. For clarity, the curves have been aligned such that the amplitude minimum occurs at 180°, rather than 270°, as it does when the signals are presented in sine phase. The *icon* indicates the changes in the stimulus waveform (see **A**) as modulation depth increases.

6.2 **The SAM stimulus**

Because the temporal variations in natural sounds tend to be complex, auditory scientists have traditionally employed much simpler sounds to characterize the neural representation of time-varying sounds at various stages of the auditory pathway. The best-studied example of this is sinusoidal amplitude modulation (SAM), in which the amplitude of a pure tone (the carrier) is modulated by another tone at lower frequency (the modulator). Just as a pure tone is the simplest stimulus in the spectral domain because it contains only a single frequency, SAM is the simplest stimulus in the modulation domain because it contains only a single modulation frequency. A SAM stimulus is fully described by four parameters: (1) the frequency of the carrier (f_c); (2) the level of the carrier (A); (3) the frequency of the modulation (f_m); and (4) the depth of the modulation (m). The equation for a SAM stimulus can be written as:

$$s(t) = A[1 + m \sin(2\pi f_m t)] \sin(2\pi f_c t).$$

When f_c substantially exceeds f_m, the term $[1 + m \sin(2\pi f_m t)]$ describes the envelope of the stimulus, and the term $\sin(2\pi f_c t)$ describes the fine structure. By rearranging the foregoing equation using the trigonometric identity $\cos(B) \sin(A) = 1/2[\sin(A+B) + \sin(A–B)]$, we obtain a simple expression for the spectrum of a SAM signal:

$$s(t) = \sin(2\pi f_c t) + m/2 [\sin(2\pi(f_c + f_m)t) + \sin(2\pi(f_c – f_m)t)].$$

The frequency spectrum of SAM contains three components: the primary peak at f_c, and sidebands at $f_c - f_m$ and $f_c + f_m$ (Fig. 6.1B). It is also worth noting that the average power of SAM signals increases with the modulation depth, m, which determines the magnitude of the sidebands. The time domain representation of the SAM signal indicated in Fig. 6.1A is perhaps more intuitive. The 'instantaneous' magnitude of the fully modulated SAM signal depicted here can be ascertained by considering the height of the fine structural changes within a narrow window. Although the modulator is sinusoidal in amplitude, it is important to note that the 'instantaneous' amplitude of the SAM signal, expressed in perceptually more appropriate logarithmic units of decibels of sound pressure level (dB SPL), is not. For a fully modulated stimulus, the signal will vary from +6 to $-\infty$ dB, relative to the unmodulated carrier level. Figure 6.1C indicates how the SPL of SAM signals varies as a function of modulation depth. These curves are useful in relating the amplitudes of SAM signals to measures of amplitude tuning, such as rate level functions for tone bursts, that are measured in dB SPL.

The modulation frequencies relevant for human perception span a range from ~1 to 1000 Hz. In fact, the modulation spectrum of natural sounds is highly constrained, so the 'acoustic biotopes' of many species overlap substantially, and low temporal modulation frequencies dominate communication sounds in many species (Singh and Theunissen, 2003). Different subregions of this range are associated with different perceptual and information-bearing domains. For human listeners, modulations below ~4 Hz are associated with the occurrence of essentially isolated acoustical events and each individual event or modulation cycle is perceived as a separate entity. In speech, this range corresponds to the occurrence rate of words and in music to the slower range of rhythm. Modulation rates between 4 and 20–30 Hz are perceived as fluctuations, i.e., individual cycles are still discernable but more difficult to count or to assign a precise moment of occurrence (Fastl et al., 1986). In speech this range is associated with the occurrence rate of syllables and phonemes, and in music it covers faster rhythms and sequences of notes. From ~30 to ~300 Hz a sensation referred to as roughness is associated with SAMs (although that sensation is not limited to SAM signals). Each stimulus cycle is not perceived individually, but the rapid sequence of events creates a continuous, uniform sensation. Maximum roughness is usually perceived around modulation rates of 70-Hz or slightly below, depending on the carrier frequency (Fastl, 1990). This range partially overlaps with that of the fundamental frequency in speech and the pitch of musical instruments. Modulation frequencies between 30 and ~800 Hz also create a percept of tonal quality, the residue or periodicity pitch, which is closely matched to the pitch produced by a pure tone with a frequency of f_m. The perceptual distinctions noted above for different ranges of the modulation spectrum underscore the notion that temporal analysis plays a critical role in identifying, segregating, and discriminating natural sounds and helps in determining the nature of the sound source, its location, and the information carried by the sound.

6.3 Analysis of neural responses to SAM: VS and MTFs

The physiological responses to SAM stimuli that have typically been measured consist of spike trains recorded from neurons at different stages of the auditory pathway. Although many methods for analyzing spike trains exist, the response measures that have been applied to SAM data almost universally are (1) the discharge rate, in spikes per second, averaged over multiple cycles of the SAM stimulus; and (2) an envelope synchronization measure that relates the time of spike occurrence to the phase of the modulating waveform. By far the most common measure of synchrony is vector strength (VS; Goldberg and Brown, 1969), which can be computed by normalizing the spectral magnitude of the peristimulus time histogram at the modulating frequency (f_m) by the average spike rate. More commonly, VS is calculated by treating each recorded spike as a unit vector that 'points' towards the phase that the modulating waveform achieved when the spike occurred (0 to 2π). The spikes ($i = 1 \ldots n$) are summed vectorially, and normalized by the total number of spikes, n, such that:

$$VS = \sqrt{\left(\sum x_i\right)^2 + \left(\sum y_i\right)^2}/n.$$

The angle of the resultant vector is the mean phase of the response. If all spikes occur at the same point in the modulation cycle, the VS will equal 1. If spike times are distributed uniformly in the modulation period, the VS will equal 0. However, there are many other ways for VS to equal 0, because spikes occurring 180° out of phase cancel each other in the vector summation. Significant synchronization is generally assessed by the Rayleigh test for circular distributions using the quantity $2nVS^2$. It is also common to report the degree of response synchronization relative to the stimulus modulation in terms of modulation gain, in decibels, as 20 log (2VS/m), where m is the modulation depth.

Because VS is integral to the vast majority of physiological studies of SAM processing, it is important to understand what aspects of the neural response VS does and does not embrace (for a more detailed discussion, see Joris *et al.*, 2004). Fundamentally, VS is a measure of how narrowly distributed spike times are within the modulation period histogram (MPH, the histogram of neural response times relative to the modulation cycle period; see Fig. 6.2). It is a measure of 'synchrony' only insofar as the spikes are understood to be synchronized to a single phase – or time point – of the modulation waveform. For example, a neuron that reliably fired spikes at two different points in the modulation waveform would yield VS values that decrease with the phase separation of those two points, reaching 0 when they are 180° out of phase. This means that higher VS values indicate 'better synchronization' only if the underlying model for the neuron's optimal encoding of SAM is a maximally peaked MPH.

Of course, there are alternatives to this underlying model. For example, the vector strength of the sinusoidal modulating waveform itself is 0.5, and that of a half-rectified sinusoid is 0.784. If the faithful representation of the modulating waveform is taken as the optimal encoding, then either of these values could be taken as 'ideal', and the shape of the MPH should be sinusoidal (with a degree of rectification set by the spontaneous rate, for example), rather than sharply peaked. Alternatively, the encoding process could be evaluated in terms of the 'instantaneous' amplitude of the SAM stimulus. For example, neurons that give sustained responses to tones might be expected to produce 'notched' MPHs in response to fully modulated SAM stimuli at low modulation frequencies, and high carrier levels; that is, the brief decrement in level occurring at 270° (for SAM modulated in sine phase) is represented faithfully by a concomitant reduction in the instantaneous probability of discharge, as shown in Fig. 6.2C, D. Despite being a faithful representation of the stimulus amplitude, VS will be very low (0.22 in the example shown in Fig. 6.2) since the cell is firing spikes at nearly all phases of the MPH. Although VS is typically used interchangeably with 'synchrony' – and we too shall uphold this convention – the reliance on VS as the sole metric for temporal encoding carries an implicit judgment that 'time-stamping' a particular phase of the modulating waveform is paramount.

A useful distinction can be drawn between the synchrony and the fidelity of the neural response. If a given SAM stimulus consistently results in an MPH with a particular shape, one would say that the given SAM stimulus is encoded with high fidelity. The foregoing 'notched' MPH is a good example of a response exhibiting high fidelity but low VS. The notion of fidelity is particularly relevant to a further distinction between the encoding of SAM generally and the encoding of modulation frequency specifically. Consider a perfect synchronizer, a neuron that always produces a VS approaching 1 for SAM stimuli. A spike-time histogram of this neuron's response

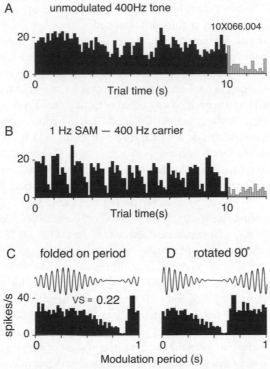

Fig. 6.2 Construction of the modulation period histogram (MPH). **A** Peristimulus time histogram (PSTH) of the responses to an unmodulated tone. Histograms of spikes occurring during the tone duration are shown in *black* and histograms of spikes occurring during the interstimulus intervals are shown in *gray*. **B** PSTH of responses to 100% modulated SAM at 1 Hz. **C** The MPH was constructed by folding the PSTH in **B** on the modulation period (1 s). The stimulus icon indicates the relative amplitude of the SAM stimulus at different phases of the modulation period. **D** The MPH shown in **C** has been rotated so that the instantaneous amplitude minimum of the stimulus is centered, and the responses at the beginning and end of the MPH in **C** appear contiguously because the time axis in this representation is circular. These data were obtained from recordings of a neuron in the primary auditory cortex of an awake rhesus monkey. (With permission of Malone *et al.*, 2007.)

would unambiguously indicate the modulation frequency of the SAM stimulus, regardless of what the modulation depth or carrier level happened to be. However, what if the goal were not discrimination of the modulation frequency but determination of the SAM stimulus itself, in the four-dimensional parameter space of all possible SAM stimuli? In this case, the perfect synchronizer would hinder discrimination of SAM parameters other than modulation frequency, unless those were somehow retained as differences in average firing rate, or in the mean phase of the MPH, because the shapes of the MPHs are highly constrained. As Joris *et al.* (2004: p.546) noted, VS 'does not capture the full harmonic content of the cycle histogram at f_m so that histograms with rather different shape can result in the same [VS] value'. Nevertheless, progressively higher values of VS do increasingly curtail the shapes of the MPHs that are compatible with them, which may constitute an important limit for encoding the shape of the envelope (Swarbrick and Whitfield, 1972), if not for modulation frequency coding. Thus, one cannot safely assume that 'better synchronization' is always equivalent to 'better encoding' of a time-varying stimulus – different aspects of the stimuli may require different codes.

Finally, we emphasize that VS is an analytical tool developed for a limited set of experimental contexts and requires knowledge of f_m, when one of the tasks of the brain, presumably, is estimation of f_m. More importantly, the notion of synchrony embodied by VS is inapplicable when the envelope of the acoustic signal is nonperiodic, as is the case for most natural sounds. Alternatives to VS and VS-based metrics have been developed recently (e.g., Kajikawa and Hackett, 2005; Joris et al., 2006; Malone et al., 2007) and we will discuss their application in a later section.

The predominant response metric for neural responses to SAM is the modulation transfer function (MTF), which describes how the response changes as a function of different modulation frequencies. Typically, responses to SAM are characterized in terms of average firing rate, VS, and mean phase; when these quantities are plotted against modulation frequency, we shall refer to them as the rate MTF (rMTF), temporal MTF (tMTF), and phase MTF (pMTF), respectively. In some cases, the average firing rate and the VS are combined, via multiplication, into what is termed the 'phase-locked rate' or 'synchronized rate'. Note that the tMTF, pMTF, and synchronizarion rate all depend on VS, and inherit its limitations.

Each MTF represents a slice through the four-dimensional SAM parameter space. MTFs are most commonly obtained for fully modulated (m = 1) SAM stimuli at the neuron's characteristic frequency and best level, or at a fixed level with respect to the neuron's response threshold. Many of the studies we review in the following sections have also reported MTFs at a range of carrier levels and modulation depths, and in a few cases carrier frequencies. A chief goal of research in this vein has been characterization of the changes in temporal coding that occur as one records from neurons at successively more central nuclei in the auditory pathway.

Analysis of corresponding changes in the shape of the MTF has been central to this endeavor. This often involves categorization of MTF in terms of filter shape categories such as lowpass, bandpass, or highpass (and, in some instances, flat or band-reject, etc.), and identification of the best modulation frequencies (BMFs) for both rate and synchrony. The representativeness of these summary measures, if derived from a single MTF, will depend on the extent to which MTF shape is invariant to changes in SAM parameters other than f_m. Importantly, MTFs have nothing to say about the reproducibility of the responses, nor do they provide an explicit means for determining how well different SAM stimuli can be discriminated from one another (Wohlgemuth and Ronacher, 2007).

In the next few sections, we will examine how the nature of SAM coding varies across different nuclei in the ascending auditory pathway, with an eye towards relating changes in temporal coding to other general changes in the response properties of more central neurons. An important confound to keep in mind is the increasing effects of anesthetics on more central structures (Ter-Mikaelian et al., 2007), as well as other factors such as the increasing prevalence of nonmonotonic tuning for SPL (Semple and Kitzes, 1993a, b; Phillips et al., 1994; Malone et al., 2007) and transient responses to tonal stimuli. Our goal is not a comprehensive review of the literature (for that see Joris et al., 2004), but rather a survey of the implications for temporal coding revealed by a selection of representative studies.

6.4 Auditory nerve

In a comprehensive study of SAM coding in cat auditory nerve (AN), Joris and Yin (1992) noted, 'To a first approximation, the behavior of AN fibers to changes in SPL of an AM signal can be predicted by considering the compressive shape of its rate-level curve as an input-output curve' (see also Yates, 1987). Since AN fibers contain all the information about the auditory signal that will ever be available to central processors, this simple model represents a baseline for evaluating central transformations in how SAM is encoded. For example, Smith and Brachman (1980) demonstrated much earlier that for some modulation frequencies (roughly 150–300 Hz) the modulation gain of AN fibers could be predicted fairly accurately by considering the slope of the rate level function in the appropriate SPL range.

The activity recorded from AN fibers in response to SAM stimuli closely resembles the actual stimulus waveform. If the carrier frequency is below a few kiloHertz, this representation includes phase locking to both the fine structure and the envelope of the modulating waveform (Joris and Yin, 1992; Fig. 6.3A). Because f_m is quite low (10 Hz, m = 0.99) in this example, the relationship with the instantaneous amplitude is particularly clear: as the carrier level is increased from 39 to 104 dB SPL, the SAM stimulus falls below the fiber's threshold for a smaller fraction of the MPH. This can be seen in the progressive narrowing of the notch near 270° (0.75 cycles), which also results in a dramatic reduction in VS. This nonmonotonic relationship between VS and stimulus level was universal in AN fibers. Note that in low CF fibers, phase locking to the carrier increased monotonically with stimulus level, indicating that the reduction in envelope VS was not a loss of temporal resolution per se. Average rate responses increased monotonically with level, as expected from the sigmoidal shape of AN rate-level functions. The mean phase of the MPH evidenced slight but measurable increases in phase lead with respect to the envelope, an effect that the authors attributed to adaptation. Finally, changes in the carrier frequency were shown to be essentially equivalent to reducing the stimulus level, since using a non-optimal f_c shifted the modulated rate and VS functions to the right on the SPL axis.

Another universal feature of AN responses to SAM is the monotonic increase in VS for increasing modulation depths. As is evident in Fig. 6.3B, MPHs obtained from AN fibers tend to be relatively isomorphic to the half-rectified SAM waveform. At low modulation depths, AN responses exhibit more modulation than the SAM envelopes (i.e., have a modulation gain > 0 dB), but all AN fibers exhibit monotonic increases in VS when the modulation depth is increased. The foregoing observations reflect the general applicability of an amplitude-based model for predicting how AN fibers will behave when SAM parameters other than f_m are varied. Historically, however, the primary motivation for most SAM studies relates to modulation frequency coding. Once again, AN fibers exhibit highly stereotyped responses to increases in modulation frequency. rMTFs are generally flat (see below), and tMTFs are lowpass, though with a shallow decline toward low f_m. As was discussed, modulation gain is highest for low modulation depths and low SPLs, so modulation gain functions (i.e., 20 $\log_{10}$ (tMTF/m)) from the same fiber but obtained at different modulation depths, or carrier levels, would be vertically displaced on a modulation frequency axis like that of Fig. 6.3C, where a single modulation gain function is shown. Because of spectral filtering, modulation gain functions from fibers that differ in CF would be horizontally displaced on the f_m axis. Recall that the spectrum of a SAM signal has sidebands at $f_c \pm f_m$ (Fig. 6.1B). As f_m increases, the sidebands become increasingly distant from f_c, and eventually fall outside of the spectral filter bandwidth of the AN fiber. Since spectral bandwidth is proportional to CF, the 3-dB corner frequency of the modulation gain function is proportional to both CF and tuning curve bandwidth, with maximal values as high as 1500 Hz. Nevertheless, there was a saturating trend that suggested that temporal factors limited synchronization at high CFs. It is also worth noting that both VS maxima and the VS cutoffs for f_c were significantly greater than those obtained for f_m, suggesting that the mechanisms limiting temporal resolution to the carrier fine structure and the modulation envelope may not be strictly equivalent (for a discussion see Joris and Yin, 1992).

The pMTFs of AN fibers were also highly stereotyped and, in this case, linear. When the cumulative phase of the response is plotted against f_m, the slope of the resulting function provides an

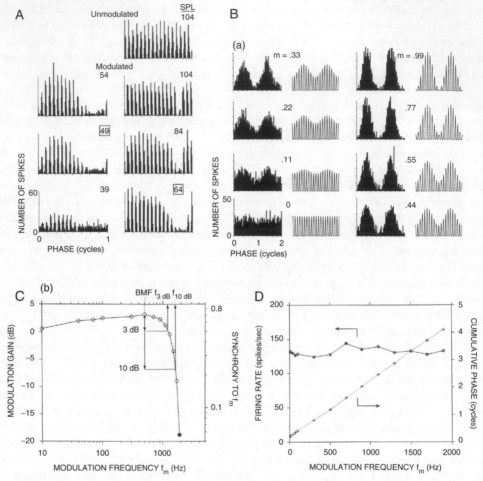

Fig. 6.3 Responses of auditory nerve (AN) fibers. **A** and **B** MPHs of the responses of an AN fiber to SAM at increasing carrier levels (indicated by the *insets*, in decibels of sound pressure level (dB SPL)). These responses exhibit phase locking to the carrier (170 Hz) and to the modulation (10 Hz). As the carrier level increases, phase locking to the carrier remains robust, and those phasic responses occupy greater portions of the modulation cycle, vanishing only during a narrow portion of the modulation period near the amplitude minimum of the stimulus (0.75 cycles, or 270°, for SAM in sine phase), as in Fig. 6.2B). MPHs comprising two modulation cycles are compared to half-wave rectified illustrations of SAM waveforms across modulation depth (f_m = 100 Hz; SPL = 49 dB; f_c = 20.2 kHz). **C** The modulation transfer function (MTF) of a typical AN fiber is shown relative to synchrony (VS; tMTF), and modulation gain (20 log (2VS/m)). The 3- and 10-dB cutoff values are indicated by *arrows*. **D** The MTF for the responses depicted in **C** is shown plotted against firing rate (rMTF) and cumulative phase (pMTF; note that a linear rather than logarithmic f_m axis is shown to indicate the linear relationship between cumulative phase and f_m). These data were obtained in the auditory nerve of anesthetized cats. (With permission of Joris and Yin, 1992.)

estimate of the cochlear group delay, which was found to vary inversely with the CF of the fibers (approximately 7 to 2 ms), as expected from the propagation of the traveling wave along the basilar membrane (Fig. 6.3D). The y-intercept of these functions converged on 0.25 cycles, which represents the instantaneous amplitude maximum for SAM signals presented in sine phase.

Thus far, we have treated AN fibers as homogenous – which, relative to central auditory neurons, they are – but AN fibers do fall into two groups, defined largely by differences in their spontaneous rates (SRs). Maximal VS values were inversely correlated with SR, as one might expect from the simple notion that spontaneous spikes distributed randomly throughout the modulation period would tend to reduce VS. In addition, low SR fibers, but not high SR fibers, typically showed a (>20%) reduction in average firing rate as f_m increased. However, Cooper *et al.* (1993) noted that the synchronized rate of high SR fibers exceeds that of low SR fibers due to their higher firing rates overall. In the absence of knowledge of how SAM is encoded – given that it is highly unlikely that VS can be computed by the brain at all – it is difficult to parse the relative contributions of high and low SR fibers to this process. Nevertheless, it does seem likely that the existence of these two fiber classes serves to extend the range of amplitude changes that can be encoded.

6.5 **Cochlear nuclei**

Møller's (1972, 1974, 1976) pioneering studies of the cochlear nuclei (CN) documented high fidelity representations of the stimulus envelopes, enhanced modulation gain (relative to the AN) over large ranges of carrier levels, higher tolerance for background noise, and impressive constancy of tMTF shapes for different stimulus types, such as SAM applied to both tones and noise carriers, and both noise-modulated tonal and noise carriers. Neurons of the CN also exhibit a striking degree of diversity in response to pure tones relative to the AN, and these physiological differences have been successfully mapped to several distinct morphological classes. Typically, the CN is subdivided into anteroventral (AVCN), posteroventral (PVCN), and dorsal (DCN) nuclei. Unsurprisingly, differences in pure tone responses among the cell classes of the CN also extend to SAM stimuli.

The different response classes, their morphologies, and their distributions within the divisions of the CN have been reviewed in detail elsewhere (see Frisina, 2001). We focus on the aspects of SAM responses in the CN that diverge most powerfully from those of AN fibers. Figure 6.4 captures a number of the differences, which have been evaluated almost entirely in the context of tMTFs. In addition to AN fiber responses (A), the seven major response classes depicted here are as follows (see Blackburn and Sachs, 1989; Rhode and Greenberg, 1992; Chapter 2, this Volume): B – primary-like (spherical bushy, AVCN); C – onset (octopus, PVCN); D – primary-like with notch (globular busy, AVCN); E – onset-chopper (multipolar stellate, PVCN); F – chopper-sustained (stellate); G – chopper-transient (stellate); and H – pauser/buildup (fusiform, DCN). At a glance, the major differences between the AN (A) and the CN (B–H) are the increased prevalence of bandpass-tuned tMTFs and the reduction in the VS cutoffs. As we will see, both of these trends remain consistent at progressively more central auditory structures.

Traditionally, the relative increase in VS has received the most attention (e.g., Frisina *et al.*, 1990), and this increase is most pronounced at higher sound levels, which significantly depress VS values in the AN. In a comprehensive study of the CN of the cat, Rhode and Greenberg (1994) ordered the various CN cell classes largely in terms of their tMTFs. Obviously, primary-like neurons responded much like (high SR) AN fibers and had the highest synchrony cutoffs. Chopper, onset-L, and pauser/buildup were described as being roughly comparable to low SR fibers, while onset-chopper and pauser/buildup neurons possessed 'considerably enhanced' phase-locking to f_m relative to other CN neurons.

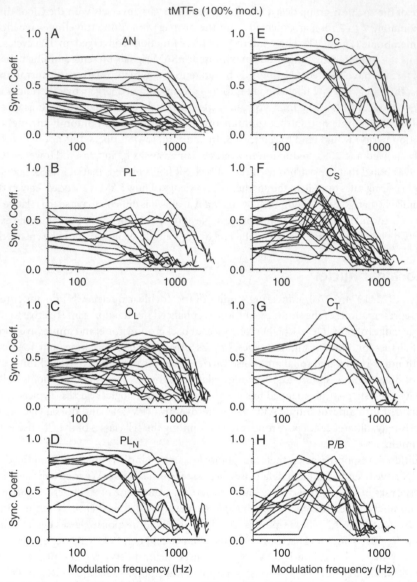

Fig. 6.4 Comparison of tMTFs obtained in the auditory nerve (AN) (**A**) and cochlear nucleus (CN) (**B–H**). The tMTFs obtained from different cell classes in the AN and CN indicate the diversity of the MTF shapes in the early auditory system. Each *curve* represents the response of a different cell, and all stimuli were 100% modulated and presented at 50 or 60 dB SPL. The cell classes were: **A** auditory nerve; **B** primary-like; **C** onset-L; **D** primary-like with notch; **E** onset-chopper; **F** chopper-sustained; **G** chopper-transient; **H** pauser/buildup. These data were obtained in the CN of anesthetized cats. (With permission of Rhode and Greenberg, 1994.)

Nevertheless, it is not entirely clear what this 'enhanced' synchrony means for temporal coding. A class of onset cells (Oi) (Rhode, 1994) shows the highest modulation gain of the CN cell classes (i.e., the amount by which modulation depth in the response exceeds the modulation depth in the stimulus). Their tMTFs also appear to be invariant to SPL, and many even exhibit sharply band-pass rMTFs with rBMFs from 300–500 Hz. Relative to AN fibers – or the primary-like neurons of the CN – Oi units appear to engage in a distinct and novel form of temporal coding. Specifically, they appear to embody the 'perfect synchronizer' discussed previously, since the invariance of their tMTFs to carrier level also implies a loss of information about carrier level. Conversely, the low VS values obtained from primary-like neurons for low depth, high level SAM signify the retention of information about 'instantaneous' SPL. The responses of onset (and onset-chopper) units, by contrast, sacrifice the encoding of amplitude in favor of encoding changes in amplitude.

The remaining cell classes in the CN fall between these extremes, and it has been proposed that this menagerie comprises a set of parallel pathways for auditory processing. It seems plausible that the different cell classes are specialized for extracting different features of acoustic signals, such as the envelope shape versus the stimulus periodicity. Before accepting the notion that higher VS values represent a true 'enhancement' of temporal coding in the CN, however, it would be instructive to perform an analysis that explicitly tests how well SAM stimuli can be identified on the basis of spike trains obtained from different cell classes in the CN, particularly for the (low) f_m ranges where low VS values for high carrier levels reflect sustained firing throughout the modulation period. It is worth noting that Rhode and Greenberg's (1994) study was restricted to f_m above 50 Hz, which is substantially higher than the modulation range (>20 Hz) most important for communication sounds, including human speech (e.g., Drullman et al., 1994; Drullman, 1995).

6.6 Superior olivary complex and lateral lemniscus

Relatively few studies have examined responses to SAM in the superior olivary complex (SOC) or the nuclei of the lateral lemniscus (NLL). Kuwada and Batra (1999) recorded from monaural units in the SOC of awake rabbits. These units were recorded within the SOC, but outside the principal binaural nuclei of the SOC and the lateral and medial superior olivary nuclei. The authors observed two distinct response types with respect to pure tones. 'Sustained' neurons responded in a sustained fashion to tones, and included a number of the response types observed in the CN (chopper, pauser, etc.). 'Off' neurons ceased to fire during tone presentation, but fired a 'rebound' response at tone offset, a discharge pattern that has rarely been observed in the CN. Both of these response classes exhibited wider dynamic ranges for sound amplitude than did the neurons of the CN.

The responses of sustained and off neurons are essentially complementary. Sustained neurons respond at the envelope maximum (0.25 cycles for signals in sine phase), which suggests that their responses reflect excitation, whereas off neurons respond immediately prior to the envelope minimum (0.75 cycles), suggesting that their responses reflect a rebound from inhibition that prevailed during the period of maximum amplitude. The differences in the shape of the sustained and off MTFs are consistent with these observations. The most obvious difference – the dramatic relative increase in VS values for off neurons – reflects the fact that the envelope trough occupies a relatively small fraction of the modulation period. As a result, off neuron VS values were very high (>0.9) even at the lowest tested f_m (25 Hz), resulting in lowpass tMTFs. Sustained neurons, by contrast, exhibited bandpass tMTFs at moderate carrier levels, and had modulation gains statistically comparable to those measured in the CN. Off neuron tMTFs were uniform across modulation depth (Fig. 6.5) because of the strong constraints on when spikes could occur (i.e., during rebounds from high amplitudes).

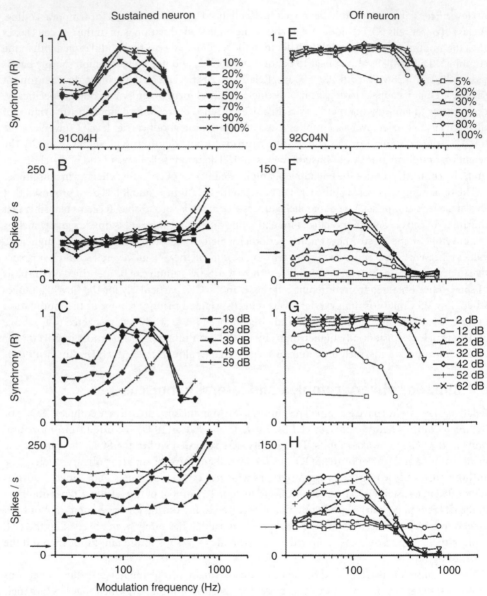

Fig. 6.5 Comparison of tMTFs (**A**, **C**, **E**, **G**) and rMTFs (**B**, **D**, **F**, **H**) obtained from a sustained (*left column*) and an off (*right column*) neuron of the superior olivary complex (SOC). The striking differences between the rMTFS and tMTFs of these two neurons indicate that the character of the response to pure tones crucially informs the responses to modulated stimuli. Modulation depth was varied as indicated in the *upper four panels* (**A**, **B**, **E**, **F**), using a stimulus intensity of 29 dB SPL for the sustained neuron and 28 dB SPL for the off neuron. Carrier level was varied as indicated in the *lower four panels* (**C**, **D**, **G**, **H**), using a modulation depth of 80%. *Horizontal arrows* indicate the spontaneous rate. These data were obtained in the SOC of awake rabbits. (With permission of Kuwada and Batra, 1999.)

Off neurons showed a strong monotonic dependence of average rate on modulation depth – at low depths the envelope troughs are rarely sufficient to release the neuron from inhibition, resulting in few spikes – but in contrast there was a nonmonotonic dependence of average rate on carrier level. Low carrier levels produce less inhibition, limiting the magnitude of a potential rebound. At sufficiently high carrier levels, envelope troughs (for m = 80%) might not be deep enough to release the neuron from inhibition (alternatively, level-related latency effects could apply, as suggested by the authors). Off-neuron tMTFs were monotonic with level. Sustained neurons, by contrast, showed monotonic increases in average firing rate with increasing carrier level, as well as the familiar lowpass to bandpass transition caused by reduction in VS at low (<100 Hz) f_ms. Interestingly, the tBMFs for sustained neurons often shifted to higher values as the level was increased. The lack of invariance of the tBMF to level changes is relevant because it is required if neurons are to function as 'modulation filterbanks' for signal envelopes.

It was only very recently that responses to SAM were recorded from the ventral nucleus of the lateral lemniscus (VNLL; Batra, 2006; unanaesthetized rabbits), a major source of monaural inhibition to the inferior colliculus. The responses there fell into two main categories: neurons with sustained responses to tones typically had flat rMTFs, and lowpass or bandpass tMTFs. Neurons with onset responses to tones, by contrast, had bandpass rMTFs and 'flat' tMTFs. Such bandpass rMTFs are reminiscent of those described for Oi neurons of the CN (weak bandpass tuning was also observed for a few onset-choppers (Rhode, 1994; Rhode and Greenberg, 1994)), and much is made of their appearance because of the notion that a conversion from a 'temporal code' to a[n] '[average] rate code' for modulation frequency occurs in the ascending auditory pathway (Langner and Schreiner, 1988; Hewitt and Meddis, 1994). Batra (2006) also cites the wide distribution of rBMFs (14–283 Hz) as being compatible with a rate-based modulation filterbank in the subcortical auditory system.

There is an obvious correspondence between tone PSTH shapes and MTF shapes, and the responses of onset neurons appear compatible with the notion that these cells fire an onset response to each cycle of the (100% modulated) SAM stimulus, as if each cycle were a separate tone. The mean response phase coincided with the rising phase of the envelope, and the population mean of the slopes of the function relating f_m to discharge rate (below the rBMF) was 1, indicating that the firing rate was roughly proportional to the number of such 'tone onsets'. Above the rBMF, however, it would appear that these pseudo-onsets occur too rapidly with regard to local integration and/or adaptation time constants to elicit spikes effectively.

In the context of this explanation, one must ask whether this represents a true 'temporal to rate' conversion for the representation of modulation frequency. Instead, one could also refer to it as an 'instantaneous' rate code for rapid amplitude increases, since the rBMF is essentially set by a temporal resolution limit for f_m. When nearly all spikes are elicited by large, rapid, excursions in amplitude, then modulation frequency tuning for SAM cannot be differentiated from sensitivity to the rise-time ('attack') of sound envelopes, which is not 'temporal' filtering as it is typically understood. More importantly, if restrictions on the carrier level or modulation depth of SAM stimuli effectively eliminate the responses of such neurons, this would complicate the argument that they encode modulation frequency, rather than simply responding to sufficiently large amplitude transients. The currently available data are not sufficient to disambiguate these competing interpretations. More fundamentally, however, it is not clear that one should describe such responses as 'encoding' the modulation envelope at high gain, since only a single feature of the envelope – its rising phase – is represented in the spike train.

6.7 **Inferior colliculus**

Setting aside the teleology of bandpass rMTFs, their prevalence in SAM responses obtained from neurons in the inferior colliculus (IC) has been extensively documented, at least in the central nucleus (ICc). As an obligatory relay of the primary lemniscal pathway, the IC performs an important integrative role, gathering inputs from subcortical and cortical areas. By the level of the IC, the response characteristics of the typical neuron are quite different from those observed in AN fibers. For example, the relationship between the CF and the synchrony cutoff no longer strictly prevails, as is true of many of the response classes in the CN, excepting the primary-like and onset-L neurons. Rees and Møller (1987) noted that the restriction of VS cutoffs to values below 360 Hz in the IC could not be explained by bandwidth limitations, and suggested instead that central limitations on VS for high f_ms were related to the 'number of synapses interposed between the sound input and the colliculus.' (p. 140). On average, VS cutoffs drop by about one half between the CN and ICc, and these authors reported modal tBMFs in a range from 100–120 Hz (anesthetized rat). In the anesthetized gerbil, only 15% of neurons had significant VS above 300 Hz (Krishna and Semple, 2000). This progressive reduction in VS cutoffs is the most obvious, and perhaps most important, trend in the ascending auditory pathway (see Joris *et al.*, 2004, their Fig. 9).

At low modulation frequencies and low modulation depths, however, the opposing trend of increased VS from AN to CN also continues in the IC. Relative to the CN, IC neurons generally showed higher maximum VS values and higher VS for low modulation depths (with the exception of CN onset-choppers), which compresses the metric's dynamic range and steepens the decline of modulation gain with increasing modulation depth (Krishna and Semple, 2000). As was true of the CN, a qualitatively similar transition from lowpass to bandpass tMTFs has been observed in the IC by a number of investigators in a number of species. The tMTFs of a few units did not exhibit this shift; in keeping with the role of the IC as an integrative center, Krishna and Semple (2000) recorded both onset neurons (their Fig. 5) and a single offset neuron (their Fig. 8) whose responses were strongly reminiscent of the SAM responses of VNLL onset and SOC offset neurons described above, albeit shifted to lower ranges of f_m.

The shapes of tMTFs are also sensitive to changes in carrier level and carrier frequency. Rees and Palmer (1989) demonstrated that it was possible to reverse the lowpass to bandpass shift in the tMTF shape by adding broadband noise (critically, however, neurons that were driven by continuous noise were excluded from this analysis). They also demonstrated that neurons with nonmonotonic tuning for sound level could also exhibit a return from bandpass to lowpass tMTFs at high levels. The increased heterogeneity of tuning for sound level in the IC (Semple and Kitzes, 1993a,b) may explain the increased heterogeneity of level-based tMTF changes there (Krishna and Semple, 2000). Changes in carrier frequency tended to reproduce changes in tMTF shape observed for changes in carrier level in a given neuron, such that mismatching the carrier frequency to the BF was roughly equivalent to reducing the SPL. Interestingly, the high f_m slope of tMTFs is relatively invariant to parametric changes in SAM stimuli, suggesting that the reduction in VS at high f_ms reflects genuine and inflexible limits on temporal resolution, rather than the 'artificial' reductions in VS that occur when neurons track amplitude changes throughout the modulation cycle at low f_ms.

Relative to other brainstem nuclei, the rMTFs of IC neurons are more commonly and more sharply tuned to f_m (Langner and Schreiner, 1988). In the anesthetized gerbil, where the shapes of rMTFs were examined in most detail, the maximum rBMF was 140 Hz and over half were less than 25 Hz (Krishna and Semple, 2000). However, in cat IC, approximately 25% of the rBMFs were above 100 Hz and as high as several hundred Hertz (Langner and Schreiner, 1988). Such differences in the overall estimate of temporal coding capacity may be influenced by species-specific differences and also by the uniformity of spatial sampling throughout a given structure due to the observation that the distribution of response preferences may not be spatially uniform (Schreiner and Langner, 1988).

The shapes of the rMTFs of the IC are also substantially more diverse (Fig. 6.6). For example, Krishna and Semple (2000) observed not only rBMFs, but also f_m ranges where the firing rate was significantly suppressed ('worst' modulation frequencies, or WMFs) in slightly less than half of IC neurons, and occasionally (eight neurons) a secondary f_m range where the average firing rate resurged, though VS was low. As was true of the VNLL, particular rMTF shapes tended to be associated with particular tone response classes: the rMTFs of onset and onset-sustained neurons contained a suppressive region more rarely (3/21) than did sustained or pauser neurons (19/24). In general, the shapes of rMTFs were constant, but scaled in magnitude as the modulation depth increased. Experiments that varied the carrier frequencies for SAM were also used to demonstrate that the suppressive regions were not related to sideband inhibition, suggesting a temporal basis for the phenomenon.

Changes in carrier level tended to produce more complex changes in IC rMTFs, including substantial variation in the rBMF. Krishna and Semple (2000) did not find a consistent trend, but did report that the variation was substantial, exceeding 66% of the mean BMF in half of the neurons tested over an SPL range of 20 dB or more. This finding poses a difficulty for theories that view the tuning of rMTFs as evidence for neural filters tuned to particular f_ms. There is a correlation between the minimum response latency to tones and the rBMF in the IC, but it appears to be different from that observed in the AN (see above), since the correlation between response latency and CF no longer prevails in the IC. There is also a correlation between the rBMF and the shape of the tMTF, such that neurons that have a clearly defined rBMF typically exhibit maximal VS at the same f_m.

Of course, it should be noted that if there is reason to believe that firing rates of neurons with transient responses to tones increase quasi-linearly up to a fixed limit of temporal resolution — as suggested by the onset neurons of the VNLL, for example – the foregoing correlation between the rBMF and tBMF is to be expected. It would be of interest to know the extent to which correlations of this sort are predictable in terms of PSTH classifications such as onset versus sustained. Similar analyses would apply to the magnitudes of lowpass to bandpass shifts with increasing SPL at low f_ms, too.

In fact, the relationship between firing rate and VS is an important one, in part because the two show increasing interdependence in the ascending auditory pathway. In the AN, where rMTFs are flat, the relationship is absent: if there is no rBMF, it cannot predict the tMTF. The relationship is likely to reflect adaptive mechanisms sensitive to recent history of stimulation (or response).

Rees and Palmer (1989) reported a similar finding –43% of IC neurons had coincident tBMFs and rBMFs. Nevertheless, they also found that modulation gain for f_ms less than 50 Hz was inversely correlated with the discharge rate elicited by either tones or SAM at equivalent levels. Generally speaking, lower discharge rates favor higher values of VS because of how VS is calculated. Krishna and Semple (2000) noted that the suppressive regions of the rMTF where firing rates were low were also often associated with high VS values. These findings seem contradictory until one considers that the typical tBMF peaked between 50 and 100 Hz (Langner and Schreiner, 1988; Rees and Palmer, 1989). The relevant metric is the spikes per modulation cycle elicited by a SAM stimulus, because every spike fired in the same modulation cycle must occur at a different phase, reducing the VS in proportion to its difference from the mean phase. As one ascends the auditory pathway, however, there is a gradual reduction in absolute discharge rates. In the f_m range where a neuron fires less than a single spike per cycle, on average, an increase in firing rate introduced by increasing the carrier level may not significantly impact the VS because the

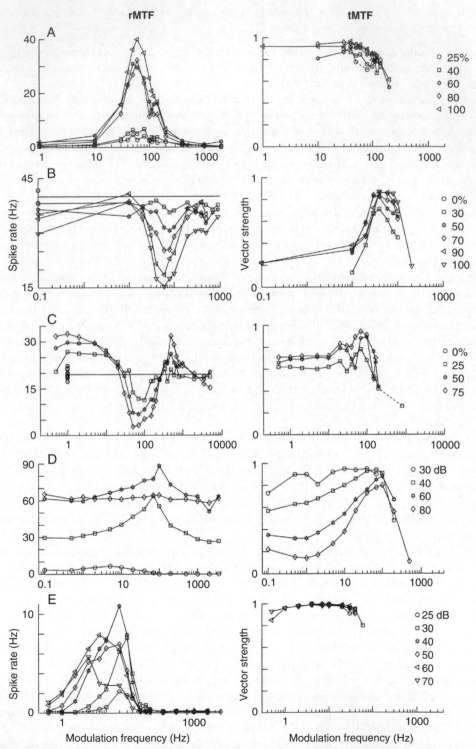

Fig. 6.6 Comparison of MTFs obtained in the inferior colliculus (IC) across modulation depth (**A–C**) and carrier level (**D** and **E**) for five single neurons. rMTFs and tMTFs are shown side by side, and the *symbols* used to plot each *curve* indicate the stimulus values. The stimulus intensities for **A**, **B**, and **C** were 50, 70, and 40 dB SPL, respectively. Modulation depth was 100% for **D** and **E**. **A–C** show cells that show bandpass enhancement and/or suppression with change in modulation depth. **D** and **E** show level dependencies in sustained neurons (**D**) and onset neurons (**E**). These data were obtained in the central nucleus of IC in anesthetized gerbils. (With permission of Krishna and Semple, 2000.)

additional spikes may fall in cycles where spikes would otherwise not have occurred. At very low modulation frequencies, however, IC neurons commonly fire multiple spikes per modulation cycle. At a minimum, refractory periods enforce a degree of scatter in phase, such that 'additional' spikes at higher levels are likely to reduce the VS. Although it is common to think of VS in terms of temporal resolution and filter bandwidths, it must be remembered that all VS calculations ultimately derive from spikes, and the number of spikes per cycle represents an ineradicable constraint on temporal coding.

6.8 Medial geniculate and auditory cortex

Relatively few studies have examined responses to SAM in the medial geniculate body (MGB). The bulk of more recent work has involved click trains or more complex dynamic stimuli. The most detailed of these (Preuss and Müller-Preuss, 1990), conducted in awake squirrel monkeys, was largely focused on MTF shape classification and tBMF determination, and reported a predominance of bandpass rMTFs and tMTFs, with tBMFs ranging from 2–128 Hz, and a mode at 32 Hz. On the other hand, SAM responses have been extensively studied in auditory cortex in a range of preparations and animal models. Because anesthetics affect cortical responses far more than those of subcortical nuclei (Ter-Merkaelian *et al.*, 2007), however, the results of studies conducted in awake and anesthetized animals differ (for a discussion of such differences see Liang *et al.*, 2002). For example, responses in awake animals extend to higher f_m ranges – VS cutoffs in awake rhesus monkeys could be as high as several hundred Hertz in a few cases (>600 Hz), and roughly one in ten neurons had significant VS at 200 Hz (Malone *et al.*, 2007). Comparable results were obtained for awake marmosets (Liang *et al.*, 2002). Nevertheless, both of the foregoing studies indicate that relative to the MGB and IC, auditory cortex does continue the trend of emphasizing very low (<20 Hz) modulation frequencies in terms of both average discharge rate and VS. Liang *et al.* (2002) reported that the vast majority (>80%) of tBMFs fell below 20 Hz; the distribution of rBMFs was wider, and distributed among higher values, with a mode at 16 Hz. Malone *et al.* (2007) found rBMF and tBMF modes at 5 Hz in macaque primary auditory cortex (AI). Different auditory cortical fields in the cat and squirrel monkey all follow the same general trend of low BMFs, but tend to have slightly different ranges of temporal encoding capacity, with BMFs in core or primary areas about twice that of belt or non-primary areas (Schreiner and Urbas, 1988; Bieser and Müller-Preuss, 1996).

The observation of progressive reduction in the upper limits of synchronized temporal encoding cannot solely be explained by an increase in the number of intervening synapses accompanied by increased temporal transmission jitter. Behavioral training of owl monkeys in an SAM discrimination task resulted in a doubling of their cortical BMFs and limiting frequencies (Beitel *et al.*, 2003). This suggests that the observed cortical emphasis on slower modulations is not a physiological limitation, but reflects specific processing strategies for different tasks as, for example, in auditory object formation and consideration of temporal contexts.

6.9 Codes of timing and codes for tasks

Having reported summary measures such as the rBMFs and tBMFs throughout the auditory pathway, it is necessary to ask again what such values mean for the encoding of time-varying sounds. In the context of a modulation filterbank hypothesis, BMFs capture the tuning of putative filters for different envelope periodicities. The relative degree of tuning expressed in the rMTF versus the tMTF has been thought to indicate the relative balance of 'temporal' and 'rate' codes for modulation frequency. The importance of (average) rate codes in the auditory pathway has been emphasized recently, and it has been postulated that two separate coding populations in auditory cortex exist: a synchronized population that encodes f_m via phase-locked responses, and a non-synchronized population that encodes f_m solely in terms of average discharge rate (for a review see Wang, 2007). In other words, the temporal-to-rate conversion is complete in the neurons of the non-synchronized population. This represents a specific instance of the more general transformation from a neural representation that is isomorphic to the stimulus, to one that is not (in principle, such a transformation could also exchange one temporal code for another). Currently, the evidence for this hypothesis is based primarily on responses to periodic click trains (Lu *et al.*, 2001). Although Liang *et al.* (2002) identified a substantial fraction (30–40%) of AI neurons in the awake marmoset as members of the non-synchronized population, neurons that exhibited rate tuning in the absence of synchrony at any tested f_m were rare (1.7%) in the cortex of rhesus monkeys (Malone *et al.*, 2007). Nevertheless, a significant percentage (16%) of such neurons did show significant variations in average discharge rate beyond their VS cutoffs, indicating that changes in firing rate were not strictly limited to modulation frequencies that elicited synchronized responses.

The suitability of different encoding schemes can be evaluated by determining the accuracy they allow for decoding stimulus information. For example, one can test the quality of 'rate' coding of SAM explicitly by asking how effectively one can guess the modulation frequency presented on a given trial based on the neural response (Foffani and Moxon, 2004).

Briefly, the responses to several different SAM frequencies are each summed and binned to create PSTH templates. Then, the response to a 'test' trial of a given SAM frequency is matched to the most similar template (e.g., using a Euclidean distance measure), and the stimulus used to generate the matching template is guessed, resulting in a confusion matrix of the actual stimuli and the guesses. For spike train classifiers of this sort, an average rate code is simply the limit case of a single bin whose width equals the 'test' duration, because the bin width determines the temporal precision of the code. Conversely, one can also eliminate average discharge rate information by normalizing the total spike counts across the templates, while preserving the relative distribution of spikes across the chosen time interval (the 'phase-only' classifier). In effect, this analysis 'flattens' the rMTF. Figure 6.7 shows the results of this analysis applied to SAM responses recorded from the cortices of awake rhesus macaques. Performance of the classifier using the full spike train is indicated along the abscissa in each panel. For modulation frequency, for example Fig. 6.7C, average firing rate information resulted in a significant improvement over chance performance in only a minority of neurons (36%), compared to 94% for the phase-only classifier. Overall, the case for average rate coding of SAM stimuli in the cortex was surprisingly weak. These data suggest that the code employed by the cortex involves spike phases, rather than spike counts – or, more properly, that the cortex counts spikes in windows narrower than a single modulation cycle for most of the tested f_ms.

The foregoing findings cast doubt on the relevance of cortical rMTFs for SAM frequency discrimination, and call into question the primacy of the MTF itself when one considers that cortical responses carried as much information about carrier level as they did about modulation frequency. This suggests that SAM encoding captures more about the stimulus envelope than its periodicity, and, as such, is fundamentally about envelope shape discrimination, rather than modulation frequency extraction. Figure 6.8 shows that the shapes of MPHs can reveal changes in f_m, depth, and level in ways that cannot be captured by VS alone. Malone *et al.* (2007) assayed the fidelity of MPH shapes by computing the 'trial similarity' (TS), which was simply the correlation between MPHs calculated from two separate SAM trials. Unlike VS, which depends on the shape (i.e., the narrowness) of the MPH, TS depends only on the reproducibility of the MPH. TS was shown to be highly predictive of the performance of the spike train classifiers discussed above, as

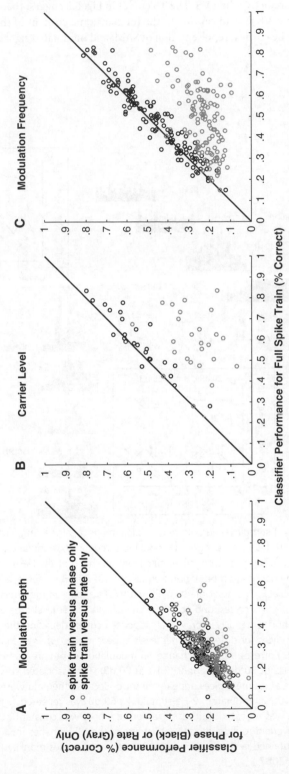

Fig. 6.7 SAM stimulus discrimination based on spike train analysis. The scatterplots compare the performance (in percent correct) of the full spike train classifier, which is plotted on the *abscissa*, to the performances of the classifiers using only information about spike phases (*black circles*) and average spike rate (*gray circles*), plotted on the *ordinate*. In **A**, the SAM stimuli varied in terms of modulation depth; in **B**, carrier level; and in **C**, modulation frequency. The *diagonal line* indicates equivalent performance. These data were obtained in the auditory cortex of awake rhesus monkeys. (With permission of Malone et al., 2007.)

well as being significantly more predictive than VS. The TS curves in Fig. 6.8 suggest that at very low modulation frequencies, what VS fails to capture – 'the full harmonic content of the cycle histogram' – is likely essential to the cortical representation of SAM, and modulated signals more generally.

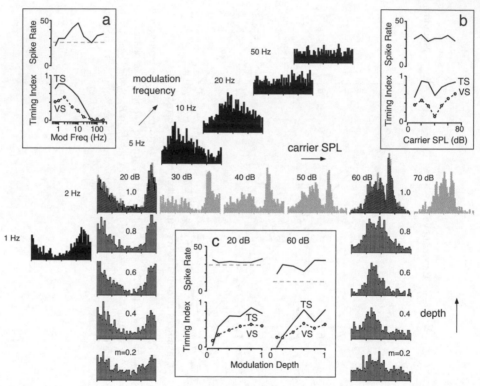

Fig. 6.8 MPH representations of SAM stimuli varying along multiple dimensions for a single neuron. The matrix of response profiles illustrates how changes in modulation frequency, modulation depth, and carrier level produce different but highly reproducible effects on the shape of the MPH. The response profiles corresponding to changes in modulation frequency for a 20-dB carrier level are aligned along the diagonal axis in *black*. The associated rMTFs and tMTFs appear in the *upper* and *lower panels* of inset **a**. Response profiles corresponding to the changes in carrier level for a 2-Hz modulation are aligned along the horizontal axis in *gray*. The associated curves depicting the changes in firing rate and timing indices for different carrier levels appear in the *upper* and *lower panels* of inset **b**. Response profiles corresponding to changes in modulation depth are shown in the *vertical columns on the left* (2 Hz at 20 dB) and *right* (2 Hz at 60 dB). The associated curves depicting the changes in firing rate and time indices appear in inset **c**. Because the data were obtained from separate runs, the 100% modulated, 2-Hz stimulus at 60 dB was repeated twice, and the analogous 20 dB stimulus was repeated thrice (the carrier frequency was constant at 700 Hz). The resulting MPHs are overlaid to illustrate the robustness of the MPH shapes for repeated trials. These data were obtained in the auditory cortex of an awake rhesus monkey. (With permission of Malone *et al.*, 2007.)

6.10 **Conclusions**

What, then, does the foregoing suggest about the transformation of the representation of SAM signals in the ascending auditory pathway? In addition to the growing systemic focus on very low modulation frequencies, there is also increasing heterogeneity in MPH shapes, which certainly must reflect, at least in part, the increased heterogeneity in level tuning among central auditory neurons. This in turn suggests that rather than abstracting information about modulation frequency, the auditory pathway instead diversifies the way in which amplitudes are encoded. Figure 6.8 demonstrates that the same cortical neuron fires to the instantaneous amplitude maximum, or minimum, of an SAM stimulus depending on the relationship between the carrier level and its preferred level. Consider also that as fewer spikes per modulation cycle are available, the range of MPH shapes becomes constrained; if we assume that there is an underlying distribution reflecting the underlying probability of discharge at each point in the modulation cycle, as the modulation frequency increases, it becomes harder to 'mark' the less preferred phases because of refractoriness relating to having recently fired a spike at the optimal phase. As a result, TS and VS values nearly always converge at a particular f_m and then decline in tandem. In fact, it is possible that the point where these metrics coincide identifies the 'hinge' value of f_m for tMTFs exhibiting a lowpass to bandpass transition with increasing carrier level. From this perspective, the average discharge rate does not encode the envelopes of modulated signals, but instead represents a limit on the resolution at which the features of envelopes can be encoded.

The timing of spikes, and not just the average spike count, clearly is an important aspect of the neural code for processing communication sounds, most of them containing many time-varying components. Neuronal synchronization to the timing of stimulus events and spike timing precision are most useful in performing periodicity analyses and improving the signal-to-noise ratios for signal detection and discrimination tasks based, for example, on information measures (Liu and Schreiner, 2007).

As is evident in our survey of various auditory stations, it is indisputable that the activity distributed across different neuronal populations represents different aspects of information regarding time-varying sounds (although there is also evidence that single neurons respond to stimulus features on multiple timescales (see Elhilali *et al.*, 2004)). These various coding strategies differ in their ability to convey particular features of time-varying sounds, such as their time of occurrence, frequency of occurrence, rate of change, and duration. It is not surprising that the panoply of auditory processing tasks has resulted in such a variety of coding schemes. An important task for future research will be the identification of the tasks that are best served by these different neuronal populations, and definition of their roles in establishing the psychophysical and perceptual capacities of the listener.

Acknowledgement

This work was supported by grants DC02260 (C.E.S.) and MH12993 (B.J.M.) from the NIH, the Coleman Fund, and Hearing Research Incorporated.

References

Batra R (2006) Responses of neurons in the ventral nucleus of the lateral lemniscus to sinusoidally amplitude modulated tones. *J Neurophysiol* **96**(5): 2388–98.

Beitel RE, Schreiner CE, Cheung SW, Wang X, Merzenich MM (2003) Reward-dependent plasticity in the primary auditory cortex of adult monkeys trained to discriminate temporally modulated signals. *Proc Natl Acad Sci USA* **100**(19): 11070–5.

Bieser A, Müller-Preuss P (1996) Auditory responsive cortex in the squirrel monkey: neural responses to amplitude-modulated sounds. *Exp Brain Res* 108: 273–84.

Blackburn CC, Sachs MB (1989) Classification of unit types in the anteroventral cochlear nucleus: PST histograms and regularity analysis. *J Neurophysiol* 62: 1303–29.

Cooper NP, Robertson D, Yates GK (1993) Cochlear nerve fiber responses to amplitude-modulated stimuli: variations with spontaneous rate and other response characteristics. *J Neurophysiol* 70(1): 370–86.

Drullman R (1995) Temporal envelope and fine structure cues for speech intelligibility. *J Acoust Soc Am* 97: 585–92.

Drullman R, Festen JM, Plomp R (1994) Effect of reducing slow temporal modulations on speech reception. *J Acoust Soc Am* 95: 2670–80.

Elhilali M, Fritz JB, Klein DJ, Simon JZ, Shamma SA (2004) Dynamics of precise spike timing in primary auditory cortex. *J Neurosci* 24: 1159–72.

Fastl H (1990) The hearing sensation, roughness and neuronal responses to AM-tones. *Hear Res* 46(3): 293–5.

Fastl H, Hesse A, Schorer E, Urbas J, Müller-Preuss P (1986) Searching for neural correlates of the hearing sensation fluctuation strength in the auditory cortex of squirrel monkeys. *Hear Res* 23(2): 199–203.

Foffani G, Moxon KA (2004) PSTH-based classification of sensory stimuli using ensembles of single neurons. *J Neurosci Meth* 135: 93–107.

Frisina RD (2001) Subcortical neural coding mechanisms for auditory temporal processing. *Hear Res* 158(1–2): 1–27.

Frisina RD, Smith RL, Chamberlain SC (1990) Encoding of amplitude modulation in the gerbil cochlear nucleus: I. A hierarchy of enhancement. *Hear Res* 44: 99–122.

Galazyuk AV, Llano D, Feng AS (2000) Temporal dynamics of acoustic stimuli enhance amplitude tuning of inferior colliculus neurons. *J Neurophysiol* 83(1): 128–38.

Goldberg J, Brown P (1969) Responses of binaural neurons of dog superior olivary complex to to dichotic tonal stimuli: some physiological mechanisms of sound localization. *J Neurophysiol* 32: 631–6.

Hartmann WH (1997) *Signals, Sound, and Sensation*. AIP Press, Woodbury.

Hewitt MJ, Meddis R (1994) A computer model of amplitude-modulation sensitivity of single units in the inferior colliculus. *J Acoust Soc Am* 95(4): 2145–59.

Kuwada S, Batra R (1999) Coding of sound envelopes by inhibitory rebound in neurons of the superior olivary complex in the unanesthetized rabbit. *J Neurosci* 19(6): 2273–87.

Langner G, Schreiner CE (1988) Periodicity coding in the inferior colliculus of the cat. I. Neuronal mechanisms. *J Neurophysiol* 60(6): 1799–822.

Liu RC, Schreiner CE (2007) Auditory cortical detection and discrimination correlates with communicative significance. *PLoS Biol* 5(7): e173.

Joris PX, Yin TC (1992) Responses to amplitude-modulated tones in the auditory nerve of the cat. *J Acoust Soc Am* 91: 215–32.

Joris PX, Schreiner CE, Rees A (2004) Neural processing of amplitude-modulated sounds. *Physiol Rev* 84: 541–77.

Joris PX, Louage DH, Cardoen L, van der Heijden M (2006) Correlation index: a new metric to quantify temporal coding. *Hear Res* 216–217: 19–30.

Kajikawa Y, Hackett TA (2005) Entropy analysis of neuronal spike train synchrony. *J Neurosci Meth* 149: 90–93.

Krishna BS, Semple MN (2000) Auditory temporal processing: responses to sinusoidally amplitude-modulated tones in the inferior colliculus. *J Neurophysiol* 84: 255–73.

Langner G, Schreiner CE (1988) Periodicity coding in the inferior colliculus of the cat. I. Neuronal mechanisms. *J Neurophysiol* 60: 1799–822.

Liang L, Lu T, Wang X (2002) Neural representations of sinusoidal amplitude and frequency modulations in the primary auditory cortex of awake primates. *J Neurophysiol* 87: 2237–61.

Lu T, Liang L, Wang X (2001) Temporal and rate representations of time-varying signals in the auditory cortex of awake primates. *Nat Neurosci* 4: 1131–8.

Malone BJ, Semple MN (2001) Effects of auditory stimulus context on the representation of frequency in the gerbil inferior colliculus. *J Neurophysiol* 86: 1113–30.

Malone BJ, Scott BH, Semple MN (2002) Context-dependent adaptive coding of interaural phase disparity in the auditory cortex of awake macaques. *J Neurosci* 22: 4625–38.

Malone BJ, Scott BH, Semple MN (2007) Dynamic amplitude coding in the auditory cortex of awake rhesus macaques. *J Neurophysiol* 98(3): 1451–74.

Møller AR (1972) Coding of amplitude and frequency modulated sounds in the cochlear nucleus of the rat. *Acta Physiol Scand* 81: 540–56.

Møller AR (1974) Responses of units in the cochlear nucleus to sinusoidally amplitude-modulated tones. *Exp Neurol* 45: 104–17.

Møller AR (1976) Dynamic properties of primary auditory fibers compared with cells in the cochlear nucleus. *Acta Physiol Scand* 98: 157–67.

Phillips DP, Semple MN, Calford MB, Kitzes LM (1994) Level-dependent representation of stimulus frequency in cat primary auditory cortex. *Exp Brain Res* 102(2): 210–26.

Preuss A, Müller-Preuss P (1990) Processing of amplitude modulated sounds in the medial geniculate body of squirrel monkeys. *Exp Brain Res* 79(1): 207–11.

Rees A, Møller AR (1987) Stimulus properties influencing the responses of inferior colliculus neurons to amplitude-modulated sounds. *Hear Res* 27: 129–43.

Rees A, Palmer AR (1989) Neuronal responses to amplitude-modulated and pure-tone stimuli in the guinea pig inferior colliculus, and their modification by broadband noise. *J Acoust Soc Am* 85: 1978–94.

Rhode WS (1994) Temporal coding of 200% amplitude modulated signals in the ventral cochlear nucleus of the cat. *Hear Res* 77: 43–68.

Rhode WS, Greenberg S (1992) Physiology of the cochlear nuclei. In: The Mammalian Auditory Pathway: Neurophysiology, Vol 2 (eds Popper AN, Fay RR), pp 94–152. Springer, New York.

Rhode WS, Greenberg S (1994) Encoding of amplitude modulation in the cochlear nucleus of the cat. *J Neurophysiol* 71(5): 1797–825.

Sanes DH, Malone BJ, Semple MN (1998) Role of synaptic inhibition in processing of dynamic binaural level stimuli. *J Neurosci* 18: 794–803.

Schreiner, CE, Langner G (1988) Periodicity coding in the inferior colliculus of the cat. II. Topographical organization. *J Neurophysiol* 60(6): 1823–40.

Schreiner CE, Urbas JV (1988) Representation of amplitude modulation in the auditory cortex of the cat. II. Comparison between cortical fields. *Hear Res* 32: 49–63.

Semple MN, Kitzes LM (1993a) Binaural processing of sound pressure level in cat primary auditory cortex: evidence for a representation based on absolute levels rather than interaural level differences. *J Neurophysiol* 69: 449–61.

Semple MN, Kitzes LM (1993b) Focal selectivity for binaural sound pressure level in cat primary auditory cortex: two-way intensity network tuning. *J Neurophysiol* 69: 462–73.

Singh NC, Theunissen FE (2003) Modulation spectra of natural sounds and ethological theories of auditory processing. *J Acoust Soc Am* 114: 3394–411.

Smith RL, Brachman ML (1980) Response modulation of auditory-nerve fibers by AM stimuli: effects of average intensity. *Hear Res* 2(2): 123–33.

Smith ZM, Delgutte B, Oxenham AJ (2002) Chimaeric sounds reveal dichotomies in auditory perception. *Nature* 416: 87–90.

Swarbrick L, Whitfield IC (1972) Auditory cortical units selectively responsive to stimulus 'shape'. *J Physiol* 224: 68P–69P.

Ter-Mikaelian M, Sanes DH, Semple MN (2007) Transformation of temporal properties between auditory midbrain and cortex in the awake Mongolian gerbil. *J Neurosci* **27**(23): 6091–102.

Ulanovsky N, Las L, Farkas D, Nelken I (2004) Multiple time scales of adaptation in auditory cortex neurons. *J Neurosci* **24**: 10440–53.

Wang X (2007) Neural coding strategies in auditory cortex. *Hear Res* **229**(1–2): 81–93.

Wohlgemuth S, Ronacher B (2007) Auditory discrimination of amplitude modulations based on metric distances of spike trains. *J Neurophysiol* **97**: 3082–92.

Yates GK (1987) Dynamic effects in the input/output relationship of auditory nerve. *Hear Res* **27**: 221–30.

Chapter 7

Pitch

Xiaoqin Wang and Daniel Bendor

7.1 Introduction

Pitch perception is crucial for speech perception, music perception, and auditory object recognition in a complex acoustic environment. Pitch is the percept that allows sounds to be ordered on a musical scale and can be evoked by either pure tones or complex sounds (Moore, 2003). The perception of the pitch of complex sounds with harmonic structures is of particular interest. A good example of how pitch is used in our daily life is our perception of music. When you listen to an orchestra, you effortlessly hear the melody of the soloist over the background of accompanying instruments. Our auditory system relies on pitch, among other things, to enable us to accomplish such tasks. Beyond our ability to segregate and perceptually group sounds, changes in pitch are used to convey information in speech (for example, prosodic information in European languages, and semantic information in tonal languages like Chinese, Vietnamese, and Thai). Pitch is closely associated with the perception of harmonically structured or periodic signals. This reflects the need of the auditory system to discriminate between environmental sounds and vocalizations. A noticeable acoustic difference between these two classes of sounds is that environmental sounds are generally aperiodic whereas most vocalizations are periodic or contain harmonic structures. Thus understanding how the auditory system processes pitch has direct implications for cochlear implant design and speech recognition technologies. In this chapter we discuss how the auditory system encodes a sound's pitch, focusing on physiological studies.

7.2 Pitch perception

7.2.1 Pitch, harmonicity, and periodicity

First and foremost, pitch is a percept defined psychophysically rather than acoustically (Plack and Oxenham, 2005). Acoustically, the information relevant for extracting pitch is available in either temporal or spectral domain and sometimes in both domains. Temporally, the repetition rate of an acoustic signal's waveform or envelope is equal to the perceived pitch. The former (periodic wave form) is referred to as the pure tone pitch and the latter (periodic envelope) as the pitch of complex sounds. Thus a waveform or envelope oscillating periodically at 100 Hz will have a pitch of 100 Hz (Fig. 7.1A, *left*). Spectrally, the perceived pitch matches the fundamental frequency ($f0$) which is the highest frequency for which each component in a harmonic complex sound is an integer multiple (Fig. 7.1A, *right*). The frequency spacing between these harmonically related components equals the fundamental frequency. Thus harmonics with frequencies of, 200, 300, and 400 Hz have a fundamental frequency of 100 Hz.

The salience of the pitch depends on several acoustic properties of sounds, including their temporal regularity. While white noise generate no pitch, repeated bursts of white noise generate a

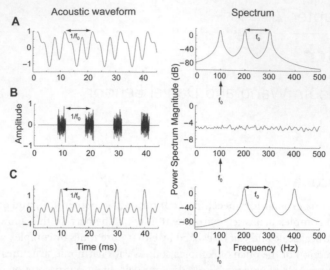

Fig. 7.1 Examples of waveform and spectrum of three different acoustic signals that have the same pitch (f_0 = 100 Hz). **A** Harmonic complex tone: composed of the 1st (fundamental), 2nd, and 3rd harmonic, each with randomized phase. **B** Repeated broadband noise burst (100 Hz repetition rate). **C** Missing fundamental harmonic complex tone: composed of the 2nd, 3rd, and 4th harmonic, all in cosine phase.

weak pitch equal to the periodic repetition rate of the bursts (Fig. 7.1B). If these noise bursts are temporally jittered so that their timing is no longer strictly periodic, the pitch salience decreases and the perceived pitch may disappear depending on the amount of jitter. Similarly, if frequency jitter is introduced to individual components of a harmonic complex, the salience of its pitch is reduced (Plack and Oxenham, 2005).

Our perception of pitch is limited to a specific range of harmonic and fundamental frequencies known as the existence region (Plack and Oxenham, 2005). Harmonic frequencies need to be below 6 kHz to generate a pitch at the fundamental frequency, lower for lower fundamental frequencies. For example, only harmonic frequencies less than 2.5 kHz will generate a pitch when the fundamental frequency is 100 Hz (Ritsma, 1962). For pure tones, musical interval discrimination and melodic pitch are lost at frequencies above 4–5k Hz (Ward, 1954; Attneave and Olson, 1971), near the highest pitch played by a piano or an orchestra. For missing fundamental sounds (see the section below), the upper limit of pitch is between 800 and 1400 Hz, depending on the number of components used (Ritsma, 1963; Plomp, 1967; Moore, 1973). The lower limit of pitch measured psychophysically is roughly 30 Hz (Krumbholz et al., 2000; Pressnitzer et al., 2001), which is near the lowest musical note found on the piano (27.5 Hz). At fundamental frequencies (or repetition rates) near or below the lower limit of pitch, we hear a stream of discretely occurring sounds known as acoustic flutter. Our ability to discriminate changes in periodicity or repetition rate within the range of acoustic flutter is substantially worse than within the range of pitch (Pollack, 1968, 1969), possibly due to differences in how these percepts are encoded by the auditory system (Bendor and Wang, 2007).

7.2.2 Missing fundamental pitch

An important phenomenon of pitch perception is the percept of the 'missing fundamental', also referred to as the residue pitch (Schouten, 1938; Licklider, 1956). When the harmonics of a fundamental frequency are played together, the pitch is still perceived as matching the fundamental frequency even if there is no spectral energy at that frequency. For example, for a fundamental frequency of 100 Hz, its harmonics are at 200, 300, 400 Hz, and so on. Playing the frequencies 200, 300, and 400 Hz together will generate a pitch of 100 Hz, even though a frequency component at 100 Hz is not physically present in the sound (Fig. 7.1C). Missing fundamental perception plays an important part in the invariance of pitch perception, allowing for the same pitch to be perceived for many different combinations of harmonics. This is particularly useful when pitch is used to convey behaviorally important information, as in the case of human speech or animal vocalizations. Sounds propagated through the environment can become spectrally degraded, losing high or low frequencies. While such spectral filtering causes the loss of spectral information, the perception of the missing fundamental is robust to the loss of some subsets of harmonics.

7.2.3 Pitch and the resolvability of the harmonics

One critical issue to consider when studying pitch is how the acoustic stimulus interacts with the cochlea's basilar membrane. If harmonics in a complex tone are spaced far apart along the basilar membrane, then no interaction between any of the harmonics occurs in the vibration patterns of the basilar membrane. Harmonics are referred to as 'resolved' in this case (Moore, 2003) and the auditory system is able to determine the frequency of each harmonic separately. However, when harmonics are close enough together in frequency, they form a single region of excitation on the basilar membrane. In this case the harmonics are referred to as 'unresolved' and the auditory system cannot determine what individual harmonics are present. Pitch salience has been shown to change with the resolvability of the harmonics. Different mechanisms are likely needed to extract the pitch from resolved versus unresolved harmonics.

7.2.4 Pitch salience

In addition to fundamental frequency and repetition rate, several other acoustic features can affect pitch. These secondary factors are important to consider when developing a complete model of how pitch is processed in the auditory system. For pure tones, sound level alters the perceived pitch: increasing sound level causes an increase in pitch for pure tones above 2 kHz and a decrease in pitch for pure tones below 2 kHz (Plack and Oxenham, 2005). Although shifts in pitch of 5–10% have been reported with changes in sound level (Stevens, 1935), later studies showed a more modest (1–2%) shift in pitch (Verschuure and van Meeteren, 1975). In addition to sound level, the mistuning of harmonics within a complex tone can influence the pitch perceived. Interestingly, the strength of the effect is not uniform among harmonics, as the 2nd, 3rd, 4th, and 5th harmonics typically show larger dominance over the shift in pitch (Plomp, 1967; Ritsma, 1967; Moore et al., 1985). When the entire complex tone is shifted in frequency, so that all of the frequency components become inharmonic (i.e. no longer integer-multiples of the fundamental frequency), more substantial changes in pitch can occur (Schouten et al., 1962). The shift in pitch decreases with the order of the harmonics, and for complex tones with very high order unresolved components, there is no longer an observable pitch shift (Moore and Moore, 2003).

Another important observation is that, for certain phase relationships between harmonics, the fundamental frequency and repetition rate can differ. In many studies, experimenters use harmonics that are all in sine or cosine phase, and in these cases the fundamental frequency and repetition rate are equal. However, if the odd harmonics are in sine phase and the even harmonics are in cosine phase (referred to as the alternating phase complex tone), the repetition rate doubles and is no longer equal to the fundamental frequency. As such, we can use this property to identify if it is temporal (repetition rate) or spectral (fundamental frequency) information that determines the perceived pitch. For lower order resolved harmonics, pitch is determined by fundamental frequency. However, when the sound is composed of only high order unresolved harmonics, the pitch matches the repetition rate (Carlyon and Shackleton, 1994; Shackleton and Carlyon, 1994). Thus when only high order unresolved harmonics are present, subjects hear the pitch of an alternating phase complex tone as one octave higher than a sine phase complex tone, even though these two sounds have identical harmonic frequencies and fundamental frequency.

7.2.5 Pitch perception in animals

The perception of the missing fundamental has been a hallmark test for the ability of an animal species to perceive pitch. Previous work has demonstrated missing fundamental perception across several vertebrate species, including birds (Cynx and Shapiro, 1986), cats (Heffner and Whitfield, 1976), and monkeys (Tomlinson and Schwarz, 1988). Repetition rate (or modulation frequency) discrimination has been demonstrated over a wider range of species, including goldfish (Fay and Passow, 1982), budgerigars (Dooling and Searcy, 1981), gerbils (Schulze and Scheich, 1999), chinchillas (Long and Clark, 1984), and monkeys (Moody, 1994). In addition to pitch perception, octave generalization (Wright *et al.*, 2000), the discrimination between consonant and dissonant sounds (Izumi, 2000), and melody discrimination (Izumi, 2001) have been shown in monkeys. It is important to note that although monkeys can discriminate between consonant and dissonant sounds, the preference humans have for consonant sounds and the appreciation for music may be unique to our species (McDermott and Hauser, 2005).

Whitfield (1980) demonstrated that in cats the perception of the missing fundamental requires auditory cortex. Cats with bilateral lesions of primary and secondary auditory cortex were still able to discriminate spectral changes (after additional training), but lost the ability to detect a change in the fundamental frequency. Similar findings have been observed in humans with lesions in auditory cortex (Zatorre, 1988; Tramo *et al.*, 2002; Warrier and Zatorre, 2004). Thus the lesion data in cats and humans are in agreement that the auditory cortex is necessary for the perception of pitch.

7.3 Models of pitch processing

7.3.1 Temporal models of pitch processing

In our definition of the pitch of pure tones and complex sounds earlier in this chapter, we stressed the importance of temporal periodicity in the acoustic waveform for a pitch to be perceived. Many models of pitch processing have utilized a temporally based mechanism that can measure this temporal periodicity and repetition rate of the acoustic waveform. Licklider (1951) proposed the use of autocorrelation, which was later realized in a computational model by Meddis and Hewitt (1991a, b). In this model, an autocorrelation function is performed on the auditory system's response in each frequency channel and then summed together. Thus the resolvability of individual harmonics is not an issue when calculating the summed autocorrelation function. A neural circuit for autocorrelation requires only delay-and-add computations. The medial superior olive uses such a delay-and-add process to compute sound location, and possibly a similar mechanism could be used for calculating the autocorrelation, though empirical evidence has not yet been found. Additionally, the naturally occurring delay between high and low frequencies along the basilar membrane could be used to calculate the autocorrelation function (Loeb *et al.*, 1983; Shamma, 1985).

7.3.2 Spectral models of pitch processing

In addition to temporal periodicity, acoustic signals with pitch (other than pure tones) are usually spectrally periodic, having a spectrum composed of harmonically related frequencies. One way to calculate the periodicity of the spectrum is the use of a harmonic template. Neural representations of pitch-evoking sounds are compared with harmonic templates representing all possible fundamental frequencies, and the best template match determines the pitch perceived (Goldstein, 1973; Wightman, 1973; Terhardt, 1974). Although these models require that harmonics are resolved, the frequency of each harmonic can be determined by using either the place of excitation or temporal pattern of activity on the basilar membrane. However, even with an input lacking harmonicity, a modeling study shows that such templates could emerge from the development of the auditory system (Shamma and Klein, 2000).

7.3.3 Unitary versus dual mechanism based pitch models

Because spectral models require resolved harmonics, they fail to explain how we can perceive the pitch of sounds containing only unresolved components. One possibility is that only a temporal pitch model is used by the auditory system (Meddis and O'Mard, 1997). Given the differences in our perception of pitch between resolved and unresolved harmonics, it has been suggested that spectral models are used for processing resolved harmonics, whereas temporal models are used for processing unresolved harmonics (Carlyon and Shackleton, 1994; Shackleton and Carlyon, 1994; Carlyon, 1998). Psychophysical and computational models have provided extensive evidence towards the validity of each of these theories. Anatomical and physiological data that examine the neural circuits responsible for extracting pitch are needed to resolve these issues.

7.4 Neural coding of pitch

Neural mechanisms for encoding pitch have been studied in nearly all auditory structures from the periphery to cortex. There are two general questions that have been asked in these physiological studies. First, how is the spectral and temporal information related to pitch represented by neural discharges? Second, where is pitch extracted from sounds that generate pitch perception? Note that we are making a distinction between 'representation' and 'extraction'. The former refers to a process that transfers the information on pitch from an acoustic signal to its corresponding neural responses. The latter refers to a process that computes pitch from the neural response of a complex sound (such as a missing fundamental harmonic complex). By these definitions, the auditory system must first be able to accurately represent the spectral and temporal information related to pitch before it could perform the extraction (or computation) of pitch at some later stages. Because pitch is a perceived quantity rather than a merely acoustic quantity, this extraction or neural computation is necessary to give rise to the perception of pitch. Currently available evidence suggests that the first stage of pitch processing takes place at the auditory periphery (cochlea and auditory nerve) and the brainstem, whereas the second stage of pitch processing may take place in the cerebral cortex (Bendor and Wang, 2006). It remains unclear how the auditory midbrain contributes to the transformation from the periphery to cortex. We therefore divide the discussions of neural processing of pitch into subcortical and cortical processing in this chapter.

7.5 Subcortical processing of pitch

7.5.1 Auditory nerve

The cochlea provides a spectral representation of the sound or combination of sounds that enter the ear. The location of activity on the basilar membrane can encode the spectral frequency of the sound. Frequency information can also be encoded by the periodicity of the basilar membrane's motion, especially when regions of excitation among several harmonics are overlapping (i.e. unresolved harmonics). Because either spectral or temporal information can be used to extract pitch, both the place and temporal representations of acoustic signals are important objects of study to understand the neural coding of pitch. These features of the basilar membrane motion are directly represented in the activity of the auditory nerve.

Frequency is represented in the auditory nerve by the place or timing of neural firings. Phase-locked discharges (neural firings that synchronize to the periodicity of the components of a sound) are later used for computing sound source information, and quite possibly are also used to extract the fundamental frequency. This idea is supported by the fact that we can hear spectral frequencies up to 20 kHz, but our upper limit of pitch perception for pure tones is near the upper limit of phase locking of auditory nerve fibers (~5 kHz) (Moore, 2003). The sufficiency of a temporal representation in the auditory nerve for the encoding of fundamental frequency was explored in a series of elegant studies by Cariani and Delgutte (1996a,b). First-order and all-order interspike interval distributions (equivalent to an autocorrelation of the spike train) were collected from auditory nerve responses in anesthetized cats to a large class of acoustic signals that differed both spectrally and in their pitch salience. The most commonly observed interspike interval in these experiments (the largest peak in the interspike interval histogram) was equal to the inverse of the fundamental frequency, thus demonstrating that temporal information is preserved well enough to support temporal pitch models (Fig. 7.2). Although all-order interspike interval distributions provided a reliable estimation of fundamental frequency, first-order interspike interval distributions were less accurate, especially across different sound levels. Interestingly, for the majority of acoustic stimuli the amplitude of the main peak of the interspike interval distribution was proportional to the pitch salience of the acoustic signal.

Cedolin and Delgutte (2005) examined the spectral resolvability of auditory nerve fibers to harmonic complex tones, and determined that a rate-place representation of harmonic frequency was sufficient to extract fundamental frequencies above 400–500 Hz (Fig. 7.3A). A temporal representation based on a pooled all-order interspike interval distribution was accurate for

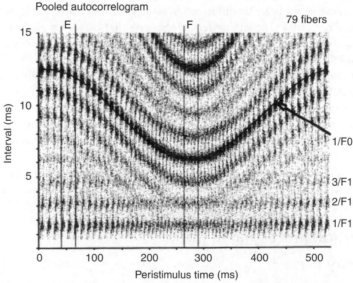

Fig. 7.2 Periodicity in auditory nerve responses. Pooled autocorrelogram in response to a variable-F_0 single-formant stimulus with $F_0 = 80–160$ Hz and $F_1 = 640$ Hz. PST binwidth = 714 μs, interval binwidth = 30 μs. *Solid line* indicates Fundamental period $1/F_0$. (From Cariani and Delgutte, 1996a.)

fundamental frequencies up to 1300 Hz (Fig. 7.3B). These data suggest that spectral or temporal pitch information is encoded by individual auditory nerve fibers, depending on the range of fundamental frequency. The two forms of representations are complementary, but neither is sufficient to account for human psychophysical data. For a subset of fundamental frequencies (~500–1300 Hz), both processing models may be used concurrently. These studies provide the first physiological evidence of dual pitch mechanisms along the ascending auditory pathway.

7.5.2 Cochlear nucleus

The cochlear nucleus is composed of three cochleotopically organized divisions, the anteroventral (AVCN), posteroventral (PVCN), and dorsal (DCN) cochlear nucleus, each receiving a parallel input from the auditory nerve (see Chapter 2). Several different types of cells exist within the cochlear nucleus, distinguishable by their morphology and response characteristics. Bushy cells (referred to as 'primary-like units' in physiology literature) in the ventral cochlear nuclei (VCN, including AVCN and PVCN) have response patterns similar to those of the auditory nerve.

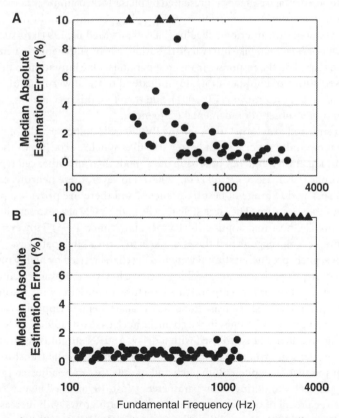

Fig. 7.3 Accuracy of pitch estimation based on cat auditory nerve responses (from Cedolin and Delgutte, 2005). Median absolute estimation error for pitch, expressed as percentage of the true F_0, is plotted as a function of F_0. **A** Pitch estimation accuracy based on rate-place profiles. Median is obtained over 100 bootstrap resamplings of the data. *Triangles* indicate data points for which the median was out of the range defined by the vertical axes. **B** Pitch estimation accuracy based on pooled all-order interspike-interval distributions. Median is obtained over 100 resampling trials. *Triangles* indicate pitch absolute estimation error exceeded 10% of the true F_0.

As such the representation of pitch-related information in primary-like units is similar to that observed in auditory nerve fibers. Primary-like units may play a role in processing pitch information in addition to their role in sound location (see Chapter 12).

Stellate cells (referred to as 'chopper units') in the VCN produce sustained responses to tones with a chopping pattern in their spiking. Compared to primary-like units, phase locking diminishes in chopper units at frequencies higher than ~2 kHz in the cat (Blackburn and Sachs, 1989). However, their rate-place representation of the spectrum is enhanced relative to the auditory nerve, and is less sensitive to changes in sound level (Blackburn and Sachs, 1990). In addition to providing a rate-place representation of the spectrum, stimulus synchronization may provide additional information related to the fundamental frequency in chopper units (Keilson *et al.*, 1997). An interesting property of chopper units is the intrinsic oscillation ('chopping') in their stimulus-driven firing that coincides with the range of pitch (~100–800 Hz) (Frisina *et al.*, 1990; Kim *et al.*, 1990). If the fundamental frequency of a sound matches the intrinsic chopping frequency of a chopper unit, there could be an enhancement of periodic firings at the fundamental frequency. It has been suggested that chopper units with a range of chopping frequencies could serve to detect fundamental frequency represented by phase-locked auditory nerve inputs (Frisina *et al.*, 1990; Kim *et al.*, 1990). The outputs of these chopper units could then be read out by neurons in the next stage, the inferior colliculus (Hewitt and Meddis, 1994). As such, a first-order (rather than an all-order) interspike interval distribution may be sufficient to calculate the fundamental frequency based on the responses from chopper units. One limitation in this model is that the intrinsic oscillations of chopper units do not extend to the lower limit of pitch (~30 Hz) (Krumbholz *et al.*, 2000; Pressnitzer *et al.*, 2001), and therefore this mechanism can only support pitch extraction over a subset of fundamental frequencies.

Octopus cells (referred to as 'onset units') in the PVCN are in some ways the opposite of stellate cells. They are temporally precise, with better stimulus synchronization to the fundamental frequency and modulation frequency of broadband sounds than any other cell types in the cochlear nucleus (Rhode, 1994, 1998; Oertel *et al.*, 2000). However, these neurons receive auditory nerve inputs across a wide range of best frequencies, and therefore provide a poor rate-place representation of the spectrum. The large stellate cells in the VCN also extract pitch information using mechanisms like those in octopus cells (Palmer and Winter, 1996). However, their status as an inhibitory interneuron suggests that this is unlikely to form a pitch pathway.

In most studies, pitch-producing stimuli were usually characterized by highly modulated envelopes and, as a consequence, it was not possible to tell if a low-CF unit was selectively responding to the envelope modulation or the temporal fine structure. In the latter case, the unit responds to the envelope modulation as well. To tease these factors apart, iterated rippled noise (IRN) stimuli have been used in a number of studies in the cochlear nucleus (Yost, 1996a). IRN is generated by iteratively adding broadband noise to itself with a delay. An IRN stimulus generates pitch sensation, but lacks regular fine structure in its waveform. It parametrically transforms a noise to a 'noise-like' stimulus that has a pitch. Both pitch and its salience can be adjusted in an IRN stimulus by changing the delay and itineration parameters (Yost, 1996a, b). The perceived pitch corresponds to the reciprocal of the delay and the pitch strength grows with increasing number of iterations. Winter *et al.* (2001) showed that all unit types in the VCN could enhance the representation of the delay of IRN using first-order interspike intervals (ISIs) over a range of periodicities (Fig. 7.4). A subset of onset units showed a clear preference for some delays of the IRN in their first-order interval statistics, and thus provide evidence for 'periodicity tuning'. Onset units also show the greatest range of best periodicities and are well suited to encode the delay of IRN for a wide range of pitches. Shofner (2008) recently showed with IRN stimuli that in chinchilla VCN primary-like instead of chopper units exhibited a neural representation of the pitch dominance region and suggested that bushy cells play a more important role in processing (relaying) pitch-related information than previously thought.

Thus onset units and a subset of chopper units appear to be the most attractive candidates for processing pitch-related information given their enhanced spectral and temporal properties (relative to the auditory nerve), whereas primary-like units seem to pass on such information to the next processing stage. Although, fundamental frequency is not yet extracted (or read out) by any of the cell types in the cochlear nucleus, the information for pitch read-out by either spectral or temporal mechanisms is still preserved at their outputs. As such, the cochlear nucleus may serve a more general role in the representation of spectral, temporal, and spatial information and relay the information necessary for extracting pitch to higher auditory processing centers.

7.5.3 Inferior colliculus

Information from the cochlear nucleus reaches the inferior colliculus by travelling either directly via monosynaptic projections or indirectly through the lateral lemniscus or superior olivary complex (see Chapter 2). Much of what we know about physiological properties of the inferior colliculus has been based on studies of the central nucleus of the inferior colliculus which is

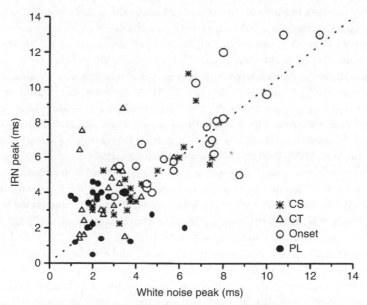

Fig. 7.4 Relationship between the peak of the first-order inter-spike interval histogram (ISIH) in response to white noise and the peak of the interval enhancement plot for single units. The interval enhancement was defined as the magnitude of the increased response at the appropriate delay, after the ISIH to the white noise was first subtracted from the ISIH to the complex pitch-producing stimulus. The peak of the first-order ISIH in response to white noise is plotted on the *abscissa*. The peak was estimated from a gamma fit to the ISIH distribution. The peak of the gamma fit to the interval enhancement plot in response to IRN is plotted on the *ordinate*. The *dotted line* indicates when the two values are equal. The correlation between the two measurements is greatest for onset chopper (Onset) and sustained chopper (CS) units. Note that onset units generally had the largest values and primary likes (PL) the smallest. Units classified as transient choppers (CT) had values similar to PL units whereas CS units had values that overlapped those of the other three unit types. (From Winter *et al.*, 2001.)

tonotopically organized. The inferior colliculus is the first stage in the auditory pathway where spatial information arising from interaural timing and level differences, spectral cues generated by the pinna, and information about sound identity are integrated (see Chapter 12).

The work on pitch processing in the inferior colliculus has primarily been focused on the coding of periodicity, which is related, but not equivalent, to the coding of pitch for the reasons explained above (i.e. spectral versus temporal pitch models). Unlike most neurons in the cochlear nucleus which only respond to temporally modulated periodic signals with variations in their synchronized rate, both the synchronized rate and the average discharge rate responses of inferior colliculus neurons give rise to bandpass functions of modulation rate, indicating that a neuron may selectively respond to particular periodicities. Langner and Schreiner (1988) showed that the average rate responses of neurons in the inferior colliculus of anesthetized cats are tuned to modulation frequency of sinusoidally amplitude modulated (sAM) tones over the range 10–1000 Hz. Although this range of 'best modulation frequency' does not cover the entire range of pure tone pitch, it does cover the range of missing fundamental pitch from sAM tones (Ritsma, 1963). In the Langner and Schreiner (1988) study, sAM tones were centered at a neuron's characteristic frequency that is usually much higher than the best modulation frequency of the neuron. Schreiner and Langner (1988) also reported that the best modulation frequency of neurons within the inferior colliculus was organized orthogonal to the tonotopic axis in the form of a map. If this is true, then summing together responses from neurons tuned to the same best modulation frequency but different characteristic frequencies can create a spectrally invariant response to modulation frequency or periodicity. The orderly organization of periodicity tuning has also been found in the inferior colliculus of awake chinchillas (Langner et al., 2002). Modulation tuning in the inferior colliculus can be characterized by neural firings synchronized to modulation waveform (Fig. 7.5A) or by average discharge rate (Fig. 7.5B). A common observation in the inferior colliculus is that neurons are synchronized to envelope modulations at lower rates than the cochlear nucleus, but at higher rates than the auditory cortex (Fig. 7.5C, D). The upper limit of the phase-locking to pure tones in the inferior colliculus is ~1000 Hz (Fig. 7.6), much lower than that of cochlear nucleus (~4000–5000 Hz) (Blackburn and Sachs, 1989).

Given that some forms of pitch perception are based on binaural cues (Plack and Oxenham, 2005), the inferior colliculus seems to be a prime location for the binaural integration of pitch-related information. It has been shown that a sound is binaurally integrated before pitch is processed (Culling et al., 1998a, b; Culling, 2000). For a harmonic complex with the fundamental frequency f0, the repetition rate of the waveform at each ear becomes 2f0 when harmonics are presented to alternate ears (e.g. old harmonics to one ear and even harmonics to the other ear). For human listeners in such dichotic listening conditions, the pitch perceived is still equivalent to f0 if the harmonics are resolved, but doubles if the harmonics are unresolved (Bernstein and Oxenham, 2003). A recent study examined both the temporal and rate-tuning of IC clusters and found no evidence for binaural integration in the central nucleus of the inferior colliculus (Shackleton et al., 2009). Therefore, the information on sound periodicity that neurons in the inferior colliculus represent may not be unique to pitch, but may reflect more general temporal processing of acoustic signals. Given that stimulus synchronization decreases to below the upper limit of missing fundamental pitch by the next stage in the auditory pathway (the medial geniculate body), this may be the last place along the auditory pathway to transform temporal information related to pitch into a firing rate-based or place-based neural code. In comparison to tuning to sAM at auditory nerve and cochlear nuclei by synchronized neural firings, at least some neurons in the inferior colliculus are tuned by firing rate to modulation frequency (Rees and Palmer, 1989; Langner et al., 2002).

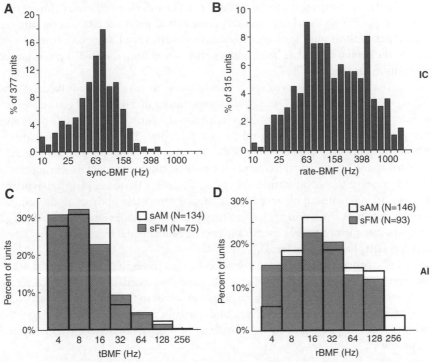

Fig. 7.5 Comparison between modulation frequency tuning in the inferior colliculus (IC) and primary auditory cortex (A1) using sinusoidal amplitude modulation (sAM) or sinusoidal frequency modulation (sFM). **A** and **B** Distributions of synchrony-based (sync-BMF) and firing rate-based (rate-BMF) best modulation frequency (BMF) of IC neurons. (From Langner *et al.*, 2002.) **C** and **D** Distributions of synchrony-based (tBMF) and firing rate-based (rBMF) best modulation frequency (BMF) of A1 neurons. (From Liang *et al.*, 2002.)

7.5.4 **Medial geniculate body**

The medial geniculate body consists of three main divisions (ventral, dorsal, and medial), with the ventral division receiving the bulk of its inputs from the central nucleus of the inferior colliculus (see Chapter 2). Of these three divisions, only the ventral division has a clear tonotopic organization. The ventral division is responsive to narrowband sounds, while the dorsal and medial divisions are generally more responsive to complex sounds (Hu, 2003). Temporal processing studies in the medial geniculate body have typically used click trains and amplitude-modulated tones as acoustic stimuli (Bartlett and Wang, 2007), and the issue of pitch (or fundamental frequency) has not been directly addressed. The type of orderly periodicity map observed in the inferior colliculus in some species (Langner *et al.*, 2002) has not been observed in the medial geniculate body.

One relevant piece of evidence for pitch processing is that the upper limit of stimulus synchronization drops considerably from the inferior colliculus to the medial geniculate body, and from the medial geniculate body to auditory cortex for both pure tones (Liu *et al.*, 2006; Wallace *et al*, 2002, 2007) and amplitude-modulated tones (Langner *et al.*, 2002; Liang *et al.*, 2002; Bartlett and Wang, 2007). In the ventral division of the medial geniculate body, the upper limit of pure tone synchronization measured in anesthetized chinchillas was between 80 and 600 Hz (Wallace *et al.*,

2007; Fig. 7.6B), in comparison to 80–1100 Hz in the inferior colliculus (Liu *et al.*, 2006; Fig. 7.6A) and 60–250 Hz in primary auditory cortex (Wallace *et al.*, 2002) of the same species. Thus the upper limit of pure tone synchronization drops about an octave from the inferior colliculus to the medial geniculate body, and another octave from the medial geniculate body to primary auditory cortex.

A similar trend has been observed for synchronization to envelope modulations (Joris *et al*, 2004; Wang *et al.*, 2008; Fig. 7.5). These observations suggest that the medial geniculate body may play an intermediate role in transforming pitch-related information to a code that represents extracted pitch, though much remains unknown at this point. The loss of temporal information representing pitch in the medial geniculate body also suggests that the conversion of neural firings synchronized to the fundamental frequency (of pure or complex tones) to a firing rate code is essential to preserve this information (Wang *et al.*, 2008). For example, non-synchronized responses to periodic stimuli observed in the medial geniculate body of awake animals may represent such a transformation at this auditory processing stage (Bartlett and Wang, 2007). However, whether such responses specifically encode fundamental frequency, pitch salience, or temporal regularity has not been tested.

If the periodicity map observed in the inferior colliculus serves the basis for representing pitch, its output must be read out in the medial geniculate body or passed on to auditory cortex. Neither periodic maps nor pitch-specific neurons have been observed in the medial geniculate body. Most physiological studies of the medial geniculate body have focused on the ventral division. Whether any periodic maps or pitch-specific neurons exist in other medial geniculate body divisions remains unknown.

7.6 Cortical processing of pitch

7.6.1 Organization of auditory cortex in humans and monkeys

The anatomical study by Brodmann (1909) suggested that the structure of the temporal lobe is largely preserved across primate species (New World monkeys, Old World monkeys, and

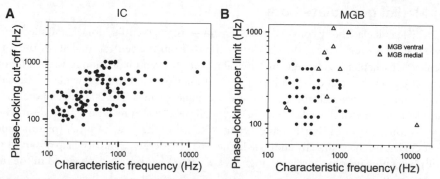

Fig. 7.6 Comparison between the upper limit of the phase-locking to pure tones in the inferior colliculus (IC) and medial geniculate body (MGB). **A** Phase-locking characteristics for all single units recorded in the IC. Plot of highest frequency where statistically significant phase-locking was still observed for units with different CFs. The phase-locking cut-off frequencies tend to increase with increasing CF up to ~1 kHz and then level out. (Adapted from Liu *et al.*, 2006.) **B** Plot of upper limit of phase-locking to pure tones against the CF of units in the ventral and medial divisions of MGB. Four of the medial units (*open triangle*) have limits higher than those of any in the ventral division (*solid circle*). (From Wallace *et al.*, 2007.)

humans). Studies in recent years have revealed distinctions between various auditory cortical areas in primates using anatomical and physiological criteria (e.g. Morel and Kass, 1992; Morel *et al.*, 1993; Kaas and Hackett, 2000; Hackett *et al.*, 2001; Formisano *et al.*, 2003). Humans and monkeys appear to share a similar organization of primary, primary-like, and secondary cortical areas (Kaas and Hackett, 2000; Hackett *et al.*, 2001), suggesting a generalizable structure and function of auditory cortex among primates. Therefore using a non-human primate model for electrophysiology offers a substantial advantage over non-primate species when attempting to bridge this research to human studies. A reasonable hypothesis is that homologous regions of auditory cortex process pitch in both monkeys and humans.

Primate auditory cortex is divided into a core region of primary and primary-like areas surrounded by a belt of multiple secondary areas (Kaas and Hackett, 2000; Figs 7.7A and 7.8A).In humans and monkeys, the core areas of auditory cortex can be distinguished from belt areas by their cytoarchitecture, namely a more prominent granular layer (Morel and Kass, 1992; Morel *et al.*, 1993; Hackett *et al.*, 2001; Chapter 2). In monkeys the core areas have been shown to receive thalamic inputs from the principal (ventral) nucleus of the medial geniculate body (Kaas and Hackett, 2000). In contrast, the belt areas receive more dominant thalamic inputs from the dorsal and medial divisions of the medial geniculate body (Kaas and Hackett, 2000). In both monkeys and humans, neurons in core areas respond strongly to narrowband sounds such as tones, whereas neurons in belt areas respond better to more spectrally complex sounds (e.g. noise, frequency modulations, spectral contours, and vocalizations) (Rauschecker *et al.*, 1995; Recanzone *et al.*, 2000; Wessinger *et al.*, 2001; Barbour and Wang, 2003; Rauschecker and Tian, 2004; Tian and Rauschecker, 2004: Recanzone, 2008). Within the core areas, for both humans (Formisano *et al.*, 2003; Fig. 7.7A) and monkeys (Morel and Kass, 1992; Morel *et al.*, 1993; Fig. 7.8A), two mirror symmetric tonotopic maps sharing a low-frequency border have been identified, corresponding to primary auditory cortex (A1) and the rostral field (R).

In humans, the core areas are generally confined to Heschl's gyrus (Hackett *et al.*, 2001), with A1 located medially to R (Fig. 7.7B). However, this is difficult to determine precisely by anatomical landmarks due to substantial intra-subject variability. Monkeys do not possess an anatomical landmark like the Heschl's gyrus, and the location of A1 must be determined physiologically or histologically. A1 is typically buried within the lateral sulcus in monkeys, except for a few New World species such as marmosets (Aitkin *et al.*, 1986; Bendor and Wang, 2008), owl monkeys (Morel and Kaas, 1992), and squirrel monkeys (Cheung *et al.*, 2001) for which the lateral portion of A1 is located on the surface of the superior temporal gyrus (Fig. 7.8A). There is anatomical and physiological evidence of a third core area, the rostrotemporal field (RT), that lies rostral to R (Morel and Kaas, 1992; Bendor and Wang, 2008; Fig. 7.8A). Kaas and Hackett (2000) have postulated that each core area is connected to a medial and lateral neighboring belt area, with additional belt areas located on the rostral and caudal ends of the core region of auditory cortex (A1, R, and RT). Three of these lateral belt areas (CL, ML, and AL) have been mapped electrophysiologically (Rauschecker and Tian, 2004; Tian and Rauschecker, 2004) as well as by the fMRI technique (Petkov *et al.*, 2006), and have been found to possess tonotopic maps in parallel to adjacent core areas. Additional higher auditory areas such as parabelt (Hackett *et al.*, 1998a,b) and the temporal pole have been defined anatomically, but little is known about their physiological properties.

7.6.2 Pitch processing in human auditory cortex

The auditory system is characterized by frequency maps (tonotopic organization), which could underlie our perception of an orderly arrangement of pure tone pitches (such as the musical scale). However, the evidence of maps of missing fundamental pitch has been lacking. Previous MEG

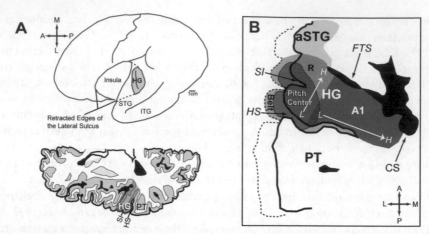

Fig. 7.7 Anatomic organization of human auditory cortex and the location of a pitch center. **A** Side view of a human brain (*top*) and a horizontal cross section of temporal lobe (*bottom*). **B** An enlarged view of Heschl's gyrus. A1 is presumed to occupy the medial portion of Heschl's gyrus (with variability between subjects). The location of neighboring areas (R, pitch center, lateral belt) is an approximation based on Patterson *et al*. (2002), Formisano *et al*. (2003), and Schneider *et al*. (2005).HG Heschl's gyrus, STG superior temporal gyrus, ITG inferior temporal gyrus, aSTG anterior superior temporal gyrus, PT planum temporale, SI intermediate sulcus, HS Heschl's sulcus, CS circular sulcus, FTS first transverse sulcus, LS lateral sulcus, STS superior temporal sulcus, A1 primary auditory cortex, R rostral field, RT rostrotemporal field.

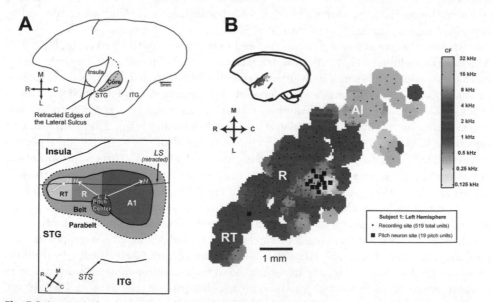

Fig. 7.8 Anatomical organization of marmoset monkey auditory cortex and the location of a pitch center. **A** Side view of the marmoset brain (*top*) and a zoomed-in view of the superior temporal gyrus (*bottom*), indicating core, belt, parabelt, and the pitch center. The borders between each auditory area are estimated based on data from Pistorio *et al*. (2004) and Bendor and Wang (2005). **B** Tonotopic maps of the auditory cortex characterized in the left hemisphere of one marmoset. Pitch-selective neurons (*black squares*) were found clustered near the anterolateral border of A1. Frequency reversals indicate the borders between A1/R and R/RT. (From Bendor and Wang, 2005.)

experiments in humans have suggested that a pitch map coexists with the tonotopic map in A1, either in parallel (Pantev *et al.*, 1989) or orthogonal (Langner *et al.*, 1997) to it. However, these topographies have not been confirmed using imaging techniques such as fMRI that directly measure spatial locations of neural activity with sufficient resolution. The existence of multiple auditory fields (and tonotopic maps) within auditory cortex exacerbates the problem of identifying sources by the MEG technique that computes, instead of directly measuring, source locations. It is possible that only a subset of neurons in A1 participate in encoding pitch, while other neurons analyze spectral and temporal properties of the sound and all the other things that make up hearing (location, sources, etc.). Alternatively, pitch may be processed within another primary-like or secondary cortical field and A1 may not be involved in extracting pitch.

Functional magnetic resonance imaging (fMRI) has become a powerful tool in neuroscience, due to its ability to non-invasively measure brain activity with better spatial acuity than any other existing human imaging methods. One issue, however, is the loud noise produced by the MRI scanner that can mask or interfere with auditory experiments. The development of techniques such as sparse imaging (Hall *et al.*, 1999), which takes advantage of the slow build-up time of the blood oxygen level dependent (BOLD) response, has helped overcome this problem. Human imaging experiments typically use a subtraction protocol, where the BOLD activity difference is taken between a stimulus with the desired feature and a second stimulus with that desired feature absent or modified (but like the first stimulus in all other respects). Thus, to find a region of the brain that responds selectively or preferentially to pitch, one must use at least two stimuli, one with pitch and the others without pitch or with weaker pitch salience, but being spectral and temporally similar in all other respects. In other words, only the spectral harmonicity or temporal periodicity is altered without varying the bandwidth, modulation frequency, frequency range of harmonics, etc. Although this limits what acoustic stimuli can be used in these experiments, several approaches are still available, such as spectrally jittering the harmonics of a random phase complex tone or temporally jittering the pulses of a regular acoustic pulse train.

Patterson and colleagues (2002) used iterated ripple noise (IRN) stimuli and found that across subjects, lateral Heschl's gyrus (bilaterally) gives a stronger BOLD signal to IRN stimuli than to noise. In contrast, A1 located in medial Heschl's gyrus and other regions within auditory cortex showed no such difference. Human auditory filters in the high-frequency range have limited spectral resolvability and therefore do not provide a basis for distinguishing IRN sounds with low-frequency pitches even though these have physically different spectra. Yet subjects hear a pitch from IRN stimuli, but not from noise. A 'pitch center' was localized to lateral Heschl's gyrus (Fig. 7.7B), and regions anterior to lateral Heschl's gyrus in the right hemisphere were found to be responsive to melodies composed of IRN stimuli (Patterson *et al.*, 2002). These results suggest a hierarchical process, whereby individual pitches are extracted within the pitch center, and then changes in pitch (relative pitch) are detected in more anterior regions of auditory cortex.

Penagos and colleagues (2004) used four harmonic complex sounds that had either a low or a high pitch and occupied either a low or high spectral range. Of these four sounds, only the sound with the low pitch and harmonics in the high spectral range had unresolved harmonics. Sounds with unresolved harmonics have a weaker pitch salience than sounds containing resolved harmonics, for which spectral cues are available (Moore, 2003). Thus, Penagos and colleagues (2004) were able to compare BOLD signals between sounds evoking a strong or weak pitch salience, but matched in their fundamental frequency or spectral range. Bilaterally, a restricted region of non-primary auditory cortex in the lateral Heschl's gyrus anterolateral to A1 was found more weakly responsive to the sound with low pitch salience than the other three sounds with high pitch salience. Furthermore, the activity in this region was not significantly different in the high pitch salience stimuli when comparing across different fundamental frequencies or frequency ranges. In addition, the inferior colliculus and cochlear nucleus showed no difference between stimuli differing in pitch salience. The study by Penagos *et al.* (2004) concluded that only lateral Heschl's gyrus was sensitive to changes in pitch salience, supporting the notion that a pitch center exists in this region of auditory cortex.

The significance of the lateral Heschl's gyrus in pitch representation was further investigated by Schneider *et al.* (2005) using a combination of psychophysics, anatomical MRI scans, and MEG measurements. For harmonic complex tones with a few components, a person may hear the pitch increasing or decreasing when the frequencies of harmonics are decreased while the fundamental frequency is increased (Moore, 2003). Schneider *et al.* (2005) found that individual subjects showed a bias towards using the fundamental frequency or spectral frequency when discriminating pitch changes. These biases were found highly correlated with hemispheric asymmetry in relative size between the right and left lateral Heschl's gyrus (and not with other regions of auditory cortex). Subjects that relied more on fundamental frequency to discriminate pitch had a larger left lateral Heschl's gyrus, whereas subjects relying on spectral frequency had a larger right lateral Heschl's gyrus. In addition, MEG responses recorded from a source estimated as lateral Heschl's gyrus showed a similar asymmetry between hemispheres. Stronger responses were obtained from the left hemisphere for subjects with a bias towards using fundamental frequency in pitch discrimination. In contrast, subjects with a bias towards using spectral frequency had larger MEG responses recorded from the right hemisphere.

Taken together, human studies published recently confirm the location of a pitch center in lateral Heschl's gyrus (Patterson *et al.*, 2002; Gutschalk *et al.*, 2004; Penagos *et al.*, 2004; Hall *et al.*, 2005; Ritter *et al.*, 2005; Schneider *et al.*, 2005; Chait *et al.*, 2006; Hall *et al.*, 2006). However, two recent studies by Hall and Plack (2007, 2009) have contradicted the notion of a general 'pitch center' in auditory cortex. In Hall and Plack's (2007) study the authors used a dichotic pitch stimulus known as a Huggin's pitch. A weak pitch percept is created by playing a broadband noise to each ear that is identical, except for a narrow frequency band (190–210 Hz in this study) in which a phase shift is introduced in one of the ears relative to the other. The Huggin's stimulus was found to evoke a weak activation of cortex and no significant activity in lateral Heschl's gyrus (Hall and Plack, 2007). These results suggest that lateral Heschl's gyrus is only involved in processing diotic rather than dichotic pitch.

In the second study, Hall and Plack (2009) played to the same listeners a variety of pitch-evoking stimuli and failed to show that all pitch is processed in a single locus in auditory cortex. Their results suggest that parts of the planum temporale are more relevant for pitch processing than lateral Heschl's gyrus. In some listeners, pitch responses occurred elsewhere, such as the temporo-parieto-occipital junction or prefrontal cortex. Hall and Plack (2009) reported a different pattern of response to the IRN stimuli and suggested the possibility that features of IRN unrelated to pitch might contribute to the earlier results (Patterson *et al.*, 2002). They concluded that it may be premature to assume that lateral Heschl's gyrus is a universal pitch center.

Taken together, the available human imaging data have shown that pitch-evoking stimuli are selectively processed in particular regions of auditory cortex, given that pitch extraction has not been observed subcortically. Evidence also shows that there may exist more than one pitch-processing center in auditory cortex, including but not limited to the lateral Heschl's gyrus. Perhaps this is not all that surprising given the complexity of pitch perception. Further studies need to investigate the specific roles played by each cortical region that has been implicated in pitch processing.

7.6.3 Pitch processing in non-human primate auditory cortex

Schwarz and Tomlinson (1990) searched for single-unit responses to the fundamental frequency of missing fundamental harmonic complex sounds in the primary auditory cortex of awake macaque monkeys. Even though these monkeys had been previously trained on a pitch discrimination task, Schwarz and Tomlinson (1990) were unable to find neurons that responded to the missing fundamental frequency. They concluded that either pitch is represented implicitly across a population of neurons in A1 or an explicit representation exists outside of A1. Consistent with these findings, Fishman *et al.* (1998) were unable to find an implicit representation for the missing fundamental in A1 based on population neuronal responses, using multi-unit recordings in awake macaque monkeys.

Bendor and Wang (2005) investigated neural representation of the missing fundamental frequency in the auditory cortex of awake marmosets (a New World primate species) using single-unit recordings. The following criteria were used to determine if a neuron can be classified as pitch-selective: (1) it responds to pure tones and is tuned in frequency with a best frequency (BF), (2) it responds to missing fundamental harmonic complex sounds with a pitch near its BF, with the harmonics being outside its excitatory frequency response area, and (3) the individual harmonics of the missing fundamental sound do not need to be more than 10 dB above the neuron's BF threshold to evoke a response (in order to avoid the confound of cochlear distortion products). Pitch-selective neurons satisfying these criteria were found in the low-frequency region of auditory cortex near the anterolateral border of A1 (Figs 7.8B and 7.9A).

In addition to meeting these criteria, a typical pitch-selective neuron responded to an array of spectrally dissimilar pitch-evoking sounds (harmonic complex tones, click trains, iterated ripple noise) when the pitch was near the neuron's preferred fundamental frequency. The tuning to the fundamental frequency in the pitch-selective neurons was similar to the neuron's tuning to pure tone frequency. Bendor and Wang (2005) also found that pitch-selective neurons increased their firing rates as the pitch salience increased and preferred temporally regular sounds (Fig. 7.9B), in agreement with the imaging studies by Patterson *et al.* (2002) and Penagos *et al.* (2004). Bendor and Wang's (2005) study showed that the pitch-processing region found in marmosets also contained non-pitch-selective neurons (spanning a similar range of BFs). Potentially, these two classes of neurons co-localized within the pitch-processing center respectively encode missing fundamental pitch and other percepts involving in low frequency spectral components. For ambiguous pitch changes, in which the fundamental frequency and spectral components shift in opposite directions, as in the study by Schneider *et al.* (2005), these two types of neurons would provide conflicting information. Unequal weighting towards one of these neuron types within the pitch-processing center (and/or between hemispheres) may be the cause of a subject's perceptual bias of hearing pitch changes based on the fundamental or spectral frequency.

Because of technical limitations in single-unit recordings, not all auditory cortex areas in non-human primates have been investigated for their possible pitch-processing functions. The similarity in the anatomic structures of auditory cortex between New World and Old World monkeys and humans suggests that the pitch center identified in marmoset monkeys may exist in other non-human primate species and that this pitch center shares similar functions to that of the lateral Heschl's gyrus in humans (Bendor and Wang, 2006).

7.6.4 Studies in non-primate species

Several studies have investigated how missing fundamental sounds are represented in the auditory cortex of non-primates species. Microelectrode recordings in gerbils showed that A1 neurons could respond to the periodicity of amplitude-modulated tones with the spectral components located outside the neuron's excitatory frequency response area, but with the periodicity ranging much higher than the pitch range found in humans (Schulze and Langner, 1997). Schulze *et al.* (2002) also reported a semi-circular shaped map of best fundamental frequency in gerbil auditory

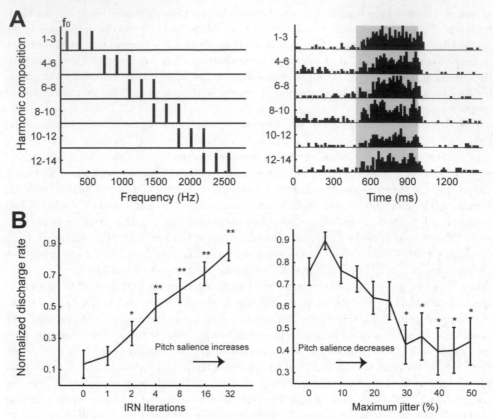

Fig. 7.9 Examples of pitch-selective responses recorded in marmoset auditory cortex. (From Bendor and Wang, 2005.) **A** *Left* Frequency spectra of a series of harmonic complex stimuli. The fundamental frequency component (f_0) and its higher harmonics have equal amplitudes of 50 dB SPL. *Right* Peristimulus time histograms of a pitch-selective neuron's responses to the harmonic complex stimuli. Harmonics 2–14 were outside the neuron's frequency response area. Stimuli were presented from 500 to 1000 ms (indicated by the *shaded region* on the plot). **B** Responses of pitch-selective neurons increases with increasing pitch salience. *Left* Averaged population response of pitch-selective neurons as a function of the iterations of IRN stimuli. The response to IRN stimuli with 0 iterations is used as a reference for statistical comparison at other iterations. *Right* Averaged population response of pitch-selective neurons to irregular click trains as a function of maximum jitter. The response to a regular click train is used as a reference for statistical comparison at other jitter values.

cortex using optical imaging techniques. Langner *et al.* (2002) reported a topographic arrangement of periodicity information in chinchilla auditory cortex that was orthogonal to the tonotopic axis.

Differences in the results from the studies in primate and non-primate species could be due to an evolutionary divergence of pitch-processing strategies within auditory cortex, or result from methodological differences. Combination tones at the fundamental frequency are produced within the cochlea by missing fundamental harmonic complex sounds, creating a potential ambiguity regarding whether a missing fundamental or combination tone is the source of the neuron's evoked response (Plack *et al.*, 2005). The use of appropriate sound levels (to ensure that combination tones are below a neuron's pure tone response threshold) (Bendor and Wang, 2005), as well as the use of noise maskers (Penagos *et al.*, 2004; Bendor and Wang, 2005) or a cancellation tone (McAlpine, 2004) are necessary to confirm that the missing fundamental response observed is not an artifact resulting from a combination tone. More generally, the observation of a missing fundamental response is not sufficient to demonstrate an encoding of pitch. If neurons only respond to missing fundamental sounds when they fall within a neuron's excitatory frequency response area, or do not show sensitivity to temporal regularity or pitch salience, then their responses may be caused by spectral or temporal acoustic features (which still could provide important information to pitch-selective neurons).

7.6.5 Further questions on pitch processing in auditory cortex

The discovery of pitch-processing regions in auditory cortex is only the first step in understanding the physiological mechanisms of pitch perception. Several important questions remain unanswered. First, what is the source of inputs to pitch-selective neurons (corticocortical or thalamocortical)? The location of the pitch center in marmoset auditory cortex (Bendor and Wang, 2005) appears to be overlapping low-frequency portions of the core areas A1, R, and lateral belt areas AL and ML. This suggests that the pitch-selective neurons may receive inputs from both ventral and dorsal divisions of the medial geniculate body that respond to narrowband and wideband sounds, respectively (Kaas and Hackett, 2000). This could be a possible source of the response to pure tones and missing fundamental sounds. Alternatively, given the extensive connectivity between A1, R, and neighboring belt areas surrounding the pitch-processing center, the pitch-selective neurons may extract the fundamental frequency using inputs from neighboring cortical areas (including A1).

Second, do pitch-selective neurons use a spectral (template) and/or temporal (periodicity) mechanism to extract the fundamental frequency of complex sounds? This is an issue that has been at the center of debate among auditory researchers for the last 60 years. Computational models and auditory nerve data support the possibility of both a purely temporal mechanism and a hybrid mechanism using both spectral and temporal information (Cariani and Delgutte, 1996a,b; Cedolin and Delgutte, 2005; Plack *et al.*, 2005). In monkeys, A1 neurons with temporal and spectral response properties potentially useful for these pitch models have been observed (Steinschneider *et al.*, 1998; Lu *et al.*, 2001; Liang *et al.*, 2002; Kadia and Wang, 2003), but whether they provide an input to pitch-selective neurons is unknown.

Finally, electrophysiological recordings need to be performed in behaving conditions so that psychophysical measurements can be directly compared with neural responses. In addition, questions such as how the cortical representation of pitch influences pitch-related stream segregation and the neural correlates of pitch ambiguity percepts will be some of the exciting future directions for this area of research.

References

Aitkin LM, Merzenich MM, Irvine DR, Clarey JC, Nelson JE (1986) Frequency representation in auditory cortex of the common marmoset (*Callithrix jacchus jacchus*). *J Comp Neurol* 252(2): 175–85.

Attneave F, Olson RK (1971) Pitch as a medium: a new approach to psychophysical scaling. *Am J Psychol* 84: 147–66.

Barbour DL, Wang X (2003) Contrast tuning in auditory cortex. *Science* 299(5609): 1073–5.

Bartlett EL, Wang X (2007) Neural representations of temporally modulated signals in the auditory thalamus of awake primates. *J Neurophysiol* 97(2): 1005–17.

Bendor D, Wang X (2005) The neuronal representation of pitch in primate auditory cortex. *Nature* 436(7054): 1161–5.

Bendor D, Wang X (2006) Cortical representations of pitch in monkeys and humans. *Curr Opin Neurobiol* **16**: 391–99.

Bendor D, Wang X (2007) Differential neural coding of acoustic flutter within primate auditory cortex. *Nat Neurosci* **10**(6): 763–71.

Bendor D, Wang X (2008) Neural response properties of primary, rostral, and rostrotemporal core fields in the auditory cortex of marmoset monkeys. *J Neurophysiol* **100**: 888–906.

Bernstein JG, Oxenham AJ (2003) Pitch discrimination of diotic and dichotic tone complexes: Harmonic resolvability or harmonic number?. *J Acoust Soc Am* **113**: 3323–34.

Blackburn CC, Sachs MB (1989) Classification of unit types in the anteroventral cochlear nucleus: PST histograms and regularity analysis. *J Neurophysiol* **62**(6): 1303–29.

Blackburn CC, Sachs MB (1990) The representations of the steady-state vowel sound /e/ in the discharge patterns of cat anteroventral cochlear nucleus neurons. *J Neurophysiol* **63**(5): 1191–212.

Brodmann K (1909) *Vergleichende Lokalisationslehre der Großhirnrinde in ihren Prinzipien dargestellt auf Grund des Zellenbaues*. Barth, Leipzig.

Cariani PA, Delgutte B (1996a) Neural correlates of the pitch of complex tones. I. Pitch and pitch salience. *J Neurophysiol* **76**: 1698–716.

Cariani PA, Delgutte B (1996b) Neural correlates of the pitch of complex tones. II. Pitch shift, pitch ambiguity, phase invariance, pitch circularity, rate pitch, and the dominance region for pitch. *J Neurophysiol* **76**(3): 1717–34.

Carlyon RP (1998) Comments on "A unitary model of pitch perception" (*J Acoust Soc Am* 102: 1811–20 (1997). *J Acoust Soc Am* **104**(2 Part 1): 1118–21.

Carlyon RP, Shackleton TM (1994) Comparing the fundamental frequency of a complex tone in the presence of a spectrally overlapping masker. *J Acoust Soc Am* **99**: 517–24.

Cedolin L, Delgutte B (2005) Pitch of complex tones: rate-place and interspike-interval representation in the auditory nerve. *J Neurophysiol* **94**(1): 347–62.

Chait M, Poeppel D, Simon JZ (2006) Neural response correlates of detection of monaurally and binaurally created pitches in humans. *Cereb Cortex* **16**(6): 835–48.

Cheung SW, Bedenbaugh PH, Nagarajan SS, Schreiner CE (2001) Functional organization of squirrel monkey primary auditory cortex: responses to pure tones. *J Neurophysiol* **85**(4): 1732.

Culling JF (2000) Dichotic pitches as illusions of binaural unmasking. III. The existence region of the Fourcin pitch. *J Acoust Soc Am* **103**: 3509–26.

Culling JF, Summerfield AQ, Marshall DH (1998a) Dichotic pitches as illusions of binaural unmasking. I. Huggins' pitch and the 'binaural edge pitch.' *J Acoust Soc Am* **103**: 3509–26.

Culling JF, Marshall DH, Summerfield AQ (1998b) Dichotic pitches as illusions of binaural unmasking. II. The Fourcin pitch and the dichotic repetition pitch. *J Acoust Soc Am* **103**: 3527–39.

Cynx J, Shapiro M (1986) Perception of missing fundamental by a species of songbird (*Sturnus vulgaris*). *J Comp Psychol* **100**: 356–60.

Dooling RJ, Searcy MH (1981) Amplitude modulation thresholds for the parakeet (*Melopsittacus undulates*). *J Comp Physiol* **143**: 383–8.

Fay RR, Passow B (1982) Temporal discrimination in the goldfish. *J Acoust Soc Am* **72**: 753–60.

Fishman YI, Reser DH, Arezzo JC, Steinschneider M (1998) Pitch vs. spectral encoding of harmonic complex tones in primary auditory cortex of the awake monkey. *Brain Res* **786**(1–2): 18–30.

Formisano E, Kim DS, Di Salle F, van de Moortele PF, Ugurbil K, Goebel R (2003) Mirror-symmetric tonotopic maps in human primary auditory cortex. *Neuron* **40**(4): 859–69.

Frisina RD, Smith RL, Chamberlain SC (1990) Encoding of amplitude modulation in the gerbil cochlear nucleus. II. Possible neural mechanisms. *Hear Res* **44**: 123–44.

Goldstein JL (1973) An optimum processor theory for the central formation of the pitch of complex tones. *J Acoust Soc Am* **54**: 1496–516.

Gutschalk A, Patterson RD, Scherg M, Uppenkamp S, Rupp A (2004) Temporal dynamics of pitch in human auditory cortex. *Neuroimage* 22(2): 755–66.

Hackett TA, Stepniewska I, Kaas JH (1998a) Thalamocortical connections of the parabelt auditory cortex in macaque monkeys. *J Comp Neurol* 400(2): 271–86.

Hackett TA, Stepniewska I, Kaas JH (1998b) Subdivisions of auditory cortex and ipsilateral cortical connections of the parabelt auditory cortex in macaque monkeys. *J Comp Neurol* 394(4): 475–95.

Hackett TA, Preuss TM, Kaas JH (2001) Architectonic identification of the core region in auditory cortex of macaques, chimpanzees, and humans. *J Comp Neurol* 441(3): 197–222.

Hall DA, Plack CJ (2007) The human 'pitch center' responds differently to iterated noise and Huggins pitch. *Neuroreport* 18(4): 323–7.

Hall DA, Plack CJ (2009) Pitch processing sites in the human auditory brain. *Cereb Cortex* 19(3): 576–85.

Hall DA, Haggard MP, Akeroyd MA, *et al.* (1999) "Sparse" temporal sampling in auditory fMRI. *Hum Brain Mapp* 7(3): 213–23.

Hall DA, Barrett DJ, Akeroyd MA, Summerfield AQ (2005) Cortical representations of temporal structure in sound. *J Neurophysiol* 94(5): 3181–91.

Hall DA, Edmondson-Jones AM, Fridriksson J (2006) Periodicity and frequency coding in human auditory cortex. *Eur J Neurosci* 24(12): 3601–10.

Heffner H, Whitfield IC (1976) Perception of the missing fundamental by cats. *J Acoust Soc Am* 59: 915–19.

Hewitt MJ, Meddis R (1994) A computer model of amplitude-modulation sensitivity of single units in the inferior colliculus. *J Acoust Soc Am* 95: 2145–59.

Hu. B (2003) Functional organization of lemniscal and nonlemniscal auditory thalamus. *Exp Brain Res* 153(4): 543–9.

Izumi A (2000) Japanese monkeys perceive sensory consonance of chords. *J Acoust Soc Am* 108: 3073–8.

Izumi A (2001) Relative pitch perception in Japanese monkeys (*Macaca fuscata*). *J Comp Psychol* 115: 127–31.

Joris PX, Schreiner CE, Rees A (2004) Neural processing of amplitude-modulated sounds. *Physiol Rev* 84(2): 541–77.

Kaas JH, Hackett TA (2000) Subdivisions of auditory cortex and processing streams in primates. *Proc Natl Acad Sci* 97(22): 11793–9.

Kadia SC, Wang X (2003) Spectral integration in A1 of awake primates: neurons with single- and multipeaked tuning characteristics. *J Neurophysiol* 89(3): 1603–22.

Keilson SE, Richards VM, Wyman BT, Young ED (1997) The representation of concurrent vowels in the cat anesthetized ventral cochlear nucleus: evidence for a periodicity-tagged spectral representation. *J Acoust Soc Am* 102(2 Part 1): 1056–71.

Kim DO, Sirianni JG, Chang SO (1990) Responses of DCN-PVCN neurons and auditory nerve fibres in unanaesthetised decerebrate cats to AM and pure tones: analysis with autocorrelation/power-spectrum. *Hear Res* 45: 95–113.

Krumbholz K, Patterson RD, Pressnitzer D (2000) The lower limit of pitch as determined by rate discrimination. *J Acoust Soc Am* 108: 1170–80.

Langner G, Schreiner CE (1988) Periodicity coding in the inferior colliculus of the cat. I. Neuronal mechanisms. *J Neurophysiol* 60: 1799–822.

Langner G, Sams M, Heil P, Schulze H (1997) Frequency and periodicity are represented in orthogonal maps in the human auditory cortex: evidence from magnetoencephalography. *J Comp Physiol A* 181: 665–76.

Langner G, Albert M, Briede T (2002) Temporal and spatial coding of periodicity information in the inferior colliculus of awake chinchilla (*Chinchilla laniger*). *Hear Res* 168(1–2): 110–30.

Liang L, Lu T, Wang X (2002) Neural representations of sinusoidal amplitude and frequency modulations in the auditory cortex of awake primates. *J Neurophysiol* 87: 2237–61.

Licklider JCR (1951) A duplex theory of pitch perception. *Experientia* 7: 128–33.

Licklider JCR (1956) Auditory frequency analysis. In: Information Theory (ed. Cherry C), pp. 253–68. Academic Press, New York.

Liu LF, Palmer AR, Wallace MN (2006) Phase-locked responses to pure tones in the inferior colliculus. *J Neurophysiol* 95(3): 1926–35.

Loeb GE, White MW, Merzenich MM (1983) Spatial cross-correlation – a proposed mechanism for acoustic pitch perception. *Biol Cybern* 47: 149–63.

Long GR, Clark WW (1984) Detection of frequency and rate modulation by the chinchilla. *J Acoust Soc Am* 75: 1184–90.

Lu T, Liang L, Wang X (2001) Temporal and rate representations of time-varying signals in the auditory cortex of awake primates. *Nat Neurosci* 4(11): 1131–8.

McAlpine D (2004) Neural sensitivity to periodicity in the inferior colliculus: evidence for the role of cochlear distortions. *J Neurophysiol* 92: 1295–311.

McDermott J, Hauser MD (2005) Probing the evolutionary origins of music perception. *Ann N Y Acad Sci* 1060: 6–16.

Meddis R, Hewitt MJ (1991a) Virtual pitch and phase sensitivity of a computer model of the auditory periphery. I: Pitch identification. *J Acoust Soc Am* 89: 2866–82.

Meddis R, Hewitt MJ (1991b) Virtual pitch and phase sensitivity of a computer model of the auditory periphery. II: Phase sensitivity. *J Acoust Soc Am* 89: 2883–94.

Meddis R, O'Mard L (1997) A unitary model of pitch perception. *J Acoust Soc Am* 102(3): 1811–20.

Moody DB (1994) Detection and discrimination of amplitude-modulated signals by macaque monkeys. *J Acoust Soc Am* 95: 3499–510.

Moore BCJ (1973) Some experiments relating to the perception of complex tones. *Q J Exp Psych* 25: 451–75.

Moore BCJ (2003) *An Introduction to the Psychology of Hearing.* Academic Press, London.

Moore BCJ, Moore GA (2003) Perception of the low pitch of frequency-shifted complexes. *J Acoust Soc Am* 113: 977–85.

Moore BCJ, Glasberg BR, Peters RW (1985) Relative dominance of individual partials in determining the pitch of complex tones. *J Acoust Soc Am* 77: 550–61.

Morel A, Kaas JH (1992) Subdivisions and connections of auditory cortex in owl monkeys. *J Comp Neurol* 318: 27–63.

Morel A, Garraghty PE, Kaas JH (1993) Tonotopic organization, architectonic fields, and connections of auditory cortex in macaque monkeys. *J Comp Neurol* 335: 437–59.

Oertel D, Bal R, Gardner SM, Smith PH, Joris PX (2000) Detection of synchrony in the activity of auditory nerve fibers by octopus cells of the mammalian cochlear nucleus. *Proc Natl Acad Sci* 97(22): 11773–9.

Palmer AR, Winter IM (1996) The temporal window of two-tone facilitation in onset units of the ventral cochlear nucleus. *Audiol Neurootol* 1(1): 12–30.

Pantev C, Hoke M, Lutkenhoner B, Lehnertz K (1989) Tonotopic organization of the auditory cortex: pitch versus frequency representation. *Science* 246: 486–8.

Patterson RD, Uppenkamp S, Johnsrude IS, Griffiths TD (2002) The processing of temporal pitch and melody information in auditory cortex. *Neuron* 36(4): 767–76.

Penagos H, Melcher JR, Oxenham AJ (2004) A neural representation of pitch salience in nonprimary human auditory cortex revealed with functional magnetic resonance imaging. *J Neurosci* 24(30): 6810–15.

Petkov CI, Kayser C, Augath M, Logothetis NK (2006) Functional imaging reveals numerous fields in the monkey auditory cortex. *PLoS Biol* 4: e215.

Pistorio A, Hendry S, Wang X (2004) *Correlation Between Electrophysiology and Anatomical Markers in the Auditory Cortex of the Common Marmoset.* Abstract # 650.13. Society for Neuroscience, Washington, DC.

Plack CJ, Oxenham AJ (2005) The psychophysics of pitch. In: Pitch: Neural Coding and Perception (eds Plack CJ, Oxenham AJ, Fay RR, Popper AN), pp 7–55. Springer, New York.

Plack CJ, Oxenham AJ, Fay RR, Popper AN (2005) *Pitch: Neural Coding and Perception.* Springer Handbook of Auditory Research. Springer, New York.

Plomp R (1967) Pitch of complex tones. *J Acoust Soc Am* 41: 1526–33.

Pollack I (1968) Discrimination of mean temporal interval within jittered auditory pulse trains. *J Acoust Soc Am* 43(5): 1107–12.

Pollack I (1969) Auditory random-walk discrimination. *J Acoust Soc Am* 46(2): 422–5.

Pressnitzer D, Patterson RD, Krumbholz K (2001) The lower limit of melodic pitch. *J Acoust Soc Am* 109: 2074–84.

Rauschecker JP, Tian B (2004) Processing of band-passed noise in the lateral auditory belt cortex of the rhesus monkey. *J Neurophysiol* 91: 2578–89.

Rauschecker JP, Tian B, Hauser M (1995) Processing of complex sounds in the macaque nonprimary auditory cortex. *Science* 268(5207): 111–14.

Recanzone GH (2008) Representation of con-specific vocalizations in the core and belt areas of the auditory cortex in the alert macaque monkey. *J Neurosci* 28(49): 13184–93.

Recanzone GH, Guard DC, Phan ML (2000) Frequency and intensity response properties of single neurons in the auditory cortex of the behaving macaque monkey. *J Neurophysiol* 83(4): 2315–31.

Rees A, Palmer AR (1989) Neuronal responses to amplitude-modulated and pure-tone stimuli in the guinea pig inferior colliculus, and their modification by broadband noise. *J Acoust Soc Am* 85(5): 1978.

Rhode WS (1994) Temporal coding of, 200% amplitude modulated signals in the ventral cochlear nucleus of cat. *Hear Res* 77: 43–68.

Rhode WS (1998) Neural encoding of single-formant stimuli in the ventral cochlear nucleus of the chinchilla. *Hear Res* 117: 39–56.

Ritsma (1962) Existence region of the tonal residue. I. *J Acoust Soc Am* 34: 1224–9.

Ritsma (1963) Existence region of the tonal residue. II. *J Acoust Soc Am* 35: 1241–5.

Ritsma (1967) Frequencies dominant in the perception of the pitch of complex sounds. *J Acoust Soc Am* 42: 191–8.

Ritter S, Gunter Dosch H, Specht HJ, Rupp A (2005) Neuromagnetic responses reflect the temporal pitch change of regular interval sounds. *Neuroimage* 3: 533–43.

Schneider P, Sluming V, Roberts N, *et al.* (2005) Structural and functional asymmetry of lateral Heschl's gyrus reflects pitch perception preference. *Nat Neurosci* 8(9): 1241–7.

Schouten JF (1938) The perception of subjective tones. *Proc Kon Akad Wetenschap* 41: 991–9.

Schouten JF, Ritsma RJ, Cardozo BL (1962) Pitch of the residue. *J Acoust Soc Am* 34: 1418–24.

Schreiner CE, Langner G (1988) Periodicity coding in the inferior colliculus of the cat. II. Topographical organization. *J Neurophysiol* 60: 1823–40.

Schulze H, Langner G (1997) Periodicity coding in the primary auditory cortex of the Mongolian gerbil (*Meriones unguiculatus*): two different coding strategies for pitch and rhythm?. *J Comp Physiol A* 181: 651–63.

Schulze H, Scheich H (1999) Discrimination learning of amplitude modulated tones in Mongolian gerbils. *Neurosci Lett* 261: 13–16.

Schulze H, Hess A, Ohl FW, Scheich H (2002) Superposition of horseshoe-like periodicity and linear tonotopic maps in auditory cortex of the Mongolian gerbil. *Eur J Neurosci* 15: 1077–84.

Schwarz DW, Tomlinson RW (1990) Spectral response patterns of auditory cortex neurons to harmonic complex tones in alert monkey (*Macaca mulatta*). *J Neurophysiol* 64(1): 282–98.

Shackleton TM, Carlyon RP (1994) The role of resolved and unresolved harmonics in pitch perception and frequency modulation discrimination. *J Acoust Soc Am* 95: 3529–40.

Shackleton TM, Liu LF, Palmer AR (2009) Responses to diotic, dichotic, and alternating phase harmonic stimuli in the inferior colliculus of guinea pigs. *J Assoc Res Otolaryngol* **10**(1): 76–90.

Shamma SA (1985) Speech processing in the auditory system II: Lateral inhibition and the central processing of speech evoked activity in the auditory nerve. *J Acoust Soc Am* **78**: 1622–32.

Shamma S, Klein D (2000) The case of the missing pitch templates: how harmonic templates emerge in the early auditory system. *J Acoust Soc Am* **107**: 2631–44.

Shofner WP (2008) Representation of the spectral dominance region of pitch in the steady-state temporal discharge patterns of cochlear nucleus units. *J Acoust Soc Am* **124**(5): 3038–52.

Steinschneider M, Reser DH, Fishman YI, Schroeder CE, Arezzo JC (1998) Click train encoding in primary auditory cortex of the awake monkey: evidence for two mechanisms subserving pitch perception. *J Acoust Soc Am* **104**(5): 2935–55.

Stevens SS (1935) The relation of pitch to intensity. *J Acoust Soc Am* **6**: 150–4.

Terhardt E (1974) Pitch, consonance and harmony. *J Acoust Soc Am* **55**: 1061–9.

Tian B, Rauschecker JP (2004) Processing of frequency-modulated sounds in the lateral auditory belt cortex of the rhesus monkey. *J Neurophysiol* **92**(5): 2993–3013.

Tomlinson RWW, Schwarz DWF (1988) Perception of the missing fundamental in non-human primates. *J Acoust Soc Am* **84**: 560–5.

Tramo MJ, Shah GD, Braida LD (2002) Functional role of auditory cortex in frequency processing and pitch perception. *J Neurophysiol* **87**(1): 122–39.

Verschuure J, van Meeteren AA (1975) The effect of intensity on pitch. *Acustica* **32**: 33–44.

Wallace MN, Shackleton TM, Palmer AR (2002) Phase-locked responses to pure tones in the primary auditory cortex. *Hear Res* **172**(1–2): 160–71.

Wallace MN, Anderson LA, Palmer AR (2007) Phase-locked responses to pure tones in the auditory thalamus. *J Neurophysiol* **98**(4): 1941–5.

Wang X, Lu T, Bendor D, Bartlett EL (2008) Neural coding of temporal information in auditory thalamus and cortex. *Neuroscience* **157**: 484–93.

Ward WD (1954) Subjective musical pitch. *J Acoust Soc Am* **26**: 369–80.

Warrier CM, Zatorre RJ (2004) Right temporal cortex is critical for utilization of melodic contextual cues in a pitch constancy task. *Brain* **127**: 1616–25.

Wessinger CM, VanMeter J, Tian B, Van Lare J, Pekar J, Rauschecker JP (2001) Hierarchical organization of the human auditory cortex revealed by functional magnetic resonance imaging. *J Cogn Neurosci* **13**(1): 1–7.

Whitfield IC (1980) Auditory cortex and the pitch of complex tones. *J Acoust Soc Am* **67**: 644–7.

Wightman FL (1973) The pattern-transformation model of pitch. *J Acoust Soc Am* **54**: 407–16.

Winter IM, Wiegrebe L, Patterson RD (2001) The temporal representation of the delay of iterated rippled noise in the ventral cochlear nucleus of the guinea-pig. *J Physiol* **537**(2): 553–66.

Wright AA, Rivera JJ, Hulse SH, Shyan M, Neiworth JJ (2000) Music perception and octave generalization in rhesus monkeys. *J Exp Psychol Gen* **129**: 291–307.

Yost WA (1996a) Pitch of iterated rippled noise. *J Acoust Soc Am* **100**: 511–18.

Yost WA (1996b) Pitch strength of iterated rippled noise. *J Acoust* **100**(5): 3329–35.

Zatorre RJ (1988) Pitch perception of complex tones and human temporal-lobe function. *J Acoust Soc Am* **84**: 566–72.

Chapter 8

Ethological stimuli

Achim Klug and Benedikt Grothe

8.1 Neural coding of ethological signals

The main purpose of sensory systems – and the auditory system is no exception – is to aid the survival of their owner in a complex world. Typical tasks of sensory systems are to help species navigate and interact with the environment, and to detect food sources and potential dangers such as predators or noxious environments. Furthermore, sensory systems assist animals in detecting signals sent by other animals about their behavioral state, and in this way help regulate the interaction between and within groups. The latter aspect relies heavily on the auditory system, where communication is of exceptional importance and was probably the driving force in the evolution of hearing. In most species, hearing and vocalization are well adapted to each other, i.e. animals hear in the same frequency spectrum in which they vocalize, and have auditory systems well tailored to processing their own vocalizations. Hearing also plays a critical role in predator–prey interactions, where some species rely heavily on their sound localization abilities to find prey. Some species, such as bats and dolphins, even use active echolocation; they emit sound signals and analyze the information contained in the returning echoes for orientation in the environment.

Besides having a well-developed sense of hearing, many species have rich repertoires of communication signals, which cover every aspect of daily life, such as progeny-raising, aggression, submission, mating, and alarm signals. Those species performing active echolocation additionally employ echolocation signals tailored to the particular ecological niche in which they live. Whenever animals listen to vocalizations, or any other type of sound, they face the task of initially receiving the signal, which consists of a complex sound wave typically containing multiple frequencies with different amplitudes and modulations. Subsequently, the individual's auditory system has to process this complex sound wave, isolate the ethologically relevant information from it, extract auditory objects, interpret them, and initiate a behaviorally appropriate response. Exactly how all this is done is still poorly understood. However, we do understand a number of principles that the auditory system employs in processing such ethologically relevant stimuli. Some of these principles can be understood best when looking at response properties of single neurons to sound, and asking how these properties are created by the interactions of the different inputs these neurons receive. Other principles only become apparent when responses of large groups of neurons are measured and compared.

In this chapter, we first discuss some common principles of vocalizations and other behaviorally relevant sound stimuli. Then we review a number of examples of how the responses of single neurons to particular components of these complex sounds are shaped through the interactions of small networks. We show how these neurons, through interaction of neural excitation and neural inhibition, analyze a complex sound wave for ethologically relevant aspects and pass information about them on to higher order auditory centers. We then turn to the question of how some behaviorally relevant cues are represented by larger networks of neurons within the auditory system. We conclude by pointing out a few examples of how the entire auditory system of an animal can be adapted to the processing of biologically relevant stimuli, and how this processing can change in a context-specific manner.

8.2 **Natural sounds have common features across animal species**

Vocalizations from different animal species can be extremely diverse. They may differ in frequency, timbre, duration, amplitude, and, particularly, in their fine structure. Some vocalizations, such as echolocation calls in bats, can be as brief as a few milliseconds (Griffin, 1958), while others, such as whale or bird songs, can be as long as several minutes and are composed of many syllables, all of which themselves consist of complex multifrequency components (Konishi, 1994). In spite of this diversity, animal vocalizations and other natural sound signals have common aspects.

Figure 8.1 shows a number of spectrograms of various animal vocalizations, which are very diverse. Nevertheless, despite the diversity, many components of these signals are identical across species and follow common principles. Each vocalization can be described as a sequence of elementary building blocks, such as constant frequency components, amplitude modulated components, or frequency-modulated components, including upward sweeps and downward sweeps. Some blocks represent broadband sounds, while others consist of almost only one pure frequency. Acoustic signals including speech and music consist of precise arrangements of such building blocks. The precise arrangement of these blocks determines a number of qualities of the sound, and guides the brain in grouping these blocks such that components originating from the same sound source are recognized as belonging together and to a particular auditory stream.

The auditory systems of most animal species contain neurons or small neural networks that respond preferentially to one or more of these elementary building blocks in complex sounds and can be considered detectors for them. Below we discuss a number of examples, many from mammals including bats. However, coding for ethological stimuli is not a bat-specific phenomenon or even a mammalian phenomenon.

One example of such feature detectors, which also illustrates that coding for ethological stimuli is not limited to mammalian or vertebrate brains, comes from insects. Noctuid moths can detect echolocation calls of their main predators, bats, and initiate avoidance responses when such calls are detected. The neural circuit detecting the call and mediating the response is, by vertebrate standards, very simple, but effective. Two sensory neurons in the tympanal organ of the moth detect the echolocation call and activate two first-order neurons in the pterothoraic ganglion. The information is subsequently processed by only a few higher-order neurons, which project directly to the motor neurons initiating the escape response (Roeder and Treat, 1957; Boyan and Miller, 1991). This simple and elegant circuit demonstrates that coding for ethologically relevant stimuli can basically be achieved by a single sensory neuron that is activated by vocalizations from the animal's main predator.

In the case of vertebrates, the processing of ethologically relevant stimuli is considerably more complex, but even here we find some surprising abilities in animals with – compared to us – relatively simple brains. Edwards *et al.* (2002) identified neurons in the frog midbrain that can count, i.e. that respond preferentially to sequences of pulses with certain repetitions and precisely timed pauses between them. As many anuran species communicate with vocalizations consisting of series of pulses differing in pulse interval and number, such 'counting' neurons might play an important role in call recognition between males and females. Edwards *et al.* demonstrated neurons that respond only when, for example, five pulses or more, with correctly timed pauses in between, are presented. In extreme cases, a single interval which is too short or too long can reset the interval counting process (Edwards *et al.*, 2002).

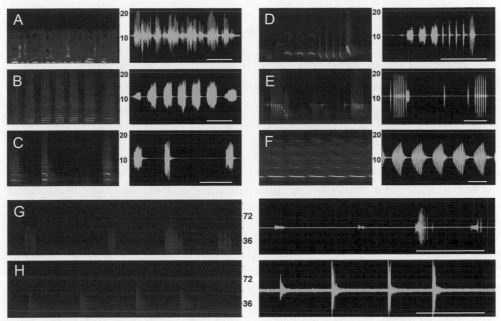

Fig. 8.1 Examples of different animal vocalizations under various behavioral conditions. For each vocalization, the spectrogram and the envelope waveform are shown. The spectrogram shows frequency as a function of time (*red*), with *colour* indicating amplitude (frequency range 0–22 kHz for **A–D** and 0–96 kHz for **G** and **H**), and the waveform shows amplitude as a function of time (*green*). The eight vocalizations are: **A** human speech; **B** Mexican hairy porcupine; **C** mink; **D** common nightingale; **E** chickadee; **F** tree cricket; **G** Mexican free tailed bat communication signals; **H** Mexican free tailed bat echolocation signals. The figure shows that natural and complex vocalizations consist of basic elements such as upward sweeps, downward sweeps, constant frequency components, amplitude modulations, and combinations of these elements. *Time bars* represent 1 s for **A–E**, 25 ms for **F**, and 100 ms for **G** and **H**. Sounds **B–F** for which spectrograms and waveforms are presented here were kindly provided by the Cornell Laboratory of Ornithology.

This example illustrates that the auditory systems of non-mammalian and non-avian species are also specialized in the coding of stimuli of ethological relevance to them. It illustrates the strategy of at least the lower auditory system to extract certain limited, and behaviorally relevant, features from the very large amount of information that is contained in the incoming sound wave. Other examples of such specializations have been found in mammals, many of them in bats.

Bat species are very common models for studying auditory neuroethology. One reason for this is that these nocturnal species rely heavily on their sense of hearing when they navigate the night skies hunting for prey (Griffin, 1958). As a result of the importance of hearing for these animals, their auditory systems are greatly hypertrophied (Pollak and Casseday, 1989), which makes them ideal models for studying auditory physiology. A second reason is that findings on their auditory physiology can easily be related to their ethological significance. A third reason for the popularity of bats in auditory research is that they vocalize intensively, both during echolocation when navigating (Schnitzler *et al.*, 1987; Surlykke and Kalko, 2008) and in a rich repertoire of communication signals which are used in various social contexts, such as mother–infant interactions, mating, and aggressive behavior (Fenton, 1985; Balcombe, 1990; Balcombe and McCracken, 1992; French *et al.*, 2003). Despite the specialized lifestyle of these animals, and the evolution of echolocation, bat auditory systems are very similar to that of other mammals, such that most findings from bats can be considered general mammalian phenomena.

8.3 Integration of excitatory and inhibitory inputs shapes selectivity for certain sound features in auditory neurons

As discussed above, bat vocalizations consist of the same basic acoustic elements as other animal vocalizations, although they are often of much higher frequencies. Echolocation calls tend to be simpler than communication calls and consist of downward frequency modulated sweeps in all bat species. However, in some species these downward sweeps are preceded by an additional constant frequency component (Neuweiler, 1984, 1990; Fig. 8.2). Not surprisingly, many neurons in the bat auditory system are tuned to downward frequency modulated sound signals. These neurons respond to downward sweeps or complex signals containing downward sweeps, but they do not respond to sweeps going in an upward direction.

Neurons with this selectivity have been found in the inferior colliculus and higher auditory centers in a number of bat species (Shannon-Hartman *et al.*, 1992; Fuzessery, 1994; Roverud, 1994, 1995; Fuzessery and Hall, 1996; Ferragamo *et al.*, 1998; O'Neill and Brimijoin, 2002; Fuzessery *et al.*, 2006; Razak and Fuzessery, 2006). It has been shown that this selectivity is created with a very simple neural circuit where neural excitation centered at a given frequency is paired with neural inhibition centered at a slightly lower frequency (Fuzessery and Hall, 1996). During downward sweeps, the excitation is activated first, followed by the inhibition, such that the neuron can respond for a brief period of time. By contrast, during upward sweeps the inhibition is activated first, followed by the excitation. In this case the neuron does not respond to the signal, since the neural inhibition, now recruited first, prevents the neuron from firing altogether.

Pharmacological blockage of neural inhibition rescues responses to upward sweeps, suggesting that the response selectivity to downward sweeps is indeed created by the interaction of the two described projections (Fuzessery and Hall, 1996). It is easy to imagine how selectivity for upward frequency modulated components can be created by reversing the timing of excitation and inhibition, or how selectivity for faster or slower frequency modulations can be achieved simply by changing the relative latencies of the two inputs. This very simple example illustrates how response selectivity for the basic building blocks of complex signals discussed above can be achieved at the level of a few neurons, and that in this case temporal interactions of excitation and inhibition are a key feature in creating selectivity. In the case of bats, the stimulus selectivity of neurons that respond to downward sweeps maps well onto the very prominent downward sweeping echolocation calls, and therefore it is reasonable to assume that the ethological role of such neurons is the coding for echolocation signals. However, we should point out that sweep selective neurons are not bat specific, just as behaviorally relevant signals with downward sweeping components are not bat specific. It is therefore not surprising that similar neurons have been found in other species, for example cats (Mendelson and Cynader, 1985; Mendelson *et al.*, 1993).

Next we turn to the discussion of another neural mechanism adapted for the detection of sinusoidal amplitude modulations (SAMs) and sinusoidal frequency modulations (SFMs). These modulations are contained in most natural sounds, and therefore the auditory systems of many species have neurons that can detect them. SAM and SFM sensitive neurons have been well described in certain bat species termed 'CF-FM' bats, where they play an important role in sound localization. CF-FM bats emit echolocation calls that consist of both a constant frequency component (CF component), followed by the brief downward frequency-modulated component described above (FM component). These CF-FM echolocation calls (or sometimes FM-CF-FM calls, as in the example in Fig. 8.2A4) are an adaptation to hunting in cluttered environments such

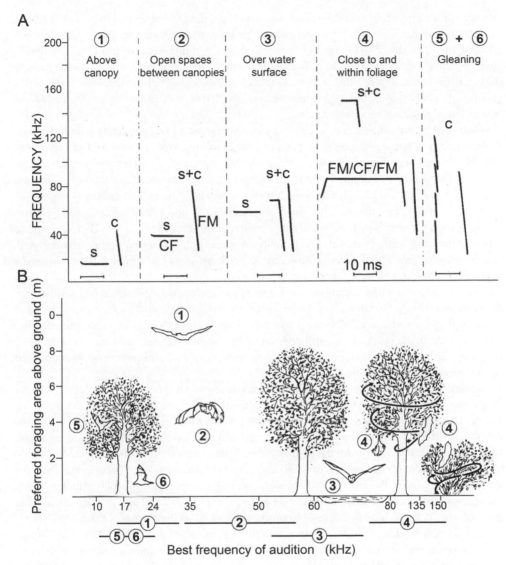

Fig. 8.2 Schematic view of echolocation calls emitted by different bat species that are adapted to different foraging situations. The atmosphere above vegetation (*1*) and between vegetation (*2*) is characterized by the absence of obstacles. Many species of molossids, emballonurids, and vespertilionids fly at high speeds in pursuit of prey. The bats typically emit shallow FM modulated sweeps during the search phase. The purpose of these longer sweeps is to obtain spectral information about interesting objects. After detecting a potential prey, the FM sweeps shorten dramatically to facilitate the computation about target distance. By contrast, bats hunting in the foliage of trees (*4*), such as rhinolophids or hipposiderids, emit an additional CF component in their echolocation calls. This component facilitates the detection of insects in the midst of a large number of other objects such as leaves and branches. Bats hunting near open water or near the ground (*3*, *5*, and *6*) emit a variety of echolocation calls, which, however, are typically simpler than the CF-FM calls that are emitted by species hunting in cluttered environments. (Adapted from Neuweiler (1989), with permission.)

as under the canopy of the rainforest, and are thus mostly used by bat species living in the foliage of trees (Neuweiler, 1984). By contrast, pure FM echolocation calls are used by FM bat species hunting the open sky. What is the significance of the CF component for hunting in cluttered environments? When echolocation calls are emitted in the foliage of trees, many echoes return to the bat, because many objects such as trees, branches, and leaves will reflect the echolocation call – a problem that bats hunting the open skies do not encounter. How can a bat recognize echoes from insects among all these background echoes?

When the CF components in echolocation calls are emitted and subsequently reflected by stationary and non-moving targets such as leaves, the returning signals are still CF components. However, if they are reflected by moving targets with fluttering wings such as insects, the returning echoes are modulated in amplitude and frequency, and thus stand out against the background (Neuweiler, 1984). A beating insect wing alternates between providing a maximal surface for sound reflection (when the wing is either completely up or down) and a minimally reflective surface (when the wing is perfectly parallel to the direction of incoming sound). Therefore, sound waves of the echolocation call will sometimes be maximally and sometimes minimally reflected, and amplitude modulations are introduced into the reflected signal. The modulations can best be detected in the echo of the CF component, as this component was emitted with a constant frequency and had a longer duration. The frequency of the amplitude modulation is, of course, the same as the wing-beat frequency of the insect. As various insect species flutter their wings at different frequencies between 30 Hz (e.g. moths, dragonflies) and 300 Hz (e.g. mosquitoes), they introduce amplitude modulations with different frequencies into the echo and thus not only distinguish themselves from background echoes, but also provide valuable information about their species identity to the hunter.

A second modulation introduced by the fluttering insect wings is frequency modulation. These frequency modulations are created as the Doppler effect shifts the frequency of the returning echolocation calls upwards in cases where the wing moves forward and approaches the bat, and introduces a downward frequency shift into the returning echolocation call during the downstroke when the wing moves away from the predator. Again, the modulation frequency introduced into the CF component of the call is identical to the wing-beat frequency of the prey item. Thus, the main purpose of the CF component of echolocation calls is to provide valuable temporal cues to the animal that would be more difficult to obtain from the very brief and multifrequency FM component. Why do bats then use FM components at all in their echolocation calls? These temporally very brief, and precise, components provide valuable information about the distance to the target, as well as data for a spectral analysis which yields information about the object's size, surface structure, and other properties (Shannon-Hartman et al., 1992; Roverud and Rabitoy, 1994; Schwartz et al., 2007).

Consistent with the information value that amplitude and frequency modulations have for bats, neurons at many levels of their auditory systems are sensitive to such modulated signals. The lowest auditory centers where neurons can recognize signals with SAMs and discriminate between different modulation frequencies were found in the medial superior olive of the mustache bat (Grothe et al., 1992; Grothe, 1994; Fig. 8.3). The neural mechanism of SAM selectivity is a combination of a sustained neural excitation with a sustained neural inhibition from the same ear (Grothe, 1994). During low SAM frequencies, each maximum in the amplitude modulation behaves like a brief tone stimulus and evokes a brief excitation. It also evokes a brief inhibition with a slightly longer latency and, thus, the neurons respond to each peak in the modulated signal until the slightly delayed inhibition turns the response off. Since the inhibition also is active for a particular duration, the neurons are unresponsive to further excitation during that time. For low SAM frequencies, the periods of excitation evoked by the peaks of the amplitude modulations are

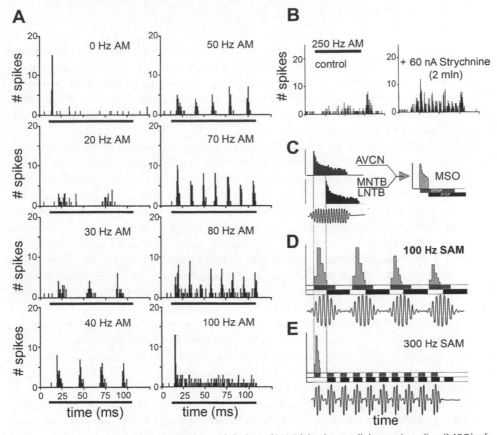

Fig. 8.3 Coding for sinusoidal amplitude modulations (SAMs) in the medial superior olive (MSO) of the mustache bat. Neurons in the MSO of the mustache bat respond to signals containing low SAM frequencies, but do not respond when signals with higher SAM frequencies are used. **A** Responses of an MSO neuron to signals with different modulation frequencies. The neuron can follow these modulations up to about 80 Hz. In these cases, the neuron responds to each peak in the SAM with a distinct response. For SAMs of 100 Hz and above, the neuron cannot follow the stimulus and instead only responds to the first cycle with a strong response, while the response to the following cycles is greatly diminished. This selective response for signals with certain modulation frequencies is created by glycinergic inhibition (**B**). For this experiment, an MSO neuron was stimulated with a tone amplitude-modulated at 250 Hz. Under control conditions, the neuron did not respond very well to the modulated stimulus. However, when glycinergic inhibition was blocked, responses to the same signal could be rescued, suggesting that glycinergic inhibition prevented the neuron from responding to the 250 Hz SAM signal. Based on these data, Grothe suggested a neural mechanism for the creation of SAM selectivity (**C**), which involves a neural excitation paired with a slightly delayed neural inhibition. For low modulation frequencies, the neuron responds to each cycle until the delayed inhibition terminates its response. The effects of the inhibition expire during the pauses between the cycles such that the neuron can respond to each consecutive cycle (**D**). However, for higher modulation frequencies, the gap between two cycles is short such that the effects of the inhibition are still active when the excitation recruited by the next cycle arrives. In this case, the neuron cannot respond to subsequent cycles of the modulated signal (**E**). As described above, neurons that code for certain SAM signals might have functional relevance in the detection of fluttering insects in the foliage of trees. However, amplitude modulations occur in virtually every natural sound such that the functional significance of such neurons goes well beyond detection of insects by bats, and might be the detection of gaps in streams of auditory information. (Adapted from Grothe (1994, 2000), with permission.)

temporally far enough apart such that the inhibition has terminated its effect. The neuron can respond to every amplitude maximum of the SAM signal. However, as the SAM frequency gets higher, the pauses between the periods of excitation get shorter and at some point will be too short to outlast the duration of the inhibition. Depending on the exact duration of that inhibition, which varies somewhat from neuron to neuron, the cells can be considered to be low pass filters for SAM signals (Grothe, 1994).

Although SAM processing and SFM processing are well understood in CF-FM bats, it is not a bat-specific phenomenon. A more general interpretation of SAM filtering neurons is that these neurons not only provide information about the wing-beat frequency of a potential prey item, but also generally detect gaps in streams of auditory information. Whenever a gap or a pause in a stream of activity gets too short, neural inhibition will prevent the neuron from responding to the following auditory event (Grothe et al., 2001). Other mammalian species have been shown to have neurons that are sensitive to these signals (Caspary et al., 2002; Godey et al., 2005; Kadner and Berrebi, 2008) and it should be emphasized that most auditory signals, including human speech, contain SAM and SFM modulations (see Fig. 8.1), and thus any processing strategy that involves the breakdown of an auditory signal into its components almost certainly has to include SAM and SFM detectors.

Detecting the duration of a sound or sound sequence appears to be another important feature in auditory processing. A duration-sensitive neuron responds maximally to sounds with a specific duration. Both shorter and longer stimuli are much less effective at exciting the neuron. Duration-sensitive neurons were initially found in the frog midbrain (Potter, 1965) and shown to code for ethologically relevant stimulus durations. Later they were found in bats, and the mechanism for the creation of duration selectivity was shown (Casseday et al., 1994, 2000; Ehrlich et al., 1997; Fig. 8.4).

Duration-sensitive neurons have a long latency and thus begin to fire only after the sound stimulus is over. The pattern of their firing is phasic and the firing rate of the response is a function of stimulus duration. In the bat midbrain, most duration-selective neurons code for stimulus durations of about 1–40 ms (Fig. 8.4A–D). Ehrlich et al. (1997) suggested that two excitatory inputs and one inhibitory input with particular properties are needed to create duration selectivity: The inhibitory input is correlated with the onset of the stimulus and is active throughout its duration. A transient excitatory input is correlated with the offset of the stimulus and a second transient excitatory input is correlated with the onset of the stimulus but delayed in time relative to the onset of inhibition. When stimuli of the preferred duration are played, the two excitatory inputs coincide at a time when the inhibition is over and the neuron can fire (Fig. 8.4E). For other stimulus durations, the timing of the three inputs is such that the two excitatory inputs do not coincide and the neuron fails to fire (Fig. 8.4F). Duration-sensitive neurons have been discovered in the mouse and guinea pig auditory system as well (Brand et al., 2000; He, 2002; Yu et al., 2004), again suggesting that this type of feature extraction is not a specialization exclusive to bats, but rather a common phenomenon that exists in mammals, and even vertebrates, and that it is used in the analysis of complex and natural sounds.

Another type of feature extraction similar to duration sensitivity is found in neurons of the inferior colliculus, medial geniculate, and auditory cortex of bats, namely range sensitivity. Range-sensitive neurons respond maximally to the time elapsed between two stimuli, in this case two FM sweeps (Suga et al., 1987; Suga, 1989; Riquimaroux et al., 1991). Recall that echolocation signals of all bat species contain temporally short and precise FM components. These components are ideally suited to provide information about how far a given target is away from the animal. The emitted sweep takes a certain amount of time to travel from the bat to the target, is reflected by the target, and travels back to be received by the bat. The elapsed time between the first sweep (the signal) and the second sweep (the echo) provides information about target distance.

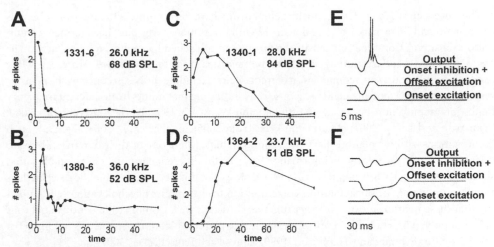

Fig. 8.4 Duration sensitivity in the inferior colliculus of the big brown bat. Four examples of such responses are shown in **A–D**. The first neuron (**A**) responds maximally to very short tones of about 1 ms. Sounds with longer durations, although they contain more sound energy, elicit fewer spikes in the neuron. The second neuron (**B**) responds optimally to tones of about 3 ms; shorter as well as longer sounds are less effective in activating it. The third and fourth neurons (**C** and **D**) respond optimally to sound durations of about 6 and 40 ms, respectively. Such duration-sensitive neurons are well suited to analyze the temporal structure of complex signals and thus might play an important role in the processing of natural and ethologically relevant sounds. The authors suggest a neural mechanism for the creation of duration sensitivity, which involved temporal coincidence of an onset inhibition, an offset excitation, and an onset excitation with a long latency (**E** and **F**). For signals of optimal duration (**E**), the termination of the onset inhibition (downward deflection in middle trace indicating an IPSP) coincides with the two excitations (upward deflections in middle and bottom traces indicating EPSPs), such that the neuron will fire (top trace indicating the occurrence of action potentials). For signals with non-optimal durations (**F**), the three inputs are unsynchronized and the neuron does not fire (absence of action potentials in top trace). (Adapted from Ehrlich *et al.* (1997) and Casseday *et al.* (2000), with permission.)

Consistent with the ethological importance of target distance, large areas of auditory cortex have been discovered in bats that represent systematically various target distances (Suga *et al.*, 1987). Large maps of range-sensitive neurons have to date not been found in other mammalian species. Therefore, out of all the examples presented above, range sensitivity might be the only one that is limited to bats. Nevertheless, it is easy to imagine that a more general role of 'range' neurons could be the detection of pauses, or the detection of repetitive elements in a complex sound signal, and thus it would not be surprising if such neurons were discovered in other animals as well.

Information processing within single frequency bands is prominent in the lower auditory system, as sound information is initially separated into its frequency components at the inner ear. This Fourier analysis is the basis for frequency selectivity among auditory neurons and the tonotopic organization of all lower auditory centers. However, one hallmark of complex and natural auditory signals is that they are multifrequency and have harmonics. In fact, the specific mix of sound energies at various frequencies gives a sound its unique qualities and makes it distinguishable from other less relevant signals that are otherwise similar. Therefore, one almost has to postulate the existence of neurons that respond to stimuli with certain frequency combinations.

The lowest auditory center in which such neurons have been found is the inferior colliculus (Mittmann and Wenstrup, 1995), and neurons with this response type have been termed 'combination sensitive'. Combination-sensitive neurons can be excited by sound presented at a single frequency, and standard tuning curves can be recorded from these neurons. However, when excited simultaneously by a combination of frequencies, including the best frequency, the neurons respond with a substantially higher response rate, indicating that inputs from different frequency bands interact in a non-linear way (Mittmann and Wenstrup, 1995; Leroy and Wenstrup, 2000; Wenstrup and Leroy, 2001; Nataraj and Wenstrup, 2005; Sanchez *et al.*, 2008; Fig. 8.5). Such combination-sensitive neurons have been found in bats, where one of their putative tasks is to integrate incoming echolocation information between the different harmonics of an echolocation sound (Suga *et al.*, 1978; Taniguchi *et al.*, 1986). However, not all of the combination sensitivities found in recordings from bat neurons correspond to the harmonics of echolocation calls, implying that these neurons must have other functional roles as well. Combination-sensitive neurons exist not only in bats but also in primates, suggesting that combination sensitivity is not just a bat specialization (Schwarz and Tomlinson, 1990; Kanwal and Rauschecker, 2007).

Presumably, combination sensitivity comes about through the non-linear interaction of several frequency channels. In this case, non-linear interaction implies that the combinatorial effect of several frequency channels is larger than the sum of the effects of each individual channel. Neurons that integrate over several frequency bands in a non-linear way are suited to detect certain motifs in complex sounds, as shown for the inferior colliculus neurons which function in echolocation (Mittmann and Wenstrup, 1995; Leroy and Wenstrup, 2000; Nataraj and Wenstrup, 2005). However, other functional roles of non-linear integration have also been described. For example, Firzlaff *et al.* found neurons in the bat auditory cortex that code for certain auditory objects, independently of the object's size (Firzlaff *et al.*, 2006).

Object constancy and the ability to recognize a new object as a member of a certain object category are obviously important characteristics of sensory systems. From our own experience, we know that we rarely have trouble recognizing a particular object as belonging to a certain group, even if we have never seen that particular object before. In the auditory world we can usually identify an unknown person's voice as male or female, although different voices of the same sex can vary dramatically in pitch, timbre, and other characteristics that may help us in the identification. The neurons described in the auditory cortex of the bat (Firzlaff *et al.*, 2006) fire in response to stimulation with a certain object, independently of the pitch or 'size' of this object. This is a deviation from the tonotopic organization of the auditory system and suggests that the different frequency channels interact with each other. Furthermore, although the exact neural circuit creating object constancy is not known, such response properties cannot be understood by simple linear integration of inputs: the neurons must perform non-linear computations.

Perhaps the most dramatic example of such non-linear integration is the existence of 'bird's own song' neurons in the avian HvC, first described by Margoliash and Konishi (1985) in white crowned sparrows. Some neurons in this nucleus only respond when stimulated with recordings of that particular bird's own song. The neurons do not respond to even very similar songs produced by conspecifics. Since the frequency components as well as the temporal properties of different bird songs are very much alike, it would be difficult to build a linear neural circuit that could discriminate between two virtually identical vocalizations. Hence, non-linearity is an important feature in signal processing, and in particular when it comes to the processing of complex signals.

8.4 **Coding for ethological stimuli is hierarchical**

While one might expect that more complex processing of sound information and feature extraction is restricted to cortical areas, the examples shown above demonstrate that this is not

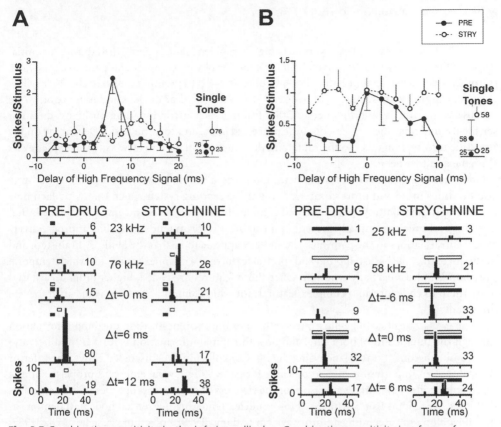

Fig. 8.5 Combination sensitivity in the inferior colliculus. Combination sensitivity is a form of non-linear interaction between different frequency channels. Non-linearity is apparent when a neuron's responses to isolated tones of different frequencies is compared to the neuron's response to the two tones presented together. For example, the neuron in **A** responded to a tone of 23 kHz with a low response of fewer than 6 spikes (*post-stimulus time (PST) histograms, top panel; number to right of histogram* denotes total spikes fired). When a pure tone of 76 kHz was presented alone, the neuron responded with about 10 spikes (*second PST histogram*). However, when both tones were presented together at the same intensity, with a delay of 6 ms between them, the neuron responded with 80 spikes. Since this response was considerably larger than the sum of spikes fired by each tone alone (6 + 10 = 16 spikes), the neuron's greatly enhanced response to the combination of the two tones can best be explained through the non-linear interaction of frequency channels. For the neuron to respond maximally, the two tones have to be presented with a specific interval between them, in this case 6 ms, with the lower-frequency tone leading. Other intervals are less effective at evoking maximal responses from the neuron. The neuron shown in **B** responded best to a combination of tones at 25 and 58 kHz presented simultaneously. Again, the number of spikes evoked by simultaneous presentation of the two sounds was much greater than the sum of the spikes fired by each tone individually. Stimulus durations are represented by *bars above the histograms*. Pharmacological application of the glycine antagonist strychnine removes the combination sensitivity. The neurons now respond to each combination of tones with about the same number of spikes, no matter at what interval the sounds were presented. In **A**, the overall response elicited by the combined tones at optimal delay is much lower when glycinergic inhibition was blocked than in control. Removal of an inhibitory input typically disinhibits a neuron and results in a greatly enhanced overall response. This effect can be observed for single stimuli and combined stimuli at non-optimal delays, but not for the optimal delay, where response was greatly diminished by blocking glycinergic inhibition. In the example shown in **B**, this effect is less dramatic, but the combination sensitivity appears to be also created by glycinergic inhibition. (Adapted from Wenstrup and Leroy (2001), copyright 2001 by the Society for Neuroscience, with permission.)

necessarily true. For example, SAM processing, or gap detection, is performed during the initial stages of the auditory pathway, namely in the superior olivary complex and paraolivary nucleus (Grothe, 1994; Kuwada and Batra, 1999; Grothe *et al.*, 2001; Kadner and Berrebi, 2008). The excitatory inputs to these nuclei come directly from the cochlear nucleus and thus are only one synapse away from the auditory nerve. Other features such as combination sensitivity, duration sensitivity, and non-linear interactions are processed in the auditory midbrain. Depending on the route the information takes to the midbrain, those inputs might be as few as two synapses away from the auditory nerve.

One emerging theme is that feature detection starts at very low levels of the auditory pathway and becomes more and more complex along the ascending system, such that with each new processing station, both specialization and complexity increase. A second emerging theme is that the temporal precision initially present in the auditory stream tends to decline at progressively more central stations in the pathway. The strategy appears to be that the auditory brainstem and midbrain extract the basic temporal and spectral features in a complex sound, for which temporal precision is at least partially required. Once those features are coded, higher order areas build upon them to code for more complex features, for which temporal precision appears to be less important.

These two strategies can be illustrated with an example of localization of sound information through the interaction of both ears, and how this initial information is further modified and refined in subsequent nuclei, including the inferior colliculus. As discussed above, the inferior colliculus is an important centre responsible for generating several emergent properties in the ascending auditory system. One reason for the richness of emergent properties in this nucleus is that it receives inputs from virtually all lower nuclei, rendering it a central node in the information flow along the ascending auditory system (Adams, 1979; Zook and Casseday, 1982, 1987; Nordeen *et al.*, 1983; Pollak *et al.*, 1986; Ross *et al.*, 1988; Chapter 2). Responses of inferior colliculus neurons are very diverse, much more so than response properties of neurons in any lower auditory nucleus. As a result, the ascending stream of auditory information that is recruited by a given complex sound stimulus creates a very heterogeneous response profile in the inferior colliculus, while in lower nuclei the same information stream recruits a very homogeneous response profile. This response diversity is the neural substrate for considerably more sophisticated response properties than neurons in lower nuclei can support. This strategy will be illustrated with an example:

Sound localization is initially performed in the nuclei of the superior olivary complex, of which the lateral nucleus (LSO) codes for the location of high-frequency sounds. This occurs through the integration of excitatory inputs projected from one ear with inhibitory inputs from the opposite ear such that an LSO neuron codes for the location of an object along the azimuth with its firing rate (Goldberg and Brown, 1969; Harnischfeger *et al.*, 1985; Chapter 12). Temporal precision plays an important role in this integration, and it has been shown that time shifts in the arrival time of excitation or inhibition in the order of microseconds can completely change the sound localization properties in LSO neurons (Pollak, 1988; Irvine and Gago, 1990; Park *et al.*, 1996; Irvine *et al.*, 2001).

The LSO has arrays of neurons in each frequency band, resulting in the nucleus as a whole performing superbly at basic sound localization. This emergent property of LSO processing is then relayed to neurons in the dorsal nucleus of the lateral lemniscus (DNLL) and in the inferior colliculus, endowing these nuclei with LSO reponse properties. The DNLL, however, receives additional binaural, i.e. spatially selective, inputs which add to the complexity of the response in these neurons. Specifically, the additional inhibitory inputs allow DNLL neurons to discriminate between inputs that originate from the original direct sound wave, and inputs that originate from echoes and reflections of the same sound wave (Yang and Pollak, 1994a, b). In closed or cluttered environments, a given sound wave is reflected by walls and objects such that in response to a given single sound, multiple sound waves from various directions arrive at the two ears.

Without the DNLL circuitry, the auditory system would localize the direction from which each sound wave arrives, and would thus be unable to localize the sound source unambiguously (Pecka *et al.*, 2007). Therefore, neurons in the LSO cannot discriminate between direct sound waves and echoes. However, neurons in the DNLL receive input from the LSO as well as a key inhibitory input which turns off neural responses in the DNLL after each original sound wave for a duration that is equivalent to that of reverberating echoes (about 30 ms). Thus, DNLL neurons build upon the property of basic sound localization by adding the ability to discriminate between the original wavefront and its echoes, such that they only respond to the original wavefront. At the same time, DNLL neurons introduce a novel temporal component into the ascending stream of information, namely an inhibitory input which operates at a time scale that is orders of magnitude slower than the inhibitory input involved in direct sound localization in the LSO (Yang and Pollak, 1994a; Pecka *et al.*, 2007). DNLL neurons project to neurons in the inferior colliculus, which also receive the original LSO inputs. The integration of LSO response properties with the newly created response properties of DNLL neurons gives inferior colliculus neurons even more complex response properties, and might facilitate our ability to hear echoes and reverberations but not localize them (Burger and Pollak, 2001; Chapter 14).

This example illustrates the general strategy of the auditory system – and also other sensory systems – in creating emergent properties which are then projected to the next higher nucleus for further refinement, such that a step-by-step processing tends to create increasingly specialized response features. It may seem intuitive that after a large number of such processing and integration steps, it is possible to obtain neurons with response properties sophisticated enough to discriminate between a bird's own song and the very similar song of a conspecific.

8.5 Representation of ethological stimuli at the systems level

Next we turn to the auditory cortex and discuss the processing of ethologically relevant stimuli by cortical circuits. Many response properties have been found in the auditory cortex that are related to the processing of such stimuli. Moreover, systematic representations for a number of ethologically relevant signal parameters have been discovered in auditory cortical areas. In the mustache bat cortex, Suga *et al.* found a large number of maps that are related to the animal's echolocation performance (Suga *et al.*, 1987; Suga, 1989; Fig. 8.6).

The mustache bat auditory system is a popular model system for the study of echolocation processing, and this bat might be the mammal with the best understood auditory cortex. Mustache bats are also excellent models for studies of auditory processing in general. One reason for the popularity of this species is the fact that mustache bats belong to the group of CF-FM bats, i.e. their echolocation calls contain a significant constant frequency component. In the case of the mustache bat, the constant frequency component is about 10–20 ms long and has a fundamental frequency of 30 kHz with harmonics at 60, 90, and 120 kHz (CF1–CF4). However, the main energy of the component is at 60 kHz (CF2), and therefore the CF component is often simply called the 60 kHz component. The FM component following the CF component is much briefer and sweeps over several kiloHertz or even several tens of kiloHertz. As is the case with the CF component, the fundamental of the FM component has three harmonics (FM1–FM4), although the main energy is again in FM2.

Due to the ethological importance of the 60 kHz CF component, a large proportion of the sensory surface in the cochlea of the mustache bat is devoted to the processing of this frequency.

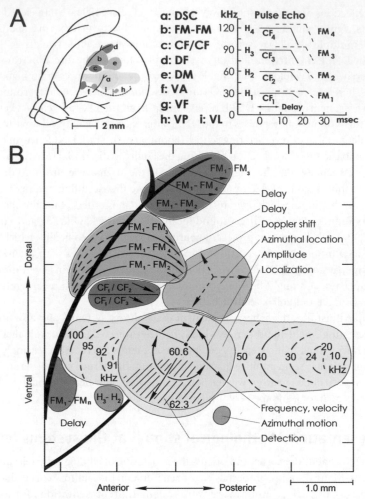

Fig. 8.6 Functional organization of the auditory cortex of the mustache bat. The mustache bat auditory system is a popular model system for the study of echolocation processing, and might be the mammal with the best understood auditory cortex. In fact, mustache bats are excellent models for studies of auditory processing in general. **A**, *left*: dorsolateral view of the left cerebral hemisphere of the mustache bat, depicting various auditory cortical areas; *right*: sketch of a spectrogram of a typical mustache bat echolocation call, consisting of a CF component followed by a FM component. **B** Magnified view of the cortical surface shown in **A** depicting the functional organization of the mustache bat auditory cortex. FM_{1-4} Frequency modulated component, harmonics 1–4; CF constant frequency component, harmonics 1–4; DSCF Doppler shifted CF processing area; DF dorsal fringe area; DM dorsal medial line area; VA ventral anterior area; VF ventral fringe area; VP ventroposterior area; VL ventrolateral area. Blood vessels are shown in *black*. (Adapted from Suga (1989), with permission of the Company of Biologists.)

This overrepresentation of a narrow frequency band has been termed 'acoustic fovea' (Neuweiler and Schmidt, 1993) and is the basis for the observation that large proportions of neurons in each nucleus of the auditory pathway as well as the auditory cortex are devoted to processing echoes signals at or near 60 kHz. Thus, the 60 kHz region in all auditory centers of the mustache bat can be considered as one greatly hypertrophied isofrequency contour.

In other CF-FM bat species, the main energy of the CF component is emitted at different frequencies, and accordingly the acoustic fovea and overrepresented frequency contour in these species is at a different frequency (e.g. 67–80 kHz in *Rhinolophus rouxi*). Furthermore, the auditory cortex of the mustache bat comprises a number of maps which contain systematic representations of various aspects of the biosonar information (Suga, 1989). One area, the Doppler-shifted CF processing area, codes for velocity. Whenever sound is emitted or reflected by moving targets, the emitted sound will be Doppler-shifted in frequency. The shift is dependent on the velocity and direction of the motion and thus can be exploited as a cue for velocity. Naturally, Doppler shifts are easier to detect in constant frequency components; therefore the CF/CF region as well as the DSCF region, which is more specialized towards processing information contained in the CF component, have neurons coding for Doppler shifts. Neurons in these areas represent velocities between –2 and +9 m/s (Suga, 1989).

It should be pointed out that during flight, bats actively adapt the frequency of the emitted CF component to ensure that the returning echoes are received by the isofrequency contour that provides the maximum resolution, i.e. the acoustic fovea and therefore the CF component of the outgoing call is adapted accordingly (Schnitzler, 1967).

By contrast, ranging is coded by FM-sensitive neurons. The neurons code for the time window between two FM components in an echolocation call. The first FM component represents the emitted call, the second component the returning echo. The elapsed time between the two is a function of the distance to the target. Neurons typically are tuned to delays between 0.4 and 18 ms, coding for ranges between 7 and 310 cm (Suga, 1989).

Note that the information represented in the cortical maps of the mustache bat maps very well onto the ethological significance of this information for this particular species. The maps illustrate that not only can single neurons be tuned to, or are specialized for, the representation of natural sounds, but also entire areas of cortex can be devoted to the task (Suga *et al.*, 1987; Suga, 1989). The maps in Fig. 8.6 illustrate the auditory cortex's strategy of separating various aspects of a complex stimulus, such as duration and frequency, and coding for these properties in different cortical areas. This strategy is in some aspects consistent with the previously described strategy of hierarchical processing, where ever higher areas exhibit progressively specialized response properties. Yet cortical processing could be considered even more specialized, since various aspects of a sound stimulus are represented by several areas of cortex such that, for each given stimulus, multiple areas of auditory cortex will be activated. Each one of these areas emphasizes a particular quality of the sound and is therefore considerably less selective, for example, than a neuron responding only to a bird's own song. The unique response of the auditory system to a unique stimulus is therefore realized in the uniquely distributed activation of multiple cortical areas.

Consistent with this view is the work of Romanski *et al.* (1999) who proposed that information is processed in the auditory system in parallel pathways, each of which specializes in a particular task. One stream of information, termed the 'where' pathway, is mainly concerned with the location of sounds in space and how to pinpoint them, while the other stream, termed the 'what' pathway, is mainly concerned with determining the ethological message in a signal. A given sound signal activates both streams, as typically an animal needs to determine both where a given sound is coming from and what message is contained in that sound.

Work by Zatorre and Belin (2001) further illustrates this point. They found that areas in the core auditory cortex respond preferentially to the temporal variation of sound signals, while the belt areas surrounding the core areas respond preferentially to spectral variations. As a result, any given sound stimulus will activate both core and belt areas in a specific pattern that corresponds to the particular temporal and spectral variations in the stimulus. A large number of groups have contributed to mapping out different cortical areas and determining the preferred stimuli of these (see Chapter 9).

The maps found by Suga *et al.*, the 'what' and 'where' pathways described by Rauschecker *et al.*, and the findings by Zatorre *et al.* of specialization in human auditory cortical areas all suggest that a particular sound signal is represented by multiple cortical areas that each code for a different aspect or quality of that sound.

8.6 Tuning of entire auditory systems to ethologically relevant stimuli

Not only are subsystems of the auditory system, such as nuclei or cortical areas, tuned to the processing of biologically relevant stimuli, but also an animal's auditory system in its entirety is obviously tuned and specialized to the processing of signals of relevance to the particular animal. This can be observed in the audiograms that can vary dramatically among species. For example, some echolocating bat species can hear sounds up to about 100 kHz and are not very good at processing signals with frequencies below 10 kHz. For humans, by contrast, hearing is most sensitive and most important at frequencies below 7 kHz, while we are completely insensitive to any sound above about 20 kHz.

The reason for these differences lies in the adaptation to a particular ecological niche and the requirements of an auditory system associated with that niche. For each animal species tested so far, the auditory adaptation to the particular demands is optimal. Echolocation signals among bat species, for example, vary in their fundamental frequencies as well as in the presence or absence of the CF components, due to their adaptation to particular ecological niches. Bats that have developed pure frequency-modulated echolocation calls live mainly in open sky environments with few obstacles, while CF-FM bats live mainly under rainforest canopies where branches and leaves provide not only obstacles, but also auditory clutter from which the signals of a prey item need to be separated (see Fig. 8.2). Their auditory systems, even at the level of the structure and function of the lower brainstem, show clear differences between species, suggesting an adaptation, even at the anatomical level, to the processing tasks a particular species has to resolve (Grothe and Park, 2000). Moreover, the auditory systems of individuals adapt to the particular circumstances that individuals have to deal with. For example, Rauschecker and Korte (1993) demonstrated that the auditory systems of cats adapt when the animals are raised blind, suggesting that other sensory systems exert influence over the auditory system to tune it optimally to the tasks a particular individual has to face.

8.7 Conclusions

This chapter has outlined the basic strategies of the auditory system in the processing of biologically relevant stimuli. These strategies can be found at the level of small networks, larger networks and systems, and at the level of the auditory system as a whole. We also highlighted areas in which our understanding is still very poor, and in which many open questions remain. Moreover, we are only now beginning to learn how complex the brain's coding for ethological stimuli can be. Three examples should illustrate this point:

Example 1: some neurons in vampire bats are specifically sensitive to the sound of an animal's breathing (Schmidt *et al.*, 1991; Groger and Wiegrebe, 2006). While the functional significance of such neurons intuitively makes sense in vampire bats, the neural circuits involved in the creation of such a response property are completely unclear.

Example 2: recently, evidence has been presented for context-dependent, dynamically changing information processing in the auditory system. One line of evidence was provided with the help of neuronal modeling and the computation of spectro-temporal response functions (STRF). An STRF can be considered as the mathematical description of the optimal stimulus for driving a given neuron (Aertsen and Johannesma, 1981). Once the STRF is obtained for a neuron, one can supposedly compute the neuron's responses to any given sound stimulus. However, recent evidence suggests that STRFs of bird auditory neurons do not remain constant, but rather change depending on whether the stimulus is a bird vocalization or other non-biologically relevant stimuli. Thus the rules these neurons use for the processing of sound can dynamically change depending on the task at hand (Sen *et al.*, 2001; Theunissen *et al.*, 2000, 2001).

Example 3: consistent with this, Nagel and Doupe (2006) and Lesica and Grothe (2008) provided evidence that temporal receptive fields in the mammalian and songbird auditory systems can also change depending on the presence or absence of noise in the sound signal. These neurons change their receptive fields in a matter of milliseconds, and adapt their processing strategy in order to code a sound signal in the most efficient way.

These examples show that there is likely to be even more complexity in the processing of ethologically relevant stimuli than shown in this chapter, and how far we are from understanding such processes completely. The examples also try to point out some exciting directions that auditory research might take in future. To date, considerable progress has been made in understanding the basic response properties and the basic representation of sound qualities. Further research will show how more complex properties can perform analyses such as the recognition of an animal's breathing or a bird's own song.

References

Adams JC (1979) Ascending projections to the inferior colliculus. *J Comp Neurol* 183: 519–38.

Aertsen AMHJ, Johannesma PIM (1981) The Spectro-temporal receptive field. *Biol Cybernetics* 42: 133–43.

Balcombe JP (1990) Vocal recognition of pups by mother Mexican free-tailed bats, *Tadarida brasiliensis mexicana. Anim Behav* 39: 960–6.

Balcombe JP, McCracken GF (1992) Vocal recognition in Mexican free-tailed bats: do pups recognize mothers?. *Anim Behav* 43: 79–87.

Boyan GS, Miller LA (1991) Parallel processing of afferent input by identified interneurones in the auditory pathway of the noctuid moth *Noctua pronuba* (L.). *J Comp Physiol [A]* 168: 727–38.

Brand A, Urban R, Grothe B (2000) Duration tuning in the mouse auditory midbrain. *J Neurophysiol* 84: 1790–9.

Burger RM, Pollak GD (2001) Reversible inactivation of the dorsal nucleus of the lateral lemniscus reveals its role in the processing of multiple sound sources in the inferior colliculus of bats. *J Neurosci* 21: 4830–43.

Caspary DM, Palombi PS, Hughes LF (2002) GABAergic inputs shape responses to amplitude modulated stimuli in the inferior colliculus. *Hear Res* 168: 163–73.

Casseday JH, Ehrlich D, Covey E (1994) Neural tuning for sound duration: role of inhibitory mechanisms in the inferior colliculus. *Science* 264: 847–50.

Casseday JH, Ehrlich D, Covey E (2000) Neural measurement of sound duration: control by excitatory-inhibitory interactions in the inferior colliculus. *J Neurophysiol* 84: 1475–87.

Edwards CJ, Alder TB, Rose GJ (2002) Auditory midbrain neurons that count. *Nat Neurosci* 5: 934–6.

Ehrlich D, Casseday JH, Covey E (1997) Neural tuning to sound duration in the inferior colliculus of the big brown bat, *Eptesicus fuscus. J Neurophysiol* 77: 2360–72.

Fenton MB (1985) *Communication in the Chiroptera*. Indiana University Press, Bloominton, p. 159.

Ferragamo MJ, Haresign T, Simmons JA (1998) Frequency tuning, latencies, and responses to frequency-modulated sweeps in the inferior colliculus of the echolocating bat, *Eptesicus fuscus*. *J Comp Physiol [A]* 182: 65–79.

Firzlaff U, Schornich S, Hoffmann S, Schuller G, Wiegrebe L (2006) A neural correlate of stochastic echo imaging. *J Neurosci* 26: 785–91.

French B, Lollar A, Ma T, Page R, Steinberg R, Xie R (2003) Library of social communication calls of the Mexican free-tailed bat (*Tadarida brasiliensis*). *Int Bat Rehab J* 1: 1–13.

Fuzessery ZM (1994) Response selectivity for multiple dimensions of frequency sweeps in the pallid bat inferior colliculus. *J Neurophysiol* 72: 1061–79.

Fuzessery ZM, Hall JC (1996) Role of GABA in shaping frequency tuning and creating FM sweep selectivity in the inferior colliculus. *J Neurophysiol* 76: 1059–73.

Fuzessery ZM, Richardson MD, Coburn MS (2006) Neural mechanisms underlying selectivity for the rate and direction of frequency-modulated sweeps in the inferior colliculus of the pallid bat. *J Neurophysiol* 96: 1320–36.

Godey B, Atencio CA, Bonham BH, Schreiner CE, Cheung SW (2005) Functional organization of squirrel monkey primary auditory cortex: responses to frequency-modulation sweeps. *J Neurophysiol* 94: 1299–311.

Goldberg JM, Brown PB (1969) Response of binaural neurons of dog superior olivary complex to dichotic tonal stimuli: some physiological mechanisms of sound localization. *J Neurophysiol* 32: 613–36.

Griffin DR (1958) *Listening in the Dark*. Yale University Press, New Haven.

Groger U, Wiegrebe L (2006) Classification of human breathing sounds by the common vampire bat, *Desmodus rotundus*. *BMC Biol* 4: 18.

Grothe B (1994) Interaction of excitation and inhibition in processing of pure tone and amplitude-modulated stimuli in the medial superior olive of the mustached bat. *J Neurophysiol* 71: 706–21.

Grothe B, Park TJ (2000) Structure and function of the bat superior olivary complex. *Microsc Res Tech* 51: 382–402.

Grothe B, Vater M, Casseday JH, Covey E (1992) Monaural interaction of excitation and inhibition in the medial superior olive of the mustached bat: an adaptation for biosonar. *Proc Natl Acad Sci USA* 89: 5108–112.

Grothe B, Covey E, Casseday JH (2001) Medial superior olive of the big brown bat: neuronal responses to pure tones, amplitude modulations, and pulse trains. *J Neurophysiol* 86: 2219–30.

Harnischfeger G, Neuweiler G, Schlegel P (1985) Interaural time and intensity coding in the superior olivary complex and inferior colliculus of the echolocating bat *Molossus ater*. *J Neurophysiol* 53: 89–109.

He J (2002) OFF responses in the auditory thalamus of the guinea pig. *J Neurophysiol* 88: 2377–86.

Irvine DR, Gago G (1990) Binaural interaction in high-frequency neurons in inferior colliculus of the cat: effects of variations in sound pressure level on sensitivity to interaural intensity differences. *J Neurophysiol* 63: 570–91.

Irvine DR, Park VN, McCormick L (2001) Mechanisms underlying the sensitivity of neurons in the lateral superior olive to interaural intensity differences. *J Neurophysiol* 86: 2647–66.

Kadner A, Berrebi AS (2008) Encoding of temporal features of auditory stimuli in the medial nucleus of the trapezoid body and superior paraolivary nucleus of the rat. *Neuroscience* 151: 868–87.

Kanwal JS, Rauschecker JP (2007) Auditory cortex of bats and primates: managing species-specific calls for social communication. *Front Biosci* 12: 4621–40.

Konishi M (1994) Pattern generation in birdsong. *Curr Opin Neurobiol* 4: 827–31.

Kuwada S, Batra R (1999) Coding of sound envelopes by inhibitory rebound in neurons of the superior olivary complex in the unanesthetized rabbit. *J Neurosci* 19: 2273–87.

Leroy SA, Wenstrup JJ (2000) Spectral integration in the inferior colliculus of the mustached bat. *J Neurosci* 20: 8533–41.

Lesica NA, Grothe B (2008) Efficient temporal processing of naturalistic sounds. *PLoS ONE* **3**: e1655.

Margoliash D, Konishi M (1985) Auditory representation of autogenous song in the song system of white-crowned sparrows. *Proc Natl Acad Sci USA* **82**: 5997–6000.

Mendelson JR, Cynader MS (1985) Sensitivity of cat primary auditory cortex (AI) neurons to the direction and rate of frequency modulation. *Brain Res* **327**: 331–5.

Mendelson JR, Schreiner CE, Sutter ML, Grasse KL (1993) Functional topography of cat primary auditory cortex: responses to frequency-modulated sweeps. *Exp Brain Res* **94**: 65–87.

Mittmann DH, Wenstrup JJ (1995) Combination-sensitive neurons in the inferior colliculus. *Hear Res* **90**: 185–91.

Nagel KI, Doupe AJ (2006) Temporal processing and adaptation in the songbird auditory forebrain. *Neuron* **51**: 845–59.

Nataraj K, Wenstrup JJ (2005) Roles of inhibition in creating complex auditory responses in the inferior colliculus: facilitated combination-sensitive neurons. *J Neurophysiol* **93**: 3294–312.

Neuweiler G (1984) Foraging, echolocation and audition in bats. *Naturwissenschaften* **71**: 446–55.

Neuweiler G (1989) Foraging, ecology and audition in echolocating bats. *Trends Ecol Evol* **4**(6): 160–6.

Neuweiler G (1990) Auditory adaptations for prey capture in echolocating bats. *Physiol Rev* **70**: 615–41.

Neuweiler G, Schmidt S (1993) Audition in echolocating bats. *Curr Opin Neurobiol* **3**: 563–9.

Nordeen KW, Killackey HP, Kitzes LM (1983) Ascending auditory projections to the inferior colliculus in the adult gerbil, *Meriones unguiculatus*. *J Comp Neurol* **214**: 131–43.

O'Neill WE, Brimijoin WO (2002) Directional selectivity for FM sweeps in the suprageniculate nucleus of the mustached bat medial geniculate body. *J Neurophysiol* **88**: 172–87.

Park TJ, Grothe B, Pollak GD, Schuller G, Koch U (1996) Neural delays shape selectivity to interaural intensity differences in the lateral superior olive. *J Neurosci* **16**: 6554–66.

Pecka M, Zahn TP, Saunier-Rebori B, *et al.* (2007) Inhibiting the inhibition: a neuronal network for sound localization in reverberant environments. *J Neurosci* **27**: 1782–90.

Pollak GD (1988) Time is traded for intensity in the bat's auditory system. *Hear Res* **36**: 107–24.

Pollak GD, Casseday JH (1989) *The Neural Basis of Echolocation in Bats*. Springer, Berlin, p. 143.

Pollak GD, Wenstrup JJ, Fuzessery ZM (1986) Auditory processing in the mustache bat's inferior colliculus. *Trend Neurosci* **9**: 556–61.

Potter HD (1965) Patterns of acoustically evoked discharges of neurons in the mesencephalon of the bullfrog. *J Neurophysiol* **28**: 1155–84.

Rauschecker JP, Korte M (1993) Auditory compensation for early blindness in cat cerebral cortex. *J Neurosci* **13**: 4538–48.

Razak KA, Fuzessery ZM (2006) Neural mechanisms underlying selectivity for the rate and direction of frequency-modulated sweeps in the auditory cortex of the pallid bat. *J Neurophysiol* **96**: 1303–19.

Riquimaroux H, Gaioni SJ, Suga N (1991) Cortical computational maps control auditory perception. *Science* **251**: 565–8.

Roeder KD, Treat AE (1957) Ultrasonic reception by the tympanic organ of noctuid moths. *J Exp Zool* **134**: 127–57.

Romanski LM, Tian B, Fritz J, Mishkin M, Goldman-Rakic PS, Rauschecker JP (1999) Dual streams of auditory afferents target multiple domains in the primate prefrontal cortex. *Nat Neurosci* **2**: 1131–6.

Ross LS, Pollak GD, Zook JM (1988) Origin of ascending projections to an isofrequency region of the mustache bat's inferior colliculus. *J Comp Neurol* **270**: 488–505.

Roverud RC (1994) Complex sound analysis in the lesser bulldog bat: evidence for a mechanism for processing frequency elements of frequency modulated signals over restricted time intervals. *J Comp Physiol [A]* **174**: 559–65.

Roverud RC (1995) Frequency modulated sound pattern analysis in the lesser bulldog bat: the role of interactions between adjacent frequency elements of complex sounds. *J Comp Physiol [A]* **176**: 1–9.

Roverud RC, Rabitoy ER (1994) Complex sound analysis in the FM bat *Eptesicus fuscus*, correlated with structural parameters of frequency modulated signals. *J Comp Physiol [A]* **174**: 567–73.

Sanchez JT, Gans D, Wenstrup JJ (2008) Glycinergic "inhibition" mediates selective excitatory responses to combinations of sounds. *J Neurosci* **28**: 80–90.

Schmidt U, Schlegel P, Schweizer H, Neuweiler G (1991) Audition in vampire bats, *Desmodus rotundus*. *J Comp Physiol A* **168**: 45–51.

Schnitzler HU (1967) Compensation of Doppler effects in horseshoe bats. *Naturwissenschaften* **54**: 523.

Schnitzler HU, Kalko E, Miller L, Surlykke A (1987) The echolocation and hunting behavior of the bat, *Pipistrellus kuhli*. *J Comp Physiol [A]* **161**: 267–74.

Schwartz C, Tressler J, Keller H, Vanzant M, Ezell S, Smotherman M (2007) The tiny difference between foraging and communication buzzes uttered by the Mexican free-tailed bat, *Tadarida brasiliensis*. *J Comp Physiol A Neuroethol Sens Neural Behav Physiol* **193**: 853–63.

Schwarz DW, Tomlinson RW (1990) Spectral response patterns of auditory cortex neurons to harmonic complex tones in alert monkey (*Macaca mulatta*). *J Neurophysiol* **64**: 282–98.

Sen K, Theunissen FE, Doupe AJ (2001) Feature analysis of natural sounds in the songbird auditory forebrain. *J Neurophysiol* **86**: 1445–58.

Shannon-Hartman S, Wong D, Maekawa M (1992) Processing of pure-tone and FM stimuli in the auditory cortex of the FM bat, *Myotis lucifugus*. *Hear Res* **61**: 179–88.

Suga N (1989) Principles of auditory information-processing derived from neuroethology. *J Exp Biol* **146**: 277–86.

Suga N, O'Neill WE, Manabe T (1978) Cortical neurons sensitive to combinations of information-bearing elements of biosonar signals in the mustache bat. *Science* **200**: 778–81.

Suga N, Niwa H, Taniguchi I, Margoliash D (1987) The personalized auditory cortex of the mustached bat: adaptation for echolocation. *J Neurophysiol* **58**: 643–54.

Surlykke A, Kalko E (2008) Echolocating bats cry out loud to detect their prey. *PLoS ONE* **3**: e2036.

Taniguchi I, Niwa H, Wong D, Suga N (1986) Response properties of FM-FM combination-sensitive neurons in the auditory cortex of the mustached bat. *J Comp Physiol [A]* **159**: 331–7.

Theunissen FE, Sen K, Doupe AJ (2000) Spectral-temporal receptive fields of nonlinear auditory neurons obtained using natural sounds. *J Neurosci* **20**: 2315–31.

Theunissen FE, David SV, Singh NC, Hsu A, Vinje WE, Gallant JL (2001) Estimating spatio-temporal receptive fields of auditory and visual neurons from their responses to natural stimuli. *Network* **12**: 289–316.

Wenstrup JJ, Leroy SA (2001) Spectral integration in the inferior colliculus: role of glycinergic inhibition in response facilitation. *J Neurosci* **21**: RC124.

Yang L, Pollak GD (1994a) Binaural inhibition in the dorsal nucleus of the lateral lemniscus of the mustache bat affects responses for multiple sounds. *Aud Neurosci* **1**: 1–17.

Yang L, Pollak GD (1994b) The roles of GABAergic and glycinergic inhibition on binaural processing in the dorsal nucleus of the lateral lemniscus of the mustache bat. *J Neurophysiol* **71**: 1999–2013.

Yu YQ, Xiong Y, Chan YS, He J (2004) In vivo intracellular responses of the medial geniculate neurones to acoustic stimuli in anaesthetized guinea pigs. *J Physiol* **560**: 191–205.

Zatorre RJ, Belin P (2001) Spectral and temporal processing in human auditory cortex. *Cereb Cortex* **11**: 946–53.

Zook JM, Casseday JH (1982) Origin of ascending projections to inferior colliculus in the mustache bat, *Pteronotus parnellii*. *J Comp Neurol* **207**: 14–28.

Zook JM, Casseday JH (1987) Convergence of ascending pathways at the inferior colliculus in the mustache bat, *Pteronotus parnellii*. *J Comp Neurol* **261**: 347–61.

Chapter 9

Speech

Sophie K. Scott and Donal G. Sinex

9.1 Introduction

Speech is arguably the most important class of sounds processed by human listeners. Understanding the representation and processing of speech is an important goal in basic auditory neuroscience, and it also has important clinical implications. The encoding and representation of speech has been studied at the level of single neurons in laboratory animals and at the highest levels of the human auditory system with non-invasive techniques. Electrophysiological studies have provided a wealth of information about the way in which the acoustic properties of speech signals are encoded at lower levels of the auditory system; that information is reviewed in Section 9.2. More recently, the availability of non-invasive techniques has enabled investigators to study mechanisms in the human brain. These techniques have extended the study of speech coding to much higher levels of the auditory system and have allowed linguistic as well as auditory processing to be studied. This work is reviewed in Section 9.3.

9.2 Processing of speech in animal models

Most studies carried out in laboratory animals have examined the representation of spectral or temporal information by primary or secondary neurons. At that level, there are only modest differences across mammalian species, and the mechanisms studied are likely to be similar to those that operate at comparable levels in the human auditory system. The representation of speech at lower levels of the auditory system has generally conformed to expectations based on characteristics of the neurons established with simpler stimuli and on acoustic details of the particular speech sounds that were studied. Possibly for that reason, there has been a decline in the rate at which new studies of the low-level representation of speech sounds appear. A few studies have examined the processing of speech sounds in the midbrain or the auditory cortex. Detailed reviews of the processing of speech have previously been provided by Sachs *et al.* (1988), Delgutte (1997), and Palmer and Shamma (2004).

9.2.1 The representation of steady-state vowels

Vowels are distinguished from one another by the shape of their spectra, and the identity of each vowel is largely determined by the locations of two to three spectral peaks. The locations of these peaks are determined by resonances of the vocal tract called formants. In reports of neurophysiological studies, the term formant is sometimes used loosely to refer to peaks in the spectrum of the stimulus. The formants, or the spectral peaks they produce, are designated in frequency order as F1, F2, F3, and so on. The first studies of the neural representation of speech examined responses to steady-state vowels; the use of sounds in which the spectrum did not vary simplified some of the data analysis (Sachs and Young, 1979). In ongoing speech, vowels rarely achieve a steady-state for more than a few milliseconds, although they are more stable than many consonants. Vowels are usually voiced, meaning that they are produced with periodic vocal fold activity that results in a harmonic or quasi-harmonic sound. When voiced, vowels have a pitch determined by the fundamental frequency (f0) of vocal fold activity. The neural representation of vowel f0 has also been studied.

9.2.2 Representation of spectral shape

The first large-scale study of the peripheral representation of vowel spectra was carried out by Sachs and Young (1979). Their experiments used the 'population' approach, in which the responses of large numbers of neurons to a small number of sounds are obtained. Measures of discharge rate or discharge synchrony (Young and Sachs, 1979) were plotted as a function of the neurons' characteristic frequencies (CF), which indicate cochlear place. Sachs and Young found that the locations of spectral peaks were represented across the spatial array of auditory nerve fibres as regions of elevated discharge rate, but only for vowels presented at relatively low levels. At higher presentation levels, peaks in the discharge rate vs place profiles were less apparent. Examples from a similar study by Miller and Sachs (1983) are shown in the right side of Fig. 9.1. Discharge rate saturation and non-linear suppression (see Chapter 5, this Volume) contributed to the loss of spectral information in the overall discharge-rate representation. At the highest levels presented, information about the locations of spectral peaks was available only in the responses of the subset of fibres with low spontaneous discharge rates, which have higher thresholds and larger dynamic ranges (Chapter 5).

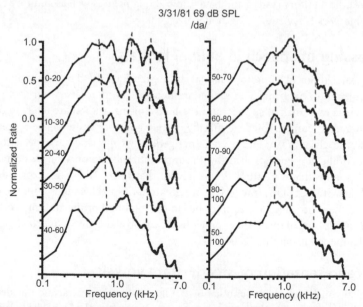

Fig. 9.1 Spatial profiles of average discharge rate elicited from cat auditory nerve fibres by a CV syllable /da/. Each rate-place profile on the left side displays average discharge rate as a function of CF. The profiles were calculated for successive 20-ms time windows during the formant transition. Spectral peaks (indicated by dashed lines) were represented as response peaks whose frequencies changed to track the changing frequencies of F1–F3. During the steady-state vowel (right side), response peaks corresponding to stimulus peaks were less apparent. (Reused with permission from Miller MI, Sachs MB (1983) Journal of the Acoustical Society of America, **74**: 502, copyright 1983, Acoustical Society of America.)

The strong level dependence and the loss of information about spectral shape at presentation levels at which speech is easily recognizable by humans raised concerns about the adequacy of average discharge rate for conveying speech information to the central auditory system. As an alternative, Young and Sachs (1979) examined potential coding mechanisms based on patterns of discharge synchrony. They reported that auditory nerve fibres synchronized strongly to larger components in the spectra of the synthesized vowels. In their stimuli, the component with the largest amplitude was always at a low frequency that corresponded to F1. Fibres with CFs near the F1 peak synchronized strongly to the peak frequency, as did a wide range of fibres with other, mostly higher, CFs. Fibres with CFs near other spectral peaks synchronized to stimulus components near those peaks. Synchronized discharge rates elicited by components near F2 or F3 were lower than those elicited by F1, consistent with the smaller amplitudes of components at F2 and above. Young and Sachs also observed that responses synchronized to stimulus components not associated with formants were suppressed.

The combination of strong synchrony at the places associated with spectral peaks and synchrony suppression at places between those peaks produced a potential spatial representation of the shape of the spectrum. Young and Sachs summarized this representation with a measure called the average localized synchronized rate (ALSR). The ALSR displayed the magnitude of the response synchronized to stimulus components near fibres' CFs as a function of CF. The ALSR combined temporal with place information, under the assumption that response components matched to CF are most relevant even though neurons may also exhibit synchrony to stimulus components remote from CF (such as those near F1). The shape of the ALSR resembled the shape of the stimulus spectrum, in that large response peaks occurred at the cochlear places that corresponded to the frequencies of spectral peaks. This shape was stable over a larger range of presentation levels than was the spatial profile of average discharge rate. Subsequent studies of the representation of vowels and vowel-like complex sounds have confirmed and extended many of the observations of Sachs and Young (Delgutte and Kiang, 1984a; Palmer et al., 1986).

The representation of vowel spectra by neurons in the cochlear nucleus (CN) has also been described. A more diverse set of responses has been observed in the CN than in the auditory nerve, consistent with the diversity of its anatomical (Chapter 2) and physiological (Chapter 5) cell types. Responses of CN primary-like neurons to speech sounds generally share features with the responses of auditory nerve fibres (Palmer et al., 1986; Blackburn and Sachs, 1990; Winter and Palmer, 1990). These features include a relatively good rate-place representation of the vowel spectrum at low presentation levels, degradation of the rate-place representation at higher presentation levels, and a representation of the frequencies of the larger spectral peaks in discharge synchrony. In contrast, the rate-place representation in CN chopper neurons is usually preserved over a larger dynamic range. Although chopper neurons convey useful information in average discharge rate, they exhibit little or no synchrony at frequencies other than f0.

9.2.3 Representation of fundamental frequency

In primary neurons, responses locked to f0 may be observed. These can be generated in either of two ways. First, neurons with very low CFs may synchronize to the f0 component of the stimulus. Second, the responses of neurons with higher CFs may be affected by two or more adjacent unresolved harmonics of f0. In this case, beating between those components will produce an envelope whose frequency matches f0 (Miller and Sachs, 1984; Palmer and Winter, 1993; Keilson et al., 1997). Chopper neurons in the CN often synchronize to envelopes in this way. Blackburn and Sachs (1990) recorded the responses of sustained (Ch-S) and transient (Ch-T) choppers in the anteroventral CN to the steady-state vowel /eh/. Strong synchrony to f0 was observed in both types of neuron, for CFs up to about 3 kHz, well above f0. Cochlear nucleus neurons with onset discharge patterns exhibit particularly robust locking to the period of f0 (Blackburn and Sachs, 1990; Palmer and Winter, 1993). For example, Kim and Leonard (1988) described the responses of an onset neuron from the posteroventral CN of the decerebrate cat that exhibited exceptionally high synchrony to f0, compared to the responses of an auditory nerve fibre with the same CF.

9.2.4 Time-varying sounds

Although studies of the representation of steady-state vowels have been extremely informative, these sounds are not representative of all ongoing speech. The next level of complexity is provided by sounds whose spectra vary over time. Syllables formed by an initial stop consonant and a vowel have been studied most often (Miller and Sachs, 1983; Sinex and Geisler, 1983; Delgutte and Kiang, 1984b, c; Carney and Geisler, 1986; Stevens and Wickesberg, 1999). A few studies have examined the representation of stop consonants in other word positions (Delgutte and Kiang, 1984c; Sinex, 1993; Sinex and Narayan, 1994; Stevens and Wickesberg 2002) and consonant-vowel (CV) syllables formed with consonants other than stops (Delgutte and Kiang, 1984b; Deng and Geisler, 1987).

9.2.5 Representation of spectral information

The representation of spectral features of consonants shares many of the characteristics observed for vowels, except of course that the representation changes over time. Miller and Sachs (1983) and Sinex and Geisler (1983) obtained responses of cat auditory nerve fibres to CV syllables differing in place of articulation. For voiced stop consonants such as /b/, /d/, and /g/, the shape of the spectrum at onset is determined by the place at which the vocal tract is completely closed by an articulator such as the lips or the tongue. The consonant /b/, for example, is produced with a closure formed by the lips, and /d/ by a closure formed by the tongue and alveolar ridge. After onset, the frequencies of spectral peaks move toward the frequencies that define the following vowel. This movement is referred to as a formant transition, and the pattern of frequency change is called the formant trajectory. Both studies found that discharge synchrony provided accurate information about the formant trajectories.

Average discharge rate has been reported to provide a better representation of the spectrum during the formant transition than during the subsequent steady-state vowel. Miller and Sachs (1983) showed that during the formant trajectories, stimulus spectral peaks were clearly represented as peaks in the spatial profiles of average discharge rate. The left side of Fig. 9.1 shows how the locations of those response peaks followed the frequencies of F1–F3. In the right side of Fig. 9.1, it can be seen that during the steady-state vowel segment of the syllable, the locations of stimulus peaks could not be identified in the responses of the same neurons, as Sachs and Young (1979) had previously shown. The average discharge rates of individual neurons vary with consonant place of articulation (Sinex and Geisler, 1983); that is because the spectrum at the onset of a consonant changes with place of articulation. Preceding sounds may affect a neuron's responses to the onset of a consonant. Delgutte and Kiang (1984c) reported that the discharge rate elicited by a /da/-like consonant decreased when the consonant followed another consonant-like sound, as often occurs in ongoing speech.

9.2.6 Representation of temporal and amplitude information

In ongoing speech, substantial changes in amplitude occur at the boundaries between vowels and consonants and in many cases within the consonants themselves. Overall amplitude may change, as when the vocal tract closure is released at the onset of a stop consonant like /b/, or within a restricted frequency band, as when voicing starts with a delay after the release of a consonant like /p/. During ongoing speech, amplitude can change by 20 dB or more within a few milliseconds, especially within restricted frequency bands.

Average discharge rate generally increases and decreases with a pattern that follows the amplitude change within the frequency band represented by the neuron's tuning curve (Sinex and McDonald, 1988; Sinex, 1993; Sinex and Narayan, 1994; Chen *et al.*, 1996; Delgutte *et al.*, 1998; Stevens and Wickesberg, 1999). This is illustrated in Fig. 9.2, which shows temporal discharge patterns elicited from auditory nerve fibres by a two-syllable VCV (vowel-consonant-vowel) nonsense word. For each neuron shown, discharge rate varied widely during the syllable, dropping to the spontaneous rate at some point during the response. The time at which rate minima and maxima were reached varied with CF; the neuron with the highest CF responded at the

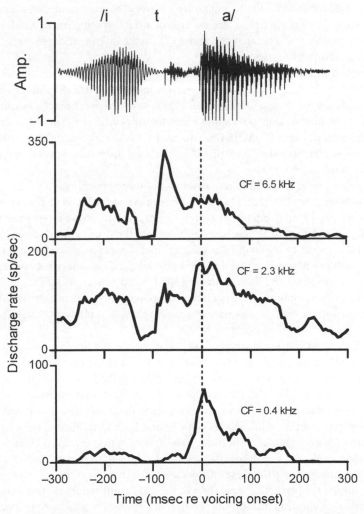

Fig. 9.2 CF-dependent differences in temporal discharge patterns evoked from auditory nerve fibres by the nonsense word /ita/. Three neurons with different CFs responded to the same stimulus with very different temporal patterns, as shown here by the variation in discharge rate with time. (Reused with permission from Sinex DG, Narayan SS (1994) *Journal of the Acoustical Society of America*, **95**: 897, copyright 1994, Acoustical Society of America.)

release of the consonant, while the lower-frequency neurons were more likely to respond to one or the other vowel. Central neurons also represent amplitude changes in CV syllables with variations in discharge rate, although the response patterns are less homogeneous than those of primary neurons (Eggermont, 1995; Chen *et al.*, 1996).

9.2.7 Representation of voice onset time

Results of several studies of the representation of consonants that differ in voice onset time (VOT) have been reported. VOT is the interval between the release of a stop consonant and the onset of vocal-fold activity; it is one of the main cues to the perceptual distinction between voiced and voiceless stop consonants produced at the same place of articulation. The distribution of VOTs produced in normal speech is highly non-uniform. For example, when speakers of English produce the voiced consonant /d/, the onset of voicing lags the consonant release by about 30 ms or less, and when they produce the voiceless consonant /t/, voicing onset is delayed by about 50 ms or more. English speakers rarely produce VOTs in the intermediate region between 30 and 50 ms (Lisker and Abramson, 1964).

Syllables from continua in which VOT varies in equal steps have received attention in neurophysiological studies because humans, monkeys, chinchillas, and birds all exhibit non-monotonic psychophysical acuity for these syllables (Kuhl, 1987). Subjects have difficulty hearing changes in VOT when VOT is short or long, but exhibit much higher acuity for the intermediate values that rarely occur in natural speech (Kuhl, 1987). This has led to the suggestion that a natural psychoacoustic or physiological boundary underlies the perceptual distinction between stop consonants produced with short or long VOT.

Sinex and colleagues measured the responses of auditory nerve fibres to tokens from synthesized VOT continua. They found that for low-CF neurons and for VOTs of 20 ms and longer, the onset of voicing produced robust increases in discharge rate whose latencies systematically increased with VOT. The rate increase was attributable to the rise in amplitude of 20 dB or more that occurs in the frequency region of F1 at voicing onset. There was no evidence in the responses of individual auditory nerve fibres for a natural physiological boundary between syllables with short VOT heard as voiced and those with long VOT heard as voiceless (Sinex and McDonald, 1988). However, when responses were pooled across populations of low-CF neurons, a relationship between the variance of the responses and psychophysical acuity was observed (Sinex *et al.*, 1991).

Figure 9.3 illustrates this pattern schematically. The syllables for which psychophysical acuity is high (VOTs of 30 and 40 ms) elicited responses with low across-neuron variability, so that the neural responses of a group of low-CF fibres to one of those syllables are easily distinguished from the responses elicited by the other. In the figure, this is illustrated by the absence of overlap between the ellipses that represent the mean responses to those syllables. In contrast, syllables for which psychophysical acuity is low (VOTs of 0–20 and 50–80 ms) elicited responses with high variability across neurons; higher response variability means that there was extensive overlap in the neural responses elicited by pairs of syllables that are difficult to resolve. This pattern of results suggests that the amplitude cues in these syllables are represented by subpopulations of neurons in a way that promotes the perceptual separation of the VOT continuum into two non-overlapping parts. There was no indication that this distribution of responses arose from any specialization on the part of the neurons to process these sounds; rather, it appeared that the patterns reflected specific acoustic properties of the syllables that varied with VOT.

The representation of stop consonants differing in VOT has also been examined in the CN (Clarey et al., 2004), the inferior colliculus (Chen et al., 1996), and the auditory cortex (Eggermont, 1995;

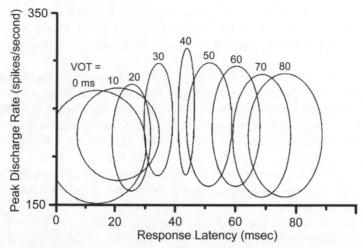

Fig. 9.3 Summary of responses of auditory nerve fibres to syllables from a VOT continuum. The *centre of each ellipse* identifies the mean response latency and mean discharge rate across a sample of low-CF fibres, for one syllable. The *width and height of the ellipse* represent the standard deviations of latency and rate. (Reused with permission from Sinex DG, McDonald LP, and Mott JB (1991) *The Journal of the Acoustical Society of America*, **90**: 2441, copyright 1991, Acoustical Society of America.)

Steinschneider et al., 1995). Cortical neurons in primates have been reported to respond categorically to syllables from an alveolar VOT continuum (Steinschneider et al., 1995). However, cortical neurons in cats studied with syllables from a bilabial VOT continuum did not exhibit comparable categorical response patterns (Eggermont, 1995). It is not likely that the use of a different consonant pair accounts for the difference in response patterns, nor does it seem likely that this is simply a species difference, given the apparent similarity of psychophysical processing of VOT by several mammalian and non-mammalian species.

The most likely explanation for the different outcomes of these two studies is that the stimuli used were not comparable. Synthesized syllables with the same nominal VOT may differ in other important properties; for example, formant transitions may be simple or complicated (Kluender, 1991). It follows that when one summarizes the response patterns elicited by a set of speech sounds, one is summarizing the responses to those particular tokens, which may or may not be representative of a larger set of instantiations of the same consonant or vowel. This has been demonstrated by a small number of studies in which several acoustically different tokens of the same phoneme were presented (Sinex, 1993; Sinex and Narayan, 1994; Stevens and Wickesberg, 2005). Generalizations from the responses to any limited set of speech sounds to larger issues in speech perception should be made with caution.

9.2.8 Evaluation of potential coding mechanisms: rate-place vs temporal representations

The results of Sachs and Young (1979) and Young and Sachs (1979) raised questions about whether the spatial profile of average discharge rate conveys enough information about the speech spectrum to account for humans' abilities to recognize speech at high presentation levels and to discriminate small changes in the frequencies of spectral peaks in vowels. Alternatives such as temporal coding have been considered, but these have shortcomings of their own. While it is clear that information about stimulus frequency is available in synchronized responses, central mechanisms to extract that information have not been identified. This is especially true of mechanisms that might identify frequency components in the manner implied by an analysis like the ALSR.

Subsequent observations of several different types indicate that average discharge rate conveys more useful information than first suspected (Sachs *et al.*, 2006). One important observation was that the olivocochlear efferent system acts to extend dynamic range (Sachs *et al.*, 1988); this feedback system can be expected to exert a greater effect on the representation of speech in awake animals or humans than it does in anesthetized animals. Also, the dynamic range of the initial, onset portion of the responses of an auditory nerve fibre is larger than the dynamic range of the same neuron's adapted response; this would be expected to improve the contrast between segments of different amplitudes. Both of these factors could improve the representation of spectral shape at high stimulus levels.

Another important observation is that small changes in the locations of spectral peaks are detectable as small changes in the discharge rates of individual auditory nerve fibres. Relative discharge rate preserves information about spectral changes that are small enough to approach the psychophysical difference limen for the frequency of a spectral peak (Conley and Keilson, 1995; Sachs *et al.*, 2006). Finally, as mentioned previously, the frequency and amplitude changes that occur over time in ongoing speech can be far more salient than those that distinguish one steady-state vowel from another, and those changes are unambiguously represented as changes in discharge rate (Sinex, 1993; Sinex and Narayan, 1994). If discharge rate can preserve spectral information down to the range of psychophysical thresholds for steady-state vowels, then it can also be expected to preserve the highly salient frequency and amplitude cues that are present in normal, time-varying speech.

Although it may not be necessary to appeal to discharge synchrony to account for the representation of spectral detail in quiet, synchrony does appear to play an important role in the representation of speech information in the presence of competing sounds. When speech sounds are presented in background noise, it is commonly observed that the noise elicits responses from all neurons, including those neurons that were not strongly driven by the speech. The result is the loss of spatial information about the locations of spectral peaks and valleys (Sachs *et al.*, 1983; Delgutte and Kiang, 1984d). Profiles of synchronized discharge rate are much more resistant to masking noise than are profiles of average rate. Discharge synchrony is also better suited to convey information about competing speech sounds (Palmer, 1990; Keilson *et al.*, 1997). These observations suggest that discharge synchrony makes its most important contribution to the representation of speech under adverse conditions.

9.3 **Cortical processing of speech**

Historically, different theoretical perspectives have emphasized different cortical structures as key to speech processing. Proponents of a motor theory of speech perception have suggested that speech is treated separately from its earliest encoded entry into the cortex (e.g. Whalen *et al.*, 2006), which would place an initial central importance on primary auditory cortex (A1), broadly corresponding to Heschl's gyrus on the supra-temporal plane (Fig. 9.4). In contrast, those coming from an anatomical perspective, focusing on structural differences in the brain, have emphasized a role for the planum temporale, posterior to A1, because it is larger on the left than on the right (Geschwind and Levitsky, 1968; Fig. 9.4). Neuropsychological approaches have tended to emphasize the left posterior temporal lobe, since lesions encompassing this area – the core of Wernicke's area – tend to be associated with receptive aphasias (e.g. Bogen and Bogen, 1976; Fig. 9.4).

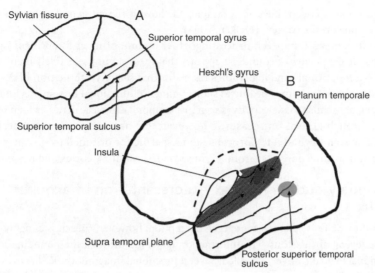

Fig. 9.4 A Lateral view of human left cerebral cortex, showing the superior temporal sulcus (STS), superior temporal gyrus (STG), and Sylvain fissure. **B** Lateral view of human left cerebral cortex, with the cortex above the Sylvian fissure removed to show temporal lobe structures on the supratemporal plane. The *coloured patches* show three different cortical fields which have been emphasized in some accounts of the neural processing of speech. *Red* represents Heschl's gyrus, which is the broad location of primary auditory cortex (A1) in humans; *pink* the planum temporale, posterior to A1 on the supratemporal plane; *turquoise* the posterior superior temporal sulcus.

Neuropsychology has in fact been very successful in providing anatomical frameworks for thinking about speech and language, linking both Wernicke's area and Broca's area (in the posterior third of the left inferior frontal cortex) to speech perception. However, the value of these terms has been called into question: Broca's area is not necessarily recruited by speech production (Wise *et al.*, 1999), and Wernicke's area appears to consist of several different functional sub-systems (Wise *et al.*, 2001).

Functional imaging techniques such as positron emission tomography (PET) and functional magnetic resonance imaging (fMRI), which allow detailed analysis of cortical responses and functional neuroanatomy, permit a more direct investigation of the cortical fields which process speech, and allow us to move beyond an uncritical reliance on Broca's and Wernicke's areas as explanatory constructs. These studies have already demonstrated that there is no selective activation of primary auditory cortex (A1) by speech (Mummery *et al.*, 1999), that the planum temporale is also not selectively activated by speech (Binder *et al.*, 1996), and that while the posterior temporal lobe is important in processing speech, it does not do so in a homogeneous or exclusive fashion (Wise *et al.*, 2001). This section uses functional imaging evidence to outline some ways in which speech is processed cortically.

9.3.1 Primary auditory cortex

There are some important differences between primary auditory cortex (A1) and primary visual cortex. As demonstrated in the first half of this chapter, there is considerable processing of the acoustic signal in the ascending auditory pathway, and many properties of the signal are represented subcortically. This has led some theorists to suggest that A1 processes auditory objects rather than invariant acoustic cues: for example, A1 shows different neural responses to acoustic stimuli, depending on the context (Nelken, 2004).

What does this mean for speech processing? If A1 is computing and representing complex, context-sensitive properties of sounds, it appears that these do not selectively include phonetic properties. No functional imaging studies have shown a selective activation of A1 by speech stimuli. A lack of selectivity may be due to shortcomings in functional imaging techniques (e.g. a lack of power), or because the selectivity is seen in a temporal dimension, rather than one that can be revealed through activation measures; however, this has not prevented speech selective responses being seen beyond A1. Cortical systems specific for or tuned to speech sounds lie at least one synaptic connection away from A1, in secondary auditory cortex and beyond.

9.3.2 Secondary auditory cortex – representation of acoustic modulations

No single auditory cue is essential for speech perception; however, speech is a highly modulated signal across several dimensions. The information conveyed through these modulations enables the speech signal to be effectively decoded. Several functional imaging studies have used modulations of basic acoustic parameters as a way of investigating the properties of the human auditory system. Both amplitude and frequency modulations elicit stronger activation (relative to continuous, unmodulated signals) of cortical fields lateral, anterior, and posterior to A1 (here termed 'early' cortical areas: Giraud et al., 2000; Hall et al., 2002; Hart et al., 2003). These findings are consistent with a heterogeneous response to changes in the acoustic signal in auditory cortical areas adjacent to A1 (Brechmann and Scheich, 2005).

Speech contains complex modulations of frequency and amplitude that occur simultaneously across multiple frequency components. These can be termed spectral modulations: for example, in the changing pattern of spectral prominences or formants as different speech sounds are produced. In a study of the neural systems recruited when stimuli with a changing spectral shape are presented (relative to stimuli with an unchanging spectral profile), there was some evidence that the peaks of activation run further forward along the temporal lobe (Thivard et al., 2000). In this study, non-speech signals with formant-like spectral prominences were used in which the activations seen when the 'formants' changed were contrasted with conditions when the 'formant' structure was constant. There is evidence therefore that spectral modulations may activate somewhat different areas to AM and FM.

The peaks of activations from three of these studies (Giraud et al., 2000; Thivard et al., 2000; Hall et al., 2002) are shown in Fig. 9.5, plotted on a representation of the left supratemporal plane, annotated with some of the auditory areas which have been described in man (Wallace et al., 2002). This shows an area lateral to A1, broadly corresponding to the lateral area (LA) area described by Wallace et al. (2002), which shows sensitivity to harmonic structure, amplitude modulation, and frequency modulation. Peak responses to spectral modulation occur yet more lateral and anterior to this.

9.3.3 Secondary auditory cortex – representation of phonetic structure

Acoustic modulations show some degree of hierarchical processing – as the stimulus modulations become more 'speech-like', the activation occurs further forward along the temporal lobe, away from A1. This might suggest that early auditory cortical areas are not selectively sensitive to speech sounds, and indeed some studies have suggested that the neural responses in early auditory association cortex, in the lateral superior temporal gyrus (STG), are not sensitive to linguistic structure (Davis and Johnsrude, 2003).

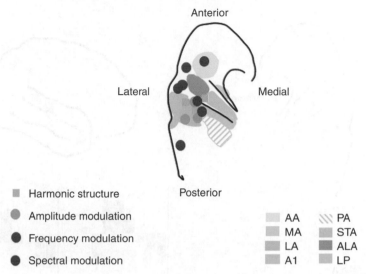

Fig. 9.5 View of the supratemporal plane on the left temporal lobe, annotated with different auditory areas (Wallace *et al.*, 2002), showing locations of activation peaks from functional imaging studies of the responses to harmonic structure (Hall *et al.*, 2002), amplitude modulation (Giraud *et al.*, 2000), frequency modulation (Hall *et al.*, 2002), and spectral modulation (Thivard *et al.*, 2000), all aligned into the same stereotaxic space.

However, there is now some evidence that there may indeed be some specialization in regions adjacent to A1 to sub-lexical properties of the speech signal. Comparisons of vowel sounds with a 'musical rain', which was matched for aspects of the temporal and spectral properties of the vowels, show responses in anterior STG, as well as further distributed along the superior temporal sulcus and beyond (Uppenkamp *et al.*, 2006).

Intriguingly, there is also evidence that quite sophisticated properties of the speech signal may be computed in the STG: Obleser *et al.* (2006) have shown that anterior STG regions discriminate between features that depend upon the place of articulation of vowels, even when the vowels are spoken by a wide range of talkers and therefore differ in their structure. This raises the possibility that maps of phonemes could be represented in these early auditory association fields. Jacquemot *et al.* (2003) demonstrated that a region of auditory association cortex, lateral to A1, showed sensitivity to the presence of linguistically relevant syllable structure, as opposed to the presence of non-linguistic acoustic variation.

A similar result was obtained in a study using noise-vocoded speech (Scott *et al.*, 2006). In this study, short sentences were noise vocoded, and the number of channels was varied between one and sixteen, to produce a range of intelligibility. As increasing the number of channels of noise vocoding also increases the spectral complexity of the stimuli, spectrally rotated versions were included at three and sixteen channels. This study revealed a peak in lateral STG that was sensitive to increases in acoustic complexity, and yet more responsive to increases in linguistic information (Fig. 9.6). Since noise vocoded speech explicitly allows us to manipulate the amplitude and spectral information in the speech signal, it may be no coincidence that this response overlaps with the locations of some of the peak responses to AM, FM, and SM seen in non-speech studies. The response to acoustic modulations seen in lateral STG may also contain some tuning to the specific early acoustic properties of one's native language. Scott *et al.* (2006) also showed that neural activity that correlated with the intelligibility measures of the noise vocoded sentence stimuli was seen

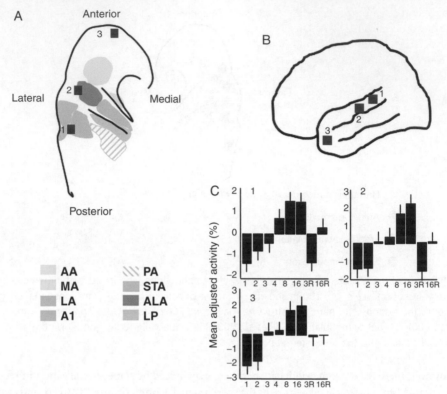

Fig. 9.6 A view of the supratemporal plane on the left temporal lobe, annotated with different auditory areas (Wallace *et al.*, 2002), with peak activations associated with speech intelligibility from Scott *et al.*, (2006). **B** The same peaks plotted on a lateral view of the left temporal lobe. **C** Profiles of activation at each peak; the *abscissa* shows the numbers of channels in noise vocoded speech (1, 2, 3, 4, 8, and 16 channels, plus 3 channel rotated (3R) and 16 channel rotated (16R)). The *ordinate* shows the effect sizes as percentage signal change. Note that further from A1, the neural responses become less linked to the acoustic structure and start to reflect the overall intelligibility of the speech.

in more anterior locations along the left temporal lobe. The further the peaks were seen from A1, the less sensitive the responses were to the acoustic properties of the noise vocoded speech, and more activated purely by lexical information (Fig. 9.6).

9.3.4 Superior temporal sulcus – representation of lexical structure, integration of cross modal information, and access for linguistic modulations

From a neurological perspective, the perception of speech is associated with the left posterior temporal lobe (Bogen and Bogen, 1976). Thus it was surprising when researchers found extensive activations along the dorsolateral temporal lobes when contrasting speech with a baseline condition such as silence or noise bursts. This led to a search for a more suitable baseline which controlled for the acoustic properties of speech. It is fair to say that a lively debate has ensued, with different baselines such as signal correlated noise (Mummery *et al.*, 1999), spectral rotation and its variants (Scott *et al.*, 2000; Narain *et al.*, 2003), and 'musical rain' (Uppenkamp *et al.*, 2006) employed in attempts to identify when and where in the system acoustic processing stops and linguistic processing begins.

Less controversially, all studies indicate that when intelligible speech is contrasted with an appropriate baseline, the dominant cortical response is seen in the superior temporal sulcus (STS). Arguably, the first cortical peak in the processing of speech where there is no sensitivity to the underlying acoustic structure is to be found in STS. While there is some variation in the extent and location of the STS activation, and whether it occurs anteriorly, posteriorly, or along its whole length, this mostly arises from differences in stimulus construction and scanning methodology. Thus fMRI tends to be less sensitive to anterior STS activation, and more sensitive to posterior STS activation (Davis and Johnsrude, 2003; Narain *et al.*, 2003), while PET is more sensitive to anterior temporal lobe activations than fMRI (Scott *et al.*, 2000). Sentences and continuous speech tend to give activation that runs most anterior, and it has been suggested that this may depend on sentence-specific processes (Hickok and Poeppel, 2007). However, it is also the case that sentences simply contain more speech information than simpler lexical sequences (like unrelated word lists), since speakers produce words more fluently in sentences than in lists of single words or syllables.

An explicit investigation of syntactic and semantic processes within the temporal lobe found no significant difference in the dorsolateral temporal lobes when semantic or syntactic violations in spoken sentences were directly compared, although differences were seen in the basal ganglia (Friederici *et al.*, 2003). Likewise, patients with anterior temporal lobe atrophy have problems understanding words, but do not show syntactic deficits. Since words are better understood in sentences than when presented alone, one might expect top-down processes to influence the response to speech in the anterior STS, if it is truly related to sentence processing.

A study attempting to identify the neural correlates of conditions when a predictable sentence really aids comprehension (Obleser *et al.*, 2007) found extensive activations in the medial frontal, inferior frontal, and parietal lobes. However, the response in anterior STS did not change. These studies suggest that lexical, contextual, and semantic influences on speech perception are mediated outwith the temporal lobes. In terms of auditory processing, the activation of the STS probably represents the end point of sub-lexical acoustic and acoustic-phonetic computations, and is the result of robust, automatic perceptual processes. One suggestion, which is consistent with this interpretation of the literature, is that the left anterior STS is the location of the auditory word form area (Cohen *et al.*, 2004). Certainly the anterior STS is well placed to have access to (and be accessed by) linguistic processes in the anterior temporal pole, ventral temporal lobe, and prefrontal cortex.

It is worth emphasizing that the STS is also extensively activated by other kinds of stimuli: it has been identified as a key area in the processing of social information such as eye gaze and gesture (Allison *et al.*, 2000). The anterior STS has also been shown to be activated by spoken or read narratives (Spitsnya *et al.*, 2006). This response to visual information is consistent with the known multiple sensory inputs to STS: visual areas as well as auditory areas project to STS. Indeed in primates, the STS is the area that divides visual and auditory areas in the temporal lobe. The response to speech along the STS may therefore relate to a generic role in representing socially relevant information, since spoken language is an exceedingly important communication tool.

9.3.5 Processing of auditory objects and attention

Speech is rarely heard in isolation, and commonly has to be streamed out from a background of masking noise. At the same time, we know that the 'unattended' masking speech is also processed to some degree for meaning (the cocktail party effect). This implies that (at least) two separate types of processing occur – one streaming out the attended signal, and one processing the unattended signal. Auditory streaming refers to a sequence of sounds being grouped into two or more percepts. How is this mediated?

Studies of how streaming processes occur have identified a role for area outside auditory cortex: the intraparietal sulcus (IPS) (Cusack, 2005). This study found that the IPS was activated when subjects reported two streams of sound in an ambiguous auditory sequence, relative to when they reported hearing only one stream. Within auditory cortex, the planum temporale has been described as a computational hub, playing an important role in the segregation of different auditory streams (Griffiths and Warren, 2002). Studies of the processing of multiple auditory sources have found activation in bilateral anterior STG, suggesting that the representation of the products of auditory streaming involves anterior auditory fields (Zatorre *et al.*, 2004). Further studies will be able to identify the way that attentional mechanisms interact with these representations.

In terms of speech processing, functional imaging has been used to dissociate the neural responses to speech in different masking contexts – specifically contrasting peripheral auditory masking (e.g. continuous white noise) with central auditory masking (e.g. a competing speaker). Scott *et al.* (2004) found that listening to speech in noise recruits areas outside auditory cortex, in the left frontal pole, left dorsolateral prefrontal cortex, and right posterior parietal lobe. These are areas that might be expected to be active in any task recruiting attentional mechanisms (such as target detection), consistent with the perceptual difficulty in listening to speech in noise.

When listening to speech in noise, we found brain areas that were sensitive to the signal to noise ratio (SNR): as the SNR decreased, there was increased activation in the left ventral prefrontal cortex and the dorsomedial prefrontal cortex. The left ventral prefrontal cortex has been associated with executive components of comprehension, such as 'top down' semantic processing and overt segmentation, and activation of the dorsomedial prefrontal cortex has been seen in association with speech production tasks. This finding indicates that as SNRs decrease, and speech becomes harder (but not impossible) to hear, brain areas associated with semantic processing and speech production are recruited – potentially indicating the use of overt strategies by the listeners (e.g. using overt articulation to try to aid comprehension). When people listen to speech in speech, however, there is extensive activation in the dorsolateral temporal lobes – activation that is exceedingly similar to the activation seen when subjects listen to speech in silence (Mummery *et al.*, 1999). This result may reflect the fact that an unattended speech masker is still processed for meaning, to some degree, and thus is processed along the same neural pathways as speech to which we are attending. This result is also consistent with the suggestion that anterior auditory fields can represent multiple auditory objects or streams (Zatorre *et al.*, 2004).

9.3.6 Speech perception–production links

Speech perception and speech production have long been linked behaviourally. For example, the language(s) that one learns to speak and understand in childhood have dramatic influences on the speech sounds that we can discriminate and produce accurately in adulthood. We might well expect speech perception and production to be linked neurally, and probably at several points in the perception/production systems. Speech perception, as we have seen, is associated with activation of the dorsolateral temporal lobes, extending down into the superior temporal sulcus. Speech production is associated with the posterior third of the left inferior frontal gyrus (Broca's area), the left anterior insula, left premotor cortex, the supplementary motor area, and primary motor cortex bilaterally, as well as several subcortical areas (Wise *et al.*, 1999).

Many of these cortical speech production areas have also been implicated in speech perception (shown in Fig. 9.7). Cortical responses in subjects listening to syllables have been reported in left premotor and primary motor cortex (Wilson *et al.*, 2004). The left anterior insula (which includes human premotor areas) shows some sensitivity to speech (Wise *et al.*, 1999). However, these responses may not be selective for the linguistic information in speech: we have demonstrated strong motor and premotor activation to non-verbal emotional vocalizations, such as laughs and screams (when contrasted with a matched acoustic baseline) (Warren *et al.*, 2006). This finding suggests that these premotor and motor responses to speech may not reflect linguistic processing of the speech signal. They may instead represent processing of any human vocalizations.

Moving into the inferior frontal lobe, there is a lively debate about the role of Broca's area in speech and language processing, with some theorists associating it directly with obligatory language perception processes (Hagoort, 2005), and others arguing that Broca's area *per se* is not specific to language or speech processing (Thompson-Schill *et al.*, 1997). It is also the case that Broca's area is not necessarily activated by speech production (Wise *et al.*, 1999).

There are other neural links between speech perception and speech production. An area of auditory cortex, posterior and medial to A1, has been demonstrated to respond to speech production, even if that speech production is silent (Hickok et al., 2000; Wise et al., 2001), shown on Fig. 9.7 as MPT. Thus, there is an area of auditory cortex that is activated by articulations. Again, this activation seems to have little to do with linguistic processing: it has been argued to reflect the representation of possible articulations (Warren et al., 2005), or the configuration of the vocal tract (Hickok and Poeppel, 2007). In contrast, in anterior auditory fields there are neural regions that are suppressed during speech production (Wise et al., 1999), shown in Fig. 9.7 as STG. Thus, the neural response to one's 'own voice' is significantly lower than the activation to the voices

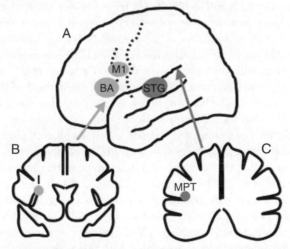

Fig. 9.7 A Lateral view of the left human cortex, with regions that show speech perception and production links. **B** and **C** Coronal slices BA through the brain, marking two further regions that do not lie on the cortical surface. *Arrows* point to the nearest cortical surface to these regions. Regions marked in *green* are in frontal cortex, and thus mostly associated with speech production; regions in *blue* are in posterior temporal cortex, and thus mostly associated with speech perception. BA Broca's area (posterior third of the left inferior frontal cortex), M1 primary motor cortex, I anterior insula, STG superior temporal gyrus (which is suppressed during speech production), and MPT medial planum temporale, posterior, and medial to A1. These regions form a potential network linking speech perception and production in a variety of ways, from sensory-motor links in speech production to activation of motor representations in perception.

of others. This may reflect the fact that monitoring of one's own voice generally occurs prior to articulation, or that one's own voice is much louder than other sounds, or that even if one is speaking, attention is directed to hear what others might be saying. It is notable that this finding is also seen in primates, and that single cell recordings show that the suppression of auditory cortical fields by 'own voice' occurs prior to articulation, which links the motor output processes to the suppression (as opposed to auditory processing).

As suggested at the start of this section, therefore, speech perception and production are linked at several points in the perception/production systems, and in several different ways: mapping sounds to articulations, mapping articulations to sounds, and suppressing the neural response to own vocalizations in brain areas associated with the processing of speech.

9.3.7 Hemispheric asymmetries

Speech and language were the first cognitive faculties to be broadly localized in the brain, with neuropsychological evidence that speech production and perception were associated with sites in the left hemisphere. Neuropsychological evidence remains compelling that speech perception deficits are associated with left hemisphere lesions, although patients with such lesions will typically recover at least single word comprehension, suggesting that some recovery of function can occur. Functional imaging has generally supported the left lateralization of speech perception: studies of speech processing that contrast speech conditions with well-designed baselines typically reveal a left temporal lobe system processing speech in the STG (Jacquemot *et al.*, 2003) and STS (Scott *et al.*, 2000, 2006; Narain *et al.*, 2003; Liebenthal *et al.*, 2005; Uppenkamp *et al.*, 2006). However, functional imaging has also revealed that the right temporal lobe is strongly activated by speech signals (Scott *et al.*, 2000). Unlike the left temporal lobe, the activation is less driven by linguistic information, and more by other properties of the speech stream, such as prosody (Scott *et al.*, 2000) and speaker identity (Belin and Zatorre, 2003). Strong activations of the right STG and STS can also be seen when non-speech stimuli are used: the presence of musical structure is also generally associated with the right temporal lobe (Patterson *et al.*, 2002). Interestingly, patients who have had a right temporal lobectomy can still detect that two tones are of different pitches, but cannot determine whether two successive tones go up or down in pitch (Johnsrude *et al.*, 2000). This suggests that the right temporal lobe is important in computing and representing pitch variation (unlike the computing of pitch itself, which is a bilateral phenomenon).

There are several competing hypotheses as to what underlies these asymmetries of processing. A common suggestion is that they are based on different acoustic processing requirements of phonetic vs pitch-based stimuli. Thus Zatorre and Belin (2001) have suggested that phonetic processing requires fast temporal processing, while pitch processing is reliant on spectral processing. Along a similar line, Poeppel and colleagues have suggested that the left hemisphere is associated with processing short temporal windows (~20–50 ms), important for segmental information in speech, and the right hemisphere is associated with processing longer temporal windows (~150–300 ms), important for processing syllable structure (e.g. Hickok and Poeppel, 2007).

A problem with these approaches is that phonetic or segmental information in speech is not expressed solely over very short time scales, nor is pitch processing solely dependent on spectral processing – pitch can also arise due to temporal properties of a signal. Indeed, given the importance of spectral structure, phonetic information in speech might be more likely linked to spectral processing. While it is clearly the case that the right dorsolateral temporal lobe can be driven by variations in pitch structure (Patterson *et al.*, 2002), and by sounds with longer durations (Belin *et al.*, 1998), it is far less common to find selective activation of the left temporal lobe by acoustic features that are not speech-based. Indeed, no modulation studies in which temporal variations are introduced into the stimuli at different rates have revealed a clear dominance for left auditory fields (Scott and Wise, 2004).

There are other possible reasons for a dominance of the left hemisphere in linguistic aspects of speech perception. One is that the left hemisphere may be better at categorizing information, and this may be particularly relevant for speech processing (Hickok and Peoppel, 2007). Another is that speech production is left lateralized, and that this may simply pull speech perception over to the left as well. However, this account does not explain why speech production itself is lateralized. Finally, there are qualitatively different processes going on in the left and the right temporal lobes, with the left processing linguistic information in speech, and the right processing all the other parallel information (Scott and Wise, 2004). Importantly, this processing asymmetry may change during development (babies do use pitch variation to segment words) and with context, for example, in non-tonal languages adults do not need pitch variation to understand speech, but will use it if the speech is hard to hear (e.g. due to background noise).

9.3.8 Streams of processing – implications for the modelling of speech perception

Some broad patterns can be seen in the speech processing systems. There is a left lateralized stream of processing associated with intelligible speech, which runs lateral and anterior to primary auditory cortex. A hierarchical pattern of processing is apparent: auditory regions adjacent to A1 respond heterogeneously to structure in sound, and also show some sensitivity to linguistic features. More lateral and anterior to A1, in the left temporal lobe, the response becomes more and more selective for the linguistic information, and less and less driven by acoustic factors (e.g. Scott *et al.*, 2006). In contrast, posterior auditory fields are associated with sensory-motor links, which may also relate to other posterior temporal fields involved in the processes of verbal working memory (Hickok *et al.*, 2000; Wise *et al.*, 2001). This dominance of anterior auditory fields for speech perception differs somewhat from the traditional view that posterior temporal lobe areas are critical for speech perception (Bogen and Bogen, 1976).

However, this pattern of results is consistent with models of auditory processing in primates. Here, neural responses running lateral to A1 are shown to be progressively more sensitive to more complex (broadband) signals (Rauschecker, 1998). There is also evidence for anatomical streams in primate auditory cortex, with one pathway running anterior to A1, forwards down the STG to STS, and up into ventral frontal cortex, and one pathway running posterior to A1, into the inferior temporal lobe and then forwards into more dorsal frontal areas (Kaas and Hackett, 1999; Romanski *et al.*, 1999). These two anatomical streams are associated with some specialization of function: the anterior stream shows a broad selectivity for conspecific vocalizations, and the posterior stream is more sensitive to the spatial location of calls (Tian *et al.*, 2001), though this distinction was not completely clear cut. Furthermore, there are regions of posterior, medial auditory cortex that show multimodal responses, being activated by both sound and touch (Fu *et al.*, 2003).

There is thus a striking consistency between the primate neuroanatomical and neurophysiological work and the human functional imaging work – the early perceptual processing of conspecific vocalizations runs lateral and anterior to A1, down the temporal lobe in both human and non-human primates. Notably, studies of spatial auditory processing in humans have similarly implicated posterior auditory fields and inferior parietal regions, as in the primate studies (e.g. Warren and Griffiths, 2003). The finding of posterior-medial auditory fields which show a response to sound and touch also shows some congruency with the sensorimotor responses seen here to speech production in humans (Hickok *et al.*, 2000; Wise *et al.*, 2001). This posterior sensorimotor area may thus form part of a 'how' stream of processing, in which sensory-motor information can be represented during speech perception and production (Warren *et al.*, 2005).

Several commentators have now put forward models of human speech perception which integrate the findings from functional imaging studies with models of primate auditory processing (e.g. Scott and Johnsrude, 2003; Hickok and Poeppel, 2007). While these differ in their anatomical framework (Scott and Johnsrude link their anterior 'what' processing stream to auditory cortex, as in the primate literature, while Hickok and Poeppel favour a 'what' processing stream that runs ventral to A1, unlike the primate models), these approaches both stress the importance of using the known neuroanatomy of primate auditory cortex as a way of interpreting data from human functional imaging studies. As functional imaging is an anatomical tool, this is an approach that helps us move beyond a simplistic linking of speech to Broca's and Wernicke's areas. It is fair to say that the concept of streams of processing in auditory cortex has attracted some criticism, but the evidence from human functional imaging studies is providing strong support.

9.4 Conclusions

Speech is the most complex sound with which we deal routinely and its social salience is exceedingly high. As infants, we spend a lot of time learning to understand speech, and how to produce it. It is therefore possible that many cortical networks are optimized for the representation and computation of speech signals. In this chapter we have addressed studies of subcortical and cortical speech processing, studies that have elaborated coding properties in the ascending auditory pathways, and streams of processing at the cortical level. As neuroscientific methods continue to develop, we predict that we will be able to investigate how these cortical and subcortical processes interact to support speech perception, and discover how they inform our understanding of coding at the cortical level.

Acknowledgements

D.G.S. was supported by grant DC00341 from the National Institute for Deafness and Other Communication Disorders. S.K.S. was supported by grant GR074414MA from the Wellcome Trust.

References

Allison T, Puce A, McCarthy G (2000) Social perception from visual cues: role of the STS region. *Trends Cogn Sci* **4**(7): 267–78.

Belin P, Zatorre RJ (2003) Adaptation to speaker's voice in right anterior temporal lobe. *Neuroreport* **14**(16): 2105–9.

Belin P, Zilbovicius M, Crozier S, *et al.* (1998) Lateralization of speech and auditory temporal processing. *J Cogn Neurosci* **10**: 536–40.

Binder JR, Frost JA, Hammeke TA, Rao SM, Cox RW (1996) Function of the left planum temporale in auditory and linguistic processing. *Brain* **119**: 1239–47.

Blackburn CC, Sachs MB (1990) The representations of the steady-state vowel sound /eh/ in the discharge patterns of cat anteroventral cochlear nucleus neurons. *J Neurophysiol* **63**: 1191–212.

Bogen JE, Bogen GM (1976) Wernicke's region – where is it?. *Ann (NY) Acad Sci* **280**: 834–43.

Brechmann A, Scheich H (2005) Hemispheric shifts of sound representation in auditory cortex with conceptual listening. *Cereb Cortex* **15**: 578–87.

Carney LH, Geisler CD (1986) A temporal analysis of auditory-nerve fiber responses to spoken stop consonant-vowel syllables. *J Acoust Soc Am* **79**: 1896–914.

Chen G, Nuding S, Narayan S, Sinex D (1996) Responses of single neurons in the chinchilla inferior colliculus to consonant-vowel syllables differing in voice-onset time. *Auditory Neuroscience* 3: 179–98.

Clarey JC, Paolini AG, Grayden DB, Burkitt AN, Clark GM (2004) Ventral cochlear nucleus coding of voice onset time in naturally spoken syllables. *Hear Res* 190: 37–59.

Cohen L, Jobert A, Le Bihan D, Dehaene S (2004) Distinct unimodal and multimodal regions for word processing in the left temporal cortex. *Neuroimage* 23(4): 1256–70.

Conley RA, Keilson SE (1995) Rate representation and discriminability of second formant frequencies for /epsilon/-like steady-state vowels in cat auditory nerve. *J Acoust Soc Am* 98: 3223–34.

Cusack R (2005) The intraparietal sulcus and perceptual organization. *J Cog Neurosci* 17(4): 641–51.

Davis MH, Johnsrude IS (2003) Hierarchical processing in spoken language comprehension. *J Neurosci* 23: 3423–31.

Delgutte B (1997) Auditory neural processing of speech. In: *The Handbook of Phonetic Sciences* (eds Hardcastle W, Laver J), pp. 507–38. Blackwell, Oxford.

Delgutte B, Kiang NY (1984a) Speech coding in the auditory nerve: I. Vowel-like sounds. *J Acoust Soc Am* 75: 866–78.

Delgutte B, Kiang NY (1984b) Speech coding in the auditory nerve: III. Voiceless fricative consonants. *J Acoust Soc Am* 75: 887–96.

Delgutte B, Kiang NY (1984c) Speech coding in the auditory nerve: IV. Sounds with consonant-like dynamic characteristics. *J Acoust Soc Am* 75: 897–907.

Delgutte B, Kiang NY (1984d) Speech coding in the auditory nerve: V. Vowels in background noise. *J Acoust Soc Am* 75: 908–18.

Delgutte B, Hammond BM, Cariani PA (1998) Neural coding of the temporal envelope of speech: relation to modulation transfer functions. In: *Psychophysical and Physiological Advances in Hearing* (eds Palmer AR, Rees A, Summerfield Q, Meddis R), pp. 595–603. Whurr, London.

Deng L, Geisler CD (1987) Responses of auditory-nerve fibers to nasal consonant-vowel syllables. *J Acoust Soc Am* 82: 1977–88.

Eggermont JJ (1995) Representation of a voice onset time continuum in primary auditory cortex of the cat. *J Acoust Soc Am* 98: 911–20.

Friederici AD, Ruschemeyer SA, Hahne A, Fiebach CJ (2003) The role of left inferior frontal and superior temporal cortex in sentence comprehension: localizing syntactic and semantic processes. *Cereb Cortex* 13: 170–7.

Fu KM, Johnston TA, Shah AS, *et al.* (2003) Auditory cortical neurons respond to somatosensory stimulation. *J Neurosci* 23: 7510–5.

Geschwind N, Levitsky W (1968) Human brain: left–right asymmetries in temporal speech regions. *Science* 161: 186–7.

Giraud AL, Lorenzi C, Ashburner J, *et al.* (2000) Representation of the temporal envelope of sounds in the human brain. *Neurophysiology* 84: 1588–98.

Griffiths TD, Warren JD (2002) The planum temporale as a computational hub. *Trends Neurosci* 25(7): 348–53.

Hagoort P (2005) On Broca, brain, and binding: a new framework. *Trends Cogn Sci* 9(9): 416–23.

Hall DA, Johnsrude IS, Haggard MP, Palmer AR, Akeroyd MA, Summerfield AQ (2002) Spectral and temporal processing in human auditory cortex. *Cereb Cortex* 12(2): 140–9.

Hart HC, Palmer AR, Hall DA (2003) Amplitude and frequency-modulated stimuli activate common regions of human auditory cortex. *Cereb Cortex* 13(7): 773–81.

Hickok G, Poeppel D (2007) Opinion – the cortical organization of speech processing. *Nat Rev Neurosci* 8(5): 393–402.

Hickok G, Erhard P, Kassubek J, *et al.* (2000) Functional magnetic resonance imaging study of the role of left posterior superior temporal gyrus in speech production: implications for the explanation of conduction aphasia. *Neurosci Lett* 287: 156–60.

Jacquemot C, Pallier C, LeBihan D, Dehaene S, Dupoux E (2003) Phonological grammar shapes the auditory cortex: a functional magnetic resonance imaging study. *J Neurosci* 23(29): 9541–6.

Johnsrude IS, Penhune VB, Zatorre RJ (2000) Functional specificity in the right human auditory cortex for perceiving pitch direction. *Brain* 123(1): 155–63.

Kaas JH, Hackett TA (1999) 'What' and 'where' processing in auditory cortex. *Nat Neurosci* 2: 1045–7.

Keilson SE, Richards VM, Wyman BT, Young ED (1997) The representation of concurrent vowels in the cat anesthetized ventral cochlear nucleus: evidence for a periodicity-tagged spectral representation. *J Acoust Soc Am* 102: 1056–71.

Kim DO, Leonard G (1988) Pitch-period following response of cat cochlear nucleus neurons to speech sounds. In: *Basic Issues in Hearing* (eds Duifhuis H, Horst JW, Wit HP), pp. 252–60. Academic Press, San Diego.

Kluender KR (1991) Effects of first formant onset properties on voicing judgments result from processes not specific to humans. *J Acoust Soc Am* 90: 83–96.

Kuhl PK (1987) The special-mechanisms debate in speech research: facts and hypotheses from animal studies. In: *Categorical Perception* (ed. Harnad S), pp. 355–86. Cambridge University Press, Cambridge.

Liebenthal E, Binder JR, Spitzer SM, Possing ET, Medler DA (2005) Neural substrates of phonemic perception. *Cereb Cortex* 15(10): 1621–31.

Lisker L, Abramson AS (1964) A cross-language study of voicing in initial stops: acoustical measurements. *Word* 20: 384–422.

Miller MI, Sachs MB (1983) Representation of stop consonants in the discharge patterns of auditory nerve fibers. *J Acoust Soc Am* 74: 502–17.

Miller MI, Sachs MB (1984) Representation of voice pitch in discharge patterns of auditory-nerve fibers. *Hear Res* 14: 257–79.

Mummery CJ, Ashburner J, Scott SK, Wise RJS (1999) Functional neuroimaging of speech perception in six normal and two aphasic patients. *J Acoust Soc Am* 106: 449–57.

Narain C, Scott SK, Wise RJ, *et al.* (2003) Defining a left-lateralized response specific to intelligible speech using fMRI. *Cereb Cortex* 13(12): 1362–8.

Nelken I (2004) Processing of complex stimuli and natural scenes in the auditory cortex. *Curr Opin Neurobiol* 14: 474–80.

Obleser J, Boecker H, Drzezga A, *et al.* (2006) Vowel sound extraction in anterior superior temporal cortex. *Hum Brain Map* 27(7): 562–71.

Obleser J, Wise RJ, Alex Dresner M, Scott SK (2007) Functional integration across brain regions improves speech perception under adverse listening conditions. *J Neurosci* 27(9): 2283–9.

Palmer AR (1990) The representation of the spectra and fundamental frequencies of steady-state single- and double-vowel sounds in the temporal discharge patterns of guinea pig cochlear-nerve fibers. *J Acoust Soc Am* 88: 1412–26.

Palmer AR, Shamma S (2004) Physiological representations of speech. In: *Speech Processing in the Auditory System* (eds Greenberg S, Ainsworth WA, Popper AN, Fay RR), pp. 163–230. Springer, New York.

Palmer AR, Winter IM (1993) Coding of the fundamental frequency of voiced speech sounds and harmonic complexes in the cochlear nerve and ventral cochlear nucleus. In: *The Mammalian Cochlear Nuclei: Organization and Function* (eds Merchan MA, Juiz JM, Godfrey DA, Mugnaini E), pp. 373–84. Plenum, New York.

Palmer AR, Winter IM, Darwin CJ (1986) The representation of steady-state vowel sounds in the temporal discharge patterns of the guinea pig cochlear nerve and primarylike cochlear nucleus neurons. *J Acoust Soc Am* 79: 100–13.

Patterson RD, Uppenkamp S, Johnsrude IS, Griffiths TD (2002) The processing of temporal pitch and melody information in auditory cortex. *Neuron* 36(4): 767–76.

Rauschecker JP (1998) Cortical processing of complex sounds. *Curr Opin Neurobiol* **8**: 516–21.

Romanski LM, Tian B, Fritz J, Mishkin M, Goldman-Rakic PS, Rauschecker JP (1999) Dual streams of auditory afferents target multiple domains in the primate prefrontal cortex. *Nat Neurosci* **2**: 1131–6.

Sachs MB, Young ED (1979) Encoding of steady state sounds vowels in the auditory nerve: representation in terms of discharge rate. *J Acoust Soc Am* **66**: 470–9.

Sachs MB, Voigt HF, Young ED (1983) Auditory nerve representation of vowels in background noise. *J Neurophysiol* **50**: 27–45.

Sachs MB, Winslow R, Blackburn C (1988) Representation of speech in the auditory periphery. In: *Auditory Function: Neurobiological Bases of Hearing* (eds Edelman G, Gall W, Cowan W), pp. 747–74. Wiley, New York.

Sachs MB, May BJ, LePrell GS, Hienz RD (2006) Adequacy of auditory nerve rate representations: comparison with behavioral measures in cat. In: *Listening to Speech: An Auditory Perspective* (eds Greenberg S, Ainsworth WA) pp. 115–27. Lawrence Erlbaum, Mahwah, New Jersey.

Scott SK, Johnsrude IS (2003) The neuroanatomical and functional organization of speech perception. *Trends Neurosci* **26**: 100–7.

Scott SK, Wise RJS (2004) The functional neuroanatomy of prelexical processing of speech. *Cognition* **92**: 13–45.

Scot SK, Blank SC, Rosen S, Wise RJS (2000) Identification of a pathway for intelligible speech in the left temporal lobe. *Brain* **123**: 2400–6.

Scott SK, Rosen S, Wickham L, Wise RJ (2004) A positron emission tomography study of the neural basis of informational and energetic masking effects in speech perception. *J Acoust Soc Am* **115**(2): 813–21.

Scott SK, Rosen S, Lang H, Wise RJ (2006) Neural correlates of intelligibility in speech investigated with noise vocoded speech – a positron emission tomography study. *J Acoust Soc Am* **120**(2): 1075–83.

Sinex DG (1993) Auditory nerve fiber representation of cues to voicing in syllable-final stop consonants. *J Acoust Soc Am* **94**: 1351–62.

Sinex DG, Geisler CD (1983) Responses of auditory nerve fibers to consonant-vowel syllables. *J Acoust Soc Am* **73**: 602–15.

Sinex DG, McDonald LP (1988) Average discharge rate representation of voice onset time in the chinchilla auditory nerve. *J Acoust Soc Am* **83**: 1817–27.

Sinex DG, Narayan SS (1994) Auditory-nerve fiber representation of temporal cues to voicing in word-medial stop consonants. *J Acoust Soc Am* **95**: 897–903.

Sinex DG, McDonald LP, Mott JB (1991) Neural correlates of nonmonotonic temporal acuity for voice onset time. *J Acoust Soc Am* **90**: 2441–9.

Spitsyna G, Warren JE, Scott SK, Turkheimer FE, Wise RJ (2006) Converging language streams in the human temporal lobe. *J Neurosci* **26**(28): 7328–36.

Steinschneider M, Schroeder CE, Arezzo JC, Vaughan HG Jr (1995) Physiologic correlates of the voice onset time boundary in primary auditory cortex (A1) of the awake monkey: temporal response patterns. *Brain Lang* **48**: 326–40.

Stevens HE, Wickesberg RE (1999) Ensemble responses of the auditory nerve to normal and whispered stop consonants. *Hear Res* **131**: 47–62.

Stevens HE, Wickesberg RE (2002) Representation of whispered word-final stop consonants in the auditory nerve. *Hear Res* **173**: 119–33.

Stevens HE, Wickesberg RE (2005) Auditory nerve representation of naturally-produced vowels with variable acoustics. *Hear Res* **205**: 21–34.

Thivard L, Belin P, Zilbovicius M, Poline JB, Samson Y (2000) A cortical region sensitive to auditory spectral motion. *Neuroreport* **11**: 2969–72.

Thompson-Schill SL, D'Esposito M, Aguirre GK, Farah MJ (1997) Role of left inferior prefrontal cortex in retrieval of semantic knowledge: a reevaluation. *Proc Natl Acad Sci USA* **94**(26): 14792–7.

Tian B, Reser D, Durham A, Kustov A, Rauschecker JP (2001) Functional specialization in rhesus monkey auditory cortex. *Science* **292**: 290–3.

Uppenkamp S, Johnsrude IS, Norris D, Marslen-Wilson W, Patterson RD (2006) Locating the initial stages of speech-sound processing in human temporal cortex. *Neuroimage* **31**: 1284–96.

Wallace MN, Johnston PW, Palmer AR (2002) Histochemical identification of cortical areas in the auditory region of the human brain. *Exp Brain Res* **143**(4): 499–508.

Warren JD, Griffiths TD (2003) Distinct mechanisms for processing spatial sequences and pitch sequences in the human auditory brain. *J Neurosci* **23**(13): 5799–804.

Warren JE, Wise RJ, Warren JD (2005) Sounds do-able: auditory-motor transformations and the posterior temporal plane. *Trends Neurosci* **28**(12): 636–43.

Warren JE, Sauter DA, Eisner F, *et al.* (2006) Positive emotions preferentially engage an auditory-motor 'mirror' system. *J Neurosci* **26**(50): 13067–75.

Whalen DH, Benson RR, Richardson M, *et al.* (2006) Differentiation of speech and nonspeech processing within primary auditory cortex. *J Acoust Soc Am* **119** (1): 575–81.

Wilson SM, Saygin AP, Sereno MI, Iacoboni M (2004) Listening to speech activates motor areas involved in speech production. *Nat Neurosci* **7**(7): 701–2.

Winter IM, Palmer AR (1990) Temporal responses of primarylike anteroventral cochlear nucleus units to the steady-state vowel /i/. *J Acoust Soc Am* **88**: 1437–41.

Wise RJS, Greene J, Buchel C, *et al.* (1999) Brain regions involved in articulation. *The Lancet* **353**: 1057–61.

Wise RJS, Scott SK, Blank SC, Mummery CJ, Warburton E (2001) Identifying separate neural sub-systems within Wernickes area. *Brain* **124**: 83–95.

Young ED, Sachs MB (1979) Representation of steady-state vowels in the temporal aspects of the discharge patterns of populations of auditory-nerve fibers. *J Acoust Soc Am* **66**: 1381–403.

Zatorre RJ, Belin P (2001) Spectral and temporal processing in human auditory cortex. *Cereb Cortex* **11**(10): 946–53.

Zatorre RJ, Bouffard M, Belin P (2004) Sensitivity to auditory object features in human temporal neocortex. *J Neurosci* **24**(14): 3637–42.

Chapter 10

Formation of auditory streams

Yonatan I. Fishman and Mitchell Steinschneider

10.1 Introduction

In everyday life, sounds generated by multiple sources impinge upon our ears simultaneously or in close succession. An essential task of the auditory system is to determine which acoustic elements in the mixture originate from which sound source, and thereby construct perceptual representations of the original sources. The ease with which the brain assigns sound components to their appropriate sources is illustrated, for example, at a cocktail party: Despite the complex acoustic signal produced by summation at the ears of sound waves emanating from multiple speakers' voices, ambient music, etc., we are easily able to perceive as a distinct 'auditory object' the voice of the person with whom we are speaking.

Auditory scene analysis refers to the processes by which the auditory system groups and segregates components of sound mixtures to construct meaningful perceptual representations of sound sources in the environment (Bregman, 1990). The auditory parsing process is thought to be governed by ecologically relevant heuristics that have evolved to exploit the acoustic properties of causally related sound-producing events (Bregman, 1990; Turgeon et al., 2002). Indeed, it has been maintained that auditory scene analysis is the *basis* of hearing (Bregman, 1990; Yost, 1991). Deficits in auditory scene analysis may partly underlie hearing difficulties encountered with aging, such as impaired discrimination of speech in noisy backgrounds, and may contribute also to deficits characteristic of some specific language disorders (Helenius et al., 1999; Sutter et al., 2000; Petkov et al., 2005; Snyder and Alain, 2005; Alain and McDonald, 2007). These considerations underscore the practical importance of understanding the neurophysiological basis of auditory scene analysis.

Scene analysis can be divided into two classes of processes dealing with the perceptual organization of simultaneously and sequentially occurring sound components, respectively (Bregman, 1990). Many of these processes are considered automatic or 'primitive', in that they do not require learning or attention and are thought to be based upon lower-level neurophysiological mechanisms. Multiple acoustic features are utilized by the auditory system in sound source determination. Acoustic components arising from different spatial locations, or that are far apart in frequency or time, tend in nature to be generated by different sources, and accordingly are perceptually segregated by the brain. In contrast, sound components that are harmonically related or that rise and fall in intensity together (i.e., are co-modulated) tend to arise from a single source, and accordingly are perceptually grouped. However, other aspects of scene analysis do appear to rely on prior learning, attention, and other 'top-down' processes that further constrain inferences made by the brain concerning the environmental sound sources giving rise to the acoustic input. These top-down processes fall under the category of 'schema-based' principles of auditory perceptual organization (Bregman, 1990).

The present chapter describes our most recent understanding of neural processes underlying auditory scene analysis. It is divided into three parts, dedicated to sequential, simultaneous, and 'schema-based' auditory perceptual segregation/grouping processes, respectively. Particular emphasis is placed on the relationship between neurophysiological studies of auditory scene analysis in humans and those involving animal models. Rather than providing an exhaustive review of the literature, the primary goal of this chapter is to highlight general physiological principles and themes that have emerged which may provide a framework for the continuing investigation of neural substrates underlying auditory perceptual organization.

Given that scalp-recorded auditory-evoked neural signals are volume-conducted reflections of the summed activation of multiple sources within the brain, non-invasive recordings in humans are limited in their ability to characterize the detailed physiological events and specific neural generators contributing to the recorded signals (Lütkenhöner, 2003; Yvert *et al.*, 2005). While they provide more direct and anatomically localized views of physiological activity within auditory cortex, extensive invasive recordings in humans are limited by obvious ethical considerations. Whereas functional magnetic resonance imaging (fMRI) is able to suggest regions of activated brain and provides better spatial resolution than event-related potentials (ERPs) and magnetic fields, it is limited in temporal resolution and is still unable to define underlying neural events. These limitations emphasize the importance of using appropriate animal models for the investigation of neural substrates of auditory perceptual organization.

10.1.1 Can neural substrates of auditory scene analysis be studied in experimental animals?

While caution must always be exercised in drawing parallels between neural responses obtained in humans and animal models and inferring the latter's potential relationship to human perception, several lines of evidence support the validity of using animal models to study neural substrates of auditory scene analysis – at least, for lower-level processes of auditory perceptual organization. Perceptual phenomena relevant for scene analysis have been demonstrated behaviorally in non-human animals and infants. For instance, auditory stream segregation (described below) has been shown in bats, birds, fish, monkeys, and newborn infants (Demany, 1982; McAdams and Bertoncini, 1997; Fay, 1998; MacDougall-Shackleton *et al.*, 1998; Izumi, 2002). Furthermore, recordings of neural activity from the scalp in humans using electroencephalography (EEG) demonstrate changes in ERP components elicited under passive listening conditions that correlate with auditory perceptual organization (see Winkler *et al.*, 2003; Alain, 2007; Snyder and Alain, 2007). These considerations suggest that many processes involved in auditory scene analysis are not specific to humans, do not require explicit learning, and likely involve pre-attentive mechanisms that can be studied in appropriate animal models under passive listening conditions.

10.2 Sequential grouping and segregation processes

The perceptual organization of sequential acoustic elements, referred to as *auditory stream segregation*, represents an important feature of scene analysis. Stream segregation denotes how interleaved sequences of acoustic elements are parsed and assigned to distinct perceptual streams. It is exemplified, for instance, by the ability to follow a melodic line in a background of other musical sounds.

Another phenomenon reflecting the perceptual organization of sound sequences is called *auditory induction* or *illusory continuity*, which describes how the brain automatically 'fills in' interruptions in sounds by occluding signals so as to maintain their perceptual continuity and stability. The perceptual psychophysics and possible neural substrates of these perceptual phenomena are considered in the following sections.

10.2.1 Auditory stream segregation

Psychophysics of auditory streams segregation Auditory stream segregation can be experimentally demonstrated by listening to a repeating sequence of temporally non-overlapping high- and low-frequency tones, 'A' and 'B', presented in an alternating pattern, 'ABAB' (Fig. 10.1a). When the frequency separation (ΔF) between the tones is small (generally less than 10%) or presentation rate (PR) is slow (generally less than 10 Hz), a single coherent alternating sequence is perceived at a tempo corresponding to the PR. At large ΔFs or rapid PRs, the sequence perceptually segregates into two auditory streams, one corresponding to 'A' tones and the other corresponding to 'B' tones, with each stream perceived at a tempo composed of half the PR. Another stimulus configuration commonly used to demonstrate stream segregation consists of a sequence in which high and low frequency tones, 'A' and 'B', are presented in a repeating triplet pattern, 'ABA_', where '_' indicates a silent gap (Fig. 10.1b). When the tones of the triplet pattern form a single auditory stream, subjects hear a galloping rhythm, whereas when the 'A' tones are perceptually segregated from the 'B' tones, the galloping rhythm disappears and subjects hear two isochronous rhythms comprised of 'A' tones and of 'B' tones, respectively. Stream segregation is facilitated by increases in ΔF, PR, and tone duration (TD). However, the effects of PR and TD on stream segregation result largely from their influence on inter-stimulus interval (ISI), i.e., the silent interval between the end of one tone and the start of the next tone in the sequence (Bregman *et al.*, 2000).

The perceptual boundaries of stream segregation are illustrated schematically as a function of ΔF and PR in Fig. 10.2. Two perceptual regions labeled 'coherent' and 'segregated' denote combinations of ΔF and PR for which perceptual fusion and segregation are reported, respectively. An 'ambiguous' region lies between them, wherein alternating sequences can be perceived as either coherent or segregated, depending upon attentional set, prior expectations, and specific task demands (see Moore and Gockel, 2002). Importantly, the tendency for segregation to occur increases over several seconds' exposure to the sound sequence (Bregman, 1978; Anstis and Saida, 1985). This 'buildup' of stream segregation suggests that the auditory system assumes the presence of a single sound source by default, and that this assumption is overridden once sufficient

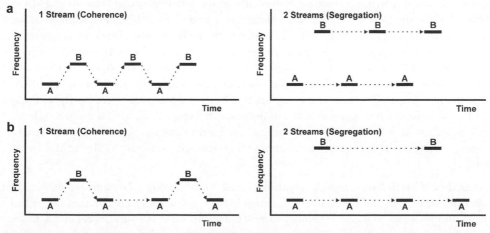

Fig. 10.1 Schematic representation of the spectrum of two types of repeating tone sequences frequently used to study auditory stream formation: **a** 'ABAB' sequence and **b** 'ABA_' sequence, where '_' indicates a silent gap.

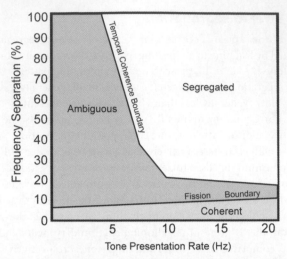

Fig. 10.2 Perceptual boundaries of auditory stream segregation (based on McAdams and Bregman, 1979). Slow presentation rates and small frequency separations between 'A' tones and 'B' tones in a repeating sequence of alternating tones, 'ABAB' or sequence of tone triplets 'ABA_' tend to promote the perception of a single auditory stream or 'coherence', whereas rapid presentation rates and large frequency separations tend to promote perceptual segregation of tones into two separate auditory streams.

evidence for two sound sources has accumulated (Moore and Gockel, 2002). While attention and learning can strongly influence stream segregation, they do not seem to be required for generating the basic phenomenon, particularly when ΔF is large and PR is rapid (McAdams and Bregman, 1979; Moore and Gockel, 2002). However, abrupt alterations in the sequence or in attention can cause a 'resetting' of the mechanisms involved in stream segregation and a return to the default perception of coherence (see Moore and Gockel, 2002; Denham and Winkler, 2006; Sussman *et al.*, 2007).

Theoretical models of stream segregation generally assume that perceptual organization of sequential sound elements is based predominantly on spectral differences (Beauvois and Meddis, 1996; McCabe and Denham, 1997). Thus, stream segregation is facilitated when sequential sound components activate separate peripheral frequency channels. However, stream segregation can occur even in the absence of spectral differences between 'A' and 'B' acoustic stimuli (for review see Moore and Gockel, 2002). For example, Vliegen and Oxenham (1999) demonstrated that subjects were able to perceptually segregate two alternating harmonic complex tones of different fundamental frequency (F0), despite the fact that both complex tones were high-pass filtered within the same spectral region so as to minimize spectral cues. Thus, while a spectral difference may be a dominant factor for stream segregation, listeners can segregate sounds into separate streams when successive sounds differ along other acoustic dimensions (Moore and Gockel, 2002).

Where in the brain does stream segregation occur? That 'buildup' of stream segregation often takes several seconds and can be reset by changes in the ear of stimulus presentation and by shifts in attention (Cusack *et al.*, 2004) strongly suggest the involvement of central mechanisms. Lesions of auditory cortex in animals and humans are associated with impairments in processing auditory temporal patterns, further implicating cortical processes in sequential stream segregation (e.g., Dewson *et al.*, 1970; Cowey and Weiskrantz, 1976; Liégeois-Chauvel *et al.*, 1998). Physiological studies demonstrate that auditory cortical neurons represent the temporal pattern of acoustic events, in part, by highly synchronized responses locked to the onset of sound components (e.g., Creutzfeldt et al., 1980; Steinschneider et al., 1994; Phillips, 1995; Wang et al., 1995; Eggermont, 2001; Fishman et al., 2001a; Nagarajan et al., 2002; Steinschneider et al., 2003). Auditory cortex may function therefore as an acoustic 'event detector', utilizing concerted activity of neural populations as a basic encoding strategy. The following sections summarize findings suggesting neural substrates of stream segregation in auditory cortex.

Neurophysiology: human studies of stream segregation Many studies have examined neural correlates of stream segregation using EEG, magnetoencephalography (MEG), and fMRI (see Denham and Winkler, 2006; Micheyl et al., 2007; Snyder and Alain, 2007). This section focuses on a representative subset of these studies to illustrate the basic processes potentially relevant for sequential stream segregation.

Neural correlates of stream segregation have been investigated using an extensively studied ERP component, the mismatch negativity (MMN), as an index of perceptual segregation of sequentially presented sounds (e.g., Sussman et al., 1999, 2007; Winkler et al., 2003). The MMN peaks at about 200 ms post-stimulus onset and is evoked by infrequent and unpredicted acoustic stimuli, referred to as 'oddballs' or 'deviants', that differ from a regular sequence of preceding sounds, referred to as 'standards' (see Näätänen and Winkler, 1999; Picton et al., 2000). The MMN is a composite ERP component likely reflecting contributions of temporally overlapping sources in the superior temporal gyrus, including auditory cortex, and in regions of frontal cortex (Javitt et al., 1994; Jemel et al., 2002; Doeller et al., 2003). Importantly, while the MMN is modulated by attention (e.g., Woldorff et al., 1991; Näätänen et al., 1993; Alain and Woods, 1994; Oades and Dittmann-Balcar, 1995; Arnott and Alain, 2002), it can be elicited even when subjects ignore auditory stimuli, thereby making the MMN a useful tool with which to examine 'automatic' processing potentially involved in the perceptual organization of sounds (Sussman et al., 1999; Winkler et al., 2003).

The general scheme used to examine stream segregation utilizes paradigms whereby deviant acoustic events may be detected and an MMN elicited only if sound sequences have been physiologically segregated. For instance, an MMN is elicited by an oddball tone embedded in a sequence when the sequence is widely separated in frequency from another perceptually segregated sequence of tones. However, no MMN is elicited under conditions where the sequences are *not* segregated, as occurs when the frequency separation between the two sequences is small. Thus, the presence or absence of an MMN may be used to indicate whether or not the brain has parsed, pre-attentively, a sequence of sounds into separate auditory streams. Using this approach, a number of studies support a pre-attentive neural process underlying auditory stream segregation that may be modulated further by attention (Sussman et al., 1999, 2007; Winkler et al., 2003). However, these studies do not directly identify neural mechanisms underlying stream segregation *per se* (see Snyder and Alain, 2007).

Potential neural substrates of stream segregation have been investigated by examining neural responses evoked by sequences of 'A' and 'B' tones in a repeating 'ABA_' pattern as a function of tonal frequency separation (e.g., Gutschalk et al., 2005; Snyder et al., 2006). The P1, N1, and P2 components of the auditory evoked potential (AEP) and magnetic field elicited by the 'B' tone increased in amplitude with increasing frequency separation in a manner that correlated with the perception of two auditory streams. The increases in 'B' tone response amplitude were not dependent on attention (Gutschalk et al., 2005; Snyder et al., 2006). Dipole source modeling suggested generators of the augmented AEP components within the superior temporal gyrus, including Heschl's gyrus, the presumed locus of primary auditory cortex in humans. The increase in 'B' tone response amplitude with increasing frequency separation may reflect a release from neural suppression, whereby the neural response to a tone is diminished by a preceding tone when the frequency separation between the tones is small and the inter-tone interval is brief (Gutschalk et al., 2005; Snyder et al., 2006; Micheyl et al., 2007; Snyder and Alain, 2007).

Snyder et al. (2006) also examined neural activity potentially related to the buildup of streaming. The investigators examined changes in ERPs evoked by a repeating 'ABA_' tone sequence over the course of 10.8 s of exposure to the sequence. The P1, N1, and P2 components of the ERP evoked by the 'B' tone were larger after 10 s of exposure to the tone sequence than during the first 2 s (Snyder et al., 2006; Snyder and Alain, 2007). Response augmentation was much more pronounced when subjects attended to the stimuli. These findings parallel modulation of stream segregation by attention and its buildup. However, the study does not reveal the mechanisms responsible for the buildup since it did not dissociate neural activity associated with the overall gain of the evoked responses resulting from attention to the signal (Hillyard et al., 1973, 1998) from that related specifically to the buildup process.

Complementary studies using fMRI suggest neural structures involved in stream segregation. For instance, an fMRI study by Cusack (2005) showed differential activation in the intraparietal sulcus depending on whether subjects heard one or two streams when listening to repeating 'ABA_' sequences. These results suggest involvement of brain areas outside of 'classical' auditory cortex. More recent studies have demonstrated an increase in activation of auditory cortex with increasing frequency separation between 'A' tones and 'B' tones in 'ABAB' sequences that correlated with subjects' perception of two streams (Wilson et al., 2007). Moreover, as frequency separation between the tones increased, the time-course of activation generally became more sustained (i.e., less phasic) and more closely resembled that of responses evoked by control sequences consisting only of 'A' tones or of 'B' tones (Wilson et al., 2007). Consistent with explanations for similar findings of EEG and MEG studies discussed earlier (Gutschalk et al., 2005; Snyder et al., 2006), Wilson et al. (2007) proposed that the increased fMRI activation in Heschl's gyrus observed with an increase in frequency separation may reflect a decrease in mutually suppressive interactions between consecutive responses to 'A' and 'B' tones.

Finally, a recent combined MEG/fMRI study by Gutschalk et al. (2007) examined neural correlates of 'non-spectral' stream segregation observed for sequences of sound elements that have similar spectra but that differ along some other acoustic or perceptual dimension. The investigators presented sequences consisting of two spectrally similar unresolved harmonic complex tones arranged in a continuously repeating 'ABBB' pattern and with a varying difference in F0 (ΔF0) between 'A' and 'B' tones. FMRI results showed enhanced sustained activity in auditory cortex evoked by sequences that were perceived as two streams (ΔF0 of 3 and 10 semitones) compared with activity evoked by sequences that were perceived as one stream (ΔF0 of 0 and 1 semitones). This response enhancement was observed in medial Heschl's gyrus corresponding to primary auditory cortex as well as in surrounding anterior and posterior non-primary areas along the superior temporal gyrus. In MEG recordings, 'A' tones elicited a P1 component under the 3- and 10-semitone ΔF0 conditions which was absent under the 0- and 1-semitone ΔF0 conditions. Thus, sequences comprised of complex sounds that differed in perceived pitch, but that stimulated the same spectral channels in the auditory system evoked similar patterns of responses to those observed in the earlier studies of Gutschalk et al. (2005) and Wilson et al. (2005) using pure tones. The results of Gutschalk et al. (2007) suggest therefore that the earlier findings reflect more general neural mechanisms underlying auditory stream segregation for sound elements that differ along a number of dimensions including frequency.

Neurophysiological investigations in humans have yielded important information regarding the possible anatomical loci and neural processes underlying stream segregation and the effects of attention on auditory perceptual organization. In general, the findings of these studies suggest greater activation of auditory cortex by tone sequences when they are perceived as two streams than when they are perceived as a single stream. However, the methodologies used are limited in their ability to identify detailed neurophysiological mechanisms involved in stream segregation. Experiments in appropriate animal models are thus required to bridge the gap between cellular neurophysiology and auditory perception.

Neurophysiology: animal models of stream segregation

Neural correlates of stream segregation were investigated in primary auditory cortex (A1) of awake macaque monkeys by Fishman *et al.* (2001a). Alternating high- and low-frequency tone sequences ('ABAB') were presented to the monkeys while neural ensemble activity, as measured by multiunit activity (MUA) and current source density of field potentials, was recorded in laminae 3–4 of A1. 'A' tones were fixed at or near the best frequency (BF) of the recorded neural populations (the tone frequency eliciting the largest neural response), while the frequency of 'B' tones differed from that of 'A' tones by an amount ΔF and PR was varied over a range of 5–40 Hz. At slow PRs neural ensembles with a BF corresponding to the 'A' tone frequency responded robustly to both 'A' tones and 'B' tones, yielding a temporal pattern of neural activity occurring at a rate equal to the overall PR. However, at rapid PRs, neural responses to 'B' tones were differentially suppressed, resulting in a temporal pattern of neural activity consisting predominantly of 'A' tone responses occurring at half the overall PR (Fig. 10.3). These changes in temporal response pattern mirrored the formation of two separate perceptual streams, one consisting of 'A' tones and the other consisting of 'B' tones. Under stimulus conditions favoring the perception of a single auditory stream, neurons responded to both BF tones and non-BF tones, whereas under

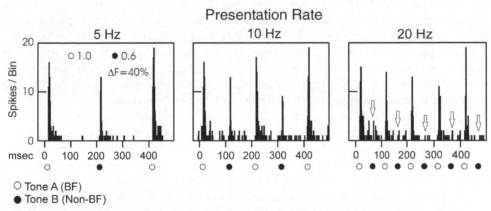

Fig. 10.3 Peri-stimulus time histograms (PSTHs) of multi-unit cluster activity evoked by alternating frequency tone sequences ('ABAB'; 60 presentations) in thalamorecipient layers of macaque primary auditory cortex (A1) under three presentation rate conditions. 'A' tones and 'B' tones are represented by the *white and black symbols*, respectively, below the timelines. Tones are 25 ms in duration (including 5 ms linear rise/fall ramps). The frequency of 'A' tones was fixed at the best frequency (BF) of the site (1.0 kHz), while the frequency of 'B' tones was set at 0.6 kHz, corresponding to a frequency separation of 40%. *Downward arrows* indicate markedly diminished or absent 'B' tone responses in the 20-Hz presentation rate condition relative to their amplitudes under the 5-Hz condition. (Adapted with permission from Fishman *et al.* (2001a), copyright 2001, *Hearing Research*, Elsevier.)

conditions favoring perception of two separate auditory streams, neurons responded only to BF tones.

The authors proposed that the differential suppression of non-BF tone responses at rapid PRs could be explained by mechanisms similar to those underlying physiological 'forward masking', i.e., the reduction in the neural response to a stimulus by the response to a preceding stimulus (Calford and Semple, 1995; Brosch and Schreiner, 1997). Forward suppression of responses to BF tones decreases with increasing frequency difference and time delay between masker and probe stimuli (Calford and Semple, 1995; Brosch and Schreiner, 1997), findings consistent with activity patterns reported by Fishman *et al.* (2001a). Differential suppression of 'B' tone responses is observed at fast PRs. Furthermore, responses to BF 'A' tones are smaller when they are preceded by other 'A' tone responses than when they are preceded by non-BF 'B' tone responses. This latter observation accords with enhanced forward masking of responses to BF tones when the preceding masker is at or near the BF (Calford and Semple, 1995; Brosch and Schreiner, 1997). Finally, responses to non-BF 'B' tones are smaller when they are preceded by responses to BF 'A' tones than when they are preceded by non-BF 'B' tones. Responses to BF tones therefore display a pattern opposite to that of responses to non-BF tones in an alternating context: non-BF tone responses are suppressed by preceding BF tone responses to a greater extent than BF tone responses are suppressed by preceding non-BF tone responses. Fishman *et al.* (2001a) proposed that this differential suppression can be explained by BF tone responses being stronger forward 'maskers' than non-BF tone responses. This differential suppression is manifested by a decrease in the ratio of non-BF response amplitude to BF response amplitude with increasing PR (Fishman *et al.*, 2001a). Consequently, stimulus conditions that promote stream segregation enhance the contrast between BF and non-BF tone responses at tonotopic locations in A1 corresponding to the frequencies of the tones in the alternating sequences.

Based on these findings, a model of neural stream segregation was proposed whereby differential suppression of non-BF tone responses by preceding BF tones would increase the spatial separation of neural activity evoked by 'A' tones and by 'B' tones along the tonotopic map in A1 (Fig. 10.4; Fishman *et al.*, 2001a, 2004). At small ΔFs, there is considerable overlap of the neural excitation patterns evoked by 'A' and 'B' tones in tonotopically organized A1. Neither tone response dominates the neural response pattern. Consequently, 'A' and 'B' tone responses are mutually suppressive to a roughly equal extent and decrease equivalently in amplitude with increasing PR. Moreover, minimal differential response suppression results in a poorly segregated distribution of activity in A1 at both slow and fast PRs. Analogously, for small ΔFs, alternating sequences are invariably perceived as one stream at all PRs. In contrast, at large ΔFs, there is minimal spatial overlap of neural activity evoked by 'A' tones and 'B' tones and minimal suppressive interactions between the tone responses. Accordingly, at both slow and fast PRs, alternating frequency tone sequences evoke two spatially well-segregated peaks of activity in A1. This physiological scenario parallels the perceptual segregation of 'A' and 'B' tones into separate auditory streams when tones are widely separated in frequency (Bregman, 1990). At intermediate ΔFs, there is considerable spatial overlap in neural activity evoked by 'A' and 'B' tones, such that neurons at corresponding tonotopic locations respond to both tones, although with BF responses dominating. Under these circumstances, the predominance of 'A' tone responses or 'B' tone responses in the resultant activity pattern is modulated by PR. At slow PRs, the tones evoke optimal responses at tonotopic sites corresponding to their frequency and sub-optimal responses at sites corresponding to the frequency of the other tone in the sequence. The intervening region responds well to both tones, and activity patterns at the 'A', 'B', and intervening tonotopic locations reflect the overall PR of the alternating tone sequence. In contrast, at fast PRs, non-BF tone responses at the 'A' tone and 'B' tone tonotopic locations are differentially suppressed, such that

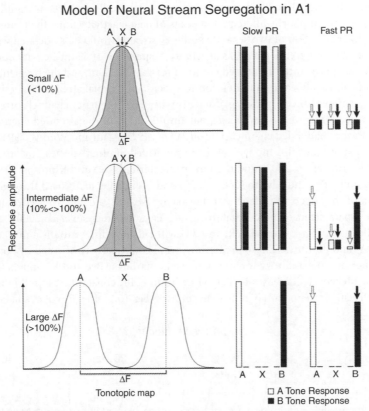

Fig. 10.4 Neurophysiological model of stream segregation in primary auditory cortex (A1). *Bell-shaped curves labeled 'A' and 'B'* represent tonotopic distributions of activity evoked by 'A' and 'B' tones comprising an alternating frequency tone sequence ('ABAB'). The region in between the tonotopic locations corresponding to the frequencies of the 'A' tones and 'B' tones is labeled 'X'. *Shaded regions* represent locations where activity patterns generated by the tones overlap. Spatial distributions of activity under three different frequency separation (ΔF) conditions are depicted (small, intermediate, and large). Hypothetical 'A' tone and 'B' tone response amplitudes at tonotopic locations 'A', 'B', and 'X', marked by *dashed vertical lines*, are represented by *white and black bars* shown in the right half of the figure under slow and fast presentation rate (PR) conditions. Bar height is proportional to response amplitude. At fast PRs, non-BF tone responses are differentially suppressed in locations 'A' and 'B', while in regions equally responsive to both tones ('X'), 'A' and 'B' tone responses are mutually suppressive to an equal extent and are equally diminished. Differential suppression of non-BF tone responses results in an effective sharpening of frequency tuning at tonotopic locations corresponding to the frequencies of the tones and the formation of two spatially discrete foci of activity along the tonotopic map which parallels the perceptual segregation of the tones into two separate streams. See text for further discussion. (Reproduced with permission from Fishman *et al.* (2001a), copyright 2001, *Hearing Research*, Elsevier.)

neurons at the 'A' tone BF site still respond vigorously to 'A' tones, but no longer respond to non-BF 'B' tones, whereas neurons at the 'B' tone BF site still respond vigorously to 'B' tones, but no longer respond to non-BF 'A' tones. This differential attenuation results in an effective sharpening of frequency tuning in A1, thereby enhancing the spatial differentiation of 'A' tone responses and 'B' tone responses along the tonotopic map.

According to the model, perception of a single, coherent auditory stream would be based in part on the presence of poorly differentiated peaks of neural activity along the tonotopic map of A1, whereas the perception of two separate auditory streams would be associated with the presence of two spatially differentiated peaks of activity. Segregation of neural activity into independent frequency channels by the combined effects of forward masking and the frequency selectivity of A1 could facilitate allocation of attention to specific perceptual streams. Selective attention could subsequently enhance processing of activity within the frequency channel corresponding to one or the other perceptual stream via signal amplification in the attended channel or signal attenuation in the unattended channel (Hillyard et al., 1973; Alain and Woods, 1994).

Findings in support of this model have been replicated in other species, including the mustached bat (Kanwal et al., 2003) and the European starling (Bee and Klump, 2004, 2005) and expanded upon by Bee and Klump (2004, 2005) and Fishman et al., (2004) through systematic examination of the effects of independently varying ΔF, PR, and TD. In accordance with the effects of these parameters on perceptual stream segregation (Bregman et al., 2000), the proposed model predicts that increasing ΔF, PR, and TD will enhance differentiation of neural activity evoked by 'A' and 'B' tones. These predictions were empirically confirmed in both A1 of the awake monkey and the auditory forebrain of awake starlings (Bee and Klump, 2004; Fishman et al., 2004). Moreover, increases in TD, while holding PR constant, resulted in a more pronounced differential attenuation of non-BF responses (Fig. 10.5). In particular, smaller ISIs led to

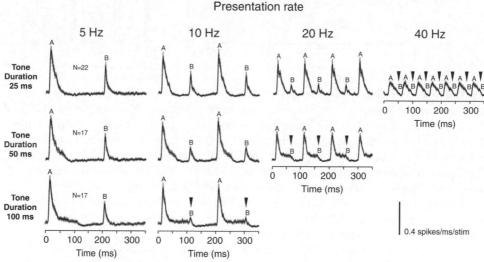

Fig. 10.5 Average peristimulus time histograms (PSTHs) of multi-unit spike activity evoked by alternating frequency tone sequences ('ABAB') in thalamorecipient layers of macaque primary auditory cortex (A1). PSTHs under four different presentation rate conditions and under three tone duration conditions are shown to illustrate the similar effects of these stimulus parameters on differential suppression of 'B' tone responses. The frequency of 'A' tones is fixed at the best frequency of the neural populations, and the frequency separation between 'A' and 'B' tones is held constant at 20% of the 'A' tone frequency across all conditions. Responses to 'A' tones and 'B' tones are labeled. The boundaries of the *gray shaded region* above and below each average PSTH (*black line*) represent +/− SEM. *Black arrowheads* indicate markedly diminished or absent 'B' tone responses. Number of sites (N) contributing to each of the average PSTHs in each row is indicated in the *far left column*. (Adapted with permission from Fishman et al. (2004) *Journal of the Acoustical Society of America*, **116**(3): 1656–70, copyright 2004, Acoustical Society of America.)

lower 'B' tone to 'A' tone response ratios (Fig. 10.6), implying that differential attenuation of non-BF tone responses depends critically not on PR or TD *per se*, but rather on ISI, which decreases with increasing TD when PR is held constant (Bee and Klump, 2004; Fishman *et al.*, 2004). These findings parallel the psychoacoustic results of Bregman *et al.* (2000) indicating that the two primary factors promoting stream segregation are increases in ΔF and decreases in ISI.

While these findings support the physiological model of stream segregation described above, they do not directly account for the buildup of stream segregation over time. To address this shortcoming, Micheyl *et al.* (2005) presented 'ABA_' sequences to awake macaques and examined changes in the pattern of responses of single neurons in A1 over a 10-s period. An advantage of this approach is that the stimulus is held constant, while only the perception changes (from hearing one stream to hearing two streams). Thus, any change in neural response patterns over time cannot be attributed simply to a change in stimulus parameters, and may be related more directly to a change in perception. As in previous studies, the frequency of 'A' tones corresponded to the BF of the recorded neurons, while the frequency of 'B' tones differed from that of 'A' tones by an amount, ΔF, which ranged from 1 to 9 semitones. The time-course of changes in the neural response pattern was found to correlate with the perceptual buildup of stream segregation in human listeners (Micheyl *et al.*, 2005). Responses to both 'A' tones and 'B' tones decreased in amplitude over a 10-s period of sequence presentation, indicative of neuronal adaptation (e.g., Ulanovsky *et al.*, 2004), but with 'B' tone response amplitudes decreasing to a greater extent. In

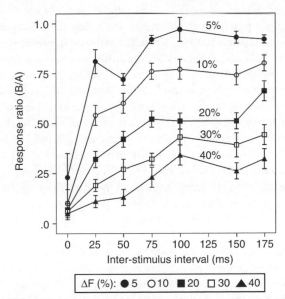

Fig. 10.6 Mean ratio of 'B' tone response amplitude to 'A' tone response amplitude plotted as a function of inter-stimulus interval (ISI) and with frequency separation (ΔF) as the parameter (*error bars* represent +/– SEM; *symbols* representing different values of the parameter are denoted in the legend). Data are based on multiunit responses evoked by alternating frequency tone sequences ('ABAB') in thalamorecipient layers of macaque primary auditory cortex (A1). The frequency of 'A' tones was fixed at the best frequency of the neural population under all stimulus conditions. The frequency of 'B' tones differed from that of 'A' tones by an amount equal to ΔF. Response ratios decrease with increasing ΔF and with decreasing ISI. (Reprinted with permission from Fishman *et al.* (2004) *Journal of the Acoustical Society of America*, **116**(3): 1656–70, copyright 2004, Acoustical Society of America.)

light of these findings, Micheyl *et al.* (2005) proposed that the buildup of perceptual stream segregation could be accounted for by the proportion of time during which the spike count evoked by the 'B' tone fails to exceed a threshold. When both 'A' and 'B' tones evoke supra-threshold neuronal spike counts at both tonotopic sites corresponding to the frequencies of the tones, a 'one stream' percept is elicited, whereas when one of the tones fails to evoke a supra-threshold spike count at both tonotopic sites a 'two stream' precept is elicited. The buildup of stream segregation is thus explained by the failure of 'B' tone responses to exceed the decision threshold as 'A' and 'B' tone response rates adapt over time. This is attributed both to the progressively lower amplitude of 'B' tone responses with increases in ΔF as the frequency of 'B' tones moves farther away from the BF of the unit and to the general response attenuation and differential attenuation of 'B' tone responses relative to 'A' tone responses over time. By offering a plausible physiological basis for 'buildup', a key feature of stream segregation, Micheyl *et al.* (2005, 2007) provide additional evidence for the relevance of temporal response patterns in A1 for the perceptual organization of sound sequences.

As noted earlier, the differential suppression of non-BF responses by preceding BF responses is consistent with the general principles of physiological forward masking (Calford and Semple, 1995; Brosch and Schreiner, 1997). By independently varying both stimulus onset-to-onset interval and the duration of masker stimuli, Brosch and Schreiner (1997) also demonstrated an increase in physiological forward suppression in A1 with decreases in masker-probe offset-to-onset interval (i.e., ISI), suggesting a role of inhibitory processes triggered by sound offsets in addition to those following sound onsets in forward masking. The cellular basis of forward suppression remain unclear, but likely include postsynaptic GABAergic inhibition (de Ribaupierre *et al.*, 1972; Cox *et al.*, 1992; Volkov and Galazyuk, 1992) as well as synaptic depression (Chung *et al.*, 2002; Ulanovsky *et al.*, 2004; Wehr and Zador, 2005). Suppressive interactions between successive tone responses observed at the level of the auditory nerve, the cochlear nucleus, and the inferior colliculus (IC) suggest additional peripheral and subcortical contributions to the forward suppression observed at the cortical level (for review see Frisina, 2001). The extent to which forward suppression at the cortex is shaped by processes at subcortical levels remains to be elucidated.

In general, the physiological results in auditory cortex are consistent with the hypothesis that pre-attentive neural mechanisms underlying frequency selectivity and differential forward masking contribute to the perceptual segregation of sequential acoustic events. Accordingly, theoretical models incorporating basic mechanisms of frequency selectivity and forward masking are sufficient to replicate many of the neural response patterns in A1 proposed to contribute to perceptual stream segregation for two-tone sequences (e.g., Kanwal *et al.*, 2003; Denham and Winkler, 2006).

Despite parallels found between neural response patterns and perceptual boundaries of stream segregation, the link between neurophysiology and perception remains tentative, particularly since behavioral studies were not conducted simultaneously with the neural recordings. An additional limitation of the neurophysiological studies is that they only used pure tones and hence do not account for stream segregation observed with sounds of similar spectral content but differing along some other perceptual dimension (see Moore and Gockel, 2002). However, these models might be able to account for 'non-spectral' stream segregation by incorporating neural elements that are selective for other, 'non-spectral' stimulus attributes.

Psychoacoustic studies have shown enhanced forward masking between broadband sounds having similar rates of amplitude modulation, suggesting the existence of modulation-rate selective neural channels in the auditory system (e.g., Wojtczak and Viemeister, 2005). Paralleling these psychoacoustic findings, forward masking studies by Bartlett and Wang (2005) in A1 of squirrel monkeys demonstrate that forward suppression of the response to amplitude-modulated

(AM) tones by the response to a preceding AM tone is maximal when both sounds have the same carrier frequency and similar rates of amplitude modulation. These results indicate that physiological forward suppression may be based upon temporal characteristics in addition to spectral characteristics of acoustic stimuli (Bartlett and Wang, 2005). Studies by Bendor and Wang (2005) suggest the existence of neurons in non-primary auditory cortex of marmosets which respond to the perceived pitch rather than the spectral content of complex sounds. Given the existence of neural populations selective for non-spectral or higher-level stimulus attributes, 'non-spectral' stream segregation might be based upon similar physiological principles to those underlying perceptual segregation based on spectral differences. Thus, in general, stream segregation would be promoted by any difference in a sequence of sounds that enhances neural selectivity for the attributes distinguishing the acoustic elements in the sequence. An enhancement in selectivity for these attributes in turn may facilitate allocation of attention to neural channels differentially sensitive to those particular stimulus attributes (Alain and Woods, 1994; Alain and Arnott, 2000).

10.2.2 Auditory induction/illusory continuity

Psychophysics of auditory induction/illusory continuity

Often a sound generated by one source may briefly overlap temporally with a sound generated by a second source. Yet listeners do not generally perceive the first sound as interrupted, even if the second sound is intense enough to completely mask a part of the first. This perceptual phenomenon, whereby a sound is perceived as complete despite its occlusion by a second sound, is called *auditory induction*, and can be used to create an illusion. When a part of a sound is omitted and replaced by a silent gap, an interruption in the sound is heard. However, if the gap is replaced by a louder burst of noise, the fainter sound is perceived as continuing behind the noise. The perception of illusory continuity represents a specific instance of auditory perceptual organization important for 'filling in' degraded acoustic information and for maintaining stable representations of auditory objects in complex or noisy acoustic environments (Warren *et al.*, 1972; Bregman and Dannenbring, 1977; Ciocca and Bregman, 1987; Petkov *et al.*, 2003, 2007). In order for illusory continuity to be perceived the following two conditions must be satisfied: (1) energy must be present at induced frequencies and (2) there should be no neural evidence of transitions, i.e., onsets or offsets in the 'occluded' sound (Bregman, 1990; Petkov *et al.*, 2007).

Neurophysiology: human studies of auditory induction/illusory continuity

One of the few neurophysiological studies investigating auditory induction used the MMN ERP component as a physiological index (Micheyl *et al.*, 2003). Standard stimuli were 500-Hz tones that were either continuous or interrupted at their middle by a 40-ms silent gap. Deviant stimuli consisted of the interrupted tone, but with the silent gap filled by a burst of band-pass-filtered noise. The spectrum of the noise occupied either the same frequency region as the tone and elicited the continuity illusion, or a remote frequency region and did not elicit the illusion. The MMN was larger in conditions where the deviants were perceived as continuous and the standards as interrupted or vice versa, than when both were perceived as continuous or both interrupted. These findings therefore suggested that neural encoding of the continuity illusion occurred prior to MMN generation. Furthermore, since subjects were instructed to ignore the tones and to watch a silent movie during the recordings, the results imply a pre-attentive neural mechanism underlying the continuity illusion.

Neurophysiology: animal models of auditory induction/illusory continuity

Behavioral evidence for auditory induction in cats (Sugita, 1997), birds (Braaten and Leary, 1999), and macaque monkeys (Miller *et al.*, 2001; Petkov *et al.*, 2003) supports the validity of studying neural substrates of the perceptual phenomenon in animal models. Neural correlates of auditory induction/illusory continuity have been investigated in A1 of cats by recording single-neuron activity evoked by frequency-modulated (FM) sweeps with spectral portions overlapping the BF of the neurons (Sugita, 1997). In one condition, the FM sweeps were continuous, whereas in a second condition they contained a brief silent gap occurring during the spectral transition that overlapped the BF of the neurons. In a third condition, the gap was filled with a burst of noise, whereas in a fourth condition the noise burst was presented alone. A significant number of neurons were found that failed to respond when the FM sweep contained a silent gap yet responded when the gap was filled with a noise burst. However, no responses were evoked by the noise burst when presented alone. These results suggest that the neurons were responding as if there were no gap in the FM sweep, analogous to the perception of auditory induction.

Similarly, Petkov et al. (2007) found neurons in macaque A1 that failed to respond during a silent gap inserted into an otherwise continuous tone set at their BF, yet responded when a noise burst was presented concurrently with the gap. As in the previously described study, these neurons did not respond to the noise burst when presented alone. Moreover, their responses did not differ appreciably when the continuous tone was presented with and without the occluding noise burst. The authors identified several types of neurons exhibiting distinctive patterns of responses to the stimuli that all correlated with the perception of auditory induction. Neurons responding in a sustained manner to tones continued to respond when a silent gap in the tones was filled with noise, while those responding in a phasic manner to transients (stimulus onsets and offsets) no longer responded to the beginning and to the end of the gap when it was filled with noise. Furthermore, simulations of auditory nerve activity evoked by the stimuli suggested a central basis for the phenomenon, as peripheral responses tended to be driven primarily by the interrupting noise burst and did not exhibit responses consistent with auditory induction (Petkov et al., 2007).

While cats and macaques show behavioral evidence for auditory induction, behavior was not monitored during the electrophysiological recordings described above, thus precluding a direct evaluation of the link between the neural response patterns and perception. Nonetheless, these studies provide support for a potential neural substrate of auditory induction in auditory cortex. Pre-attentive mechanisms underlying neural response patterns correlating with auditory induction may be similar to those proposed to account for primitive auditory stream segregation. Indeed, psychoacoustic studies suggest that stream segregation and illusory continuity may share common mechanisms (Bregman et al., 1999). For instance, the absence of a phasic response to the onset of the tone occurring after the gap might be due to forward masking by the prior response to the noise filling the gap. This might occur even if there is no excitatory response to the noise burst, as forward masking of responses to BF tones can be observed even when masker frequencies are outside the excitatory frequency response area of the neuron (Calford and Semple, 1995).

10.3 **Simultaneous grouping and segregation processes**

The two most prominent cues utilized by the auditory system for grouping together acoustic components are *common temporal onsets* and *harmonicity*. Conversely, the perceptual segregation of sound components is promoted by stimulus onset asynchrony (SOA) and inharmonicity (Bregman, 1990; Yost, 1991; Turgeon et al., 2002, 2005). Weaker segregation cues include spectral and spatial separation of acoustic elements. These cues reinforce each other in a synergistic manner (Turgeon et al., 2002, 2005). It is statistically unlikely that acoustic components generated by two different sound sources would turn on and off simultaneously or be harmonically related, thereby making onset asynchrony and inharmonicity reliable cues indicating the presence of two or more sound sources in the environment. The psychoacoustics and neural encoding of common temporal onsets/SOA and harmonicity/inharmonicity are considered in the following sections.

10.3.1 Grouping/segregation based on harmonicity/inharmonicity

Psychophysics of harmonicity/inharmonicity

When a single component of a harmonic complex tone is mistuned from its harmonic value by a sufficient amount (usually greater than 3%), it is heard as a separate tone, standing out from the complex as a whole (Moore *et al.*, 1985, 1986; Bregman, 1990; Hartmann *et al.*, 1990; Hartmann, 1996). This phenomenon exemplifies perceptual grouping/segregation based on harmonicity/ inharmonicity (Bregman, 1990; Yost, 1991; Hartmann, 1996). Detection of inharmonicity is facilitated by the perception of 'beats', particularly for higher, spectrally unresolved harmonics (Moore *et al.*, 1985; Hartmann *et al.*, 1990; Lee and Green, 1994). These beats correspond to amplitude modulations in the temporal envelope of the stimulus waveform arising from the mis-tuning. Threshold for detection of a mistuned partial decreases as mistuning increases from 3% to 16% and as the duration of the stimulus is extended beyond 50 ms (Moore *et al.*, 1985, 1986; Alain *et al.*, 2001, 2002). A difference in F0 between two simultaneous vowels or harmonic complex tones also greatly enhances perceptual segregation, discrimination, and individual identification (Chalikia and Bregman, 1989, 1993; Assmann and Summerfield, 1990; Culling and Darwin, 1993). Generally, identification accuracy improves as the difference in F0 between simultaneous vowels or harmonic complex tones increases up to about 1 semitone and then asymptotes for larger F0 differences.

Neurophysiology: human studies of harmonicity/inharmonicity

Enhancement of early and late ERP components evoked by complex tones occurs when a partial is mistuned from its harmonic relationship to the other components by an amount sufficient for it to stand out perceptually from the rest of the complex (reviewed in Alain, 2007). Further, sub-traction of ERPs evoked by harmonic complexes from ERPs elicited by inharmonic stimuli reveals a negative component referred to as the 'object related negativity' (ORN) that overlaps the obligatory N1 and P2 components (Alain *et al.*, 2001, 2002). The ORN can be elicited under passive listening conditions, thus supporting a pre-attentive mechanism underlying detection of inharmonicity (Bregman, 1990; Alain *et al.*, 2001, 2002). The ORN is augmented and a later ERP component (the P400) emerges under active listening conditions in which subjects are instructed to report whether they heard one or two sound objects (Alain *et al.*, 2001, 2002; Dyson and Alain, 2004; McDonald and Alain, 2005; Alain, 2007). An ORN-like component is evoked by concurrent vowels when their F0s differ by 4 semitones but not when their F0s are identical. This component parallels the perceptual segregation of the concurrent sounds and is elicited even when the subjects are instructed to ignore the auditory stimuli (Alain *et al.*, 2002). Enhancement of a later ERP component (the 'sustained potential') correlating with the perception of the mistuned harmonic as a separate sound is observed for long-duration mistuned harmonic complexes under active listening conditions, suggesting recruitment of longer-latency neural processes in the perceptual segregation of concurrent sounds (Alain *et al.*, 2002; Alain, 2007). Augmentation of the ORN is observed under active but not passive conditions when a slightly (i.e., 2%) mistuned partial is presented from a different location from the remaining harmonics, paralleling the increased likeli-hood of hearing the mistuned partial as a separate object (McDonald and Alain, 2005). These find-ings suggest that sound segregation is based on both pre-attentive and attentional mechanisms.

While the early ERP components modulated by inharmonicity have been attributed to sources within the superior temporal gyrus (Alain *et al.*, 2001, 2002; Dyson and Alain, 2004), the specific neural generators of the other ERP components and detailed neural mechanisms underlying concurrent sound segregation based on inharmonicity remain unclear. However, invasive studies in animal models are beginning to shed some light on these issues.

Neurophysiology: animal models of harmonicity/inharmonicity

Few studies in animals have investigated potential neural processes underlying the perceptual segregation of simultaneous sounds based on harmonic relations. One notable study examined responses in the IC of chinchillas to harmonic complex tones with F0s equal to 250 or 400 Hz (Sinex *et al.*, 2002). The complex tones were either 'in-tune' or had one of the lower partials mistuned by varying amounts (3–12%). Generally, the spectral components of the complex sounds all fell within the excitatory response area of the neurons studied. Harmonic complexes with a mistuned partial evoked synchronized periodic temporal discharges which were largely absent in responses to in-tune harmonic complexes (Sinex *et al.*, 2002; Fig. 10.7). The periodicity of these discharges roughly corresponded with the period of 'beats' corresponding to the difference in frequency between adjacent stimulus components. The temporal pattern of discharges was dramatically modulated by the degree of mistuning of the partial. Temporal discharge patterns evoked by mistuned harmonic complexes were also associated with an overall increase in firing rate, thus paralleling the perceptual 'pop-out' of the mistuned component in human listeners. The appearance of periodic temporal discharge patterns was largely independent of the relationship between the frequency of the mistuned component and the BF of the recorded neurons.

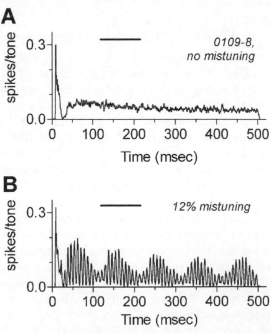

Fig. 10.7 A Response of an inferior colliculus neuron (characteristic frequency = 1.7 kHz) elicited by a harmonic complex tone consisting of eight partials (60 dB SPL per component) with a fundamental frequency of 250 Hz. **B** Response of the same neuron to the complex tone when the 4th harmonic is mistuned by 12%. (Reproduced with permission from Sinex *et al.* (2002), copyright 2002, *Hearing Research*, Elsevier.)

Finally, the authors demonstrated that the overall discharge rate of IC neurons was modulated by changes in the relative level of a single partial only if that partial was mistuned from its harmonic relationship to the other partials in the complex. This finding is consistent with the psychoacoustic observation that components in harmonic complex tones are not generally perceived individually (Plomp, 1976). In contrast to the IC, periodic temporal discharge patterns of auditory nerve fibers failed to differentiate harmonic from mistuned complexes and reflected instead the F0 of the harmonic complexes and the frequency of individual stimulus components, thus suggesting the importance of central auditory structures for inharmonicity detection (Sinex *et al.*, 2003).

Based on this work, a reasonable hypothesis is that neural responses evoked by harmonic complexes with a mistuned partial will be enhanced relative to responses evoked by in-tune harmonic complexes, thus correlating with the perceptual 'pop-out' of the mistuned partial. Moreover, given psychoacoustic findings that detection of inharmonicity in harmonic complexes containing high-numbered, spectrally unresolved mistuned harmonics is correlated with the perception of 'beats' arising from interactions between adjacent partials within the same auditory filter, an additional prediction is that complex tones with high-numbered mistuned harmonics will evoke periodic neuronal discharges phase-locked to beat frequencies corresponding to the difference in frequency between stimulus components.

Preliminary observations from our laboratory support both of these predictions (Fishman and Steinschneider, 2005). Neural responses in A1 of awake macaques evoked by complex tones with mistuned harmonics placed at or near the BF of the recorded neural populations are often increased relative to responses evoked by in-tune harmonic complex tones (Fig. 10.8a). Moreover, periodic temporal response patterns are observed when the unresolved 9th harmonic is mistuned relative to the other partials in the complex tone (Fig. 10.8b). Furthermore, AEPs recorded from superficial laminae of macaque A1 display a similar 'object-related negativity' observed in human ERPs evoked by harmonic complexes containing mistuned partials (data not shown). These parallels suggest that the neural responses recorded in animals may provide insights into neurophysiological mechanisms underlying auditory perceptual organization based on harmonic relations.

In order for response enhancement to represent a potential neural correlate of the enhanced perceptual salience of a mistuned component, it is reasonable to expect this enhancement to be maximal for neurons with a BF that corresponds to the frequency of the mistuned component. However, the response enhancements and changes in temporal discharge patterns evoked by mistuned complexes in the IC were observed even when the frequency of the mistuned component did not correspond to the BF of the recorded neurons (Sinex *et al.*, 2002). Thus, while the non-specific global response modulations reported by Sinex *et al.* (2002) may represent neural correlates of *inharmonicity detection*, they cannot presently account for *perceptual segregation* of sounds based on inharmonicity. Whether response enhancements observed in monkey A1 are global or spectrally local remains to be clarified in future studies.

The perceptual segregation of a mistuned partial from an otherwise harmonic complex represents a specific case of auditory stream formation based on inharmonicity. More typically, two or more periodic complex signals, such as voiced speech sounds, are present. Several theoretical models have been proposed to account for how the auditory system might segregate sounds based on F0 differences (for reviews see Darwin, 2005; de Cheveigné, 2005). One such model relies on local computations of periodicity using autocorrelation, which are then pooled across active frequency channels to yield a global estimate of the dominant F0 in the mixture. The F0 of additional sounds is then derived by analysis of the residual activity that remains once the frequency channels associated with the F0 of the dominant sound have been identified (Meddis and Hewitt, 1992).

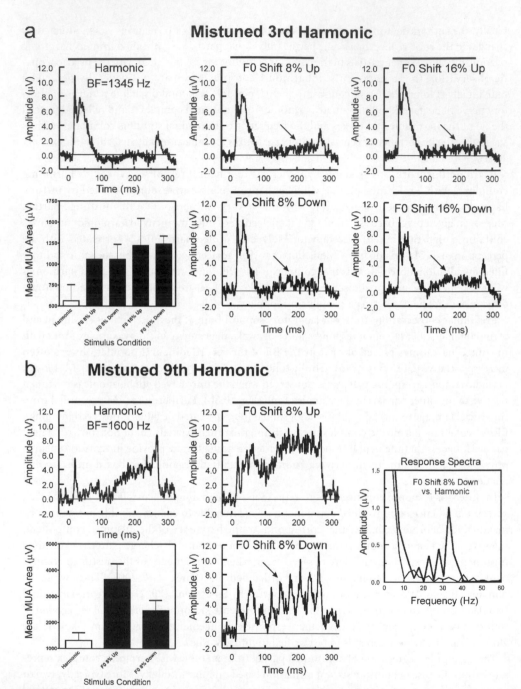

Fig. 10.8 Multiunit activity (MUA) evoked by in-tune and mistuned harmonic complex tones within thalamorecipient layers of primary auditory cortex (A1) in an awake macaque monkey. Harmonic complexes consisted of ten equal-amplitude harmonics and were presented at a total intensity of 70 dB SPL via a free-field speaker located contralateral to the recorded hemisphere. In **a** the 3rd harmonic was fixed at the best frequency (BF) of the neural population (1345 Hz) and mistuned from its harmonic relationship to the other partials by shifting the fundamental frequency (F0 = 448 Hz) and the other harmonics up or down by 8% or 16% of their value under the in-tune (harmonic) condition, as indicated.

Fig. 10.8 (*continued*) In **b** the 9th harmonic was fixed at the BF of the neural population (1600 Hz) and mistuned from its harmonic relationship to the other partials by shifting the F0 (178 Hz) and the other harmonics up or down by 8% of their value under the in-tune (harmonic) condition, as indicated. All MUA waveforms represent mean responses to 50 presentations of each stimulus and averaged over five separate blocks of stimulus presentation. Stimulus duration is 250 ms, represented by the *horizontal line* above the waveforms. Mean area under MUA waveforms from 0–250 ms under each stimulus condition is shown in the *bar graphs*. *Error bars* indicate +/– SEM. (N = 5). *Arrows* denote enhanced sustained MUA evoked under the mistuned conditions relative to that evoked under the harmonic condition. Oscillations are evident in the MUA evoked by the complex tones with a mistuned 9th harmonic (F0 shift 8% down condition) and are reflected by a peak in the response spectrum shown on the *right* in **b**. Spectra of responses under the mistuned and the harmonic conditions are represented by the *thick and thin lines*, respectively. The frequency of oscillatory activity (34 Hz) is close to the predicted stimulus beat frequency of approximately 38 Hz.

Other models include neural delay lines or recurrent timing networks consisting of delay loops that are tuned to either suppress or extract neural activity associated with particular periodicities in a sound mixture (de Cheveigné, 1998; Cariani, 2001). While these models have demonstrated some success in replicating psychoacoustic data, there is presently little empirical evidence supporting the processes required by these models (see de Cheveigné, 2005).

A recent study aimed to clarify potential neural mechanisms underlying the perceptual segregation of simultaneous complex sounds based on differences in their F0s (Sinex and Li, 2007). The investigators examined neural responses in the IC of chinchillas evoked by harmonic complex tones, presented alone and in the presence of a second harmonic complex with a different F0. Responses to single harmonic tones either exhibited no stimulus-related temporal pattern or displayed a periodic modulation at the F0. Responses to double harmonic tones exhibited complex temporal discharge patterns that varied with the difference in F0, the BF of the neurons, and with the relative levels of the two complex tones. These response modulations were attributed to beats arising from interactions between responses synchronized to adjacent components in the spectrum of the composite stimulus. Thus, IC neurons convey information about simultaneous sounds, at least in part, via temporal discharge patterns produced by interactions between adjacent components in the stimulus. Analogous temporal response patterns are evoked by dissonant musical chords in the auditory cortex of monkeys and humans (Fishman *et al.*, 2001b).

While these findings suggest a means by which the auditory system may detect the *presence* of two or more complex sounds based upon inharmonicity, it is unclear whether they can account for their *segregation* based upon differences in F0. A potential solution to this problem is suggested by a study reporting the existence of neurons in non-primary auditory cortex of marmoset monkeys that are specifically responsive to the missing F0 and thus the global pitch of complex tones (Bendor and Wang, 2005). Several MEG and fMRI studies (reviewed in Bendor and Wang, 2006) provide support for a homologous region of non-primary auditory cortex in humans specifically involved in processing pitch. As these promising findings in marmosets await further confirmation, an intriguing possibility is that such 'pitch cells' could provide a physiological basis for the segregation and improved identification of sounds based on differences in F0. Important questions remain concerning the neurophysiological means by which these neurons acquire their pitch-selective properties.

10.3.2 Grouping/segregation based on onset synchrony/asynchrony

Psychophysics of onset synchrony/asynchrony

The relative contributions of SOA, spectral separation, and spatial separation in the perceptual organization of sound components have been investigated using a rhythmic masking release

(RMR) paradigm (Turgeon *et al.*, 2002, 2005). When a regular sequence of sounds ('Rhythm') is presented in isolation, a simple rhythm is heard (Fig. 10.9). Perception of this simple rhythm is interrupted, however, when an additional sequence of identical sounds, designated as 'Maskers', is intermingled among those of the regular sequence. Perception of the rhythm of the original sequence can be restored, i.e., released from 'masking', by the addition of narrowband noise or tone 'Flankers' placed in frequency regions adjacent to those of the Maskers. RMR is maximal when Maskers and Flankers are synchronous, are spectrally adjacent, are harmonically related, and originate from the same spatial location (Turgeon *et al.*, 2002, 2005). By far the most powerful factor influencing RMR is the degree of synchrony between the onsets of Maskers and Flankers, thus highlighting the key role of common temporal onsets in the perceptual grouping of acoustic components of complex sound mixtures (Turgeon *et al.*, 2005). The RMR studies by Turgeon and colleagues suggest that the asynchrony needed for the perceptual segregation of brief acoustic events with abrupt onsets and offsets is about 20–40 ms (Turgeon *et al.*, 2002, 2005). This range of asynchrony thresholds is consistent with findings of other psychoacoustic studies of auditory grouping showing that an asynchrony of 20–40 ms is required for eliminating the contribution of a partial to the overall timbre, to the lateralization, and to the vowel quality of a complex sound (Turgeon *et al.*, 2002). The limited contribution of spatial separation to segregation of sound sources, at least when examined with the RMR paradigm, suggests that temporal coincidence is a more robust cue than a common location in space for sound-source determination. This is not altogether surprising given that spatial information about a sound source is often unreliable or

Fig. 10.9 Schematic representation of stimuli used to study rhythmic masking release (RMR). The 'Rhythm' consists of a regular sequence of tones or narrow band noise bursts (*white rectangles* in **A**). Perception of this simple rhythm is interrupted, however, when identical sounds, designated as 'Maskers', are interspersed among those of the Rhythm sequence (*black rectangles* in **B**). Perception of the rhythm of the original sequence can be restored, i.e., released from 'masking', by the addition of simultaneous tone or narrow band noise 'Flankers' placed in frequency regions adjacent to those of the Maskers (*gray rectangles* in **C**).

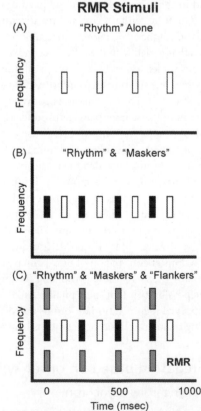

RMR Stimuli

(A) "Rhythm" Alone

(B) "Rhythm" & "Maskers"

(C) "Rhythm" & "Maskers" & "Flankers"

RMR

Time (msec)

ambiguous, owing to the combined effects of diffraction, echoes, and reverberation (Bregman, 1990; Turgeon *et al.*, 2005).

Neurophysiology: human studies of onset synchrony/asynchrony

To our knowledge, there have been no published studies in humans specifically examining neurophysiological correlates of auditory perceptual organization using an RMR paradigm. Several studies support a physiological encoding of rapid acoustic transients by robust onset responses within auditory cortex (e.g., Liégeois-Chauvel *et al.*, 1999; Steinschneider *et al.*, 1999, 2005). Synchronous responses to acoustic transients are therefore a robust feature of temporal information processing at the cortical level with potential relevance to auditory perceptual organization. MEG studies demonstrate single evoked responses to double-click stimuli when the interval between clicks is less than 20 ms and two responses when the inter-click interval exceeds this threshold (Joliot *et al.*, 1994). The appearance of a second response coincides with subjects' perception of a second distinct auditory stimulus (Joliot *et al.*, 1994). Similarly, AEPs recorded directly from auditory cortex display categorical-like 'double-on' temporal response patterns when the voice onset time (VOT) of stop-consonant syllables exceeds about 20 ms (Steinschneider *et al.*, 1999, 2005). The presence of one versus two onset responses in auditory cortex has been proposed as a physiological determinant of the categorical perception of stop-consonant VOTs and of determining the order of two sequential acoustic events (e.g., Steinschneider *et al.*, 1999, 2005). Thus, the generation of two discrete onset responses in human auditory cortex typically requires an SOA on the order of 20–40 ms between two acoustic elements, in agreement with the perceptual thresholds for the segregation of sounds based on onset asynchrony.

Neurophysiology: animal models of onset synchrony/asynchrony

Neurophysiological studies in animals demonstrate that temporal discontinuities in sounds are encoded by prominent onset responses synchronized across tonotopically distributed neural populations in auditory cortex (e.g., Creutzfeldt *et al.*, 1980; Wang *et al.*, 1995; Gehr *et al.*, 2000; Eggermont, 2001; Nagarajan *et al.*, 2002). Synchronized onset responses might provide a physiological means of representing the beginning of new auditory objects (Eggermont, 2001; Steinschneider *et al.*, 2003, 2005) and for grouping together acoustic elements that originate from the same sound source. Accordingly, synchronized onset responses across A1 may contribute to the perceptual grouping of Maskers and Flankers and to their resulting segregation from the Rhythm sequence in RMR. Both enhancement and suppression of stimulus-evoked onset responses in A1 occur when sounds are presented concurrently (e.g., Shamma and Symmes, 1985; Phillips and Hall, 1992; Fitzpatrick *et al.*, 1993; Nelken *et al.*, 1994; Kadia and Wang, 2003; Fishman and Steinschneider, 2006). Thus, enhancement or suppression of responses to Maskers by the presence of the synchronous Flankers may distinguish Masker responses from those evoked by the Rhythm sequence, and thereby provide a potential neural basis for their perceptual segregation.

Preliminary recordings in macaque A1 from our laboratory using an RMR stimulus paradigm provide support for this idea. Rhythm and Masker stimuli were comprised of 50-ms tones with a frequency corresponding to the BF of the recorded neural populations. Two Flanker tones were presented simultaneously with Masker tones and were separated in frequency from Maskers by varying amounts. In the presence of Flankers, responses to Masker tones were diminished relative to those evoked by Rhythm tones, thus enhancing the saliency of the Rhythm responses (Fig. 10.10). The difference between Rhythm and Masker responses induced by the introduction of the Flankers provides a possible basis for distinguishing Rhythm and Masker responses, and thus represents a potential neural correlate of RMR. Although based upon well-documented

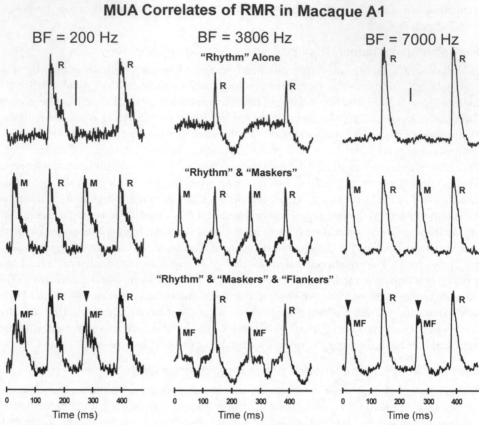

Fig. 10.10 Neural correlates of rhythmic masking release (RMR) reflected by multiunit activity recorded within thalamorecipient laminae of primary auditory cortex (A1) in an awake macaque monkey. Responses to continuous stimuli consisting of Rhythm (*top row*), Rhythm & Masker (*middle row*), and Rhythm & Masker & Flanker (*bottom row*) tones are shown at three sites with different best frequencies (BFs) (see Fig. 10.9 for a schematic description of the RMR stimuli). The frequency of Rhythm and Masker tones corresponded to the BF of the neural populations. The frequencies of Flanker tones were 100 and 300 Hz at the site with a BF of 200 Hz, 2691 and 5382 Hz at the site with a BF of 3806 Hz, and 3500 and 14,000 Hz at the site with a BF of 7000 Hz. All tones were 50 ms in duration and presented at 60-dB SPL via a free-field speaker located contralateral to the recorded hemisphere. Responses to Rhythm tones, Masker tones, and Masker tones presented with concurrent Flanker tones are labeled 'R', 'M', and 'MF', respectively. *Downward black arrowheads* indicate diminished responses to the Masker tones in the presence of the concurrent Flanker tones. (*Vertical scale bars* = 5 μV).

physiological phenomena, the model of RMR described here is still speculative and requires further investigation. Considering that RMR represents a paradigmatic case of auditory perceptual grouping by temporal coincidence of acoustic elements, elucidation of neural substrates underlying RMR is likely to provide a general framework applicable to understanding the physiological underpinnings of other auditory perceptual grouping phenomena based on common temporal onsets.

10.4 'Schema-based' auditory scene analysis

Many of the phenomena considered in this chapter appear to be based in part on pre-attentive processes of auditory perceptual organization that do not require prior learning or focused attention to the sounds. However, much of our auditory experience is influenced by top-down processes of learning and attention. According to Bregman (1990), such top-down or 'schema-based' processes are not directly involved in the grouping and segregation of acoustic elements that underlie the formation of auditory perceptual streams; rather, they govern the selection of information that has already been partitioned by lower-level primitive mechanisms of auditory scene analysis.

10.4.1 Learning, cortical plasticity, and auditory scene analysis

Studies in animals and humans have demonstrated rapid and long-lasting stimulus-specific changes in neural response magnitude, tuning selectivity, and extent of activation in auditory cortex associated with learning (e.g., Recanzone *et al.*, 1993; Cansino and Williamson, 1997; Menning *et al.*, 2000; Weinberger, 2004; Polley *et al.*, 2006). For instance, extensive musical training is associated with enhanced neuronal responses to acoustic stimuli (e.g., Schneider *et al.*, 2002; Pantev *et al.*, 2003; Shahin *et al.*, 2003; Kuriki *et al.*, 2006) and with alterations in how the brain parses auditory input, as indexed by the MMN (e.g., Koelsch *et al.*, 1999; Russeler *et al.*, 2001; Lopez *et al.*, 2003; van Zuijen *et al.*, 2004). How these experience- and learning-induced changes might modulate neural processes underlying auditory scene analysis is just beginning to be explored (e.g., Reinke *et al*, 2003; Alain, 2007; Alain *et al.*, 2007).

10.4.2 Attention and auditory scene analysis

Many studies have reported attention-induced enhancements in the amplitude and selectivity of auditory ERP components attributed to sources in human auditory cortex (for reviews see Hillyard and Picton, 1987; Näätänen, 1990). In general, effects of attention include modulation of obligatory AEP components and the introduction of new, longer latency processing-contingent waves such as Nd and N2 (e.g., see Näätänen, 1990). These findings suggest the involvement of top-down processes in the *selection* of auditory streams rather than in the initial formation of the auditory streams themselves, the latter being accomplished by lower-level mechanisms of perceptual organization (Bregman, 1990; Alain and Arnott, 2000). Support for this interpretation is provided by studies showing enhancement of ERPs indexing perceptual segregation of acoustic elements when subjects are instructed to report whether they heard one or two auditory objects (Alain *et al.*, 2001, 2002) or to attend to particular frequency channels (Alain and Woods, 1994). For instance, Alain and Woods (1994) showed that ERPs were larger when subjects attended to a sequence of tones occupying a different frequency region from that occupied by two other 'distracter' tone sequences. ERPs elicited by tones of the attended sequence were further enhanced when the two distracter sequences were clustered together in frequency. These attention effects correlated with improved behavioral performance on a task involving discrimination of longer tones embedded within the attended sequence. However, attention effects were diminished when the frequency separation between the attended and the distracter tone sequences was reduced so as to minimize their perceptual segregation. Thus, the results suggested that signal clustering promoted the formation of separate auditory perceptual streams and facilitated stream-specific modulation by attention, which accentuated the contrast between physiological representations of attended and unattended auditory perceptual streams (Alain and Woods, 1994). While the detailed neural mechanisms underlying modulation of auditory cortical responses by attention are still not well understood, these ERP studies suggest how stream-specific enhancement of neural responses by attention may contribute to schema-based processes of auditory scene analysis.

Role of attention in the buildup of stream segregation

While it is clear that attention modulates cortical processing relevant to auditory stream segregation, it is not clear whether it is *required* for the initial formation and buildup of auditory streams. Carlyon *et al.* (2001) examined the role of attention in the buildup of stream segregation by assessing whether listeners judged a previously unattended sequence of sounds as containing one or two streams. In one ear, the subjects were presented with a 21-s sequence containing high- and low-frequency pure tones in a triplet pattern ('ABA_'). In the other ear, noise bursts were presented once every second, and the participants were instructed to identify each noise burst as either continuously increasing or continuously decreasing in intensity. Ten seconds into the 21-s train, the subjects were cued to switch their attention to the tone sequence. At the switch, they reported whether they heard the tones as one stream or as two separate streams. The authors found that after attention switching, subjects tended to initially perceive the tone sequence as a single stream and, only later, as two streams. Thus, the authors concluded that focused attention is required for the formation of auditory streams (however, for an alternative interpretation see Macken *et al.*, 2003).

On the other hand, physiological evidence based on MMN suggests that focused attention is not required for the buildup of stream segregation (Sussman *et al.*, 2007). ERPs evoked by short trains of tones were recorded while subjects' attention was diverted to the simultaneous performance of a difficult noise intensity change detection task. Trains of tones of varying intensity of 3.55 s in duration were separated by 4.05 s of silence. This silent interval acted to reset the stream segregation process every time the stimulus train was presented. Segregation was promoted by increasing the frequency separation between subsets of the tones comprising the sequences in which were embedded probe tones of different intensity. The stimuli were designed so that when the tones comprising the train are part of the same frequency stream, the intensity variation of the tones prevents the perception of a regular pattern of iso-intensity tones. Since perceptual regularity is absent, and such regularity is a prerequisite for eliciting an MMN, the probe tones do not elicit an MMN. In contrast, when the tones are segregated into separate streams, a regularity of intensity emerges in one of the streams, such that the probe tones, which differ in intensity from the standard tones, violate the intensity regularity and elicit the MMN. An MMN was elicited by probe tones only when the tones were perceptually segregated into two separate streams. Moreover, the MMN was elicited by probe tones occurring only at the end of the train of tones but not near the beginning, thus indicating that pre-attentive ERP indices of auditory perceptual organization paralleled the buildup of stream segregation over time and suggesting that the silent interval in between the tone sequences was sufficient to reset the stream segregation process (Sussman *et al.*, 2007). Given the diversion of attention away from the tone sequences, the findings strongly suggest that focused attention is not required to initiate the formation of auditory streams.

10.5 **Conclusions**

The general picture emerging from the literature examining putative neural mechanisms underlying sequential and simultaneous auditory perceptual organization is consistent with the object-based account of Bregman (1990) and Alain and Arnott (2000), according to which attention is allocated to auditory objects after an initial pre-attentive or 'primitive' neural process has partitioned the acoustic input into distinct streams. However, it is likely that this view is oversimplified and that the formation and maintenance of auditory streams depend upon a dynamic interplay between attentive/top-down and pre-attentive/bottom-up processes (Denham and Winkler, 2006). Many important questions remain to fuel future investigations of neural substrates of auditory scene analysis, the significance of which is highlighted by findings suggesting impairments in auditory scene analysis with aging (Snyder and Alain, 2005, 2007; Alain and McDonald, 2007) and in some individuals with developmental language disorders (Helenius *et al.*, 1999; Sutter *et al.*, 2000; Petkov *et al.*, 2005). Indeed, a greater understanding of neural mechanisms involved in processes of auditory perceptual organization might suggest additional therapies or other forms of intervention to ameliorate deficits contributing to developmental language disorders.

References

Alain C (2007) Breaking the wave: effects of attention and learning on concurrent sound perception. *Hear Res* 229: 225–36.

Alain C, Arnott SR (2000) Selectively attending to auditory objects. *Front Biosci* 5: 202–12.

Alain C, McDonald KL (2007) Age-related differences in neuromagnetic brain activity underlying concurrent sound perception. *J Neurosci* 27: 1308–14.

Alain C, Woods DL (1994) Signal clustering modulates auditory cortical activity in humans. *Percept Psychophys* 56: 501–16.

Alain C, Arnott SR, Picton TW (2001) Bottom-up and top-down influences on auditory scene analysis: evidence from event-related brain potentials. *J Exp Psychol Hum Percept Perform* 27: 1072–89.

Alain C, Schuler BM, McDonald KL (2002) Neural activity associated with distinguishing concurrent auditory objects. *J Acoust Soc Am* 111: 990–5.

Alain C, Snyder JS, He Y, Reinke KS (2007) Changes in auditory cortex parallel rapid perceptual learning. *Cereb Cortex* 17: 1074–84.

Anstis S, Saida S (1985) Adaptation to auditory streaming of frequency-modulated tones. *J Exp Psychol Hum Percept Perform* 11: 257–71.

Arnott SR, Alain C (2002) Stepping out of the spotlight: MMN attenuation as a function of distance from the attended location. *Neuroreport* 13: 2209–12.

Assmann PF, Summerfield Q (1990) Modeling the perception of concurrent vowels: vowels with different fundamental frequencies. *J Acoust Soc Am* 88: 680–97.

Bartlett EL, Wang X (2005) Long-lasting modulation by stimulus context in primate auditory cortex. *J Neurophysiol* 94: 83–104.

Beauvois MW, Meddis R (1996) Computer simulation of auditory stream segregation in alternating-tone sequences. *J Acoust Soc Am* 99: 2270–80.

Bee MA, Klump GM (2004) Primitive auditory stream segregation: a neurophysiological study in the songbird forebrain. *J Neurophysiol* 92: 1088–104.

Bee MA, Klump GM (2005) Auditory stream segregation in the songbird forebrain: effects of time intervals on responses to interleaved tone sequences. *Brain Behav Evol* 66: 197–214.

Bendor D, Wang X (2005) The neuronal representation of pitch in primate auditory cortex. *Nature* 436: 1161–5.

Bendor D, Wang X (2006) Cortical representations of pitch in monkeys and humans. *Curr Opin Neurobiol* 16: 391–9.

Braaten RF, Leary JC (1999) Temporal induction of missing birdsong segments in European starlings. *Psychol Sci* 10: 162–6.

Bregman AS (1978) Auditory streaming is cumulative. *J Exp Psychol Hum Percept Perform* 4: 380–7.

Bregman AS (1990) *Auditory Scene Analysis: The Perceptual Organization of Sound*. MIT Press, Cambridge, Massachusetts.

Bregman AS, Dannenbring GL (1977) Auditory continuity and amplitude edges. *Can J Psychol* 31: 151–9.

Bregman AS, Colantonio C, Ahad PA (1999) Is a common grouping mechanism involved in the phenomena of illusory continuity and stream segregation?. *Percept Psychophys* 61: 195–205.

Bregman AS, Ahad PA, Crum PA, O'Reilly J (2000) Effects of time intervals and tone durations on auditory stream segregation. *Percept Psychophys* 62: 626–36.

Brosch M, Schreiner CE (1997) Time course of forward masking tuning curves in cat primary auditory cortex. *J Neurophysiol* 77: 923–43.

Calford MB, Semple MN (1995) Monaural inhibition in cat auditory cortex. *J Neurophysiol* 73: 1876–91.

Cansino S, Williamson SJ (1997) Neuromagnetic fields reveal cortical plasticity when learning an auditory discrimination task. *Brain Res* 764: 53–66.

Cariani PA (2001) Neural timing nets. *Neural Netw* 14: 737–53.

Carlyon RP, Cusack R, Foxton JM, Robertson IH (2001) Effects of attention and unilateral neglect on auditory stream segregation. *J Exp Psychol Hum Percept Perform* 27: 115–27.

Chalikia MH, Bregman AS (1989) The perceptual segregation of simultaneous auditory signals: pulse train segregation and vowel segregation. *Percept Psychophys* 46: 487–96.

Chalikia MH, Bregman AS (1993) The perceptual segregation of simultaneous vowels with harmonic, shifted, or random components. *Percept Psychophys* 53: 125–33.

Chung S, Li X, Nelson SB (2002) Short-term depression at thalamocortical synapses contributes to rapid adaptation of cortical sensory responses in vivo. *Neuron* 34: 437–46.

Ciocca V, Bregman AS (1987) Perceived continuity of gliding and steady-state tones through interrupting noise. *Percept Psychophys* 42: 476–84.

Cowey A, Weiskrantz L (1976) Auditory sequence discrimination in macaca mulatta: the role of the superior temporal cortex. *Neuropsychologia* 14: 1–10.

Cox CL, Metherate R, Weinberger NM, Ashe JH (1992) Synaptic potentials and effects of amino acid antagonists in the auditory cortex. *Brain Res Bull* 28: 401–10.

Creutzfeldt O, Hellweg FC, Schreiner C (1980) Thalamocortical transformation of responses to complex auditory stimuli. *Exp Brain Res* 39: 87–104.

Culling JF, Darwin CJ (1993) Perceptual separation of simultaneous vowels: within and across-formant grouping by F0. *J Acoust Soc Am* 93: 3454–67.

Cusack R (2005) The intraparietal sulcus and perceptual organization. *J Cogn Neurosci* 17: 641–51.

Cusack R, Deeks J, Aikman G, Carlyon RP (2004) Effects of location, frequency region, and time course of selective attention on auditory scene analysis. *J Exp Psychol Hum Percept Perform* 30: 643–56.

Darwin CJ (2005) Pitch and auditory grouping. In: *Pitch: Neural Coding and Perception* (eds Plack CJ, Oxenham AJ, Fay RR, Popper AN). Springer, New York.

de Cheveigné A (1998) Cancellation model of pitch perception. *J Acoust Soc Am* 103: 1261–71.

de Cheveigné A (2005) Pitch perception models. In: *Pitch: Neural Coding and Perception* (eds Plack CJ, Oxenham AJ, Fay RR, Popper AN). Springer, New York.

De Ribaupierre F, Goldstein MH Jr, Yeni-Komshian G (1972) Intracellular study of the cat's primary auditory cortex. *Brain Res* 48: 185–204.

Demany L (1982) Auditory stream segregation in infancy. *Infant Behav Dev* 5: 261–76.

Denham SL, Winkler I (2006) The role of predictive models in the formation of auditory streams. *J Physiol Paris* 100: 154–70.

Dewson JH 3rd, Cowey A, Weiskrantz L (1970) Disruptions of auditory sequence discrimination by unilateral and bilateral cortical ablations of superior temporal gyrus in the monkey. *Exp Neurol* 28: 529–48.

Doeller BF, Opitz B, Mecklinger A, Krick C, Reith W, Schroger E (2003) Prefrontal cortex involvement in preattentive auditory deviance detection: neuroimaging and electrophysiological evidence. *Neuroimage* 20: 1270–82.

Dyson BJ, Alain C (2004) Representation of concurrent acoustic objects in primary auditory cortex. *J Acoust Soc Am* **115**: 280–8.

Eggermont JJ (2001) Between sound and perception: reviewing the search for a neural code. *Hear Res* **157**: 1–42.

Fay RR (1998) Auditory stream segregation in goldfish (*Carassius auratus*). *Hear Res* **120**: 69–76.

Fishman YI, Steinschneider M (2005) *Initial observations reflecting representation of inharmonicity in auditory cortex of the awake monkey*. Society for Neuroscience Conference; Advances and Perspectives in Auditory Neurophysiology (APAN II), November, Washington Convention Centre.

Fishman YI, Steinschneider M (2006) Spectral resolution of monkey primary auditory cortex (A1) revealed with two-noise masking. *J Neurophysiol* **96**: 1105–15.

Fishman YI, Reser DH, Arezzo JC, Steinschneider M (2001a) Neural correlates of auditory stream segregation in primary auditory cortex of the awake monkey. *Hear Res* **151**: 167–87.

Fishman YI, Volkov IO, Noh MD, *et al.* (2001b) Consonance and dissonance of musical chords: neural correlates in auditory cortex of monkeys and humans. *J Neurophysiol* **86**: 2761–88.

Fishman YI, Arezzo JC, Steinschneider M (2004) Auditory stream segregation in monkey auditory cortex: effects of frequency separation, presentation rate, and tone duration. *J Acoust Soc Am* **116**: 1656–70.

Fitzpatrick DC, Kanwal JS, Butman JA, Suga N (1993) Combination-sensitive neurons in the primary auditory cortex of the mustached bat. *J Neurosci* **13**: 931–40.

Frisina RD (2001) Subcortical neural coding mechanisms for auditory temporal processing. *Hear Res* **158**: 1–27.

Gehr DD, Komiya H, Eggermont JJ (2000) Neuronal responses in cat primary auditory cortex to natural and altered species-specific calls. *Hear Res* **150**: 27–42.

Gutschalk A, Micheyl C, Melcher JR, Rupp A, Scherg M, Oxenham AJ (2005) Neuromagnetic correlates of streaming in human auditory cortex. *J Neurosci* **25**: 5382–8.

Gutschalk A, Oxenham AJ, Micheyl C, Wilson EC, Melcher JR (2007) Human cortical activity during streaming without spectral cues suggests a general neural substrate for auditory stream segregation. *J Neurosci* **27**: 13074–81.

Hartmann WM (1996) Pitch, periodicity, and auditory organization. *J Acoust Soc Am* **100**: 3491–502.

Hartmann WM, McAdams S, Smith BK (1990) Hearing a mistuned harmonic in an otherwise periodic complex tone. *J Acoust Soc Am* **88**: 1712–24.

Helenius P, Uutela K, Hari R (1999) Auditory stream segregation in dyslexic adults. *Brain* **122**: 907–13.

Hillyard SA, Picton TW (1987) Electrophysiology of cognition. In: *Handbook of Physiology, Section I: The Nervous System* (eds Mountcastle VB, Blum F, Geiger SR), pp. 519–38. American Physiological Society, Bethesda.

Hillyard SA, Hink RF, Schwent VL, Picton TW (1973) Electrical signs of selective attention in the human brain. *Science* **182**: 177–80.

Hillyard SA, Teder-Salejarvi WA, Munte TF (1998) Temporal dynamics of early perceptual processing. *Curr Opin Neurobiol* **8**: 202–10.

Izumi A (2002) Auditory stream segregation in japanese monkeys. *Cognition* **82**: B113–22.

Javitt DC, Steinschneider M, Schroeder CE, Vaughan HG Jr, Arezzo JC (1994) Detection of stimulus deviance within primate primary auditory cortex: intracortical mechanisms of mismatch negativity (MMN) generation. *Brain Res* **667**: 192–200.

Jemel B, Achenbach C, Muller BW, Ropcke B, Oades RD (2002) Mismatch negativity results from bilateral asymmetric dipole sources in the frontal and temporal lobes. *Brain Topogr* **15**: 13–27.

Joliot M, Ribary U, Llinas R (1994) Human oscillatory brain activity near 40 Hz coexists with cognitive temporal binding. *Proc Natl Acad Sci USA* **91**: 11748–51.

Kadia SC, Wang X (2003) Spectral integration in A1 of awake primates: neurons with single- and multipeaked tuning characteristics. *J Neurophysiol* **89**: 1603–22.

Kanwal JS, Medvedev AV, Micheyl C (2003) Neurodynamics for auditory stream segregation: tracking sounds in the mustached bat's natural environment. *Network* 14: 413–35.

Koelsch S, Schroger E, Tervaniemi M (1999) Superior pre-attentive auditory processing in musicians. *Neuroreport* 10: 1309–13.

Kuriki S, Kanda S, Hirata Y (2006) Effects of musical experience on different components of MEG responses elicited by sequential piano-tones and chords. *J Neurosci* 26: 4046–53.

Lee J, Green DM (1994) Detection of a mistuned component in a harmonic complex. *J Acoust Soc Am* 96: 716–25.

Liégeois-Chauvel C, Peretz I, Babai M, Laguitton V, Chauvel P (1998) Contribution of different cortical areas in the temporal lobes to music processing. *Brain* 121: 1853–67.

Liégeois-Chauvel C, de Graaf JB, Laguitton V, Chauvel P (1999) Specialization of left auditory cortex for speech perception in man depends on temporal coding. *Cereb Cortex* 9: 484–96.

Lopez L, Jurgens R, Diekmann V, *et al.* (2003) Musicians versus nonmusicians. a neurophysiological approach. *Ann N Y Acad Sci* 999: 124–30.

Lütkenhöner B (2003) Magnetoencephalography and its Achilles' heel. *J Physiol Paris* 97: 641–58.

MacDougall-Shackleton SA, Hulse SH, Gentner TQ, White W (1998) Auditory scene analysis by European starlings (*Sturnus vulgaris*): perceptual segregation of tone sequences. *J Acoust Soc Am* 103: 3581–7.

Macken WJ, Tremblay S, Houghton RJ, Nicholls AP, Jones DM (2003) Does auditory streaming require attention? Evidence from attentional selectivity in short-term memory. *J Exp Psychol Hum Percept Perform* 29: 43–51.

McAdams S, Bertoncini J (1997) Organization and discrimination of repeating sound sequences by newborn infants. *J Acoust Soc Am* 102: 2945–53.

McAdams S, Bregman AS (1979) Hearing musical streams. *Comp Music J* 3: 23–43.

McCabe SL, Denham MJ (1997) A model of auditory streaming. *J Acoust Soc Am* 101: 1611–21.

McDonald KL, Alain C (2005) Contribution of harmonicity and location to auditory object formation in free field: evidence from event-related brain potentials. *J Acoust Soc Am* 118: 1593–604.

Meddis R, Hewitt MJ (1992) Modeling the identification of concurrent vowels with different fundamental frequencies. *J Acoust Soc Am* 91: 233–45.

Menning H, Roberts LE, Pantev C (2000) Plastic changes in the auditory cortex induced by intensive frequency discrimination training. *Neuroreport* 11: 817–22.

Micheyl C, Carlyon RP, Shtyrov Y, Hauk O, Dodson T, Pullvermuller F (2003) The neurophysiological basis of the auditory continuity illusion: a mismatch negativity study. *J Cogn Neurosci* 15: 747–58.

Micheyl C, Tian B, Carlyon RP, Rauschecker JP (2005) Perceptual organization of tone sequences in the auditory cortex of awake macaques. *Neuron* 48: 139–48.

Micheyl C, Carlyon RP, Gutschalk A, *et al.* (2007) The role of auditory cortex in the formation of auditory streams. *Hear Res* 229: 116–31.

Miller CT, Dibble E, Hauser MD (2001) Amodal completion of acoustic signals by a nonhuman primate. *Nat Neurosci* 4: 783–4.

Moore BCJ, Gockel H (2002) Factors influencing sequential stream segregation. *Acta Acust Acust* 88: 320–32.

Moore BC, Peters RW, Glasberg BR (1985) Thresholds for the detection of inharmonicity in complex tones. *J Acoust Soc Am* 77: 1861–7.

Moore BC, Glasberg BR, Peters RW (1986) Thresholds for hearing mistuned partials as separate tones in harmonic complexes. *J Acoust Soc Am* 80: 479–83.

Näätänen R (1990) The role of attention in auditory information processing as revealed by event-related potentials and other brain measures of cognitive function. *Behav Brain Sci* 13: 201–88.

Näätänen R, Winkler I (1999) The concept of auditory stimulus representation in cognitive neuroscience. *Psychol Bull* 125: 826–59.

Näätänen R, Paavilainen P, Tiitinen H, Jiang D, Alho K (1993) Attention and mismatch negativity. *Psychophysiology* **30**: 436–50.

Nagarajan SS, Cheung SW, Bedenbaugh P, Beitel RE, Schreiner CE, Merzenich MM (2002) Representation of spectral and temporal envelope of twitter vocalizations in common marmoset primary auditory cortex. *J Neurophysiol* **87**: 1723–37.

Nelken I, Prut Y, Vaadia E, Abeles M (1994) Population responses to multifrequency sounds in the cat auditory cortex: one- and two-parameter families of sounds. *Hear Res* **72**: 206–22.

Oades RD, Dittmann-Balcar A (1995) Mismatch negativity (MMN) is altered by directing attention. *Neuroreport* **6**: 1187–90.

Pantev C, Ross B, Fujioka T, Trainor LJ, Schulte M, Schulz M (2003) Music and learning-induced cortical plasticity. *Ann N Y Acad Sci* **999**: 438–50.

Petkov CI, O'Connor KN, Sutter ML (2003) Illusory sound perception in macaque monkeys. *J Neurosci* **23**: 9155–61.

Petkov CI, O'Connor KN, Benmoshe G, Baynes K, Sutter ML (2005) Auditory perceptual grouping and attention in dyslexia. *Brain Res Cogn Brain Res* **24**: 343–54.

Petkov CI, O'Connor KN, Sutter ML (2007) Encoding of illusory continuity in primary auditory cortex. *Neuron* **54**: 153–65.

Phillips DP (1995) Central auditory processing: a view from auditory neuroscience. *Am J Otol* **16**: 338–52.

Phillips DP, Hall SE (1992) Multiplicity of inputs in the afferent path to cat auditory cortex neurons revealed by tone-on-tone masking. *Cereb Cortex* **2**: 425–33.

Picton TW, Alain C, Otten L, Ritter W, Achim A (2000) Mismatch negativity: different water in the same river. *Audiol Neurootol* **5**: 111–39.

Plomp R. (1976) *Aspects of Tone Sensation*. Academic Press, London.

Polley DB, Steinberg EE, Merzenich MM (2006) Perceptual learning directs auditory cortical map reorganization through top-down influences. *J Neurosci* **26**: 4970–82.

Recanzone GH, Schreiner CE, Merzenich MM (1993) Plasticity in the frequency representation of primary auditory cortex following discrimination training in adult owl monkeys. *J Neurosci* **13**: 87–103.

Reinke KS, He Y, Wang C, Alain C (2003) Perceptual learning modulates sensory evoked response during vowel segregation. *Brain Res Cogn Brain Res* **17**: 781–91.

Russeler J, Altenmuller E, Nager W, Kohlmetz C, Munte TF (2001) Event-related brain potentials to sound omissions differ in musicians and non-musicians. *Neurosci Lett* **308**: 33–6.

Schneider P, Scherg M, Dosch HG, Specht HJ, Gutschalk A, Rupp A (2002) Morphology of Heschl's gyrus reflects enhanced activation in the auditory cortex of musicians. *Nat Neurosci* **5**: 688–94.

Shahin A, Bosnyak DJ, Trainor LJ, Roberts LE (2003) Enhancement of neuroplastic P2 and N1c auditory evoked potentials in musicians. *J Neurosci* **23**: 5545–52.

Shamma SA, Symmes D (1985) Patterns of inhibition in auditory cortical cells in awake squirrel monkeys. *Hear Res* **19**: 1–13.

Sinex DG, Li H (2007) Responses of inferior colliculus neurons to double harmonic tones. *J Neurophysiol* **98**: 3171–84.

Sinex DG, Sabes JH, Li H (2002) Responses of inferior colliculus neurons to harmonic and mistuned complex tones. *Hear Res* **168**: 150–62.

Sinex DG, Guzik H, Li H, Henderson Sabes J (2003) Responses of auditory nerve fibers to harmonic and mistuned complex tones. *Hear Res* **182**: 130–9.

Snyder JS, Alain C (2005) Age-related changes in neural activity associated with concurrent vowel segregation. *Brain Res Cogn Brain Res* **24**: 492–9.

Snyder JS, Alain C (2007) Toward a neurophysiological theory of auditory stream segregation. *Psychol Bull* **133**: 780–99.

Snyder JS, Alain C, Picton TW (2006) Effects of attention on neuroelectric correlates of auditory stream segregation. *J Cogn Neurosci* **18**: 1–13.

Steinschneider M, Schroeder CE, Arezzo JC, Vaughan HG Jr (1994) Speech-evoked activity in primary auditory cortex: effects of voice onset time. *Electroencephalogr Clin Neurophysiol* **92**: 30–43.

Steinschneider M, Volkov IO, Noh MD, Garell PC, Howard MA 3rd (1999) Temporal encoding of the voice onset time phonetic parameter by field potentials recorded directly from human auditory cortex. *J Neurophysiol* **82**: 2346–57.

Steinschneider M, Fishman YI, Arezzo JC (2003) Representation of the voice onset time (VOT) speech parameter in population responses within primary auditory cortex of the awake monkey. *J Acoust Soc Am* **114**: 307–21.

Steinschneider M, Volkov IO, Fishman YI, Oya H, Arezzo JC, Howard MA 3rd (2005) Intracortical responses in human and monkey primary auditory cortex support a temporal processing mechanism for encoding of the voice onset time phonetic parameter. *Cereb Cortex* **15**: 170–86.

Sugita Y (1997) Neuronal correlates of auditory induction in the cat cortex. *Neuroreport* **8**: 1155–9.

Sussman E, Ritter W, Vaughan HG Jr (1999) An investigation of the auditory streaming effect using event-related brain potentials. *Psychophysiology* **36**: 22–34.

Sussman ES, Horvath J, Winkler I, Orr M (2007) The role of attention in the formation of auditory streams. *Percept Psychophys* **69**: 136–52.

Sutter ML, Petkov C, Baynes K, O'Connor KN (2000) Auditory scene analysis in dyslexics. *Neuroreport* **11**: 1967–71.

Turgeon M, Bregman AS, Ahad PA (2002) Rhythmic masking release: contribution of cues for perceptual organization to the cross-spectral fusion of concurrent narrow-band noises. *J Acoust Soc Am* **111**: 1819–31.

Turgeon M, Bregman AS, Roberts B (2005) Rhythmic masking release: effects of asynchrony, temporal overlap, harmonic relations, and source separation on cross-spectral grouping. *J Exp Psychol Hum Percept Perform* **31**: 939–53.

Ulanovsky N, Las L, Farkas D, Nelken I (2004) Multiple time scales of adaptation in auditory cortex neurons. *J Neurosci* **24**: 10440–53.

van Zuijen TL, Sussman E, Winkler I, Näätänen R, Tervaniemi M (2004) Grouping of sequential sounds – an event-related potential study comparing musicians and nonmusicians. *J Cogn Neurosci* **16**: 331–8.

Vliegen J, Oxenham AJ (1999) Sequential stream segregation in the absence of spectral cues. *J Acoust Soc Am* **105**: 339–46.

Volkov IO, Galazyuk AV (1992) Peculiarities of inhibition in cat auditory cortex neurons evoked by tonal stimuli of various durations. *Exp Brain Res* **91**: 115–20.

Wang X, Merzenich MM, Beitel R, Schreiner CE (1995) Representation of a species-specific vocalization in the primary auditory cortex of the common marmoset: temporal and spectral characteristics. *J Neurophysiol* **74**: 2685–706.

Warren RM, Obusek CJ, Ackroff JM (1972) Auditory induction: perceptual synthesis of absent sounds. *Science* **176**: 1149–51.

Wehr M, Zador AM (2005) Synaptic mechanisms of forward suppression in rat auditory cortex. *Neuron* **47**: 437–45.

Weinberger NM (2004) Specific long-term memory traces in primary auditory cortex. *Nat Rev Neurosci* **5**: 279–90.

Wilson EC, Melcher JR, Micheyl C, Gutschalk A, Oxenham AJ (2007) Cortical FMRI activation to sequences of tones alternating in frequency: relationship to perceived rate and streaming. *J Neurophysiol* **97**: 2230–8.

Winkler I, Sussman E, Tervaniemi M, Horvath J, Ritter W, Näätänen R (2003) Preattentive auditory context effects. *Cogn Affect Behav Neurosci* **3**: 57–77.

Wojtczak M, Viemeister NF (2005) Forward masking of amplitude modulation: basic characteristics. *J Acoust Soc Am* **118**: 3198–210.

Woldorff MG, Hackley SA, Hillyard SA (1991) The effects of channel-selective attention on the mismatch negativity wave elicited by deviant tones. *Psychophysiology* 28: 30–42.

Yost WA (1991) Auditory image perception and analysis: the basis for hearing. *Hear Res* 56: 8–18.

Yvert B, Fischer C, Bertrand O, Pernier J (2005) Localization of human supratemporal auditory areas from intracerebral auditory evoked potentials using distributed source models. *Neuroimage* 28: 140–53.

Chapter 11

Role of descending control in the auditory pathway

Jufang He and Yanqin Yu

In this chapter we summarize our understanding of the mechanisms of corticofugal modulation on the auditory pathways. The chapter is organized as follows: (1) a review of the anatomy and physiology of the medial geniculate body (MGB; the auditory division of the thalamus) which is the main target of the corticofugal system and (2) a discussion of corticofugal modulation of subcortical nuclei, including the MGB, thalamic reticular nucleus (TRN), inferior colliculus (IC), and brainstem nuclei, including non-auditory brainstem sites.

11.1 Descending cortical projections

It is now clear that the profuse descending connections of the auditory cortex to the thalamus, midbrain, and brainstem demand a re-evaluation of the simple hierarchical model of ascending auditory processing.

11.1.1 Roles of the auditory corticofugal systems

At the outset it is useful to enumerate some candidate processes that are influenced by auditory corticofugal systems. Most of the data that follow have been obtained chiefly from the cat, with additional data from rodents, bats, and primates.

Physiological studies demonstrate that the descending pathways can affect many aspects of subcortical auditory performance, including sharpness of tuning, neural plasticity in subcortical structures, and integration with other sensory and motor systems.

As well as targeting auditory structures, the auditory corticofugal systems target several other non-auditory brain centers including some involved in motor control, emotions, and learning. For the motor system these include the basal ganglia and other premotor structures, and the pontine nuclei whose output ultimately reaches the cerebellum. This implies that preparation for motor performance also involves integration of auditory corticofugal signals.

The auditory cortex also projects to the amygdala and central gray. These polysynaptic routes to the hypothalamus and to tegmental structures are implicated in the control of smooth muscle tone and may affect behaviors as diverse as milk ejection and startle reflexes (Yeomans and Frankland, 1996).

11.2 Functional anatomy and connections of the auditory thalamus

The MGB of the thalamus is the major target of the corticofugal system. The MGB consists of three divisions: ventral (MGBv), dorsal (MGBd), and medial (MGBm). The MGBv, the largest division, contains a densely packed aggregate of medium-sized and small neurons, in which the former predominate. In MGBd, the neurons have slightly smaller somata and are more dispersed, while MGBm has a broad range of somatic sizes, including the largest cells in the MGB, and a lower neuronal density than the other two divisions (Winer, 1992).

The MGB in the guinea pig is ovoid in shape and about 3 mm long in the rostrocaudal direction, with a mediolateral diameter of maximally 2.5 mm and a vertical diameter of 2–2.5 mm. The guinea pig's MGB has been divided into four subnuclei (Redies and Brandner, 1991). The MGBv is located lateroventrally in the rostral two-thirds of the MGB and projects to two tonotopic fields (anterior and dorso-caudal) of the auditory cortex. The cells in MGBv are densely packed and do not stain very deeply in neutral red preparations. The shell nucleus (MGBs) surrounds MGBv in a continuous shell dorsally, laterally, and ventrally. Neurons in MGBs project to a non-tonotopic cortical field situated in the ventrocaudal belt, and are cytoarchitectonically similar to those in MGBv, although MGBs is not immediately apparent in Nissl material. Two more MGB subnuclei have been identified in this species. One is the caudomedial nucleus (MGBcm) which consists in Nissl preparations of less densely packed and deeply stained large cells which send sparse projections to nearly the entire auditory cortex. The other is the rostromedial nucleus (MGBrm) which lies medial to MGBv in the rostral half of the MGB and projects to a small tonotopic cortical field (field s), which is not innervated by MGBv. It can be distinguished from MGBv by its less densely packed and deeper-stained cells.

In the cat, MGBv is regarded as the lemniscal projection nucleus. It is tonotopically organized with the low-frequency region located laterally, middle-frequency region caudomedially, and high-frequency region rostromedially (Aitkin and Webster, 1972). In the guinea pig, the tonotopic map runs rostrocaudally, with high frequencies located rostrally and low frequencies caudally (Redies and Brandner, 1991; He et al., 2002; Zhang et al., 2008b). Neurons in non-MGBv nuclei typically have long latency, show bursting firing patterns, broadly tuned frequency response properties, and are not tonotopically organized. Thus the non-MGBv nuclei are regarded as the non-lemniscal projection nuclei. Some cells in the non-lemniscal divisions respond not only to auditory stimuli, but also to other sensory modalities (Redies and Brandner, 1991; Winer et al., 1992, 1999; Rauschecker et al., 1997; He and Hashikawa, 1998; He and Hu, 2002). Neurons in the cat MGBv project primarily to the primary auditory cortex (AI) and the anterior auditory field (AAF). The equivalent auditory fields in the guinea pig are the anterior (A) and the dorsocaudal (DC) fields.

The MGBd of the cat, which corresponds to the guinea pig's MGBs and partial MGBcm, projects to areas of auditory cortex surrounding the primary cortex, while the MGBm projects to all auditory cortices, including its association cortex (Imig and Morel, 1983). The non-lemniscal MGBm, which is approximately equivalent to the caudomedial nucleus (MGBcm) of the guinea pig, also projects to and receives input from the amygdala and the basal ganglia (Shinonaga et al., 1994). The cortical projection of MGBv is mainly to cortical layers IV and IIIb, while many MGBm cells project to layer I from where neurons in all layers receive input (Winer, 1992; Hashikawa et al., 1995).

Thalamic nuclei receive reciprocal projections from those same cortical areas to which they project. Corticothalamic neurons originate from layer VI as well as the lower part of layer V and are known to be glutaminergic and aspartergic. They are quite different from corticofugal neurons projecting to the brainstem or spinal cord. The auditory cortex projects to the MGB and the IC (Rouiller and Welker, 2000). In the cat, about half of all layer VI pyramidal cells contribute to the corticogeniculate pathway. It has been estimated that each geniculate relay cell receives convergent input from at least ten cortical cells and most likely many more (Montero, 1991; Ojima, 1994; Liu et al., 1995a).

In the cat, each auditory cortical area projects reciprocally to the MGB: AI and AAF project to the MGBv, AII to MGBd, and all fields to MGBm. However, the reciprocity of the thalamocortical and corticothalamic projections is not quantitatively rigid (Winer and Larue, 1987; He and Hashikawa, 1998). The corticothalamic projection terminates over a region in the thalamus that is wider than the region sending an ascending projection to the same cortical field (Winer and Larue, 1987). In addition, the corticothalamic projection does not appear to be equally dense in all regions of MGB.

Injection of a bi-directional tracer into the cortex labeled a large number of MGBv and MGBd cell bodies and corticothalamic terminals. In contrast, the same injections retrogradely labeled many neurons in MGBm, but very few corticothalamic terminals (He and Hashikawa, 1998), hinting that MGBm receives a relatively weaker modulation from the cortex than other divisions. The ascending fibers of the thalamic relay neurons send collateral projections to the large GABAergic neurons of the TRN before reaching the cortex (Crabtree, 1998). The TRN also receives feedback projections from the cortex and projects back to the thalamus. Neurons in different areas of the TRN project to different regions of the thalamus (Liu *et al.*, 1995b).

The thalamus is at the crossroads of the brainstem, basal ganglia, and telencephalic circuits, and it is much more than a set of nuclei that relay afferent impulses to the cerebral cortex. The modulation of the corticothalamic projection and the inhibition from TRN changes the firing modes of thalamic neurons which are proposed to mediate global oscillations, and modulates discharge synchrony and oscillation frequency, and may participate in the process of changing vigilance (Steriade and Deschênes, 1988; Steriade, 2000). The thalamus is actively involved in shaping afferent signals through both facilitatory and inhibitory processes. It selectively facilitates or inhibits frequency channels, amplifies or attenuates signals depending on their intensity, and minimizes the interference from other sensory inputs. It participates in highly complex integrative functions, and is crucial for shifting the functional mode of the brain between an adaptive behavioral state, open to the outside world, and a disconnected state such as in slow-wave sleep when thalamic gates are closed (He, 2003b).

11.3 Corticofugal modulation of subcortical auditory nuclei

11.3.1 Corticofugal modulation of the nuclei of the MGB

Both corticofugal facilitatory and inhibitory effects are observed in the MGB with electrical stimulation or deactivation by cooling of the auditory cortex (Aitkin and Webster, 1972; Villa *et al.*, 1991). Recently, Suga and colleagues (2000) investigated the corticofugal modulatory effects on the thalamus and midbrain of the bat. They found that corticofugal feedback could sharpen the frequency-tuning curves of thalamic neurons, and facilitate the time-domain processing of biosonar information.

Effects of corticofugal modulation on MGBv are mainly facilitatory

Corticofugal activation of the most effective facilitatory cortical site usually increases spontaneous firing in cat MGBv neurons (Villa *et al.*, 1991) and enhances their responses to sound stimuli (Fig. 11.1; He, 1997). In a minority of cat MGBv neurons it induces a small reduction in spontaneous firing and the maximal responses to pure tones or noise-burst stimuli.

The areas of auditory cortex that give rise to corticofugal modulation of the MGB form patch-like patterns on the cortical topography. The size of these patches ranges from 600–1900 µm, with an average of 1130 µm (He, 1997). This is larger than the spread of the terminal projections of thalamocortical neurons in the cortex, but roughly the same size as the terminal projections of reciprocal corticothalamic neurons in the MGB. Thus, the large functional patches observed in AI appear to reflect the effects of the widely ramifying corticothalamic projections (He, 1997).

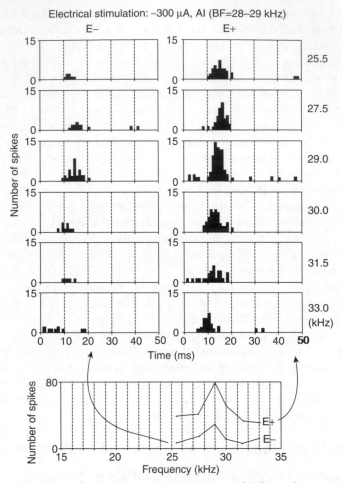

Fig. 11.1 Neuronal responses of an MGB neuron to pure tones of different frequencies at sound intensity of 50 dB SPL. *Above* Peristimulus time histograms (PSTHs); *below* frequency response functions, which were defined to be the responses to pure tones at a certain intensity as a function of frequency under two conditions, with (E+) and without (E−) electrical activation of the primary auditory cortex (AI). The PSTH of the neuronal responses for each frequency tested is shown. The PSTHs were formed by summing spikes for 20 repeated trials. *In the lower figure* the *lower curve* shows the neuronal responses to pure tones in the control condition and the *upper curve* shows those to the same pure tones when an AI site having the same best frequency (BF) was activated. The MGB neuron was tuned to 29 kHz and the BF of the activation site in AI was about 28 kHz. *E−* Control, i.e., without electrical stimulation of AI; *E+* AI was activated by pulse trains (99 pulses, 300 Hz) of negative current (−300 µA) 100 ms (delay interval) before the acoustic stimulus. The order of sampling points was pseudo-random, e.g., E− of 30 kHz, E+ of 33 kHz, E+ of 29 kHz, E− of 31.5 kHz, etc. (Data from the cat; He, 1997.)

In the thalamus of the guinea pig, where, in contrast to that of the cat, interneurons only account for about 1% of the cell population, cortical activation results in both facilitatory and inhibitory effects on neuronal responses of auditory thalamic neurons, but the great majority of the effects are excitatory. Compared to the cat, a higher percentage of MGBv neurons in the guinea pig are affected by corticofugal activation. Of the MGBv neurons recorded, 72% were corticofugally modulated. Of these responses, 95% were facilitated and only 5% were inhibited (He *et al.*, 2002).

Corticofugal modulation of MGBd and MGBm

In contrast to MGBv, where activation of either the auditory field A or DC of the guinea pig caused a mainly facilitatory effect on its neurons, activation of the same areas caused large inhibitory effects on neurons in MGBcm and MGBrm, and smaller inhibitory effects on neurons in the shell nucleus (MGBs). Examples are shown in Fig. 11.2 (He, 2003a). The MGBcm neuron in Fig. 11.2B was completely switched off by cortical activation.

Eighty-five percent of the cells seen in MGBcm and 73% of the cells in MGBrm showed an inhibitory effect of cortical activation. Only in 12% of neurons in MGBrm were responses inhibited by more than 50%, while the proportion in MGBcm was 36%. In MGBs, 77% of neurons sampled showed inhibitory effects, but only 14% showed inhibitory effects of more than 50%.

Thus the inhibitory effect of the cortex on the non-lemniscal MGB is generally widespread, with inhibition generated, in many cases, by stimulation at each of three cortical sites in the primary fields A and DC of the guinea pig (He, 2003a). Besides cortical stimulation, cortical

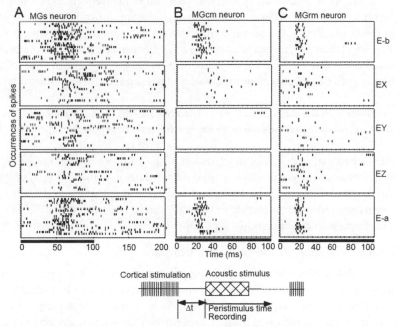

Fig. 11.2 Effects of cortical activation on non-lemniscal MGB neurons. Raster displays show three typical examples of neuronal responses to repeated noise-bursts while different sites in the auditory cortex were electrically activated: **A** a shell nucleus (MGBs) neuron; **B** a caudomedial nucleus (MGBcm) neuron; **C** a rostromedial nucleus (MGBrm) neuron. A noise burst was repeated over 19 trials at 1.0-s intervals for each condition. E-b and E-a represent control measurements, taken before or after the experimental conditions, during which only an acoustic stimulus was delivered to the subjects. EX, EY, and EZ indicate the experimental conditions in which an electrical stimulation was applied to the auditory cortex at one of three different sites prior to the acoustic stimulus. Only the first 100–200 ms of the responses are shown in the figure. The time interval (Δt) between the electrical stimulation and the acoustic stimulus was 100 ms. The experimental paradigm is shown in the *inset* below the raster displays. (Data from the guinea pig; He, 2003a.)

deactivation by cooling can also affect corticofugal influences. Villa *et al.* (1991) reported increased spontaneous firing in the MGB when the auditory cortex was cooled, with more neurons in the medial division of the MGB showing increased spontaneous firing rate than in other subdivisions. It is also interesting to note that neurons with tonic responses showed more corticofugal inhibition than excitation.

MGBcm is involved in the integration of multisensory afferents (Edeline and Weinberger, 1992). The finding that primary auditory cortex strongly inhibits MGBcm while strongly facilitating MGBv provides a possible explanation for the selective gating of auditory information through the lemniscal MGB. This 'switching off' of other unwanted sensory signals and interference from the limbic system would leave the auditory cortex prepared to process only the auditory signal.

11.3.2 Corticofugal modulation of sound coding

Corticofugal modulation in the frequency domain

As shown in Fig. 11.1, AI activation modulates the frequency-response functions of MGB neurons. The influence on frequency-response functions depends on sound intensity, as shown in the example in Fig. 11.3. In this case, frequency-response functions were facilitated when AI was activated (Fig. 11.3A). The facilitatory effect was defined as the frequency-gain function. The frequency-gain functions for different stimulus intensities are shown in Fig. 11.3B. When the stimulus intensity was 30 dB, AI activation enhanced responses to the best frequency (BF) to a much greater extent than it enhanced responses to other frequencies. Such 'BF-enhancement' for at least one sound intensity was found in about half of the neurons tested, and of these BF-enhanced neurons, half showed BF-enhancement for all sound intensities tested, as in the example shown in Fig. 11.3.

When the AI site with the same BF as the recorded MGB neuron was activated, the gains of the MGB neuronal responses to sounds are modulated differently depending on the frequency of the stimuli.

In the mustached bat, widespread inactivation of the auditory cortex, including neurons matched to subcortical neurons, results in a sunstantial reduction in the responses of the subcortical neurons to sounds (Yan and Suga, 1999); matched here means that the electrically stimulated cortical neurons and recorded subcortical or cortical neurons are tuned to the same value of the acoustic parameter under consideration.

Corticofugal modulation in the temporal domain

Corticofugal modulation on the temporal firing pattern The corticofugal pathway modulates not only firing rate but also a neuron's temporal firing pattern (Fig. 11.4; He *et al.*, 2002). Cortical activation increases the first spike latency and lengthens the duration of the response. The mean latency of the first spike was increased from 11.2 ms without cortical stimulation to 17.1 ms when the cortex was activated by a single pulse, and to 16.0 ms with 30 pulses.

The temporal firing pattern is widely believed to encode information in sensory signal transmission. For example, using an artificial neural network, Middlebrooks and colleagues (1994) demonstrated that a single cortical neuron could more accurately distinguish a sound from a different direction when they used information about both spike number and spike timing than when they used only spike number.

Recent data clearly show that corticofugal modulation changes the temporal firing pattern of thalamic relay neurons (Figs 1 and 3 of He, 2003a), and we speculate that if one applied a similar method to that of Middlebrooks *et al.* (1994), neurons with different temporal firing patterns would reveal different patterns of corticofugal modulation. It will be interesting to investigate

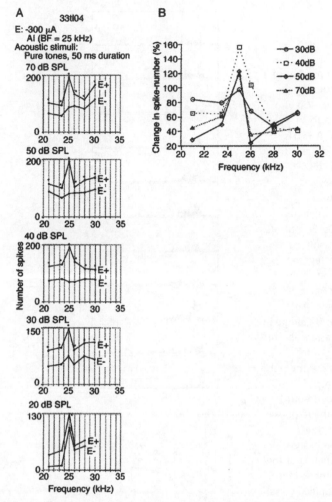

Fig. 11.3 Effects of cortical electrical stimulation on the responses of an MGBv neuron to pure tones of different frequencies and sound intensities (frequency-response functions). **A** Curves for the E– and E+ conditions. AI was activated by pulse trains of –300 μA at the site representing the best frequency (BF = 25 kHz). **B** Gain functions, defined as the change in the frequency-response functions between E– and E+, are shown for sound intensities between 30 and 70 dB SPL. *Asterisk* denotes $P < 0.05$. (Data from the cat; He, 1997.)

whether thalamic neurons can detect different acoustic stimuli more accurately when corticofugal modulation is activated. On the other hand, Ryugo and Weinberger (1976) demonstrated that cooling the cortex suppressed the long-latency rhythmic discharges of MGB neurons. These changes in temporal patterns of the rhythmic and rebound discharges (discharges after a period of silence) might represent another dimension of the encoding of sensory information, or a change in the mode of transmission of sensory information in the thalamus. However, this speculation awaits further investigation.

Corticofugal modulation of OFF and ON-OFF neurons 'OFF' responses are defined as responses that always occur following the offset of the stimulus, while 'ON-OFF' responses are defined as responses with a time locked increase at both tone onset and tone offset. OFF and ON-OFF

Fig. 11.4 Effect of number of pulses in the electrical stimulation on the MGB neuronal response to an acoustic stimulus. **A** PSTHs show neuronal responses to noise bursts of 60 dB SPL while the auditory cortex was activated by electrical stimulation with different numbers of pulses. E– indicates control measurement taken either before or after the experimental conditions; N is the total number of onset responses; L is the mean first-spike latency. **B** Change in spike number as a function of the pulse number of the electrical stimulation. The pulse number of the electrical stimulation changed from 1 to 200. Changes in the responses to noise bursts of three neurons (a, b, and c) are illustrated as a function of the pulse number of the electrical stimulation. Stimulation current was 200 μA. (Data from the guinea pig; He *et al.*, 2002.)

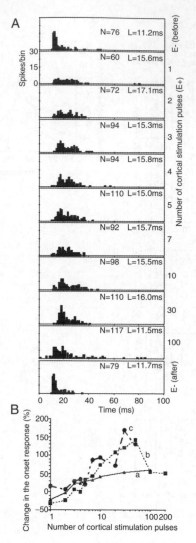

neurons account for 10–20% of the total MGB neurons. Most OFF and ON-OFF neurons tend to be found on the border between the MGBv and other subdivisions and outside the MGBv, respectively (He, 2001, 2002). Corticofugal activation appeared to facilitate the OFF responses of most neurons (Fig. 11.5A, B), while it inhibited or had no effect on others (Fig. 11.5C; He, 2003a).

For ON responses in ON-OFF neurons, two different effects were seen. For ON-OFF cells in and around the border region of the MGBv, corticofugal modulation facilitated the ON response. For ON-OFF cells located in the MGBs and MGBcm, corticofugal effects were mainly inhibitory. Similar results have been reported for cat MGBm neurons. An early report showing that cortical *inactivation* caused an increase in the ON response and a decrease in the OFF response of cat MGBm neurons agrees with our results. It is reasonable to conclude that the OFF response is produced at the offset of the inhibitory input generated by the auditory stimulus (Villa *et al.*, 1991). Intracellular studies showed that OFF responses often occurred in hyperpolarized neurons with low-threshold calcium spikes (Yu *et al.*, 2004a). A further hyperpolarization caused by the cortical stimulation creates a stronger rebound at the OFF response, causing an increase in the spike rate.

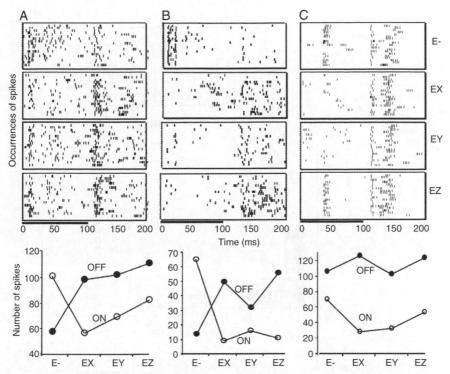

Fig. 11.5 Modulatory effects of cortical activation on ON-OFF neurons in the guinea pig MGBcm. Raster displays show the responses for three neurons to noise-burst stimuli in the control condition (E−) and while the cortex was activated at sites X (field A, BF = 2.8 kHz, EX), Y (12.5 kHz, EY), and Z (16 kHz, EZ). Noise bursts of 60 dB SPL and 100-ms duration were repeated at 1-s interstimulus intervals. *Below* Spike counts of ON and OFF responses as a function of the stimulation site compared with the control condition E− for each neuron. (Data from the guinea pig; He, 2003a.)

Corticofugal modulation in the intensity domain

Activation of a site in AI with the same best frequency as the cells recorded in the MGB showed non-homogeneous effects on neuronal responses to pure tones at different sound intensities (He, 1997). Half the neurons tested showed a larger effect at low sound intensity, and smaller or no effects at high sound intensities (Fig. 11.6); these were named low-sound-intensity effective (LIE) neurons. More than 20% of the neurons showed larger effects on responses to acoustic stimuli of higher intensity than at lower intensity, and were named high-sound-intensity effective (HIE) neurons. The remainder was non-intensity specific, showing effects over a wide range of sound intensities or a complicated pattern of response to sound intensity. Most of the LIE neurons had monotonic rate-intensity functions (discharge rate plotted as a function of sound pressure level (SPL)). Neurons of other types showed monotonic and non-monotonic functions of SPL. The selectivity of the facilitatory effect for low-sound-intensities suggests that, in many cases, cortical feedback to the MGB may act to amplify the response of the MGB cell to weak sounds.

11.3.3 Functional implications of corticothalamic modulation

The central auditory system contains many physiologically distinct types of neurons for auditory signal processing. Their response properties have been interpreted as being produced by divergent and convergent interactions between neurons in the ascending auditory system. The corticofugal

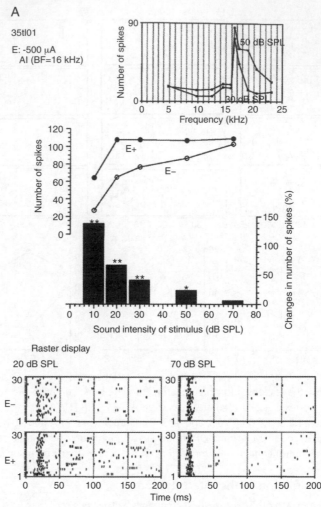

Fig. 11.6 Cortical modulation of neuronal responses to pure tones as a function of sound intensity. **A** Neuronal responses plotted in terms of spike number for two conditions, showing changes when AI was activated in comparison with the control. *Inset* Two frequency tuning curves at 30 and 50 dB SPL, showing that the BF of the neuron was 16.5 kHz. The neuron shows a large facilitatory effect to low-intensity sound, but not to high-intensity sound, and therefore was classified as a low sound intensity effective (LIE) neuron. **B** Raster displays comparing neuronal responses to pure tones at 16 kHz at 20 and 70 dB SPL for two conditions: E− control, and E+ with electrical stimulation of AI. The BF of the effective cortical activation site in AI was at 16 kHz, and the stimulation current was −500 μA. The Pure tones for sound stimulation were 16.5 kHz. (Data from the cat; He, 1997.)

system plays a significant role in generating or refining the response properties of auditory neurons, and in reorganizing maps of frequency and, for example, echo-delay (Crick, 1984; Villa *et al.*, 1991; He, 1997; He *et al.*, 2002; Jen and Zhou, 2003).

Studies have shown that the massive corticofugal system adjusts subcortical auditory signal processing in the frequency, amplitude, time, and spatial domains (Villa *et al.*, 1991; He, 1997; Palmer *et al.*, 2007). The corticofugal modulation likely plays a role in binding the different features of sounds. It may also mediate aspects of auditory attention and be affected by other modalities. For example, in humans, visual attention has been shown to reduce cochlear output (for review see Suga *et al.*, 2000). If we suppose there are dynamic attentional filters that selectively gate the signals in the auditory system, then according to signal processing theory this filter array should be placed at the earliest possible stage in the auditory pathway, and the gains of the filters would need to be controlled from the cerebral cortex (Zhang and He, 2006). Either or both the corticothalamic and corticocollicular systems are candidates for this filtering processing. Such dynamic filtering is likely to be a universal feature for the visual and other sensory systems. However, the corticocollicular system is unique to the auditory system, and may be specialized for other functions such as plasticity (Zhou and Jen, 2000) and sound localization. Thus the more likely candidate for the filtering mechanism is the corticothalamic system.

Summarizing the above results, we conclude that the corticothalamic system selectively facilitates or inhibits frequency-specific responses of neurons in the MGBv, amplifies or attenuates signals with weak or strong intensity, and minimizes the interference of other sensory inputs.

11.3.4 Corticofugal modulation of the thalamic reticular nucleus

Modulation of auditory responses through the TRN

Corticothalamic fibers make excitatory synaptic contacts on the distal dendrites of thalamic principal cells (Liu *et al.*, 1995a), as well as on inhibitory local circuit cells (Golgi type 2, inhibitory interneurons) of the main thalamic sensory nuclei and the TRN. The ascending fibers of the thalamic relay neurons send collateral projections to the TRN en route to the cortex (Crabtree, 1998). The TRN also receives feedback projections from the cortex and projects back to the thalamus. The collateral thalamocortical and corticothalamic inputs display a topographical distribution of their terminals with respect to best frequency in the TRN. The TRN neurons of all species are large and GABAergic (Montero and Singer, 1984). Neurons in different areas of the TRN project to local inhibitory neurons in different regions of the thalamus (Liu *et al.*, 1995b; Cox *et al.*, 1997; Crabtree, 1998). The incidence of these local inhibitory neurons is species-specific and varies across the different sensory thalamic subdivisions. In the MGB of rat or guinea pig, the relative frequency of local inhibitory neurons is 0–3%, while in the cat it is 25–30% (Peruzzi *et al.*, 1997).

Activation of the auditory cortex results in a strong and long-lasting inhibition on non-lemniscal MGB neurons in contrast to a strong facilitation and a small inhibitory effect on the lemniscal MGB neurons (Yu *et al.*, 2004a, b). Three possible pathways might contribute to the corticofugal inhibition of the non-lemniscal MGB:

1 Via thalamic interneurons: anatomical studies have revealed very few interneurons in the MGB of the guinea pig and rabbit: <1%. Therefore, corticofugal activation of thalamic interneurons is an unlikely candidate for the strong corticofugal inhibitory pathway. Another possible source of inhibition is from the pre-synaptic dendrites (PSDs) of the interneurons on the thalamic relay neurons (Liu *et al.*, 1995a; He, 1997). However, in the guinea pig, the PSDs account for <6% of the total terminals, compared with an average of 35% inhibitory terminals in the cat where interneurons account for 24–27% of the total population (Liu *et al.*, 1995a). With so few interneurons in the guinea pig thalamus, it is unlikely that the strong nucleus-specific inhibition is primarily caused by the PSDs. The interneurons and PSDs might account for the low levels of inhibition in the MGBv (He, 1997).

2 Via IC GABAergic neurons: the auditory cortex projects to the IC and the projections are excitatory (Ojima, 1994). In the cat, about 20% of the neurons in the central nucleus of the IC are GABAergic. Among the tectothalamic projection neurons in the IC, GABAergic neurons account for 14–36% in the cat and 20–45% in the rat (Peruzzi *et al.*, 1997). However, in

a recent *in-vivo* intracellular recording, we could still record a strong, long-lasting inhibition in the MGB while electrically stimulating the auditory cortex with a pulse train after sectioning the tectothalamic fibers. This suggests that the strong inhibition was not mediated by the IC pathway (Fujimoto *et al.*, 2002; Zhang *et al.*, 2008a).

3 Via TRN neurons: as mentioned earlier, thalamocortical and corticothalamic pathways are not rigidly reciprocally connected. The majority of the excitatory inputs to the TRN neurons are derived from the cerebral cortex, confirming that the corticofugal fibers to the TRN neurons exert a strong control over the excitability of TRN neurons (Golshani *et al.*, 2001). Studies by Crabtree and colleagues have revealed that the interconnections between the TRN and the dorsal thalamus are cross-nucleus and cross-modality (Crabtree, 1999). The TRN neurons also project to the contralateral TRN in the rat. The TRN neurons extend dendrites within the thin reticular sheet, which enable them to receive projections from a wide cortical region, and project to widespread areas in the ventroposterior nucleus of the thalamus (Liu *et al.*, 1995b). This, together with the results of other studies, leads to the reasonable conclusion that the control of the thalamus via the TRN is widespread (Liu *et al.*, 1995b; Cox *et al.*, 1997; Crabtree, 1998).

The corticofugal inhibitory pathway was identified by examining the response of the membrane potential of MGB neurons to electrical stimulation of the auditory cortex (AC), with (1) bilateral ICs ablated and (2) a selective lesion of the TRN neurons. The guinea pig, in which only very few interneurons (<1%) are found in the MGB, was used as the experimental model. The amplitude, latency, and duration of IPSPs of MGB neurons in the IC-ablated animals were not statistically different from those in control animals, as in Fig. 11.7. After chemical lesion of the TRN, corticofugally induced EPSPs or spikes were observed in MGB neurons, but no IPSPs. This result strongly suggests that the strong inhibition was not mediated by the IC pathway, but by TRN (Fujimoto *et al.*, 2002; Zhang *et al.*, 2008a).

Giant GABAergic terminals of unknown origin have been found mainly in the non-lemniscal nuclei of the MGB, but not in the MGBv of the cat (Winer *et al.*, 1999). This location in the non-lemniscal nuclei may in part explain the observation of stronger corticofugal inhibition in these regions of the guinea pig MGB.

In summary, activation of the corticothalamic fibers directly generates excitatory inputs to the MGB neurons including both lemniscal and on-lemniscal neurons, and also activates the TRN neurons. These TRN neurons inhibit the MGB neurons mainly in non-lemniscal regions.

Corticofugal modulation of thalamic oscillations through the TRN

The corticothalamic system likely has a central role in the switching of thalamic neurons from burst-to-tonic firing modes. This change of firing mode is proposed to mediate global oscillations through the inhibitory involvement of TRN, which, in turn, modulates discharge synchrony and may embody changes in vigilance (Steriade, 2000; Winer, 2006; Guo *et al.*, 2007, Zhang *et al.*, 2008a).

Thus the TRN may also play a significant role in sleep oscillations and the global regulation of the sleep–waking cycle (Destexhe *et al.*, 1999). The long-lasting strong inhibition from the TRN to the dorsal thalamus could hyperpolarize the membrane potential of the thalamocortical neurons in that region, leading to bursts of low-threshold calcium spikes (Steriade, 2001) and thus switching the thalamus from working mode to sleeping mode. Although many thalamocortical oscillations are initiated in or involve the TRN, the TRN could also be a passive follower of the rhythm of an external stimulus (Xu *et al.*, 2007). Rhythmic electrical activation of the cortex resulted in a rhythmic oscillation at the same frequency in the TRN for 20 s after the activation (Xu *et al.*, 2007).

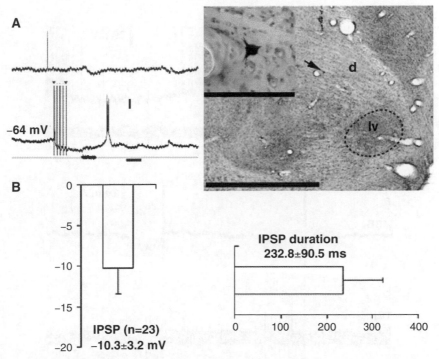

Fig. 11.7 Electrical stimulation caused inhibition in non-lemniscal MGB neurons. **A** *Left panel* shows neuronal responses to an auditory stimulus and to electrical AC stimulation (*triangles* point to stimulus artifacts). The resting membrane potential is indicated on the *left* of the recording traces. *Right panel* shows the location of the neurobiotin labeled neuron (*arrow*) in a low magnification Nissl counterstained section, and enlarged in the *inset*. **B** Means and SDs of the amplitudes and durations of the IPSPs in MGB neurons caused by electrical stimulation of the cortex. *Vertical scale bars* 20 mV; *horizontal scale bars* 100 ms. (Data from the guinea pig; Zhang *et al.*, 2008a.)

Figure 11.8A shows simultaneous intracellular recordings of MGB neurons and extracellular activity in the TRN. Inhibitory membrane potentials in the MGB neurons were preceded by extracellular discharges of the TRN neurons. In both control and IC-ablated animals, many GABAergic TRN neurons responded to the AC electrical stimulation with oscillatory discharges (Fig. 11.8Ba). In separate experiments, an oscillation-like IPSP triggered by cortical stimulation was observed in the MGB neuron. The TRN activity and MGB inhibitory oscillation had similar time courses (Fig. 11.8Bb).

11.3.5 Corticofugal modulation of the inferior colliculus

The corticocollicular auditory system: anatomy

Neurons in the deep layers of the AC send tonotopically organized projections to the MGB, the IC, and to subcollicular auditory nuclei (Huffman and Henson, 1990). Corticothalamic fibers only project to the thalamic reticular nucleus and the ipsilateral MGB (Huffman and Henson, 1990; Ojima, 1994), whereas, corticocollicular fibers project bilaterally to the IC. The ipsilateral projection is more profuse and shows greater topographical organization than the contralateral projection (Saldaña *et al.*, 1996) and, therefore, ipsilateral corticofugal modulation of the IC is expected to be much stronger than contralateral corticofugal modulation.

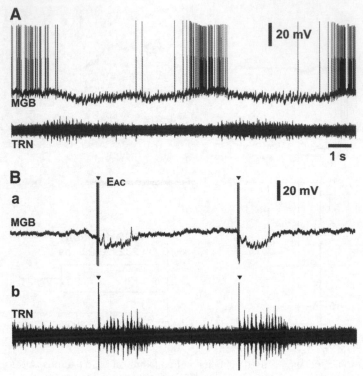

Fig. 11.8 Electrical stimulation of the AC triggered burst discharges in TRN and IPSP oscillations in MGB. **A** Traces show the simultaneous recording intercellular signals of a medial geniculate (MGB) neuron and extracellular signals of thalamic reticular nucleus (TRN) neurons in a control animal under Nembutal anaesthesia. **B** Electrical stimulation of the AC caused burst discharges in TRN neurons of control animals, and spindle-like IPSP oscillation in MGB neurons in IC ablated animals. *Vertical scale bars* 20 mV; *horizontal scale bars* 1 s. (Data from the guinea pig; Zhang *et al.*, 2008a.)

Modulation of sound coding in the IC and comparison with that in the MGB

Corticocollicular modulation of sound coding Electrical stimulation of the auditory cortex, combined with low-repetition acoustic stimulation, reduced the responses of corticofugally inhibited neurons in the central nucleus of the inferior colliculus (ICc) and increased their spatial and frequency selectivity, but had the opposite effect on corticofugally facilitated collicular neurons (Zhou and Jen, 2000). This corticofugal modulation which typically vanished within 5–10 s after stimulation was called brief corticofugal modulation (Zhou and Jen, 2000). When cortical electrical stimulation was delivered at a high repetition rate, synchronized with acoustic stimulation at the BF of a single neuron or a cluster of cortical neurons, the BFs of collicular neurons were shifted toward the BFs of the stimulated cortical neurons. Such corticofugal modulation reorganized the collicular frequency map by increasing the representation of the frequency corresponding to the site stimulated in the cortex. This effect lasted for as long as 3 hours (Suga *et al.*, 2000) and was called short-term corticofugal modulation (Zhou and Jen, 2000).

While the time course of corticofugal modulation of collicular auditory responses varies with the stimulus parameters, the functional significance of brief and short-term corticofugal modulations remains to be determined, as do the neural mechanisms that underlie them. Furthermore, the neural circuits and synaptic mechanisms that produce the corticofugal inhibition and facilitation of responses in the colliculus remain to be explored.

The cortical feedback has been termed 'egocentric selection' since it adjusts and improves subcortical signal processing. It reorganizes the frequency map in the central nucleus of the IC, enhancing the neural representation of frequently occurring signals. When cortical neurons are activated with high-repetition rate electrical stimulation, they produce tightly focused facilitation of subcortical neurons that are 'matched' in a specific acoustic parameter, and extensive inhibition to 'unmatched' neurons (Suga *et al.*, 2000). Subcortical information processing is affected by auditory experience involving associative learning and attention and such effects could be mediated by the corticofugal system (Suga *et al.*, 2000).

Comparison of corticocollicular and corticothalamic modulation The corticocollicular system differs from the corticothalamic projection in almost all respects. Where the latter is massive and closely associated with the lemniscal thalamic nuclei, the former is weak and concentrated mainly in the extralemniscal IC subdivisions. However, extensive local connections may faciltate interactions between subdivisions of the IC; such pathways are absent in the MGB (Morest, 1975).

The specificity of corticocollicular projections has some similarities to that of the corticothalamic system. For example, in the ferret, input to layers II–III of the non-lemniscal dorsal cortex of the IC arises principally from the five tonotopic areas of auditory cortex (Bajo *et al.*, 2007). Tonotopic fields in AC send more projections to the IC than non-primary, limbic-related cortical areas, which have more limited and specific IC targets.

The laminar origin of the corticollicular projections complements those of the corticothalamic system. The corticocollicular cells of origin occupy the central and deep part of layer V where corticothalamic cells are absent. Corticothalamic projections originate in layer VI. Thus, these corticofugal projections occupy layers V and VI and originate from the largest pyramidal cells (Winer, 2006). There are several neuronal types with either single spiking or bursting modes of discharge, patterns whose role in information processing likely differs. This supports the view that the corticothalamic and corticocollicular systems are independent, as does the sparse population of corticofugal neurons that project jointly to both the IC and MGB.

Finally, the axons of corticocollicular and corticothalamic neurons are different: corticocollicular axons are more homogeneous, with fine preterminal segments and small terminal boutons (Saldaña *et al.*, 1996).

Using Fos protein as an activity marker with immunohistochemical techniques, Sun and colleagues (2007) investigated the corticofugal modulation of acoustic information ascending through the auditory pathway of the rat. With auditory stimulation at different frequencies, Fos expression in the MGB, IC, superior olivary complex, and cochlear nucleus was examined and the extent of Fos expression on either side of the brain was compared. Strikingly, they found densely Fos-labeled neurons in MGBv only after both presentation of an auditory stimulus and administration of a $GABA_A$ antagonist (bicuculline methobromide, BIM) to the AC. The location of Fos-labeled neurons in the MGBv after acoustic stimulation at different frequencies was in agreement with the known tonotopic organization. That no Fos-labeled neurons were found in the MGBv with acoustic stimuli alone suggests that the transmission of ascending thalamocortical information is critically governed by corticofugal modulation. The dorsal (DCIC) and external cortices (ECIC) of the IC ipsilateral to the BIM-injected cortex showed a significantly higher number of Fos-labeled neurons than the contralateral IC. However, no difference in the number of Fos-labeled neurons was found between the central nucleus of the IC on either side, indicating that direct corticofugal modulation only occurs in the ECIC and DCIC. Further investigations are needed to assess the functional implications of the morphological differences observed between the descending corticofugal projections to the thalamus and the IC (Sun *et al.*, 2007).

Corticofugal facilitation of plastic changes in the IC

Various factors such as focal cortical electrical stimulation, conditioning, and learning of a discrimination task can change the maps in central auditory nuclei (including the cortex) and can affect the response properties of the neurons (Suga *et al.*, 2000). However, until quite recently the contribution to such central auditory plasticity of the corticofugal system was largely unexplored (Krupa *et al.*, 1999). The importance of the corticofugal system for plasticity is clear from the data from the big brown bat obtained by Gao and Suga (2000).

Collicular and cortical neurons show asymmetrical shifts in their BFs towards the BF of electrically stimulated neurons (centripetal) when focal electrical stimulation is applied to the AC and for repetitive auditory stimuli. Thus, egocentric selection operates as an intrinsic mechanism for reorganizing the auditory system.

Some acoustic stimuli alone do not evoke a BF shift; however, when a train of acoustic stimuli is delivered as a conditioned stimulus followed by an unconditioned electrical stimulation to the leg, large BF shifts are evoked that are asymmetrical and centripetal. Neither electrical stimulation of the leg alone nor acoustic stimuli delivered after electrical stimulation of the leg (backward conditioning) evokes a BF shift. These data indicate that behavioral relevance is determined by the auditory and non-auditory systems, through associative learning. Stimuli that have behavioral significance for the animal evoke plastic changes in central auditory nuclei.

Electrical stimulation of the somatosensory cortex enhances the BF shifts evoked in the colliculus and thalamus by the electrical stimulation of the AC (Ma and Suga, 2001). This demonstrates that the AC and the somatosensory cortex are both necessary for the BF shifts in the IC and AC caused by the conditioning. The cholinergic basal forebrain is also involved in the plasticity of the AC (Suga *et al.*, 2000).

Cortical and collicular BF shifts evoked by 30-min repetitive electric stimulation of the AC are similar in magnitude and recovery time (Fig. 11.9). However, a 30-min conditioning session evoked changes that were quite different in IC and cortex (Fig. 11.9A, curves c and d). The collicular BF shift reaches a maximum at the end of conditioning, and still exceeds the cortical shift even 45 min after termination of the conditioning. At 180 min after the termination of the conditioning the collicular BF shift has fully recovered, as does that evoked by electric stimulation of the AC (compare curves c with a in Fig. 11.9A).

On the other hand, the cortical BF shift gradually increases after the conditioning, reaches a plateau at the time when the collicular BF shift almost recovers, and then persists over many hours (Fig. 11.9A, curve d). This is quite different from the cortical BF shift evoked by electric stimulation of the AC (Fig. 11.9A, curve b). A second conditioning session following the recovery of the collicular BF shift produces another collicular BF shift which is similar to the first. In contrast, the cortical shift evoked by the second conditioning gradually increases over 3 hours to a new plateau.

These findings indicate that the collicular BF shift is not a direct consequence of the cortical BF shift, and it always precedes the BF shift seen in the cortex. The cortical BF shift appears to be enhanced by the BF shift in the colliculus (Gao and Suga, 2000).

Weinberger pointed out the importance of the amygdala and the cholinergic basal forebrain in plasticity of the AC evoked by fear conditioning (Chernyshev and Weinberger, 1998). Application of acetylcholine to the AC during auditory conditioning in the big brown bat enhances both collicular and cortical BF shifts. Blocking the action of acetylcholine by application of atropine to the AC during a conditioning session prevents the cortical BF shift and reduces the BF shift in the

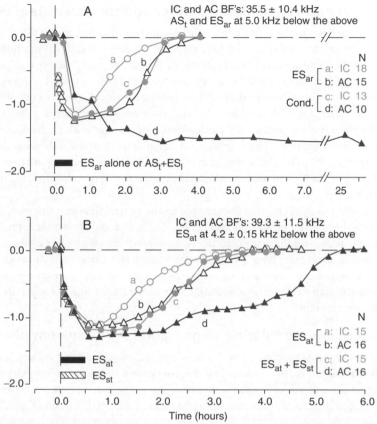

Fig. 11.9 A Shifts in the neural BF in the inferior colliculus (IC) and auditory cortex (AC) of the big brown bat evoked by focal electrical stimulation of the cortex (ES_{ar} *a* and *b*) or auditory conditioning ($AS_t + ES_l$ *c* and *d*). Conditioning consisted of a 1-s train of tone bursts (AS_t) followed by an unconditioned electrical stimulus to the leg (ES_l). Cortical neurons showed a slower recovery of their BF than did collicular neurons in response to electrical stimulation of the AC (*a* vs *b*). Following conditioning, the time course of the BF shift in collicular neurons was similar to that by repetitive electrical stimulation; however, the BF shift of cortical neurons changed slowly and did not recover within 1 day (*c* vs *d*). **B** Duration of the collicular (*a*) and cortical (*b*) BF shifts evoked by trains of electrical stimuli delivered to the AC (ES_{at}) was augmented by electrical stimulation of the somatosensory cortex (ES_{st} *c* and *d*). These electrical stimuli mimicked the conditioned (acoustic) and unconditioned (somatosensory) stimuli. The mean BF of collicular and cortical neurons was 35.5±10.4 kHz for **A** and 39.3±11.5 kHz for **B**. The acoustic stimuli were 5.0 kHz below the recorded BFs of the collicular and cortical neurons. The BFs of cortical neurons stimulated or electrical stimuli delivered to the AC (ES_{ar} and ES_{at}) were 4.2±0.15 kHz lower than the BFs of the recorded neurons. BF shifts were measured with tone bursts at 10 dB above minimum threshold of individual collicular or cortical neurons. *N* Number of neurons recorded. (From Suga *et al.*, 2000.)

colliculus (Ji *et al.*, 2001). Thus the cholinergic system augments the plasticity evoked by the AC and the corticofugal system, but the collicular BF shift can still be evoked in part in the absence of a cortical BF shift. These observations suggest that the subcortical short-term (less than 3 hours) change caused by egocentric selection elicits a long-term (longer than 3 hours) change in the cortex in the presence of acetycholine.

11.3.6 Corticofugal connections to other auditory brainstem nuclei

Corticofugal projections to the subcollicular nuclei, superior olivary complex (SOC), and cochlear nucleus (CN) are also bilateral (Saldaña et al., 1996), and corticofugal modulation could operate even in the cochlea via olivocochlear neurons in the superior olivary complex. The IC projects not only to the MGB and the superior colliculus, but also to medial olivocochlear neurons, which mostly project to contralateral cochlear outer hair cells. In general, olivocochlear neurons project bilaterally to the cochlea, although there are some differences in olivocochlear projections between species. Because the corticofugal system forms multiple feedback loops, the exploration of corticofugal functions is ongoing at different levels of the auditory system.

The proportion of AC cells terminating in the SOC or CN is estimated to be no more than 10% of that projecting to the IC, and while corticofugal input to the IC is mainly ipsilateral, it is more bilateral for the olivary targets.

AC axons ending in the SOC are concentrated in the ventral nucleus of the trapezoid body bilaterally, with the heaviest projection ipsilaterally. In the CN, the projection is predominantly ipsilateral with labeled boutons in the granule cell areas of the dorsal cochlear nucleus. This input to the granule cells arises from layer V of the primary and secondary cortex, which also gives rise to the projections to the SOC (bilaterally). The vast majority of these cortical cells projected to only one brainstem target (Doucet et al., 2003). Other AC targets include the sagulum and associated paralemniscal regions.

11.3.7 Descending modulation to non-auditory brainstem nuclei

All subdivisions of the AC project to the pons, where the principal target is the lateral pontine nucleus. The individual corticopontine axons form narrow sheets just a few cells wide which contain clusters of hundreds of boutons. These endings in the pons are quite different from the smaller, more divergent, and more numerous endings in the MGB, IC, and CN. The pontine axonal laminae are discrete, separated by terminal-free spaces even after large cortical injections that produce extensive and more continuous labeling in the MGB and IC (Winer, 2006).

Input to the claustrum and entopeduncular nucleus arises from all subdivisions of the auditory cortex. The projections to the dorsal putamen and nearby caudate nucleus are topographic projections from tonotopic areas and form zones of dense input among weaker projections. The axons of these projection pathways are thinner and more delicate than those to the pons or to the thalamus (Winer et al., 1999). The functional significance of these projections remains to be investigated.

11.4 Functional segregation of different descending projections

In summary, the corticofugal projection to the core region of the MGBv is likely to act as an executive circuit in the dynamic filter for auditory attention (Fig. 11.10). This circuit may operate as a gain-controlled multichannel filter that provides selective amplification. The corticofugal projection to other MGB subnuclei is probably more related to temporal features of the auditory signal and may also be related to directional tuning (Palmer et al., 2007).

The corticofugal projections to the non-lemniscal MGB involve a much wider area of the cortex and are able to switch the firing patterns of thalamic neurons, suggesting that they are probably more related to switch states of vigilance (He and Hu, 2002; He, 2003a; Xu et al., 2007). This projection also involves the TRN which imposes lasting inhibition on the non-lemniscal MGB (Xu et al., 2007; Zhang et al., 2008a).

The corticocollicular projection counts for only a small proportion of the corticofugal projections. Their functions possibly include (1) facilitating neuronal plasticity in the IC, and

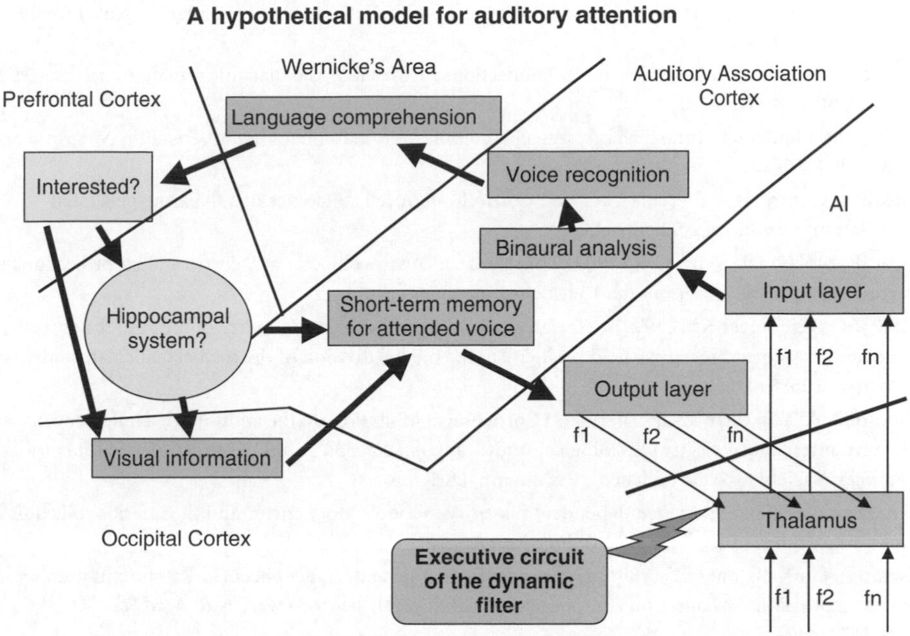

A hypothetical model for auditory attention

Fig. 11.10 A hypothetic model of the dynamic filter for auditory attention. In hearing, we can selectively attend to a particular speaker at a noisy party (the well-known 'cocktail party phenomenon'). In the proposed model, the filter is located between the thalamus and the cortex (Cx). Spatial and spectral cues are used to identify the specific speaker. The cue information is stored in the cortex and refreshed all the time. As recognition and memory are required here, the AC and/or other cortical areas must be involved in this process. The corticothalamic pathways are used to form the dynamic filter array in the auditory system, termed as executive circuit of the dynamic filter. Besides auditory sensory, visual sensory are used to supplement the switching of the filter, though more experimental evidence is needed to consolidate such a notion (Zhang *et al.*, 2006). f1, f2, ..., fn represent parallel channels of the ascending and descending pathways. AI Primary auditory cortex (Modified from Zhang *et al.*, 2006).

(2) influencing behaviors ranging from the startle reflex to the genesis of sound-induced seizures (Ma and Suga, 2001).

The corticofugal projection to the brainstem could possibly contribute to the modulation of the cochlear hair cells through the activation of the olivocochlear system. The function of this projection awaits further investigation.

References

Aitkin LM, Webster WR (1972) Medial geniculate body of the cat: organization and responses to tonal stimuli of neurons in ventral division. *J Neurophysiol* **35**: 365–80.

Bajo VM, Nodal FR, Bizley JK, Moore DR, King AJ (2007) The ferret auditory cortex: descending projections to the inferior colliculus. *Cereb Cortex* **17**(2): 475–91.

Chernyshev BV, Weinberger NM (1998) Acoustic frequency tuning of neurons in the basal forebrain of the waking guinea pig. *Brain Res* **793**(1–2): 79–94.

Cox CL, Huguenard JR, Price DA (1997) Nucleus reticularis neurons mediate diverse inhibitory effects in thalamus. *Proc Natl Acad Sci USA* **94**: 8854–9.

Crabtree JW (1998) Organization in the auditory sector of the cat's thalamic reticular nucleus. *J Comp Neurol* **390**: 167–82.

Crabtree JW (1999) Intrathalamic sensory connections mediated by the thalamic reticular nucleus. *Cell Mol Life Sci* **56**(7–8): 683–700.

Crick F (1984) Function of the thalamic reticular complex: the searchlight hypothesis. *Proc Natl Acad Sci USA* **81**: 4586–90.

Destexhe A, Contreras D, Steriade M (1999) Cortically-induced coherence of a thalamic-generated oscillation. *Neuroscience* **92**: 427–43.

Doucet JR, Molavi DL, Ryugo DK (2003) The source of corticocollicular and corticobulbar projections in area Te1 of the rat. *Exp Brain Res* **153**(4): 461–6.

Edeline JM, Weinberger NM (1992) Associative retuning in the thalamic source of input to the amygdala and auditory cortex: receptive field plasticity in the medial division of the medial geniculate body. *Behav Neurosci* **106**: 81–105.

Fujimoto K, Yu YQ, Chan YS, He JF (2002) Corticofugal inhibition on the auditory thalamic neurons: an in-vivo intracellular electrophysiological study. *Program No. 354.3. 2002 Abstract Viewer/Itinerary Planner*. Society for Neuroscience, Washington, DC.

Gao E, Suga N (2000) Experience-dependent plasticity in the auditory cortex and the inferior colliculus of bats: role of the corticofugal system. *Proc Natl Acad Sci USA* **97**: 8081–6.

Golshani P, Liu X-B, Jones EG (2001) Differences in quantal amplitude reflect GluR4-subunit number at corticothalamic synapses on two populations of thalamic neurons. *Proc Natl Acad Sci USA* **98**, 4172–4177.

Guo YP, Sun X, Li C, Wang NQ, Chan YS, He J (2007) Corticothalamic synchronization leads to c-fos expression in the auditory thalamus. *Proc Natl Acad Sci USA* **104**(28): 11802–7.

Hashikawa T, Molinari M, Rausell E, Jones EG (1995) Patchy and laminar terminations of medial geniculate axons in monkey auditory cortex. *J Comp Neurol* **362**(2): 195–208.

He J (1997) Modulatory effects of regional cortical activation on the onset responses of the cat medial geniculate neurons. *J Neurophysiol* **77**: 896–908.

He J (2001) ON and OFF pathways segregated at the auditory thalamus of the guinea pig. *J Neurosci* **21**: 8672–9.

He J (2002) OFF responses in the auditory thalamus of the guinea pig. *J Neurophysiol* **88**: 2377–86.

He J (2003a) Corticofugal modulation on both ON and OFF responses in the nonlemniscal auditory thalamus of the guinea pig. *J Neurophysiol* **89**: 367–81.

He J (2003b) Corticofugal modulation of the auditory thalamus. *Exp Brain Res* **153**(4): 579–90.

He J, Hashikawa T (1998) Connections of the dorsal zone of cat auditory cortex. *J Comp Neurol* **400**: 334–48.

He J, Hu B (2002) Differential distribution of burst and single-spike responses in auditory thalamus. *J Neurophysiol* **88**: 2152–6.

He J, Yu YQ, Xiong Y, Hashikawa T, Chan YS (2002) Modulatory effect of cortical activation on the lemniscal auditory thalamus of the guinea pig. *J Neurophysiol* **88**: 1040–50.

Huffman RF, Henson OW Jr (1990) The descending auditory pathway and acousticomotor systems: connections with the inferior colliculus. *Brain Res Brain Res Rev* **15** (3): 295–323.

Imig TJ, Morel A (1983) Organization of the thalamocortical auditory system in the cat. *Annu Rev Neurosci* **6**: 95–120.

Jen PH, Zhou X (2003) Corticofugal modulation of amplitude domain processing in the midbrain of the big brown bat, *Eptesicus fuscus*. *Hear Res* **184**(1–2): 91–106.

Ji W, Gao E, Suga N (2001) Effects of acetylcholine and atropine on plasticity of central auditory neurons caused by conditioning in bats. *J Neurophysiol* **86**(1): 211–25.

Krupa DJ, Ghazanfar AA, Nicolelis MA (1999) Immediate thalamic sensory plasticity depends on corticothalamic feedback. *Proc Natl Acad Sci USA* **96**(14): 8200–5.

Liu XB, Honda CN, Jones EG (1995a) Distribution of four types of synapse on physiologically identified relay neurons in the ventral posterior thalamic nucleus of the cat. *J Comp Neurol* 352: 69–91.

Liu XB, Warren RA, Jones EG (1995b) Synaptic distribution of afferents from reticular nucleus in ventroposterior nucleus of cat thalamus. *J Comp Neurol* 352: 187–202.

Ma X, Suga N (2001) Corticofugal modulation of duration-tuned neurons in the midbrain auditory nucleus in bats. *Proc Natl Acad Sci USA* 98: 14060–5.

Middlebrooks JC, Clock AE, Xu L, Green DM (1994) A panoramic code for sound location by cortical neurons. *Science* 264: 842–4.

Montero VM (1991) A quantitative study of synaptic contacts on interneurons and relay cells of the cat lateral geniculate nucleus. *Exp Brain Res* 86(2): 257–70.

Montero VM, Singer W (1984) Ultrastructure and synaptic relations of neural elements containing glutamic acid decarboxylase (GAD) in the perigeniculate nucleus of the cat. A light and electron microscopic immunocytochemical study. *Exp Brain Res* 56(1): 115–25.

Morest DK (1975) Synaptic relationships of Golgi type II cells in the medial geniculate body of the cat. *J Comp Neurol* 162: 157–94.

Ojima H (1994) Terminal morphology and distribution of corticothalamic fibers originating from layers 5 and 6 of cat primary auditory cortex. *Cereb Cortex* 4: 646–63.

Palmer AR, Hall DA, Sumner C, Barrett DJ, Jones S, Nakamoto K, Moore DR (2007) Some investigations into non-passive listening. *Hear Res* 229(1–2): 148–57.

Peruzzi D, Bartlett E, Smith PH, Oliver DL (1997) A monosynaptic GABAergic input from the inferior colliculus to the medial geniculate body in rat. *J Neurosci* 17: 3766–77.

Rauschecker JP, Tian B, Pons T, Mishkin M (1997) Serial and parallel processing in rhesus monkey auditory cortex. *J Comp Neurol* 382: 89–103.

Redies H, Brandner S (1991) Functional organization of the auditory thalamus in the guinea pig. *Exp Brain Res* 86(2): 384–92.

Rouiller EM, Welker E (2000) A comparative analysis of the morphology of corticothalamic projections in mammals. *Brain Res Bull* 53: 727–41.

Ryugo DK, Weinberger NM (1976) Corticofugal modulation of the medial geniculate body. *Exp Neurol* 51(2): 377–91.

Saldaña E, Feliciano M, Mugnaini E (1996) Distribution of descending projections from primary auditory neocortex to inferior colliculus mimics the topography of intracollicular projections. *J Comp Neurol* 371(1): 15–40.

Shinonaga Y, Takada M, Mizuno N (1994) Direct projections from the non-laminated divisions of the medial geniculate nucleus to the temporal polar cortex and amygdala in the cat. *J Comp Neurol* 340: 405–26.

Steriade M (2000) Corticothalamic resonance, states of vigilance and mentation. *Neuroscience* 101: 243–76.

Steriade M (2001) The GABAergic reticular nucleus: a preferential target of corticothalamic projections. *Proc Natl Acad Sci USA* 98: 3625–7.

Steriade M, Deschênes M (1988) Intrathalamic and brain stem-thalamic networks involved in resting and alert states. In: Cellular Thalamic Mechanisms (eds Bentivolglio M and Spreafico R) pp 51–76. Elsevier, Amsterdam.

Suga N, Gao E, Zhang Y, Ma X, Olsen JF (2000) The corticofugal system for hearing: recent progress. *Proc Natl Acad Sci USA* 97(22): 11807–14.

Sun X, Xia Q, Lai CH, Shum DK, Chan YS, He J (2007) Corticofugal modulation of acoustically induced Fos expression in the rat auditory pathway. *J Comp Neurol* 501(4): 509–25.

Villa AE, Rouiller EM, Simm GM, Zurita P, de Ribaupierre Y, de Ribaupierre F (1991) Corticofugal modulation of the information processing in the auditory thalamus of the cat. *Exp Brain Res* 86: 506–17.

Winer JA (1992) The functional architecture of the medial geniculate body and the primary auditory cortex. In: The Mammaliam Auditory Pathway: Neuroanatomy (eds Webster DB, Popper AN, Fay RR), pp 222–409. Springer, New York.

Winer JA (2006) Decoding the auditory corticofugal systems. *Hear Res* **212**(1–2): 1–8.

Winer JA, Larue DT (1987) Patterns of reciprocity in auditory thalamocortical and corticothalamic connections: study with horseradish peroxidase and autoradiographic methods in the rat medial geniculate body. *J Comp Neurol* **257**: 282–315.

Winer JA, Wenstrup JJ, Larue DT (1992) Patterns of GABAergic immunoreactivity define subdivisions of mustached bat's medial geniculate body. *J Comp Neurol* **319**: 172–90.

Winer JA, Larue DT, Huang CL (1999) Two systems of giant axon terminals in the cat medial geniculate body: convergence of cortical and GABAergic inputs. *J Comp Neurol* **413**: 181–97.

Xu M, Liu CH, Xiong Y, He JF (2007) Corticofugal modulation of the auditory thalamic reticular nucleus of the guinea pig. *J Physiol (Lond)* **585**: 15–28.

Yan J, Suga N (1999) Corticofugal amplification of facilitative auditory responses of subcortical combination-sensitive neurons in the mustached bat. *J Neurophysiol* **81**: 817–24.

Yeomans JS, Frankland PW (1996) The acoustic startle reflex: neurons and connections. *Brain Res Rev* **21**: 301–14.

Yu YQ, Xiong Y, Chan YS, He J (2004a) *In vivo* intracellular responses of the medial geniculate neurones to acoustic stimuli in anaesthetized guinea pigs. *J Physiol* **560**(1): 191–205.

Yu YQ, Xiong Y, Chan YS, He J (2004b) Corticofugal gating of auditory information in the thalamus: an *in vivo* intracellular recording study. *J Neurosci* **24**(12): 3060–9.

Zhang Z, Chan YS, He JF (2006) Thalamocortical and corticothalamic interaction in the auditory system. *Neuroembryol Aging* **3**: 239–48.

Zhang Z, Liu CH, Yu YQ, Fujimoto K, Chan YS, He JF (2008a) Corticofugal projection inhibits the auditory thalamus through the thalamic reticular nucleus. *J Neurophysiol* **99**: 2938–45.

Zhang Z, Yu YQ, Liu CH, Chan YS, He JF (2008b) Frequency tuning and firing pattern properties of auditory thalamic neurons: an *in-vivo* intracellular recording from the guinea pig. *Neuroscience* **151**: 293–302.

Zhou X, Jen PH (2000) Brief and short-term corticofugal modulation of subcortical auditory responses in the big brown bat, *Eptesicus fuscus*. *J Neurophysiol* **84**: 3083–7.

Section 3

Information coding in the auditory brain: sound location

Chapter 12

Binaural localization cues

Tom C.T. Yin and Shigeyuki Kuwada

12.1 Introduction

Why do we have two ears when we can hear perfectly well with one, e.g., when carrying on a conversation on the telephone? The answer to this question is largely the same as the analogous and perhaps better known problem in the visual system. The spatial information provided by each eye is essentially two dimensional while binocular vision yields information in another dimension, i.e., in depth. In the auditory system, without binaural cues there is little spatial information because it is the frequency of the sound, not its spatial location, that is topographically represented over the sensory epithelium (cochlea), unlike the other two major sensory systems, vision and touch, where the spatial location of the stimulus is topographically represented on the retina and skin surfaces, respectively. Integrating inputs from the two ears then gives the auditory system spatial information about the location of the sound source along the horizontal dimension. In this chapter we discuss the neural processing of the binaural localization cues in mammals.

A crucial aspect of a sound stimulus is its panoramic properties and its ability to convey information at a distance, even when the source of the stimulus is out of sight. It has been known for over a century (Rayleigh, 1907) that the important interaural cues for localizing a sound source along the horizontal plane are interaural time (ITDs) and interaural level disparities (ILDs). These cues are illustrated in Fig. 12.1, which shows recordings, now commonly called head-related transfer functions (HRTFs), made by Musicant *et al.* (1990), near the eardrum from the left (blue) and right (red) ears of a cat in response to a click stimulus from five different positions in space along the horizontal meridian in the frontal sound field. For each of the five stimulus conditions, the upper traces show the time waveform and the lower traces the power spectrum recorded at the two ears. When the stimulus is directly opposite the left ear, as expected, the left ear signal arrives before the right ear, creating an ITD, and it is louder to the left ear than the right, creating a frequency-dependent ILD, which is evident in the differences in the amplitudes of the time waveforms and gain of the power spectrum signals.

The two interaural cues, ITD and ILD, are not equally effective over all frequencies. Indeed, according to Rayleigh's classic duplex theory, ITDs are only used at low frequencies while ILDs are only effective at high frequencies. There are several reasons for this dichotomy between ITD and ILD. In order to encode ITDs, it is obviously necessary to have timing information available to the binaural comparator. For pure tones the ongoing time information is encoded by the phase locking of auditory nerve fibers which is limited to low frequencies (in mammals below about 3–4 kHz). Thus ITD information is not available for tones at high frequencies. On the other hand, ILDs are only created when the wavelengths of the sound are less than the dimensions of the head and external ears, i.e., at high frequencies, thereby creating an acoustic shadow at the far ear. Thus, at low frequencies ILDs are small and not effective cues. A caveat here is that large ILDs can be created by low frequency sounds if the source is close to the head.

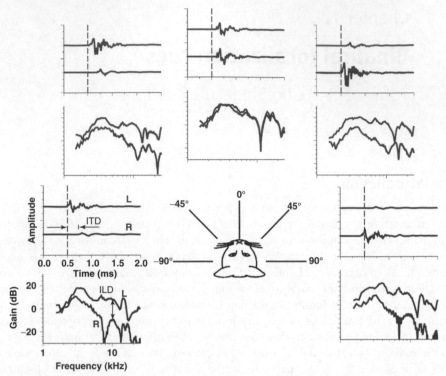

Fig. 12.1 Recordings made near the tympanic membrane of both ears of a cat to a click stimulus from five different spatial locations along the horizontal meridian. *Upper panels* depict the time waveform from the left (*blue*) and right (*red*) ear and corresponding *lower panels* depict the power spectrum. (Adapted from data of Musicant *et al.* 1990.)

The range of ITDs and ILDs that an animal encounters is called its physiological range. The magnitude of these cues is dependent on head size and shape, pinna size and shape, body size and shape, and head and body surfaces (e.g., hair, fur, clothing). Measurements using a human manikin show that for a sound source positioned at 0° elevation and away from the midline, ITD increases with decreasing frequency (Kuhn, 1977) of the sound source. The ITD dependence with frequency has also been demonstrated in other animals (e.g., Sterbing *et al.*, 2003). In contrast, ILD increases with increasing frequency and reaches about 20 dB for signals in the 8–10 kHz frequency band. As the sound source approaches the ear the ILD can increase substantially, e.g., ~30 dB for high frequency signals (e.g., 3 kHz) and even by ~10 dB for low frequency (e.g., 500 Hz) signals (Brungart and Rabinowitz, 1999). So, the physiological range changes appreciably with frequency and distance of the sound source. The fact that the perception of the azimuthal location of the sound source does not change with frequency or distance attests to the adaptive plasticity of the brain.

When the stimulus is on the midline, there are no interaural disparities as the left and right ear signals are essentially identical. Localization of sounds in the vertical dimension depends upon the monaural spectral cues that result from the filtering properties of the external ears and head. We will not discuss the coding of these spectral cues as they are the subject of the next chapter.

12.2 Interaural time disparities (ITDs)

12.2.1 Psychophysical evidence

Sensitivity to ITDs in the fine structure of sounds

The primary method for studying ITD sensitivity is through earphones since this allows for precise control of the interaural disparities reaching the two ears. Using this method, it has been shown that ongoing ITDs in the fine structure of low frequency sounds, and not the onset ITD, is the primary cue for lateralization in humans (Buell *et al.*, 1991). The binaural system is exquisitely sensitive to small changes in ITD and this sensitivity is dependent on the stimulus frequency, i.e., the threshold for detecting a change in ITD is lowest (~10 µs) near 1000 Hz and increases systematically to about 60 µs at 125 Hz (Zwislocki and Feldman, 1956). Sensitivity to ITDs in humans falls off rapidly above about 1200 Hz. The potency of the ITD cue was demonstrated in experiments where virtual sound sources were manipulated such that the ITD cue signaled one direction whereas the ILD and pinna cues signaled the opposite direction. The apparent direction almost always followed the ITD cue provided that the wideband sound contained low frequencies (Wightman and Kistler, 1992).

Sensitivity to ITDs in the envelopes of amplitude modulated sounds

The duplex theory only holds for pure tone stimuli: the ITDs of a high frequency stimulus that carries timing information in its low frequency (<300 Hz) envelope, e.g., sinusoidally amplitude modulated (SAM) tones, can be discriminated by human subjects (Klumpp and Eady, 1956). This finding is important because many naturally occurring sounds have time-varying envelopes. Although human listeners were sensitive to ITDs of the envelopes in such stimuli, their ability to detect changes in ITDs of envelopes was much poorer compared to ITDs in low frequency tones (Bernstein, 2001). However, recent research indicates that ITDs conveyed by envelopes created by multiplying a half wave rectified low frequency tone by a high frequency carrier (i.e., so-called transposed envelopes), a stimulus whose temporal structure mimics the temporal structure of low frequency signals as processed by the auditory periphery, can be as effective as ITDs conveyed by low frequency tones (Bernstein and Trahiotis, 2002). ITD sensitivity to envelopes of high frequency signals is limited to below 200 Hz, considerably lower than the limit for sensitivity to fine structure of low frequency signals (~1200 Hz).

12.2.2 Anatomical and physiological substrates

Peripheral coding

Auditory nerve fibers bifurcate after entering the cochlear nucleus: one branch projects to the dorsal and posteroventral cochlear nuclei where it makes synapses with ordinary bouton-like endings on the various cells types there, while the other branch projects to the ventral cochlear nucleus where it contacts bushy cells with large, specialized synaptic endings known as the end bulbs of Held. Bushy cells are named for their unusual dendritic morphology: a single or even non-existent bushy dendritic tree. The secure and large end bulb endings enable excitatory neurotransmitter to be released quickly and synchronously to the postsynaptic receptors so that the precise temporal information carried in the auditory nerve fibers is faithfully preserved in the bushy cells. Not only are the synaptic endings uncommon, but also the intrinsic biophysical properties of the bushy cells are highly unusual; their receptors are abnormally rapid with low threshold potassium conductances and low input impedances so that their membrane time constant is very short, making them especially fast acting (Oertel, 1983). Two types of bushy cells have been described, spherical and globular, which differ in their location in the VCN, their central projections, and the size and number of end bulb endings that they receive (spherical bushy cells receive larger and fewer end bulbs).

Figure 12.2 compares the responses of an auditory nerve fiber (upper) and a bushy cell (lower) to similar low frequency tone bursts. Each dot reflects the time of occurrence of an action potential, and each row of dots reflects the action potentials evoked by a presentation of a tone burst. Viewed over multiple presentations of this stimulus, it is clear that the action potentials tend to occur at intervals that match the period of the stimulating frequency. The lower panel depicts the responses of a bushy cell to a 340-Hz tone burst. Compared with the response of the auditory nerve fiber to a similar 350-Hz tone burst (upper panel), the jitter in the phase-locked responses of the bushy cell is considerably reduced. The neuron fired to almost each cycle of the tone, and consequently the spike rate remained near constant over the duration of the tone burst. This transformation between phase-locking in the nerve and cochlear nucleus is consistent with the convergence of more than one auditory nerve fibers onto a cochlear nucleus neuron which responds like a coincidence detector (Joris *et al.*, 1994).

Binaural processing in the MSO and LSO

Medial superior olive The inputs to the primary binaural comparators, the medial superior olive (MSO) and the lateral superior olive (LSO), are shown in Fig. 12.3A and B, respectively. In most mammals the MSO is composed of a thin sheet of neurons with the narrow axis in the mediolateral direction. Low to high frequencies are represented in the dorsoventral axis with a disproportionately large area devoted to low frequencies (Osen, 1969). The axons of spherical bushy cells, which relay precise temporal information from the auditory nerve (Fig. 12.2), leave the cochlear nucleus by way of the trapezoid body, to provide excitatory inputs to MSO neurons on each side (Harrison and Warr, 1962; Cant and Casseday, 1986; Fig. 12.3A). The MSO neurons act like coincidence detectors and fire maximally when the inputs from the two sides arrive simultaneously.

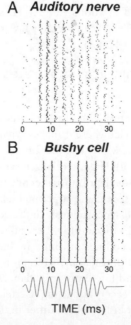

A *Auditory nerve*

B *Bushy cell*

TIME (ms)

Fig. 12.2 Dot rasters depicting phase-locked discharges of an auditory nerve fiber (panel A) and a bushy cell (panel B) to multiple presentations of similar low frequency tone bursts (350-Hz in A and 340-Hz in B). A schematic of the tone burst in B is shown at the bottom of panel B. (From Joris *et al.*, 1994.)

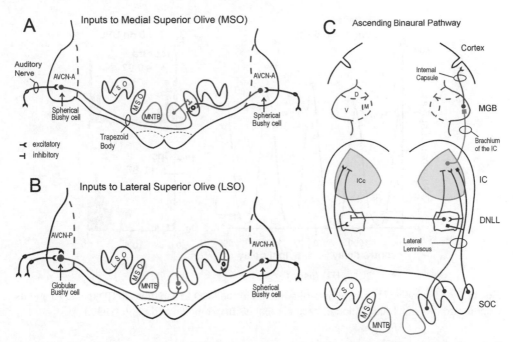

Fig. 12.3 Schematic representation of the inputs to the medial (**A**) and lateral (**B**) superior olives and their ascending projections (**C**). AVCN-A Anterior part of the anteroventral cochlear nucleus; AVCN-P posterior part of the anteroventral cochlear nucleus; MNTB medial nucleus of the trapezoid body; DNLL dorsal nucleus of the lateral lemniscus; ICc central nucleus of the inferior colliculus; MGB medial geniculate body; D dorsal division; V ventral division; M medial division.

Figure 12.4 shows the typical response of an ITD-sensitive MSO neuron and evidence of a coincidence mechanism. A 1000-Hz tone was delivered to each ear with ITDs ranging from 2000 µs delay to the contralateral ear (negative ITDs in our convention) with respect to the recording site to 2000 µs delay to the ipsilateral ear (positive ITDs). Because tones are perfectly periodic, the ITD function will display multiple peaks, with the interval between peaks equal to the period of the stimulation frequency (viz 1 ms; Fig. 12.4, left panel). The right panels display the monaural phase-locked responses of this neuron in the form of period histograms when each ear was stimulated separately with the same tone. Note that the response to ipsilateral stimulation leads the response to contralateral stimulation by a small fraction of a cycle. Based on the mean phase responses, the tone to the ipsilateral ear would have to be delayed by 0.15 cycles (1.02–0.87 cycles), or equivalently a 150-µs delay, in order to bring the responses from each ear into coincidence. This predicted value is close to the peak of the actual mean phase of the ITD function when the neuron is stimulated binaurally (Fig. 12.4, left panel, 90-µs delay to the ipsilateral ear). The correspondence between the optimal interaural phase predicted from monaural stimulation of each ear alone with the actual best ITD obtained under binaural stimulation was first described by Goldberg and Brown (1969) and confirmed by nearly all MSO recordings to date (Yin and Chan, 1990; Spitzer and Semple, 1995; Batra *et al.*, 1997b) and constitutes the definitive test of coincidence in the MSO.

In addition to the excitatory inputs, there is also good evidence for inhibitory inputs to the MSO from both anatomical and physiological studies. The MSO receives inputs from glycinergic

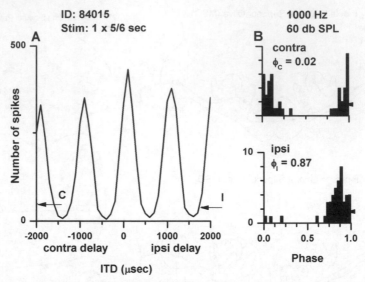

Fig. 12.4 An example of the responses of a neuron in the MSO to variations in ITD (*panel* **A**) and its response to monaural stimulation of each ear (*panels* **B**). (From Yin and Chan, 1990.)

neurons in the ipsilateral medial nucleus of the trapezoid body (MNTB) (Fig. 12.3) and ipsilateral lateral nucleus of the trapezoid body (LNTB; not shown in Fig. 12.3) (Saint Marie *et al.*, 1989; Cant and Hyson, 1992). Electrical stimulation involving these tracts evoked inhibition in nearly all cells in the gerbil MSO and it was usually able to block synaptically evoked action potentials (Grothe and Sanes, 1993). Application of strychnine, a glycinergic antagonist, affects ITD sensitivity of MSO cells (Brand *et al.*, 2002).

For a single tone, due to phase-locking of its inputs, an ITD-sensitive neuron would display a periodic function at intervals equal to the period of the stimulating frequency for as long as the tones to each ear overlapped in time. When the stimulation frequency is varied and the responses of the same neuron plotted on a common ITD axis, then the neuron's preferred or best ITD emerges (Fig. 12.5A). Summing these delay functions results in a composite tone function which predicts the response of the cell to a wide band stimulus (Fig. 12.5B). When compared with this neuron's actual response to ITDs of a wideband noise stimulus, the similarity in the ITD sensitivities suggests that a simple linear summation of the tonal ITDs can predict the noise ITD function. If the mean interaural phase derived from each tonal ITD function is plotted as a function of stimulating frequency (e.g., Fig. 12.5C, 500–1700 Hz), then the linearity demonstrates that the neuron satisfies the requirements of 'characteristic delay' (CD) (Rose *et al.*, 1966) where the slope of this function estimates the neuron's CD and the phase intercept at 0 Hz estimates its characteristic phase (CP) (Yin and Kuwada, 1983b). The CD is an estimate of the difference in conduction times from each ear to the binaural coincidence detector, i.e., the ITD required for coincident arrival of the inputs at each frequency. The CP is a measure of whether the alignment of the tonal ITD functions occurs at the peak (CP near 0 or 1.0 cycles) or the trough (CP near 0.5 cycles). For this neuron, the CP is 0.063 cycles, indicating alignment at the peaks of the ITD function and a CD of 33 μs. The CP estimate fits well with the alignment of peaks seen in Fig. 12.5A and the CD closely approximates the best ITD estimated from the neuron's composite tone and noise functions (Fig. 12.5B).

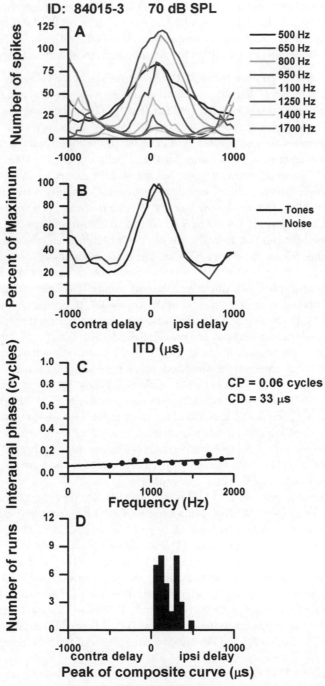

Fig. 12.5 Responses of an MSO neuron to ITDs in tones and noise. **A** ITD functions to tones from 500–1700 Hz at 70 dB SPL. **B** Normalized comparison of the summed response to tones in **A** (composite curve) to ITD function to noise. **C** Interaural phase versus stimulating frequency calculated from the ITD functions in **A**. CP Characteristic phase; CD characteristic delay; **D** distribution of best ITDs measured from the peak of composite curves for MSO neurons recorded in the cat. (From Yin and Chan, 1990.)

The CDs and best ITDs of neurons in the MSO are biased to ipsilateral delays, i.e., those created by a sound source in the contralateral sound field. Figure 12.5D plots the distribution of best ITD (peak of the composite curve) for MSO neurons recorded in the cat. All of the best ITDs are to ipsilateral delays and all but one fall within the physiological range of the cat ($\sim \pm 360$ μs).

Lateral superior olive In contrast to the MSO, the narrow axis of the LSO is in the rostrocaudal direction. In the cat it is an S-shaped structure where neurons tuned to low and high frequencies are represented along a lateral to medial gradient. The LSO has a disproportionately large area devoted to high frequencies. It receives input that is derived from both ears via cells that are excited by stimulation of the ipsilateral ear and inhibited by the contralateral ear, which is why it has traditionally been considered a center for the initial processing of ILDs (Boudreau and Tsuchitani, 1968). However, its circuitry also has many of the elements of the MSO circuit, i.e., bushy cells and calyceal-type synapses, suggesting that the LSO circuitry is also designed to process timing information. Indeed, low-frequency cells sensitive to ITDs in the fine structure (Finlayson and Caspary, 1991; Tollin and Yin, 2005) and high-frequency cells sensitive to the ITDs in envelopes (Joris and Yin, 1995; Batra *et al.*, 1997a,b) have been found in the LSO.

The inputs to the LSO are shown in Fig. 12.3B. The ipsilateral pathway is similar to that of the MSO, while the contralateral pathway is unique, with the largest synapse in the nervous system. Like the MSO, axons of spherical bushy cells in the anteroventral cochlear nucleus (AVCN) travel via the trapezoid body to synapse in the LSO of the same side (Harrison and Warr, 1962). These excitatory inputs tend to be segregated to the distal dendrites, while the inhibitory endings from the MNTB are located on the cell body and proximal dendrites (Helfert *et al.*, 1989).

The contralateral input begins with the axons of globular bushy cells in the posterior part of the contralateral AVCN that enter the trapezoid body, cross the midline, and synapse upon principal cells in the MNTB (Tolbert *et al.*, 1982). Morphologically these MNTB neurons resemble the bushy cells of the AVCN with giant calyceal-type endings (calyx of Held) (Harrison and Warr, 1962). The excitatory presynaptic terminal of the calyx of Held is so large that it has become a model system for biophysical studies of neurotransmission as it allows simultaneous recording from both the pre- and post-synaptic elements (Barnes-Davies and Forsythe, 1995). The axons of principal cells in the MNTB make inhibitory glycinergic (Moore and Caspary, 1983) synapses onto LSO neurons of the same side (Spangler *et al.*, 1985).

The ITD sensitivity to pure tones of LSO neurons is the converse of MSO neurons, reflecting the difference in their inputs. Whereas MSO neurons display a maximum (peak) response at a common ITD across stimulating frequencies (Figs 12.5A and 12.6A), LSO neurons display a minimum (trough) response at a common ITD (Fig. 12.6B). This is consistent with MSO neurons receiving excitatory inputs from each side and LSO neurons receiving excitatory and inhibitory inputs from the ipsilateral and contralateral side, respectively. Consequently, MSO neurons commonly show a CP near 0 cycles (Fig. 12.6A, right panel) whereas LSO neurons show a CP half a cycle away (i.e., near 0.5 cycles; Fig. 12.6B, right panel). Tollin and Yin (2005) demonstrated that like their high frequency counterparts, low frequency, ITD-sensitive LSO neurons were excited by stimulation of the ipsilateral ear and inhibited by stimulation of the contralateral ear with CPs near 0.5 cycles.

The differences in ITD sensitivity between MSO and LSO neurons to ongoing ITDs (Fig. 12.6A, B) are also seen to envelope ITDs (Fig. 12.6C,D). The neuron in Fig. 12.6C was recorded in the vicinity of the MSO and displayed peak-type ITD sensitivity to amplitude modulation (AM; envelope) frequencies from 50–800 Hz. In contrast, the neuron in Fig. 12.6D was recorded in the vicinity of the LSO and displayed trough-type ITD sensitivity to envelope frequencies over a similar range. An often overlooked type of ITD sensitivity in the superior

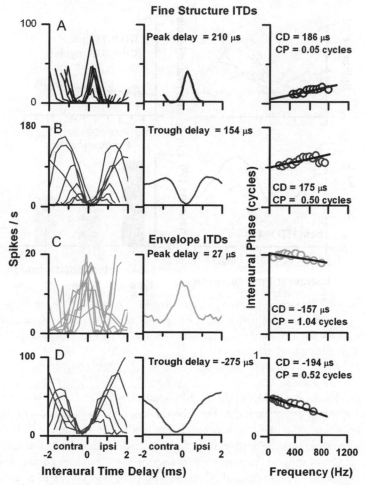

Fig. 12.6 Types of ITD sensitivity seen in the SOC. **A** Peak-type response to tones. **B** Trough-type response to tones. **C** Peak-type response to envelopes of sinusoidally amplitude modulated (SAM) tones. **D** Trough-type response to SAM tones. *Left column* Response to individual tones or envelope frequencies. *Middle column* Composite curves derived from averaging the responses in *left column*. *Right column* Interaural phase versus stimulating frequency calculated from the ITD functions in *left column*. (Adapted from Batra *et al.*, 1997a.)

olivary complex (SOC) is the so-called irregular or intermediate response pattern. For these neurons, the ITD curves across frequency align neither at the peak nor at the trough, but at some point in between (e.g., Fig. 12.7A–C). Such neurons show a CP intermediate between 0 (or 1; peak-type) and 0.5 cycles (trough-type). The example in Fig. 12.7 displays a CP of –0.21 cycles and a best ITD (–434 μs) that is about four times greater than its CD (–112 μs). Dividing the CP axis (0–1 cycles) into thirds to equally represent peak-type, trough-type, and intermediate-type neurons yields estimates of intermediate-type neurons from ~27% (16/60 neurons) in the SOC of rabbits (Fig. 12.7D) to ~12% (25/210 runs) in the MSO of cats (Yin and Chan, 1990), and ~ 23% (8/34 neurons) in the gerbil SOC (Spitzer and Semple, 1995).

A model mechanism for creating intermediate-type responses in the SOC was proposed by Batra *et al.* (1997a) where a contralateral input was added to the normal ipsilateral and contralateral

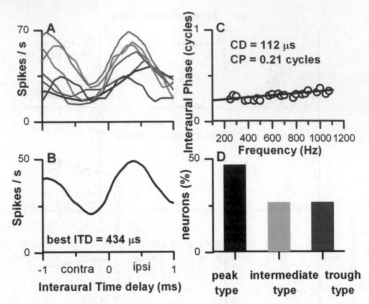

Fig. 12.7 Example of an intermediate-type neuron in the SOC. **A** ITD functions to frequencies from 375–1050 Hz. **B** Composite curve derived from averaging the responses in **A**. **C** Interaural phase vs stimulating frequency calculated from the ITD functions in **A**. **D** Distribution of characteristic phase (CP) in the SOC of rabbits (n = 60 neurons).

inputs of a model neuron. For MSO cells the additional contralateral input would be inhibitory, while for LSO it would be excitatory. As described above, there is anatomical evidence for such additional inputs onto MSO and LSO neurons. In the model, the addition of such inputs created intermediate-type responses, the relative strengths of which determined the value of CP. Moreover, Fitzpatrick et al. (2002) showed that systematic changes in the CP create a continuous representation of best ITDs from the MSO-like to LSO-like. Viewed in this way, the CPs create a continuum of best ITD from small to large. Consistent with this theme, blocking inhibition in the MSO has been reported to shift the peak ITD towards the midline, suggesting that ITD tuning involves inhibitory mechanisms (Brand et al., 2002).

The ITD pathway from the superior olivary complex to the auditory cortex

The pathway by which ITD information is carried from the MSO and LSO to higher centers is outlined in Fig. 12.3C. The MSO projects to the dorsal nucleus of the lateral lemniscus (DNLL) (Glendenning et al., 1981) and central nucleus of the inferior colliculus (ICc) on the same side (Fig. 12.3; Rockel and Jones, 1973; Glendenning and Masterton, 1983; Morest and Oliver, 1984) with excitatory, glutamatergic synapses (Helfert et al., 1989; Glendenning et al., 1992). In contrast, the LSO projects almost equally to both the ipsi- and contralateral DNLL and ICc (Glendenning and Masterton, 1983). The contralateral LSO projection is excitatory (glutamatergic), whereas the ipsilateral projection can be excitatory or inhibitory (glycinergic) (Saint Marie et al., 1989; Glendenning et al., 1992). Loftus et al. (2004) showed that the projections of trough-type neurons in the ipsilateral LSO and peak-type neurons in the ipsilateral MSO show some overlap in the ICc.

Almost all neurons in the DNLL are immunoreactive to gamma-aminobutyric acid (GABA) and glutamic acid decarboxylase (Penney et al., 1984) and thus provide inhibitory inputs to their projection sites. The major targets of the DNLL are the contralateral DNLL and the ICc of both sides (Li and Kelly, 1992b).

In addition to the ITD-sensitive inputs from the MSO, LSO, and DNLL, the ICc receives inputs from the contralateral cochlear nucleus from stellate cells, contralateral ICc via the commissure of the IC, and also by intrinsic connections within the ICc. Most, if not all, neurons in the ICc have extensive intrinsic axon collaterals (Oliver et al., 1991). Finally, descending influences may also provide the ICc with ITD information. The primary auditory cortex provides a direct input to the dorsal cortex of the IC (Rockel and Jones, 1973).

The ICc projects to the auditory thalamus via the brachium of the IC. The auditory thalamus consists of the medial geniculate body (MGB) and the lateral part of the posterior thalamic group. The MGB is comprised of ventral, dorsal, and medial divisions. Although all divisions receive some inputs from the ICc, the ventral division receives its primary input from the ipsilateral ICc in the form of strong, topographic projections (Moore and Goldberg, 1963). The ICc also provides the primary input to the lateral part of the posterior thalamic group (Moore and Goldberg, 1963; Kudo and Niimi, 1980). The posterior group and the ventral MGB have reciprocal connections with the primary auditory cortex. Thus, corticofugal projections could help to shape the ITD sensitivity of neurons in the auditory thalamus.

ITD coding beyond the superior olivary complex

Sensitivity to ITDs in the fine structure and envelopes of sounds in the SOC is seen in all major, higher structures. Although phase-locking to monaural stimulation has been reported in the DNLL (Kuwada et al., 2006), ICc (Kuwada et al., 1984), and thalamus (Stanford et al., 1992), it is generally confined to very low frequencies and is too weak to be a primary site for generating sensitivity to ITDs. Thus, it is generally agreed that most, if not all, ITD sensitivity is generated in the SOC and that ITD sensitivity seen at these higher centers reflects binaural interactions from the SOC modulated by convergence and other processes.

Higher structures reflect convergent inputs from the SOC. All ITD neurons at suprathreshold sound levels exhibit sensitivity over a range of frequencies. At the level of the SOC in the rabbit, this frequency range on average is 1.4 octaves. In contrast, for equivalent sound levels in all structures above the SOC this frequency range increases to at least 1.8 octaves (Fig. 12.8A). The increased frequency range suggests convergence of inputs from ITD-sensitive neurons in the SOC tuned to different frequencies. This convergence was also thought to be the basis for neurons in the ICc that displayed non-linear or intermediate-type interaural phase vs frequency plots (e.g., Fig. 12.7). McAlpine et al. (1998) introduced a suppressive ITD in the frequency domain of a non-linear segment and showed that the remaining segment had a linear phase vs frequency plot, suggesting that neurons in the ICc receive convergent input from brainstem coincidence detectors (i.e., MSO and LSO) and that these inputs onto a neuron can have different CDs and/or CPs.

The ITD tuning widths from the SOC to the thalamus become sharper, and then broaden at the auditory cortex. Figure 12.8B plots the mean peak width (in cycles) and standard error of the ITD curves as a function of stimulus frequency for neurons in the SOC, DNLL, ICc, thalamus, and auditory cortex of the rabbit. The ITD functions were generated from the responses to binaural beats that create a dynamically changing ITD (Yin and Kuwada, 1983a) and the width measured 50% down from the peak response. For the measure of peak width, ITD functions become progressively sharper from the SOC to the thalamus. However, at the cortex the ITD functions broaden and approach the widths of tuning seen in the ICc. The sharpest cortical ITD functions are almost identical to the sharpest seen in the thalamus, so this feature is preserved by some cortical neurons (Fitzpatrick et al., 2000). Broadening in tuning from the thalamus to the cortex is also seen in the visual system. In the lateral geniculate nucleus, visual receptive fields are small.

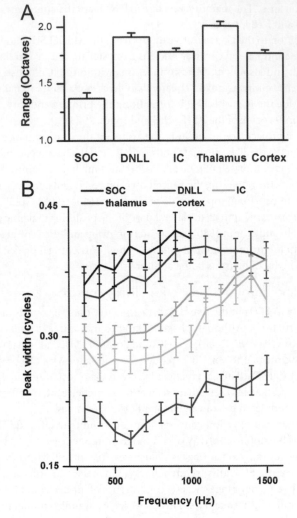

Fig. 12.8 Mean range of frequencies in octaves for ITD sensitivity (**A**) and the peak width of ITD functions measured in cycles as a function of frequency (**B**) for different auditory structures (SOC, DNLL, ICc, auditory thalamus, and cortex). (From Kuwada *et al.*, 2006.)

These cells project to the visual cortex where small receptive fields are found in layer IV, the input layer of the cortex. However, beyond layer IV, cells show larger receptive fields known as simple and complex cells. These cells are specialized for features such as oriented bars or moving edges. Using an ordered array of ITD functions to create a population code, Fitzpatrick *et al.* (1997) showed that sharper ITD tuning increases the efficiency of the population code in that fewer neurons are required to achieve a given acuity.

Sharpening in the ICc is related to GABA-ergic mechanisms. The anesthetic sodium pentobarbital, a potentiator of GABA, reduced the peak width of ICc neurons (Kuwada *et al.*, 1989). When GABA was applied to ICc neurons, the peak width could be substantially reduced and, conversely, blocking GABA could increase the peak width (D'Angelo *et al.*, 2005). As noted above, the contralateral DNLL is a primary source of GABA-ergic input to the ICc and may function as a sharpening mechanism for ITD-sensitive neurons in the ICc.

A neuron's sensitivity to ITDs can match perceptual measures in human subjects. Skottun *et al.* (2001) and Shackleton *et al.* (2003) measured the response variability as a function of ITD for several neurons in the ICc of the guinea pig and determined that their steep slopes could signal

ITD differences as small as 10 μs, the psychophysical threshold for humans. These findings show that there is sufficient information in the ITD response of a single neuron to match the ITD sensitivity seen in humans.

A consistent finding in almost all studies is a strong contralateral bias: most cells respond maximally when the ITDs favor the contralateral ear, i.e., when the sound is delayed to the ipsilateral ear. Intuitively, this makes sense given the coincidence requirement in the MSO: since the projection from the contralateral AVCN to the MSO must travel a longer distance, a sound source in the contralateral sound field arrives earlier to the contralateral ear and thus can compensate for the conduction delay (see Fig. 12.5D). However, the proportion of best ITDs tuned to delays of the contralateral ear increases from the midbrain to the cortex.

Figure 12.9 plots the distribution of best ITDs for one side and its mirror image on the other side as well as the sum of the two sides for the DNLL, ICc, thalamus, and cortex. In all structures the majority of neurons are tuned to ipsilateral delays, i.e., those created by sound in the contralateral sound field At the level of the midbrain (DNLL and ICc), the ratio of those tuned to ipsilateral and contralateral delays is ~2.8 whereas in the auditory thalamus and cortex this ratio reduces to ~1.8. Moreover, summing the distribution on the two sides indicates that in all structures, and in particular the auditory cortex, there is a robust representation of best ITDs near the midline. Finally, the distribution of best ITDs in the cortex is nearly flat and encompasses the largest ITD measured in the rabbit (~400 μs; Kuwada and Kim, unpublished observation).

Combining ongoing and envelope ITDs

The proportion of neurons that showed ITD sensitivity to tones or modulation frequencies in the rabbit is plotted in Fig. 12.10. These curves show that the range of frequencies or modulation frequencies to which a large number of neurons were sensitive extended from 50 to nearly 2000 Hz.

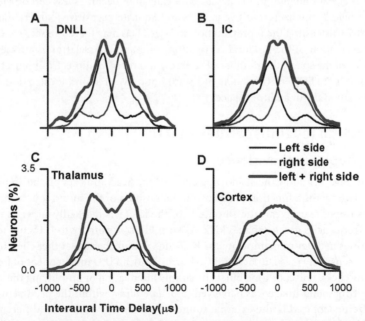

Fig. 12.9 Distribution of best ITDs in the DNLL, ICc, auditory thalamus, and cortex. The distributions for the left (*black lines*) and right (*red lines*) structures are mirror images of each other and these are summed (*blue lines*) to depict the combined distribution of best ITDs.

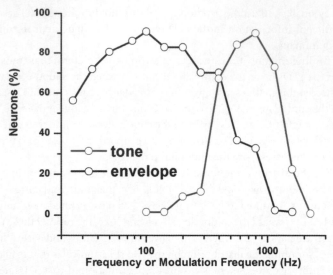

Fig. 12.10 Proportion of neurons in the auditory cortex that showed significant ITD sensitivity to tones or modulation frequencies. (From Fitzpatrick *et al.*, 2000.)

Fitztpatrick *et al.* (2000) suggested that such an array of ITDs ranging from microseconds to milliseconds could be used to create a continuous representation of binaural correlation. The relationship between ITD sensitivity and the correlation of signals at the ears has long been known (Colburn and Durlach, 1978). Highly correlated signals with small ITDs create a compact intracranial sound image with a strong perception of azimuthal location. As the correlation declines, the image broadens and the perceived localization becomes less certain (Jeffress *et al.*, 1962). Physiologically, neurons sensitive to ITDs are exquisitely sensitive to interaural correlation (Yin *et al.*, 1987). Extending the representation to large ITDs may therefore serve to create a continuous representation of the binaural correlation. Interaural correlation is affected by factors such as the size of the space, the number of sources, and reverberations from reflective surfaces, and the large axis of ITD sensitivity may be useful not only for sound localization, but also for gaining information about auditory space.

12.3 **Interaural level disparities (ILDs)**

12.3.1 **Psychophysical evidence**

The HRTFs in Fig. 12.1 show the shadowing effect of the head and ears on the amplitude of the signals to the two ears as a function of the azimuthal position of the sound source in space: at the two positions opposite each ear, the amplitude of the HRTF is markedly larger in the near ear, especially at frequencies greater than 3 kHz. As with ITDs, sensitivity to ILDs has to be studied with headphones in order to manipulate the ILD cue without changing other cues. In traditional studies of ILD sensitivity (see Durlach and Colburn, 1978), an ILD independent of frequency was imposed upon clicks, noise, or tone bursts by simply attenuating or amplifying the signal to one ear. The resulting sound image was perceived to be *lateralized* within the head between the ears rather than being *localized* in the external sound field. The just noticeable difference (jnd) for ILDs studied in this manner is usually reported to be between 0.5 and 1.0 dB across all frequencies (Mills, 1960). It is noteworthy that at low frequencies we are sensitive to ILDs that are smaller than those we would typically encounter in the free field.

A common objective of early studies of ILD sensitivity was to examine time-intensity trading, by displacing the image from the midline with a given ILD to see what ITD favoring the opposite ear would bring the image back to the midline. Such trading experiments could be done with any number of different stimuli, e.g., tones, noise, clicks. The trading ratios measured in a large number of different studies showed considerable variability, ranging from 1–300 µs/dB, due to differences in the signals used, the way in which the ratio was measured, the parameter space explored by each study, and inter-subject variability (Durlach and Colburn, 1978). The variability suggests that the concept of being able to 'trade' time for intensity is too simplistic.

The development of digital technology in the 1970s allowed HRTFs to be recorded in the ear canals of human subjects. The same subjects could then listen to sounds filtered by their own HRTFs to simulate sounds originating from different spatial positions. Kulkarni and Colburn (1998) showed that when subjects hear sounds filtered through their individualized HRTFs, their judgments of spatial position of virtual sounds are indistinguishable from real sounds and they have difficulty discriminating a free field sound from a virtual sound. An important aspect of such virtual sounds is that they are no longer perceived inside the head but instead are externalized in space like real sound sources.

Anatomical circuit for encoding ILDs

Many physiological studies in the central auditory system have reported cells that show sensitivity to ILDs. The primary site of binaural interaction for encoding ILDs is at the level of the superior olivary complex in the LSO (Fig. 12.3B). Cells in the LSO are inhibited by stimulation of the contralateral ear and excited by stimulation of the ipsilateral ear, which is designated as IE binaural interaction. The IE interaction at the LSO is converted to EI interaction at levels above the LSO by a combination of two processes: an excitatory projection of LSO cells to the contralateral ICc and nuclei of the lateral lemniscus along with a predominantly inhibitory projection of LSO cells to the ipsilateral ICc (Glendenning and Masterton, 1983; Saint Marie et al., 1989; Glendenning et al., 1992). When the stimulus is delivered in free field, these EI cells will respond when the sound source is in the contralateral sound field (where the level to the contralateral, excitatory ear exceeds that to the ipsilateral, inhibitory ear) and are suppressed when the source is moved to the ipsilateral sound field. Thus, the neural mechanism for ILD sensitivity involves a subtractive process, unlike the case for ITD sensitivity where the mechanism is more similar to cross correlation, or multiplication.

Given that the LSO is important for encoding ILDs, not ITDs, it is not immediately obvious why there should be in this circuit such extraordinary anatomical and physiological specializations like the calyx of Held which appears to be dedicated to sharpening temporal processing. It is often argued that the calyx of Held provides sharp temporal precision in the transmission of information from the AVCN globular bushy cell to the MNTB (Barnes-Davies and Forsythe, 1995). However, the precise temporal information carried by auditory nerve fibers in the form of phase-locked responses to tones is not present at frequencies above about 3–4 kHz where ILD cues are present. As mentioned above, high frequency auditory nerve fibers and higher order auditory neurons also carry temporal information about amplitude modulated sounds. However, the phase locking in the auditory nerve to the modulation frequency of AM sounds is more than an octave lower than phase locking to the fine structure of pure tones (Joris and Yin, 1992). So what is the reason for calyceal synapses in this circuit?

The answer to this conundrum probably lies in the physiological observation first made in the early studies of the LSO by Boudreau and Tsuchitani (1968). They found that the latency of the inhibitory input is comparable to that of the excitatory input, despite the longer anatomical path length to reach the contralateral side and the additional synapse. The near coincidence of excitation and inhibition in the LSO has been confirmed by other investigators by measurements using a number of different metrics (Sanes and Rubel, 1988). Joris and Yin (1998) estimated the difference in latency using three different independent measures and arrived at an estimate that the inhibition is slower on average by ~ 200 µs relative to the excitation. The need for having a near coincidence of excitation and inhibition arises because many natural sounds are composed of transients rather than the long duration steady state signals that are usually used in the laboratory. With short transient sounds the computation of ILD requires that the excitation and inhibition arrive at the LSO at approximately the same time. The need for an additional sign-changing synapse on the inhibitory side and the position of the LSO on the lateral aspect of the superior olivary complex apparently dictated neuronal mechanisms for speeding up the inhibitory pathway. The large calyceal ending in the MNTB, fast post-synaptic responses of the bushy and MNTB cells, and large caliber axons of the globular bushy cells all serve this purpose. In this regard the reason for the development of the calyceal ending is for speed rather than temporal fidelity.

Physiological coding of ILDs

Classically, two different methods have been used to study ILD sensitivity. In one case ILDs are varied by holding the level to the excitatory ear constant and varying the level of sound to the inhibitory ear. This is a useful technique to determine whether increasing the level to the inhibitory side causes increased binaural suppression, i.e., if the non-excitatory side is indeed inhibitory. In the other case, ILDs are varied by choosing some average level for the two sides and increasing the level to one ear while decreasing the level to the other side by an equal amount. This procedure, sometimes referred to as average binaural intensity (ABI), more closely mimics, but does not simulate precisely, the levels produced when a real sound source is moved around the head in the horizontal plane. However, it is difficult to infer the neural mechanism, since the inputs to both ears are varying, i.e., a decrease in the binaural response could be due to increased inhibition from one side and/or decreased excitation from the other.

Goldberg and Brown (1968, 1969) first described the sensitivity of cells to changes in ILD in the SOC of the dog. They also provided the initial classification scheme for binaural interaction by classifying cells that received excitation from one ear and inhibition from the other as EI and cells that received excitation from both ears as EE. Furthermore, they proposed that EI cells would be useful for encoding spatial location, while EE cells would be useful for coding overall sound pressure level (SPL). The standard, though not universal convention, is to designate EI as an excitatory response to the contralateral ear and inhibitory to the ipsilateral ear, while IE cells have the opposite characteristic. Many authors have also adopted a more detailed classification scheme whereby, for example, E0/f would be a cell that responds to monaural stimulation of the contralateral ear, unresponsive to monaural stimulation of the ipsilateral ear, but facilitated (with a response greater than monaural contralateral) when binaurally stimulated. Other classes of cells that have been described include E0/I and 00/f. The latter class is interesting since they tend to have ILD functions that are peaked near 0 ILD and would be expected to have spatial receptive fields limited to the frontal field (Irvine and Gago, 1990; Irvine et al., 1996).

The classical physiological studies of the LSO (Boudreau and Tsuchitani, 1968) were all done using dichotic stimulation which permitted independent stimulation of the two ears. These studies showed IE binaural interaction: stimulation of the contralateral ear was inhibitory and stimulation of the ipsilateral ear was excitatory. The responses to binaural stimulation were then dependent upon the relative strength of excitation and inhibition.

Figure 12.11 shows the responses of an LSO cell to binaural stimulation at a best frequency tone of 16 kHz at different ILDs (Tollin and Yin, 2002a). In Fig. 12.11A–D each row of the dot raster shows the response of individual trials to the 300-ms duration tone and the histogram below

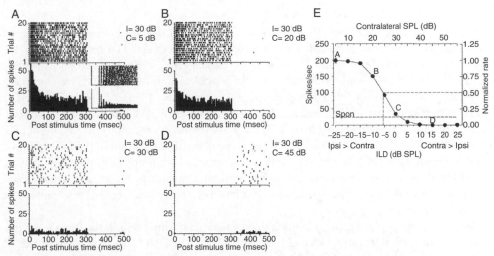

Fig. 12.11 Responses of an LSO neuron to ILDs of tones at CF. **A–D** show dot rasters and post-stimulus time histograms of responses at four different ILDs. The *inset* in **A** shows the dot rasters and PST histogram for the first 40 ms of the response, showing the characteristic 'chopping' response of LSO cells. **E** Plot of response rate vs ILD for the same LSO cell. Points labeled *A–D* correspond to the data shown to the *left*. (From Tollin and Yin, 2002a.)

shows the summed responses over the 20 trials. The SPL of the excitatory, ipsilateral ear was held at 30 dB while the SPL to the inhibitory, contralateral ear was increased from 5 dB (Fig. 12.11A) to 45 dB (Fig. 12.11D). The inhibitory effect of the contralateral input is clear as it suppresses the excitatory response as the contralateral SPL rises above 20 dB or so. Figure 12.11E shows the response plotted as a function of the ILD, defined as the difference between the SPL of the tone to the contralateral ear minus the SPL of the tone to the ipsilateral ear. Since SPL is a logarithmic measure, the difference in log values means that the ILD is a ratio of sound levels, with positive ILDs defined in this case as favoring the contralateral ear.

The ILD sensitivity of LSO cells has been studied by numerous investigators in different species (Sanes and Rubel, 1988; Joris and Yin, 1995; Irvine *et al.*, 2001; Tollin and Yin, 2002a, b). With few exceptions the effect of stimulating the contralateral ear was purely inhibitory, i.e., the binaural response is always less than the ipsilateral-alone response. These studies clearly show the IE binaural interaction, but most of them have used BF tones rather than more natural broadband stimuli. Curiously there are no studies in which recordings have been made with free field sound sources varying in spatial location to directly measure spatial receptive fields of LSO cells other than those using virtual space technology (see below).

As discussed above, psychophysical evidence shows that human subjects are sensitive to ILDs of high frequency sounds in accordance with the classical duplex theory, but are also sensitive to ITDs of AM high-frequency sounds. Physiological studies show a correlate of the psychophysical findings: high frequency LSO cells that are sensitive to ILDs are also sensitive to ITDs of AM tones (Joris and Yin, 1995, 1998). When the modulation frequency is varied, LSO cells also show characteristic delay as evidenced by a linear interaural phase vs modulation frequency function, similar to that described above for MSO cells except that the characteristic phase values cluster near 0.5 cycles, reflecting the IE nature of binaural interaction (see 'Binaural processing in the MSO and LSO' above). The response of LSO cells to ITDs of AM sounds can be viewed as the response to a time-varying ILD (Joris and Yin, 1995).

ILD coding beyond the SOC

Above the level of the LSO most cells that exhibit sensitivity to ILDs show EI binaural interaction. Such cells have been studied by many investigators working in the DNLL (Brugge *et al.*, 1970), ICc (Rose *et al.*, 1966; Semple and Kitzes, 1987; Irvine and Gago, 1990; Park and Pollak, 1993), superior colliculus (Wise and Irvine, 1985), medial geniculate body (Aitkin, 1973; Ivarsson *et al.*, 1988), and auditory cortex (Phillips and Irvine, 1983; Irvine *et al.*, 1996). At the level of the ICc, which is the major nexus for ascending information from the SOC to the cortex, this, at least partly, reflects binaural processing in the LSO that is transmitted by excitatory projections of LSO to the contralateral DNLL and ICc, thereby converting the IE interaction in the LSO to EI. In addition, most studies of ILD sensitivity at these higher levels have found more complex binaural processing than the pure ipsilateral excitatory, contralateral inhibitory properties seen in the LSO. These complexities reflect additional binaural interactions that modulate the basic framework established in the LSO.

There are three primary sources of inhibition to the ICc: intrinsic cells in the ICc, the ventral nucleus of the lateral lemniscus (VNLL), and the DNLL. The DNLL is a prominent source of GABA-ergic inhibition to the ICc, with strong projections to the contralateral side and weaker projections to the ipsilateral side (Brunso-Bechtold *et al.*, 1981) as well as to the opposite DNLL (Fig. 12.3C). In a classic study Brugge *et al.* (1970) showed that many high-frequency cells of the DNLL are sensitive to ILDs and show EI binaural interaction. The effect of this EI inhibitory input onto cells in the ICc will be complex, depending upon the relative threshold of the inhibitory effect and to which side it projects.

A common finding in the ICc and higher centers is that some cells show a mixed input from the ipsilateral side: facilitation at low SPLs and inhibition at high SPLs (Semple and Kitzes, 1987; Irvine and Gago, 1990; Park and Pollak, 1993). This binaural interaction is often called EI/f or E0/f, and the associated ILD functions become non-monotonic rather than sigmoidal in shape, with a peak sensitivity usually near 0 ILD (Fig. 12.12A). As Park and Pollak (1993) pointed out, it is possible to generate E0/f sensitivity in the ICc by starting with a cell that receives IE excitatory input from the contralateral LSO (thereby becoming EI) and adding an inhibitory input from another cell that also has an EI (as referenced to the ICc neuron) interaction. An additional requirement is that the threshold for inhibition of the inhibitory cell must be lower than that of the ICc neuron. Figure 12.12B shows a simplified model that illustrates this mechanism for generating the E0/f binaural interaction. The neuron in the ICc receives excitatory input from the contralateral LSO and inhibitory input from a cell in the DNLL, both of which are ILD sensitive. By varying the strength of the DNLL inhibition, a variety of ILD sensitivity profiles are possible in the ICc, from an E0/f response (Fig 12.12B, blue line) similar to that in Fig. 12.12A to a peaked 00/f or primarily binaural response (green line). Note that the asymptotic values of the ILD function essentially show the monaural responses to the two ears and that the inhibitory cell to the ICc can also be monaural and driven by the contralateral ear.

Park and Pollak (1993, 1994) and Pollak *et al.* (2002) provided evidence for this model by blocking GABA-ergic inhibition on EI/f neurons in the ICc and showing that the facilitation (i.e., non-monotonic ILD function) was eliminated and the ILD function became sigmoidal after blocking inhibition. That ICc neurons receive direct inhibitory input was demonstrated by the presence of inhibitory post-synaptic potentials (IPSPs) in intracellular recordings from ICc cells (Kuwada *et al.*, 1997) and from studies that showed increased firing in ICc neurons when GABA-ergic inhibition was blocked (Park and Pollak, 1993, 1994; D'Angelo *et al.*, 2005). That the contralateral DNLL is one important source of the inhibition to the ICc was shown by studying the effects of inactivating it while recording from the ICc (Li and Kelly, 1992b; Burger and Pollak, 2001).

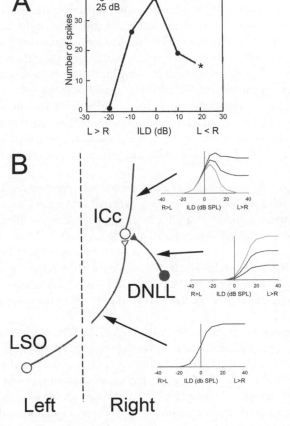

Fig. 12.12 A ILD functions of a cell in the hypertrophied 60-kHz region of the inferior colliculus of the mustache bat. The level of the tone to the contralateral (right) ear was held at 25 dB SPL while the level of the ipsilateral (left) ear was varied from 5–45 dB corresponding to 20 to −20 dB ILD. The *asterisk* shows the monaural contralateral response at 25 dB. (From Park and Pollak, 1993.) **B** A model of how IE responses in the LSO can be converted to E0/f (blue) or 00/f (green) responses in the inferior colliculus.

In the rat, kainic acid lesions of the SOC did not abolish EI sensitivity in the ICc (Li and Kelly, 1992a) and evidence for direct inhibitory input to the ICc suggests that EI sensitivity may also be generated in the ICc itself.

The two general classes of cells, EI and EE, first identified by Goldberg and Brown (1969), have been found at all levels of the ascending auditory system. In the primary auditory cortex these cells are often found clustered together in a patchy or strip-like distribution with columnar bands of EI and EE cells (Imig and Adrian, 1977). In some cases the columns of binaural interaction run perpendicular to the isofrequency lines in the cortex. The bands or clusters of EI and EE cells were correlated with the presence of strong ipsilateral and contralateral cortico-cortical connections, respectively.

A critical parameter of ILD sensitivity is the ILD where the inhibition is effective, usually measured at the level where the response is half-maximal. In terms of azimuthal sensitivity, this would determine the edge of the receptive field with increasing responses in one direction and decreasing responses in the other direction. An obvious parameter of interest is whether there is a spatial map of ILDs as reflected in the point of half-maximal sensitivity. There is compelling evidence in several structures for such a map (see below) but also apparent lack of spatial maps of ILD in many prominent auditory structures.

The earliest description of such a map of ILDs was obtained from the superior colliculus (SC), a structure usually associated with visuomotor processing. While the superficial layers of the SC receive visual input, early studies had found cells in the deep and intermediate layers that responded to acoustic stimulation (Gordon, 1973). Moreover, the spatial receptive fields of these cells were in rough alignment with the well-known retinotopic organization in the superficial layers: cells in the rostral pole of the SC had receptive fields located straight ahead of the animal and cells further caudally had receptive fields further laterally in the contralateral sound field. Using dichotic stimulation, deep SC neurons were found to have high BFs, predominantly onset responses, at least in the anesthetized animal, and to derive their spatial receptive fields from ILD sensitivity (Wise and Irvine, 1985). The topography in spatial receptive fields was mirrored by a systematic variation in the border of the ILD function moving from ILDs favoring the ipsilateral side toward those favoring the contralateral side as one moves from rostral to caudal in the SC (Wise and Irvine, 1985). Moreover, cells with peaked facilitatory responses were usually found in the rostral pole of the SC.

In the ICc of the mustached bat there is a hypertrophied region that represents 60 kHz, the second harmonic of the bat echolocation call. EI cells are segregated into a subdivision of the 60 kHz representation and are topographically arrayed according to their ILD sensitivity: dorsal cells are suppressed only when the ipsilateral sound is considerably louder than the contralateral sound, whereas more ventrally located cells are suppressed when the contralateral sound is considerably louder than the ipsilateral sound (Wenstrup *et al.*, 1986). There is the suggestion of a similar topography in the cat ICc, with cells located more caudally having half-maximal cutoffs at ILDs where the ipsilateral sound is louder relative to rostral cells where the reverse is true (Irvine and Gago, 1990).

A question of considerable interest in several studies at the level of the SOC, ICc, and cortex is whether the ILD functions are stable with variations in overall SPL. Usually these experiments have been done by holding the ABI constant. Generally speaking, studies of the variation of ILD sensitivity with changes in overall SPL have found that most cells are not invariant with level in the ICc (Semple and Kitzes, 1987; Irvine and Gago, 1990) or auditory cortex (Irvine *et al.*, 1996).

An additional complication was studied in the SC where several sensory modalities with different coordinate frames have to deal with a common motor system. Not only are the visual receptive fields in the superficial and deep layers of the SC aligned with the auditory and somatosensory receptive fields in the deep and intermediate layers (Gordon, 1973), but also there is a corresponding motor map in the deep layers which is also in alignment. Stimulation of cells in the rostral pole elicits eye movements directed straight ahead, while stimulation more caudally elicits movements into the contralateral fields. This seemed to be a natural substrate for sensorimotor integration in which activation of one or more of the sensory modalities caused activity to be propagated ventrally to the deep layers where an eye or head movement would be made to the corresponding spatial location due to the alignment of the motor map with the sensory ones. However, the alignment of visual and auditory maps would only hold when the eyes and head are directed straight ahead, since the coordinate systems of the two modalities are different. Visual maps are retinotopic while auditory maps are head-centered. Jay and Sparks (1987) showed in the awake behaving monkey that the auditory spatial receptive fields are modulated by eye position, i.e., the auditory receptive field shifted with eye position.

12.4 **Putting ITDs and ILDs together**

As we have seen, most studies have varied either ITDs or ILDs in isolation in order to determine the effectiveness of each cue. While the classical duplex theory implies that the cues are independent and effective over different frequency ranges, we have noted above that the theory only holds for pure tones and not for more natural broadband stimuli. For natural sound sources in free field, both ITD and ILD co-vary in ways that are not captured well by experiments using ABI or that only manipulate a single cue. Furthermore it is difficult to relate these results to spatial sensitivity for sounds in free field since ILD and ITD both vary in a complex way with frequency (Fig. 12.1).

With the virtual space technique, it is possible to simulate free field broadband sounds through earphones by stimulating the subject with the convolution of the HRTFs (Fig. 12.1) with a broadband stimulus. Additionally, the cues can be manipulated by holding one or more cue constant while varying the other(s).

Figure 12.13 shows responses from the same LSO neuron (Tollin and Yin, 2002a) as in Fig. 12.11 stimulated with 200-ms duration broadband sounds filtered by the HRTFs to simulate a sound source in free field varying in azimuth from –90 (ipsilateral sound field) to +90 degrees. In Fig. 12.13A and B the responses are shown as dot rasters. Azimuth is varied in 9-degree steps and the 20 trials at each virtual azimuthal position are plotted between tic marks on the y-axis with stimulus onset at 0 ms. The response of the LSO neuron to binaural stimulation shows the expected shape of the spatial receptive field (Fig. 12.13A and C, filled circles): it peaks in the ipsilateral sound field near the pinna axis where the excitatory input is maximal, and is suppressed strongly in the contralateral sound field where the inhibition dominates. By turning off the input

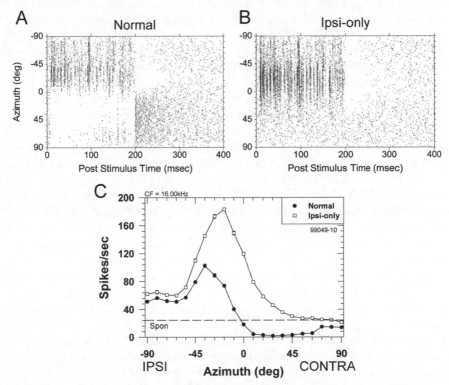

Fig. 12.13 Responses of an LSO neuron to ILDs of virtual space stimuli simulating stimuli varying in azimuth in the frontal sound field. **A** Dot rasters showing responses to the virtual space stimuli varying in azimuth (*ordinate*) as a function of time (*abscissa*) with binaural stimulation. Stimulus was turned on at time 0 for a duration of 200 ms. **B** Same format as in **A** but with the stimulus to the contralateral ear turned off. **C** Plots of the responses in **A** and **B** as a function of azimuth. (From Tollin and Yin, 2002a.)

to the contralateral ear, it is possible to see the influence of the inhibitory input in suppressing responses when the sound source is in the contralateral sound field (Fig. 12.13B). In the LSO the contribution of the contralateral ear appears to be purely inhibitory as the binaural response is never greater than the ipsilateral alone response. The inhibition provides a strong suppression of the response in the contralateral sound field which sharpens the border of the receptive field.

As described above, studies using the average binaural intensity method have tried to simulate natural changes in ILD by linearly increasing the level to one ear while decreasing by the same amount to the other ear. The large variation in discharge rate when only the ipsilateral ear is stimulated is presumably due to the particular interaction of the shape of the HRTF at the CF of the cell (Fig. 12.13C, open circles) and shows the necessity of using the virtual space technique for simulating natural stimuli.

Using the virtual space technique it is also possible to explore the relative potency of the three localization cues by manipulating each cue independently while keeping the other cues constant (Tollin and Yin, 2002b). Usually when cues are kept constant, those appropriate for the position straight ahead are used (ITD = 0, or ILD = 0, spectra corresponding to the straight ahead position). For example, to explore the importance of ITD as a cue to localization along the azimuthal dimension, one can either vary ITDs while keeping the other cues constant (Δ-ITD condition) or set ITDs to zero (0-ITD condition) while letting the other cues vary naturally for different azimuthal positions. To implement the ΔITD condition, Tollin and Yin (2002b) varied the onset of the HRTF signal to one ear relative to the other with values appropriate to different azimuthal positions while keeping the ILD and spectra constant appropriate to the straight-ahead position. If ITDs were a potent cue for localization, then this manipulation would be expected to cause little difference in the perceived location. On the other hand, if ITDs play only a small role, then this manipulation will dramatically disrupt localization performance. Similarly one can set ITDs to be zero, equivalent to the straight-ahead position, by eliminating the difference in the time of onset of the signal to the two ears while letting the ILDs and spectral differences vary naturally with azimuthal position.

Figure 12.14 shows the responses of an LSO cell to manipulations in localization cues. The curves labeled 'Normal' show the responses to a full complement of HRTFs, i.e., they reflect its spatial receptive field. Figure 12.14A shows that when the ITD cue is set to zero while ILDs and spectra are varied ('0-ITD' condition), the cell's response is virtually unchanged from 'Normal'. In contrast, when ITDs are varied while ILDs and spectra are kept constant ('Δ-ITD' condition), the modulation with azimuth disappears. Similar changes are seen when the spectra (here labeled interaural spectral difference or ISD) are manipulated (Fig. 12.14B). Both of these sets of manipulations strongly suggest that neither ITD nor spectra are playing important roles in the azimuthal sensitivity seen in the 'Normal' condition. If this is true, then it must be that ILD is the major determinant of azimuthal sensitivity. This is demonstrated in Fig. 12.14C where the 'Normal' and 'Δ-ILD' conditions are nearly identical while the '0-ILD' condition shows no modulation.

While different LSO cells showed different degrees of modulation with the cue manipulations illustrated in Fig. 12.14, the same general result was found for the population of 24 cells studied (Tollin and Yin, 2002b). The results were quantified by computing the RMS error between each cue manipulation condition and the 'Normal' condition, which is shown as the 'Error' in Fig. 12.14. Overall, the mean RMS error was largest in the 0-ILD condition and smallest in the Δ-ILD condition of the three conditions in which only one cue was varied. These results show the dominant role of ILD in determining the sensitivity of LSO cells to azimuthal localization cues and by elimination the diminished role of ITDs and spectra. Similar studies using cue manipulation in the SC showed that ITDs were not an effective cue (Campbell *et al.*, 2006).

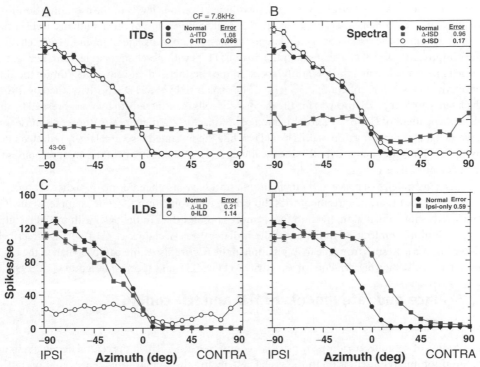

Fig. 12.14 Spatial receptive fields in azimuth for an LSO cell (CF = 7.8 kHz) to cue manipulations of the HRTFs. In all graphs the 'Normal' (*filled circles*) response is that recorded with all localization cues varied naturally. **A** ITD manipulations. Responses obtained when the ITD cue was varied normally (Δ-ITD) while ILD and spectra were kept constant are shown by *filled squares*, while responses when the ITD cue was held constant (0-ITD) are shown by *open circles*. **B** Spectral manipulations. Analogous manipulations as in **A** except the spectral cue was manipulated. **C** ILD manipulations. Same as in **A** except ILD was manipulated. **D** Comparison of the 'Normal' and ipsilateral stimulus alone responses. (From Tollin and Yin, 2002b.)

However, a caveat in drawing the conclusion that only ILDs are pertinent to LSO cells in the experiment of Tollin and Yin (2002b) is that the stimuli were long duration (200 ms) wide band noise. We have argued above that the specializations seen in the LSO circuitry may arise from the need to handle the transient stimuli which may be more common in our environment. Several studies have shown an important role for ITDs for transient stimuli (Park *et al.*, 1996; Irvine *et al.*, 2001). Because of the small anechoic room in which the measurements were made, the HRTFs in the Musicant *et al.* (1990) study are not valid for frequencies below 2 kHz and are filtered, so there is minimal energy at those frequencies where ITDs are most effective.

In Jeffress' (1948) classic work, he suggested the possibility that sensitivity to ILDs might arise through the changes in timing of responses that naturally occur when the level of a sound is varied, the so-called latency hypothesis. Under this formulation the changes in level of sound to either ear will cause either shorter (at high levels) or longer (at low levels) latencies for the excitatory and inhibitory postsynaptic potentials to reach the binaural cell. The variation of latency with sound level is normally in the order of several milliseconds, well above the ITDs naturally encountered in HRTFs. ILD sensitivity then depends upon coincidence of excitation and inhibition with a coincidence window of several milliseconds. Support for this latency hypothesis has been reported by a number of investigators working at various levels of the ascending auditory system (Yin *et al.*, 1985; Park *et al.*, 1996). In the most complete test of the hypothesis, Irvine *et al.* (2001) measured the actual changes in latency of the excitatory ipsilateral input of LSO cells and then imposed those latency changes in the form of ITDs with no changes in level or eliminated those ITDs while keeping the level differences. In the anesthetized rat using click stimuli the ILD sensitivity of a small number of neurons could be explained by the ITD sensitivity, thereby fitting the latency hypothesis. However, for the majority of cells the ILD sensitivity was governed by the SPL independent of ITD or by a combination of both factors. Using tones, the onset response was governed for a higher fraction of cells by ITDs, while the sustained response largely reflected relative levels. Thus the latency hypothesis contributes to the ILD sensitivity of the onset responses in the LSO, but this is not the only factor.

Studies using virtual space and cue manipulation have also been done in higher centers. In general, the results are in agreement with those done with tones or noise. For example, in the ICc many cells show binaural interaction that is more complex than in the SOC with mixed facilitation and inhibition from stimulation of the ipsilateral ear (Delgutte *et al.*, 1999), as described above for tones. Results from cue manipulation in the ICc are also more complex than in the LSO, with many cells showing evidence of sensitivity to ITD, ILD, and spectra (Delgutte *et al.*, 1999).

12.5 Place and rate models of ITD and ILD coding

12.5.1 Place code

The coding of stimulus attributes by place is a common mechanism in the central nervous system. The retinotopic representation in the visual system and the somatotopic representation in the somatosensory system are two examples. In the auditory system, cochleotopic representation of frequency is seen in all major ascending structures including the auditory cortex. A place coding of sound localization by ITDs was proposed 60 years ago by Jeffress (1948). Through an array of coincidence detectors each with its own set of neural delay lines from each ear that offset the acoustic delays created between the ears from a sound source along the azimuthal plane, an interaural time code (ITD) was transformed into a place code for sound localization (Fig. 12.15). Many of the anatomical and physiological features of the MSO and its inputs have been found to be consistent with the Jeffress model (Goldberg and Brown, 1969; Yin and Chan, 1990; Smith *et al.*, 1993; Spitzer and Semple, 1995; Batra *et al.*, 1997b; Joris *et al.*, 1998; Beckius *et al.*, 1999).

Jeffress postulated an array of coincidence detectors (tertiary fibers) on the left and right side of the brain (Fig. 12.15, 1–7 and 7–1) that receive inputs from each cochlear nucleus (secondary fibers). These inputs form a ladder-like pattern such that each coincidence detector receives a different combination of neural delays from each side. These are reflected as different path lengths. So, for example, the path lengths for detector 4 on each side are equal and this detector would then respond optimally to a sound directly in front of the animal. In contrast, detector 1 on each side would respond optimally to a sound in the contralateral sound field since the contralateral path length is longer than the ipsilateral. Thus the difference in neural path length compensates for the difference in acoustic path length. Detectors 5–7 would respond to sound source locations in the ipsilateral sound field. Since experimental evidence indicates that each MSO prefers delays of sounds in the contralateral sound field, detectors 5–7 on each side of the Jeffress model are not necessary.

Another possible source of internal delay lines is the traveling wave in the cochlea. Because the traveling wave starts at the basal, high frequency, end of the cochlea and propagates to the apical end, the latency for low frequency auditory fibers is longer than for higher frequency fibers. While the inputs to any MSO cell appears to derive from bushy cells of similar frequency, even small

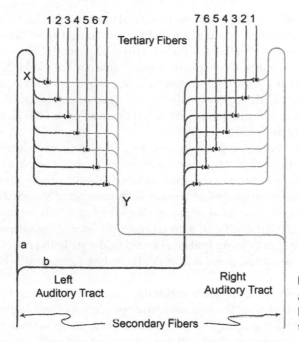

Fig. 12.15 Jeffress delay line as a mechanism for the localization of low frequency tones. (From Jeffress, 1948.)

differences in frequency (e.g., 0.2 octaves for frequencies between 250 and 2500 Hz) can produce substantial delays (e.g., 400 µs) (Joris *et al.*, 2006). Although it is reasonable to assume that the binaural comparator may receive inputs from neurons tuned to slightly different frequencies, there are problems with proposing that cochlear delays are the sole source of internal delay lines. For example, to account for the contralateral bias in MSO cells, the disparate frequency inputs would have to be always in the same direction (Joris *et al.*, 2006).

In mammals the best evidence for a place code for sound location is in the deep layers of the superior colliculus (Palmer and King, 1982; Wise and Irvine, 1985). The map in the superior colliculus appears to be based on ILDs, with no evidence of ITD processing in this structure. It is perhaps understandable that a place code has not been shown in the ICc and thalamus because of the complex geometry of these structures. However, there is also no evidence in the auditory cortex for a place representation for sound location (e.g., Brugge *et al.*, 1996; Middlebrooks *et al.*, 1998). These studies found that although neurons in the auditory cortex preferred sounds presented in the contralateral sound field, this preference was modest and could vanish with increases in the intensity of the sound source. Such features are not consistent with a place code mechanism or behavioral performance. The spatial tuning was sharper and the effect of sound intensity was weaker when anesthesia was not a factor (Mickey and Middlebrooks, 2003), but still there was no support for a place code.

12.5.2 Rate code

Rate models of sound localization commonly involve comparison of activity in a structure on one side of the brain with the activity of the equivalent structure on the other side (von Bekesy, 1930; van Bergeijk, 1962). Such count comparison models received little attention but were recently resurrected as a mechanism for low frequency sound location in the ICc of the guinea pig, where there appears to be a relationship between a neuron's best ITD and its characteristic frequency (McAlpine *et al.*, 2001). Moreover, the peaks of the ITD functions were considered to be outside the range that the guinea pig would naturally encounter (estimated to be ±150 but later measured at ±330 μs) (Sterbing *et al.*, 2003) and there was a dearth of neurons tuned to a midline source (i.e., 0-ITD). These features are not compatible with the Jeffress place model. However, the medial slope of the ITD functions, independent of characteristic frequency, fell within the physiological range of the guinea pig and showed rapid changes in response rate with ITD (also see Skottun *et al.*, 2001). Brand *et al.* (2002) provided evidence in the MSO of gerbils that inhibitory mechanisms could shift the peaks of the ITD functions so that the steep part of this function is within the physiological range of the animal.

One way that a rate code could be used to derive the exact location of the sound source would be to compare the activity of the relevant neurons on each side of the brain. A pitfall of this scheme is that lesions of the auditory structures above the SOC on one side create sound localization deficits in the contralateral, but not the ipsilateral sound field (Jenkins and Merzenich, 1984; Malhotra *et al.*, 2004). Removing the comparison structure should lead to deficits in both sound fields. However, Stecker *et al.* (2005) showed that in the cat auditory cortex of one side, neurons preferring sounds from the contralateral and ipsilateral sound field were both present, albeit biased for those tuned to the contralateral sound field. A similar finding is presented in Fig. 12.9 for the rabbit.

This dual representation alleviates the requirement that the comparisons be across the brain hemispheres. Furthermore, Las *et al.* (2008) have found a larger percentage of ipsilaterally tuned neurons in the anterior ectosylvian sulcus (AES) of the anesthetized cat as well as relatively high proportions of cells tuned to the frontal hemifield in the posterior aspect of the AES. On the other hand, while computations indicate that a count comparison or opponent channel code is feasible (Stecker *et al.*, 2005), neurons that actually do this computation have not been demonstrated in the cortex. The place code versus a rate code mechanism for sound localization is far from resolved (Joris and Yin, 2007).

12.6 **Cortical representation of auditory space**

Despite the paucity of evidence for a systematic map of auditory space at the level of the auditory cortex, it is nonetheless clear from studies with selective lesions of the cortex that the cortex is important for the representation of auditory space. One of the clearest examples is from Jenkins and Merzenich (1984) who showed that a unilateral lesion of the auditory cortex in cats led to a selective loss of sound localization ability in the contralateral sound field and that this loss could show frequency selectivity when specific tonotopic bands were lesioned. More recently this methodology has been improved by using selective cooling of cortical areas using small cryoloops, which has the big advantage of being able to rewarm the cortex so that comparisons can be made between responses before and after inactivation of the cortical area (Malhotra *et al.*, 2004).

In studies of the extrastriate visual cortex a major unifying theme has been the concept of two divergent streams emerging from the primary visual area: a dorsal 'where' and a ventral 'what' stream (Ungerleider and Mishkin, 1982). A number of studies show evidence for a similar organization in the auditory system. Physiological recordings (Tian *et al.*, 2001) and anatomical tract tracing (Romanski *et al.*, 1999) in anesthetized monkeys suggest the possibility of two pathways emanating from the caudal and rostral divisions of the auditory cortex and projecting to spatial and non-spatial regions, respectively, in the prefrontal cortex. Perhaps the most convincing evidence of 'what' and 'where' streams comes from a behavioral double dissociation experiment in the cat in which the effects of reversible cooling of the posterior auditory field (PAF) and anterior auditory field (AAF) were shown to affect a spatial localization task and a temporal pattern discrimination task, respectively (Lomber and Malhotra, 2008). Cooling of the PAF produced deficits in localization but not pattern discrimination, while cooling of the AAF had the opposite effect. The dramatic and clearcut results from the cryoloop, reversible lesion study are not reflected as clearly in physiological recordings from the same areas in cats or homologous areas in monkeys. One of the reasons for this might be that most cortical physiological studies are not done in awake behaving animals where the effects of anesthesia and behavioral state are likely to be important.

Acknowledgements

It is a pleasure to acknowledge the many wonderful colleagues who did the bulk of the work in our laboratories over many years. These studies would not have been possible without the hard work and seminal contributions of Ranjan Batra, Theo Buunen, Laurel Carney, Joseph Chan, Bill D'Angelo, Bertrand Delgutte, Doug Fitzpatrick, Lew Haberly, Philip Joris, Doug Oliver, Mike Ostapoff, Phil Smith, Terry Stanford, Joseph Syka, Susanne Sterbing-D'Angelo, Dan Tollin, and Robert Wickesberg. Our laboratories were supported by funding from NIH for many years from grants NS12732, EY02606, DC0016, DC02840, DC01366, and DC002178, for which we are very grateful.

References

Aitkin LM (1973) Medial geniculate body of the cat: responses to tonal stimuli of neurons in the medial division. *J Neurophysiol* **36**: 275–83.

Barnes-Davies M, Forsythe ID (1995) Pre- and postsynaptic glutamate receptors at a giant excitatory synapse in rat auditory brainstem slices. *J Physiol* **488**(2): 387–406.

Batra R, Kuwada S, Fitzpatrick DC (1997a) Sensitivity to interaural temporal disparities of low- and high-frequency neurons in the superior olivary complex. I. Heterogeneity of responses. *J Neurophysiol* **78**: 1222–36.

Batra R, Kuwada S, Fitzpatrick DC (1997b) Sensitivity to interaural temporal disparities of low- and high-frequency neurons in the superior olivary complex. II. Coincidence detection. *J Neurophysiol* **78**: 1237–47.

Beckius GE, Batra R, Oliver DL (1999) Axons from anteroventral cochlear nucleus that terminate in medial superior olive of cat: observations related to delay lines. *J Neurosci* **19**: 3146–61.

Bernstein LR (2001) Auditory processing of interaural timing information: new insights. *J Neurosci Res* **66**: 1035–46.

Bernstein LR, Trahiotis C (2002) Enhancing sensitivity to interaural delays at high frequencies by using "transposed stimuli". *J Acoust Sci Am* **112**: 1026–36.

Boudreau JC, Tsuchitani C (1968) Binaural interaction in the cat superior olive S segment. *J Neurophysiol* **31**: 442–54.

Brand A, Behrend O, Marquardt T, McAlpine D, Grothe B (2002) Precise inhibition is essential for microsecond interaural time difference coding. *Nature* **417**: 543–7.

Brugge JF, Anderson DJ, Aitkin LM (1970) Responses of neurons in the dorsal nucleus of the lateral lemniscus of cat to binaural tonal stimulation. *J Neurophysiol* **33**: 441–58.

Brugge JF, Reale RA, Hind JE (1996) The structure of spatial receptive field of neurons in primary auditory cortex of the cat. *J Neurosci* **16**: 4420–37.

Brungart DS, Rabinowitz WM (1999) Auditory localization of nearby sources. Head-related transfer functions. *J Acoust Soc Am* **106**: 1465–79.

Brunso-Bechtold JK, Thompson GC, Masterton, RB (1981) HRP study of the organization of auditory afferents ascending to central nucleus of inferior colliculus of the cat. *J Comp Neurol* **197**: 705–22.

Buell TN, Trahiotis C, Bernstein LR (1991) Lateralization of low-frequency tones: relative potency of gating and ongoing interaural delays. *J Acoust Soc Am* **90**: 3077–85.

Burger RM, Pollak GD (2001) Reversible inactivation of the dorsal nucleus of the lateral lemniscus reveals its role in the processing of multiple sound sources in the inferior colliculus of bats. *J Neurosci* **21**: 4830–43.

Campbell RA, Doubell TP, Nodal FR, Schnupp JW, King AJ (2006) Interaural timing cues do not contribute to the map of space in the ferret superior colliculus: a virtual acoustic space study. *J Neurophysiol* **95**: 242–54.

Cant NB, Casseday JH (1986) Projections from the anteroventral cochlear nucleus to the lateral and medial superior olivary nuclei. *J Comp Neurol* **247**: 447–76.

Cant NB, Hyson RL (1992) Projections from the lateral nucleus of the trapezoid body to the medial superior olivary nucleus in the gerbil. *Hearing Res* **58**: 26–34.

Colburn HS, Durlach NI (1978) Models of binaural interaction. In: Handbook of Perception, Volume IV, Hearing (eds Carterette EC, Friedman MP), pp. 467–518. Academic Press, New York.

D'Angelo WR, Sterbing SJ, Ostapoff EM, Kuwada S (2005) Role of GABAergic inhibition in the coding of interaural time differences of low-frequency sounds in the inferior colliculus. *J Neurophysiol* **93**: 3390–400.

Delgutte B, Joris PX, Litovsky RY, Yin TCT (1999) Receptive fields and binaural interactions for virtual-space stimuli in the cat inferior colliculus. *J Neurophysiol* **81**: 2833–51.

Durlach NI, Colburn HS (1978) Binaural phenomena. In: Handbook of Perception, Volume IV, Hearing (eds Carterette EC, Friedman MP), pp. 365–466. Academic Press, New York.

Finlayson PG, Caspary DM (1991) Low-frequency neurons in the lateral superior olive exhibit phase-sensitive binaural inhibition. *J Neurophysiol* **65**: 598–605.

Fitzpatrick DC, Batra R, Stanford TR, Kuwada S (1997) A neuronal population code for sound localization. *Nature* **388**: 871–4.

Fitzpatrick DC, Kuwada S, Batra R (2000) Neural sensitivity to interaural time differences: beyond the Jeffress model. *J Neurosci* **20**: 1605–15.

Fitzpatrick DC, Kuwada S, Batra R (2002) Transformations in processing interaural time differences between the superior olivary complex and inferior colliculus: beyond the Jeffress model. *Hear Res* **168**: 79–89.

Glendenning KK, Masterton RB (1983) Acoustic chiasm: efferent projections of the lateral superior olive. *J Neurosci* **3**: 1521–37.

Glendenning KK, Brunso-Bechtold JK, Thompson GC, Masterton RB (1981) Ascending auditory afferents to the nuclei of the lateral lemniscus. *J Comp Neurol* **197**: 673–703.

Glendenning KK, Baker BN, Hutson KA, Masterton RB (1992) Acoustic chiasm V: inhibition and excitation in the ipsilateral and contralateral projections of LSO. *J Comp Neurol* **319**: 100–22.

Goldberg JM, Brown PB (1968) Functional organization of the dog superior olivary complex: an anatomical and electrophysiological study. *J Neurophysiol* **31**: 639–56.

Goldberg JM, Brown PB (1969) Response properties of binaural neurons of dog superior olivary complex to dichotic tonal stimuli: some physiological mechanisms of sound localization. *J Neurophysiol* **32**: 613–36.

Gordon B (1973) Receptive fields in deep layers of cat superior colliculus. *J Neurophysiol* **36**: 157–78.

Grothe B, Sanes DH (1993) Bilateral inhibition by glycinergic afferents in the medial superior olive. *J Neurophysiol* **69**: 1192–6.

Harrison JM, Warr WB (1962) A study of the cochlear nuclei and ascending auditory pathways of the medulla. *J Comp Neurol* **119**: 341–80.

Helfert RH, Bonneau JM, Wenthold RJ, Altshsculer RA (1989) GABA and glycine immunoreactivity in the guinea pig superior olivary nucleus. *Brain Res* **501**: 269–86.

Imig TJ, Adrian HO (1977) Binaural columns in the primary field (A1) of cat auditory cortex. *Brain Res* **138**: 241–57.

Irvine DR, Gago G (1990) Binaural interaction in high-frequency neurons in inferior colliculus of the cat: effects of variations in sound pressure level on sensitivity to interaural intensity differences. *J Neurophysiol* **63**: 570–91.

Irvine DR, Rajan R, Aitkin LM (1996) Sensitivity to interaural intensity differences of neurons in primary auditory cortex of the cat. *I*. Types of sensitivity and effects of variations in sound pressure level. *J Neurophysiol* **75**: 75–96.

Irvine DR, Park VN, McCormick L (2001) Mechanisms underlying the sensitivity of neurons in the lateral superior olive to interaural intensity differences. *J Neurophysiol* **86**: 2647–66.

Ivarsson C, De Ribaupierre Y, De Ribaupierre F (1988) Influence of auditory localization cues on neuronal activity in the auditory thalamus of the cat. *J Neurophysiol* **59**: 586–606.

Jay MF, Sparks DL (1987) Sensorimotor integration in the primate superior colliculus. II. Coordinates of auditory signals. *J Neurophysiol* **57**: 35–55.

Jeffress LA (1948) A place code theory of sound localization. *J Comp Physiol Psych* **41**: 35–9.

Jeffress LA, Blodgett HC, Deatherage BH (1962) Effect of interaural correlation on the precision of centering a noise. *J Acoust Soc Am* **34**: 1122–3.

Jenkins WM, Merzenich MM (1984) Role of cat primary auditory cortex for sound-localization behavior. *J Neurophysiol* **52**: 819–47.

Joris PX, Yin TCT (1992) Responses to amplitude-modulated tones in the auditory nerve of the cat. *J Acoust Soc Am* **91**: 215–32.

Joris PX, Yin TC (1995) Envelope coding in the lateral superior olive. I. Sensitivity to interaural time differences. *J Neurophysiol* **73**: 1043–62.

Joris PX, Yin TCT (1998) Envelope coding in the lateral superior olive. III. Comparison with afferent pathways. *J Neurophysiol* **79**: 253–69.

Joris P, Yin TC (2007) A matter of time: internal delays in binaural processing. *Trends Neurosci* **30**: 70–8.

Joris PX, Carney LH, Smith PH, Yin TC (1994) Enhancement of neural synchronization in the anteroventral cochlear nucleus. I. Responses to tones at the characteristic frequency. *J Neurophysiol* **71**: 1022–36.

Joris PX, Smith PH, Yin TC (1998) Coincidence detection in the auditory system: 50 years after Jeffress. *Neuron* **21**: 1235–8.

Joris PX, Van de Sande B, Louage DH, van der Heijden M (2006) Binaural and cochlear disparities. *Proc Natl Acad Sci USA* **103**: 12917–22.

Klumpp R, Eady H (1956) Some measurement of interaural time difference thresholds. *J Acoust Soc Am* **28**: 859–60.

Kudo M, Niimi K (1980) Ascending projections of the inferior colliculus in the cat: an autoradiography study. *J Comp Neurol* **191**: 545–66.

Kuhn G (1977) Model for the interaural time differences in the azimuthal plane. *J Acoust Soc Am* **82**: 157–67.

Kulkarni A, Colburn HS (1998) Role of spectral detail in sound-source localization. *Nature* **396**: 747–9.

Kuwada S, Yin TC, Syka J, Buunen TJ, Wickesberg RE (1984) Binaural interaction in low-frequency neurons in inferior colliculus of the cat. IV. Comparison of monaural and binaural response properties. *J Neurophysiol* **51**: 1306–25.

Kuwada S, Batra R, Stanford TR (1989) Monaural and binaural response properties of neurons in the inferior colliculus of the rabbit: effects of sodium pentobarbital. *J Neurophysiol* **61**: 269–82.

Kuwada S, Batra R, Yin TCT, Oliver DL, Haberly LB, Stanford TR (1997) Intracellular recordings in response to monaural and binaural stimulation of neurons in the inferior colliculus of the cat. *J Neurosci* **17**: 7565–81.

Kuwada S, Fitzpatrick DC, Batra R, Ostapoff EM (2006) Sensitivity to interaural time differences in the dorsal nucleus of the lateral lemniscus of the unanesthetized rabbit: comparison with other structures. *J Neurophysiol* **95**: 1309–22.

Las L, Shapira AH, Nelken I (2008) Functional gradients of auditory sensitivity along the anterior ectosylvian sulcus of the cat. *J Neurosci* **28**: 3657–67.

Li L, Kelly JB (1992a) Binaural responses in rat inferior colliculus following kainic acid lesions of the superior olive: interaural intensity difference functions. *Hearing Res* **61**: 73–85.

Li L, Kelly JB (1992b) Inhibitory influence of the dorsal nucleus of the lateral lemniscus on binaural responses in the rat's inferior colliculus. *J Neurosci* 12: 4530–9.

Loftus WC, Bishop DC, Saint Marie RL, Oliver DL (2004) Organization of binaural excitatory and inhibitory inputs to the inferior colliculus from the superior olive. *J Comp Neurol* 472: 330–44.

Lomber SG, Malhotra S (2008) Double dissociation of 'what' and 'where' processing in auditory cortex. *Nat Neurosci* 11: 609–16.

Malhotra S, Hall AJ, Lomber SG (2004) Cortical control of sound localization in the cat: unilateral cooling deactivation of 19 cerebral areas. *J Neurophysiol* 92: 1625–43.

McAlpine D, Jiang D, Shackleton TM, Palmer AR (1998) Convergent input from brainstem coincidence detectors onto delay-sensitive neurons in the inferior colliculus. *J Neurosci* 18: 6026–39.

McAlpine D, Jiang D, Palmer AR (2001) A neural code for low-frequency sound localization in mammals. *Nature Neurosci* 4: 396–401.

Mickey BJ, Middlebrooks, JC (2003) Representation of auditory space by cortical neurons in awake cats. *J Neurosci* 23: 8649–63.

Middlebrooks JC, Xu L, Eddins AC, Green D (1998) Codes for sound-source location in nontonotopic auditory cortex. *J Neurophysiol* 80: 863–81.

Mills AW (1960) Lateralization of high-frequency tones. *J Acoust Soc Am* 32: 132–4.

Moore MJ, Caspary DM (1983) Strychnine blocks binaural inhibition in lateral superior olivary neurons. *J Neurosci* 3: 237–42.

Moore RY, Goldberg JM (1963) Ascending projections of the inferior colliculus in the cat. *J Comp Neurol* 121: 109–36.

Morest DK, Oliver DL (1984) The neuronal architecture of the inferior colliculus in the cat: defining the functional anatomy of the auditory midbrain. *J Comp Neurol* 222: 209–36.

Musicant AD, Chan JC, Hind JE (1990) Direction-dependent spectral properties of cat external ear: new data and cross-species comparisons. *J Acous Soc Am* 87: 757–81.

Oertel D (1983) Synaptic responses and electrical properties of cells in brain slices of the mouse anteroventral cochlear nucleus. *J Neurosci B*: 2043–53.

Oliver DL, Kuwada S, Yin TCT, Haberly L, Henkel CK (1991) Dendritic and axonal morphology of HRP-injected neurons in the inferior colliculus of the cat. *J Comp Neurol* 303: 75–100.

Osen KK (1969) Cytoarchitecture of the cochlear nuclei in the cat. *J Comp Neurol* 136: 453–84.

Palmer AR, King AJ (1982) The representation of auditory space in the mammalian superior colliculus. *Nature* 299: 248–9.

Park TJ, Pollak GD (1993) GABA shapes sensitivity to interaural intensity disparities in the mustache bat's inferior colliculus: implications for encoding sound location. *J Neurosci* 13: 2050–67.

Park TJ, Pollak GD (1994) Azimuthal receptive fields are shaped by GABAergic inhibition in the inferior colliculus of the mustache bat. *J Neurophysiol* 72: 1080–102.

Park TJ, Grothe B, Pollak GD, Schuller G, Koch U (1996) Neural delays shape selectivity to interaural intensity differences in the lateral superior olive. *J Neurosci* 16: 6554–66.

Penney GR, Conley M, Schmechel DE, Diamond IT (1984) The distribution of glutamic acid decarboxylase immunoreactivity in the diencephalon of the opposum and rabbit. *J Comp Neurol* 228: 38–56.

Phillips DP, Irvine DR (1983) Some features of binaural input to single neurons in physiologically defined area AI of cat cerebral cortex. *J Neurophysiol* 49: 383–95.

Pollak GD, Burger RM, Park TJ, Klug A, Bauer EE (2002) Roles of inhibition for transforming binaural properties in the brainstem auditory system. *Hear Res* 168: 60–78.

Rayleigh Lord (1907) On our perception of sound direction. *Phil Mag* 3: 456–64.

Rockel AJ, Jones E (1973) The neuronal organization of the inferior colliculus of the adult cat. II. The pericentral nucleus. *J Comp Neurol* 149: 301–34.

Romanski LM, Tian B, Fritz J, Mishkin M, Goldman-Rakic PS, Rauschecker JP (1999) Dual streams of auditory afferents target multiple domains in the primate prefrontal cortex. *Nature Neurosci* 2: 1131–6.

Rose JE, Gross NB, Geisler CD, Hind JE (1966) Some neural mechanisms in the inferior colliculus of the cat which may be relevant to localization of a sound source. *J Neurophysiol* **29**: 288–314.

Saint Marie RL, Ostapoff EM, Morest DK, Wenthold RJ (1989) Glycine-immunoreactive projection of the cat lateral superior olive: possible role in midbrain ear dominance. *J Comp Neurol* **279**: 382–96.

Sanes DH, Rubel EW (1988) The ontogeny of inhibition and excitation in the gerbil lateral superior olive. *J Neurosci* **8**: 682–700.

Semple MN, Kitzes LM (1987) Binaural processing of sound pressure level in the inferior colliculus. *J Neurophysiol* **57**: 1130–147.

Shackleton TM, Skottun BC, Arnott RH, Palmer AR (2003) Interaural time difference discrimination thresholds for single neurons in the inferior colliculus of guinea pigs. *J Neurosci* **23**: 716–24.

Skottun BC, Shackleton TM, Arnott RH, Palmer AR (2001) The ability of inferior colliculus neurons to signal differences in interaural delay. *Proc Natl Acad Sci USA* **98**: 14050–4.

Smith PH, Joris PX, Yin TC (1993) Projections of physiologically characterized spherical bushy cell axons from the cochlear nucleus of the cat: evidence for delay lines to the medial superior olive. *J Comp Neurol* **331**: 245–60.

Spangler KM, Warr WB, Henkel CK (1985) The projections of principal cells of the medial nucleus of the trapezoid body in the cat. *J Comp Neurol* **238**: 249–62.

Spitzer MW, Semple MN (1995) Neurons sensitive to interaural phase disparity in gerbil superior olive: diverse monaural and temporal response properties. *J Neurophysiol* **73**: 1668–90.

Stanford TR, Kuwada S, Batra R (1992) A comparison of the interaural time sensitivity of neurons in the inferior colliculus and thalamus of the unanesthetized rabbit. *J Neurosci* **12**: 3200–16.

Stecker GC, Harrington IA, Middlebrooks JC (2005) Location coding by opponent neural populations in the auditory cortex. *PLoS Biol* **3**: e78.

Sterbing SJ, Hartung K, Hoffmann KP (2003) Spatial tuning to virtual sounds in the inferior colliculus of the guinea pig. *J Neurophysiol* **90**: 2648–59.

Tian B, Reser D, Durham A, Kustov A, Rauschecker JP (2001) Functional specialization in rhesus monkey auditory cortex. *Science* **292**: 290–3.

Tolbert LP, Morest DK, Yurgelun-Todd DA (1982) The neuronal architecture of the anteroventral cochlear nucleus of the cat in the region of the cochlear nerve root: horseradish peroxidase labelling of identified cell types. *Neuroscience* **7**: 3031–52.

Tollin DJ, Yin TC (2002a) The coding of spatial location by single units in the lateral superior olive of the cat. I. Spatial receptive fields in azimuth. *J Neurosci* **22**: 1454–67.

Tollin DJ, Yin TCT (2002b) The coding of spatial location by single units in the lateral superior olive of the cat. II. The determinants of spatial receptive fields in azimuth. *J Neurosci* **22**: 1468–79.

Tollin DJ, Yin TC (2005) Interaural phase and level difference sensitivity in low-frequency neurons in the lateral superior olive. *J Neurosci* **25**: 10648–57.

Ungerleider LG, Mishkin M (1982) Two cortical visual systems. In: Analysis of Visual Behavior (eds Ingle Dj, Goodale ma, Mansfield RJW), pp. 486–549. M.I.T. Press, Cambridge.

van Bergeijk WA (1962) Variation on a theme of Bekesy: a model of binaural interaction. *J Acoust Sci Am* **34**: 1431–7.

von Bekesy G (1930) *Experiments in Hearing*, translated into English 1960 (ed. Wever EG). McGraw-Hill, New York.

Wenstrup JJ, Ross LS, Pollak GD (1986) Binaural response organization within a frequency-band representation of the inferior colliculus: implications for sound localization. *J Neurosci* **6**: 962–73.

Wightman FL, Kistler DJ (1992) The dominant role of low-frequency interaural time differences in sound localization. *J Acoust Soc Am* **91**: 1648–61.

Wise LZ, Irvine DR (1985) Topographic organization of interaural intensity difference sensitivity in deep layers of cat superior colliculus: implications for auditory spatial representation. *J Neurophysiol* **54**: 185–211.

Yin TC, Chan JC (1990) Interaural time sensitivity in medial superior olive of cat. *J Neurophysiol* **64**: 465–88.

Yin TC, Kuwada S (1983a) Binaural interaction in low-frequency neurons in inferior colliculus of the cat. II. Effects of changing rate and direction of interaural phase. *J Neurophysiol* **50**: 1000–119.

Yin TC, Kuwada S (1983b) Binaural interaction in low-frequency neurons in inferior colliculus of the cat. III. Effects of changing frequency. *J Neurophysiol* **50**: 1020–42.

Yin TCT, Hirsch JA, Chan JC (1985) Responses of neurons in the cat's superior colliculus to acoustic stimuli. II. A model of interaural intensity sensitivity. *J Neurophysiol* **53**: 746–58.

Yin TCT, Chan JCK, Carney LH (1987) Effects of interaural time delays of noise stimuli on low-frequency cells in the cat's inferior colliculus. III. Evidence for cross correlation. *J Neurophysiol* **58**: 562–83.

Zwislocki JJ, Feldman RS (1956) Just noticeable dichotic phase difference. *J Acoust Soc Am* **28**: 152–4.

Chapter 13

Sound location: monaural cues and spectral cues for elevation

Bradford J. May

The processes that govern sound localization are traditionally distinguished by their reliance on binaural or monaural directional information. Binaural cues are based on interaural time and level differences (ITDs and ILDs) that reflect the horizontal position, or azimuth (AZ), of a sound source. Monaural cues are derived from the effects of elevation (EL), or front-back locations, on the spectral filtering properties of the head-related transfer function (HRTF: the filter shape describing the transformation of a free-field sound to energy at the tympanic membrane). Although both forms of localization must merge to evoke a coherent spatial identity, this chapter focuses on the acoustic cues, perceptual behaviors, and physiological mechanisms that relate most directly to monaural sound localization.

An extensive literature defines the domain of monaural sound localization not by listening contexts, where spectral information contributes to directional hearing, but by instances where binaural cues are assumed to be least effective. Important areas of research include monaural deafness, ear occlusion, locations in the median plane, and virtual sound fields where cue strength is manipulated under closed-field conditions. In keeping with those conventions, this chapter will use the term 'monaural localization' to differentiate spectral processing from binaural comparisons of ITD and ILD cues that are described elsewhere in this book (see Chapter12). Ample psychoacoustic and physiological evidence suggests that binaural and monaural localization pathways converge within the central auditory system to enhance spatial tuning in the dimensions of both elevation and azimuth. Consequently, once spatial representations exit the auditory brainstem, it is an oversimplification to regard any localization process as functionally independent, or exclusively monaural.

This chapter begins by summarizing the acoustic basis of monaural sound localization (section 13.2). Human HRTFs describe the rich content of monaural spectral information that exists at high frequencies, changes rapidly with location, and is easily distorted by acoustic probes. The reliability of measurements of these acoustic phenomena is verified by our ability to create the illusion of directionality by synthesizing HRTF-based filtering effects under closed-field conditions. Directional transfer functions (DTFs) move beyond absolute physical specifications of the HRTF to emphasize the spectral information that is uniquely associated with spatial locations. These statistically defined directional properties often predict perceptual experience more accurately than absolute localization cues.

The psychoacoustic factors that shape spatial hearing are explored in detail in section 13.3. Plugging one ear, distorting the acoustic properties of the pinna, or altering the spectral content of auditory stimuli induces systematic errors that help isolate the meaningful dimensions of sound and the mechanisms for encoding directional information.

The ascending auditory representations of spectral cues for sound localization are followed as they change from generalized population codes in the auditory nerve (section 13.4) to directionally sensitive neural integration patterns in the dorsal cochlear nucleus (section 13.5) and on to spatially tuned receptive fields in the inferior colliculus (section 13.6). The functional implications of these transformations are examined by comparing basic response properties, spatial tuning, and the impact of surgical lesions on the major nuclei of the auditory brainstem. The concept of a spectral processing pathway is introduced as an organizing principle for this extensive literature.

Laboratory experiments in domestic cats are a rich source of evidence for the existence of an auditory pathway that is dedicated to the processing of monaural localization cues. The Conclusions (section 13.7) point out some important qualifications of this influential animal model, then propose new directions for research on monaural localization and spectral processing.

13.2 **The acoustic basis of monaural sound localization**

When a measuring instrument is applied to any physical event, the presence of the device alters the properties to be observed. This 'observer effect' can be minimized by calibrating the instrument, which is simply knowing *a priori* the nature of the distortion and removing it from the computed signal. These principles apply to any physical system, including how the brain derives the elevation of a sound from spectral alterations that are introduced by the outer ear.

When sound propagates to the eardrum, it is shaped by the filtering properties of the HRTF. The HRTF describes the linear alteration of the sound's amplitude and phase spectrum by the reflective, dispersive, and diffractive properties of the torso, head, and pinna (Kuhn, 1987). The resulting patterns of interference combine to increase and decrease sound energy entering the ear canal. The constructive or destructive nature of the interference is determined by the wavelength of the sound and the angle of incidence upon which it reaches the ear; consequently, the spectral shape of the HRTF changes with the direction of the sound source. Psychoacoustic studies in human observers and physiological studies in animals suggest that specialized neurons in the central auditory pathways are endowed with the capacity to decode the directionality of this spectral information.

13.2.1 **Head-related transfer functions**

Early detailed descriptions of the HRTF were provided by Wiener and Ross (1946), who obtained their acoustic data by inserting a miniaturized probe microphone deeply into the ear canal of human subjects. Directional filtering effects were determined by calculating the gain in sound pressure near the eardrum relative to the source spectrum in free field. Examples of their measures are presented in Fig. 13.1, which compares the average gain of adult men at three locations in the interaural horizontal plane.

Positive gains are observed at all but a few frequencies because the funnel-shaped outer ear acts as a sound collector. Signal levels are increased by almost 20 dB at frequencies between 2 and 5 kHz, where the resonances of the ear canal and the surrounding concha are most effective (Shaw, 1974). A similar gain profile is observed at the three locations. These monaural acoustic properties, therefore, exert stronger influences on signal detection than localization.

Two-directional patterns may be isolated from the HRTF shapes in Fig. 13.1. Higher gains are observed when the location of the sound source moves from in front of the observer (0° AZ) to opposite the ear with the probe microphone (90°AZ). The increase is produced by a lessening of the head's sound shadow; that is, the obstructive influence of head reflections. The contralateral ear would show lower gains because the same movement would increase head shadowing.

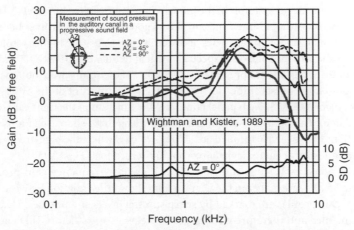

Fig. 13.1 Gain of the head-related transfer function at three azimuths (AZs) in the horizontal plane. Each function represents the average of 6–12 adult men. Variations between subjects are indicated by the standard deviation (SD) at 0° AZ (*bottom*). More recent measures are represented by the 0° AZ function of Wightman and Kistler (1989b) (*red*). (Adapted from Wiener and Ross, 1946.)

The resulting interaural level difference (ILD) is an important binaural cue for localization in the horizontal plane.

A second directional cue is communicated by changes in spectral shape. As the sound source moves through space, each location is associated with a unique maximum gain. The frequency of the prominent null at 0° AZ is similarly affected by changes in elevation that are not shown here. Because these spectral peaks and notches are only fully represented in broadband sounds, sound localization accuracy is altered by manipulations of stimulus bandwidth (Butler and Flannery, 1980; Flannery and Butler, 1981). Locations in the median vertical plane minimize binaural disparity cues, making narrowband sounds virtually impossible to localize (Blauert, 1969/1970; Middlebrooks and Green, 1992).

The consistency of HRTF-based localization cues across human subjects is indicated by standard deviations (SDs) at the bottom of Fig. 13.1. The statistical analysis was applied to HRTFs from different subjects at the same location (0° AZ). Individual differences are small at low frequencies, but progressively increase at high frequencies. The variability at high frequencies arises from individualized features of the HRTF resulting from differences in the size and shape of the head and ears (Middlebrooks, 1999b), as well as the difficulties of acoustic measures (Wightman and Kistler, 1989b).

Early recordings of the human HRTF provided faithful descriptions of low-frequency directional effects, but were limited by existing sampling techniques to frequencies well below the upper bounds of human hearing. Often, the transfer functions were discretely sampled with pure tones. This combined lack of content and resolution obscured the perceptual significance of sharp spectral features that populate high frequencies of the HRTF.

Modern sampling procedures have expanded the characterization of the HRTF at high frequencies. Psychoacoustic validation is a defining characteristic of these recent studies (Wightman and Kistler, 1989a). The process of validation proceeds in three stages (Wightman *et al.*, 1987). The directional properties of the HRTF are measured in free field. They are imposed upon headphone stimuli to simulate directional properties. Then, the fidelity of the 'virtual sound field' is verified by asking subjects to identify the perceived free-field location of the synthetic stimuli.

Figure 13.1 also provides an example of the modern description of the human HRTF (Wightman and Kistler, 1989a, b). Although the function shows good agreement with earlier recordings at lower frequencies, it deviates at frequencies above 2.5 kHz because the higher resolution characterization reveals the presence of a deep spectral notch at frequencies between 7 and 10 kHz.

The HRTFs of three subjects are presented in Fig. 13.2. These results were obtained by presenting pseudorandom noise bursts at locations that ranged from in front of the observer (0° AZ) to behind the observer (180° AZ). Each panel compares the function of the right ear (solid line) and left ear (dashed line). The right ear is the near ear for the lateralized source locations (45° and 135° AZ). The functions have been partitioned at 2.5 kHz, which is where the high-frequency measures of Wightman and Kistler begin to deviate from earlier recordings (Fig. 13.1).

As previously noted by Wiener and Ross (1946), the low-frequency gain profiles rise to a maximum near 2.5 kHz, are higher in the near ear, and show little variation between subjects. The high-frequency gain profiles are marked by sharp spectral peaks and notches. Head-shadowing effects are augmented and therefore yield larger ILD cues. Contradictory ILD cues are created when a spectral notch decreases gain in the near ear or a spectral peak increases gain in the far ear. Individuals show clear differences in these spectral features.

When Wightman and Kistler (1989a) validated their acoustic measures with headphone stimuli, localization errors in the azimuth dimension only slightly exceeded those for natural sounds. By contrast, the subjects exhibited front-back confusions and displayed elevation responses that were inaccurate and variable. Similar patterns of error can be produced with free-field stimuli by

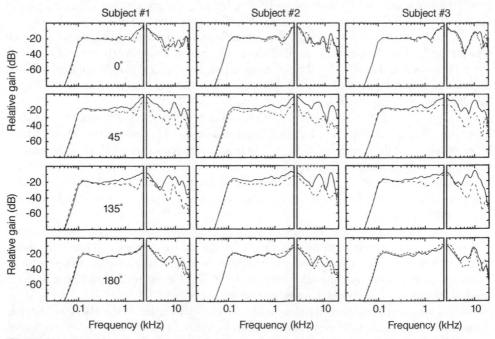

Fig. 13.2 Head-related transfer functions for three subjects at four azimuths in the horizontal plane. *Numerical labels* state sound source azimuth. *Solid curves* indicate responses from each subject's right ear (near the speaker). *Dashed curves* show responses from the left ear. The functions are separated at 2.5 kHz to emphasize inter-subject differences at high frequencies. (Adapted from Wightman et al., 1987.)

narrowing stimulus bandwidth (Blauert, 1969/1970; Oldfield and Parker, 1986), suggesting that the simulations failed to capture the full complement of spectral cues for sound localization.

13.2.2 **Directional transfer functions**

A directional transfer function (DTF) reveals the dynamic spectral cues that are associated with changing sound source locations. It is the spectral shape that remains after non-directional components, such as the large 2.5-kHz ear canal resonance (Figs 13.1 and 13.2), are removed from the HRTF by statistical methods (Middlebrooks and Green, 1990). The DTF is calculated by dividing the spectrum that reaches the ear canal from a particular location by the average ear-canal spectrum for many sampled locations. What remains are the unique spectral features that distinguish the individual HRTF from 'non-directional' properties of the outer ear and distortions that are introduced by the acoustic measurement.

Figure 13.3 illustrates how the HRTF and DTF are differentially affected by microphone placement. Two probe microphones have been placed in the proximal and distal ear canal of a human subject. The unprocessed magnitude spectra in Fig. 13.3A differ by as much as 24 dB between the recording sites. These pressure differences are produced by standing waves in the ear canal that may cancel or amplify select wavelengths according to insertion depth. This non-directional component would be retained if the raw microphone recordings were divided by the source spectrum to create the HRTF.

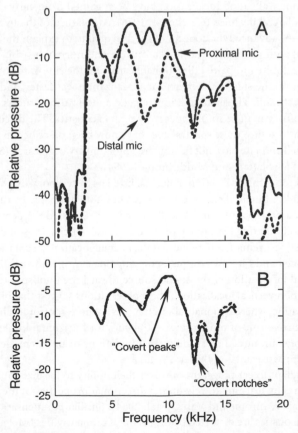

Fig. 13.3 Effects of microphone position on measures of outer ear acoustics. **A** Unprocessed spectra recorded from two microphones with 9-mm separation in the ear canal. The source was broadband noise at 0° AZ, 0° EL. **B** Directional transfer functions derived by dividing the microphone responses by the stimulus spectrum and the common transfer function (see text). Localized gains well above or below the common transfer function are known as covert peaks and notches. (Adapted from Middlebrooks and Green, 1990.)

The DTFs in Fig. 13.3B illustrate the effects of removing the common elements of the transfer function from the disparate HRTFs. The remaining directional components are virtually identical. Unlike the deep spectral notch at 7–10 kHz in the HRTF of Wightman and Kistler (Fig. 13.1), the DTF exhibits a prominent peak at the same frequencies. These differences exist because the spectral notch is a non-directional component that is eliminated when the microphone recording is divided by the common transfer function. Frontal locations have smaller than average notches yielding a 'covert' peak after calculation of the DTF. These subtle acoustic features exert powerful effects on the perception of sound location (Musicant and Butler, 1984b). Consequently, the directional cues conveyed by the HRTF must be evaluated in relation to the global statistics of the transfer functions and then confirmed with perceptual measures. This process typically involves altering localization behavior by manipulating the acoustic properties of auditory stimuli.

13.3 Acoustic manipulations of the spectral processing pathway

Multiple sources of sensory information come together to create the spatial identity of the events that impact our auditory experience. To isolate the critical role of monaural sound localization, veritical directional cues are altered by manipulating the acoustic properties of the ear or the spectral content of the stimulus. The perceptual significance of spectral information is demonstrated by ensuing errors in localization behavior.

13.3.1 Altering the acoustic properties of the outer ear

Informative descriptions of monaural sound localization have been gained from early clinical assessments of humans with unilateral deafness (Gatehouse, 1976). At the turn of the twentieth century, Angell and Fite (1901a, b) advanced the concept of spectral quality to explain the localization abilities of an individual with profound deafness in one ear and normal hearing in the other. Although the individual exhibited impaired directional hearing on the side of the affected ear, he retained normal abilities on the side of the intact ear. Localization was faster, and more accurate, for spectrally complex stimuli. These observations suggest a localization process that is based on the damping and reinforcement of sound energy by pinna acoustics. The directional properties of the human ear that produce these spectral cues have now been described in detail, but the essential findings of Angell and Fite have not been altered by a century of research (Starch, 1908; Viehweg and Campbell, 1960; Slattery and Middlebrooks, 1994).

Investigators have simulated monaural localization in normal listeners by temporarily plugging one ear (Oldfield and Parker, 1986). Binaural cues are attenuated but not eliminated by the procedure (Wightman and Kistler, 1997). Slattery and Middlebrooks (1994) tested the perceptual ramifications of ear plugging by comparing temporary versus congenital deficits. Most individuals with congenital unilateral deafness remarkably replicated the normal localization abilities that were originally reported by Angell and Fite. By contrast, plugging one ear of a normal listener skewed the perceived horizontal localization of the sound source toward the unobstructed ear. The manipulation had less effect on vertical localization. These observations suggest that binaural cues dominate horizontal localization, whereas monaural spectral cues are necessary for localization in the vertical plane. The supportive role of monaural spectral cues for horizontal localization expands when binaural cues are confounded by stimulus manipulations or unilateral deafness (Batteau, 1967; Searle *et al.*, 1975; Musicant and Butler, 1984a).

If listeners are given time to adapt to ear plugs, they recover their ability to localize sounds in the horizontal and vertical planes by learning to rely on the directional properties of the pinna (Musicant and Butler, 1980; Van Wanrooij and Van Opstal, 2004). Similar compensation has been observed when outer ear acoustics are distorted by occlusion of pinna cavities (McPartland *et al.*, 1997; Hofman *et al.*, 1998; Van Wanrooij and Van Opstal, 2005), when supernormal localization cues are added to the source spectrum (Shinn-Cunningham *et al.*, 1998), or when binaural processing is unbalanced by conductive hearing loss (Kawase *et al.*, 1999).

13.3.2 Altering the spectral content of auditory stimuli

The importance of monaural directional cues may also be identified by manipulating the spectral content of auditory stimuli. This approach includes localization of pure tones, which may be viewed as a radical reduction of spectral content.

Pratt (1930) noted that the frequency of a tone imparted an illusionary percept of front–back location. These effects have been replicated with narrow bands of noise (Blauert, 1969/1970, 1997). As the frequency of the tone or noise band increases from 1 to 5 kHz, the perceived source moves from a rearward to a frontal location regardless of its actual position. The spatial illusions are correlated with regions of high gain in the DTF (Fig. 13.3B). Actual rearward locations produce 'covert peaks' at frequencies near 1–2 kHz, while frontal locations are associated with peaks near 4–5 kHz (Musicant and Butler, 1984b).

Implicit in the concept a 'covert peak' is a template that stores the statistical properties of outer ear directional effects. The existence of such a template matching process has been tested by correlating the localization of noise bands with the spectral shape of DTFs (Middlebrooks, 1992). Figure 13.4 relates the actual and perceived locations of noise bands with a center frequency of 12 kHz. The limited horizontal spread of the data suggests that source azimuth was accurately localized by attending to interaural level difference cues (Fig. 13.4A). Large elevation errors and front–back confusions were generated because the sound sources were assigned locations in the frontal horizontal plane (Fig. 13.4B).

The directional effects that dictate these systematic errors are shown in Fig. 13.4C. The four DTFs correspond to the preferred response locations for 6, 8, 10, and 12-kHz noise bursts. Each function displays a 'covert peak' that closely matches the spectral content of the noise band. This relationship suggests a localization strategy in which statistically unique features of the HRTF contribute disproportionately to the perceived location of the stimulus.

Hebrank and Wright (1974) evaluated the effects of spectral notches on vertical localization by adding synthetic notches to flat spectrum noise. Accurate localization of the natural spectrum required content between 4 and 16 kHz, which is where natural notches are introduced by pinna acoustics. When an artificial notch was added to these frequencies, the perceived azimuth of the noise bands shifted to a frontal location. The perceived elevation of the sound source could be altered by manipulating the lower cutoff of the notch.

Bloom (1977) used an unorthodox psychophysical approach to investigate the acoustic basis of auditory spatial illusions. Instead of placing a microphone in the ear, he used the ear itself as the measuring device under the assumption that free-field detection thresholds would manifest the directional filtering effects of the outer ear. His audiometric methods required a battery of pure tones with fine frequency resolution, a monaural presentation mode, and the elimination of head movements. After collecting the thresholds at different elevations in the median plane, he subtracted the average sensitivity curve of all locations from the results from each location. This derivation of the directional transfer function revealed 'covert notches' that changed systematically in frequency with sound source elevation.

Bloom validated his psychoacoustic measures by adding synthetic notches to free-field sounds. The potential conflict between natural and synthetic spectral cues was avoided by presenting the stimulus from a location where natural cues were weak. Subjects listened to unmodified stimuli from actual elevations in the median plane and created the perceptual illusion of a matching

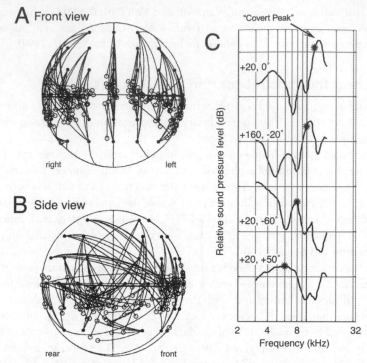

Fig. 13.4 Significance of covert peaks for localization of narrowband noise. **A** and **B** Localization errors generated by a noise band with a center frequency of 12 kHz. Stimulus locations (*filled circles*) and response locations (*open circles*) are joined by lines. **C** Directional transfer functions for the same subject. Numerical labels state the azimuth and elevation of each function. *Stars* mark the frequency of noise that generated responses near the four locations. The *arrow* points to a covert peak in the +20° AZ, 0° EL function. (Adapted from Middlebrooks, 1992.)

location by adjusting the frequency of the synthetic notch. Notch frequency was highly correlated between natural and simulated source locations.

Animal subjects also rely on spectral cues for sound localization in the median plane. The HRTFs in Fig. 13.5A have been selected to illustrate how spectral energy in the ear canal of the domestic cat is influenced by the elevation of a sound source (Rice *et al.*, 1992). The large collection of HRTFs in Fig. 13.5B summarizes the combined effects of azimuth and elevation. Three types of localization cues are suggested. Frequencies below 5 kHz display a broad resonance that varies in level with sound source azimuth. This directional effect is not seen in Fig. 13.5A because it is created by the sound shadow of the head at locations outside the median plane. Frequencies between 5 and 20 kHz exhibit directionally dependent notches that are systematically related to elevation and azimuth. The gain of the HRTF decreases at frequencies above 20 kHz and is marked with a complex pattern of peaks and notches.

The perceptual significance of mid-frequency cues has been investigated by measuring the effects of spectral manipulations on localization in the median plane. Cats make accurate head orientation responses to bursts of broadband noise (May and Huang, 1996), or band-passed noise if the spectrum is truncated in a manner that preserves mid-frequency cues (Huang and May, 1996). Stimuli lacking this spectral information elicit large elevation errors.

Spatial illusions are created when the auditory system misinterprets synthetic spectral peaks and notches as directional filtering effects of the outer ear (Tollin and Yin, 2003). These systematic

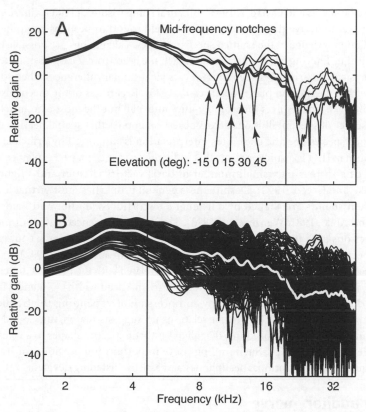

Fig. 13.5 Directional filtering properties of the cat's outer ear. **A** HRTFs at five elevations in the median plane (*numerical labels* state elevation). **B** HRTFs encompassing additional locations in the frontal sound field. The average spectrum of all HRTFs is indicated by the *bold line* in **A** and the *white line* in **B**. (Adapted from May *et al.*, 2008.)

errors suggest that the natural process of localization demands the capacity to distinguish spectral features that are introduced by the ear from features that exist in the source spectrum. Consequently, there is a learning dimension for monaural spectral cues that enhances the localization of familiar sounds.

Spectral learning has been investigated by training listeners to identify noise bands that contain synthetic peaks and notches at different frequencies (Rakerd *et al.*, 1999). Near-perfect performance was observed after a brief training period with stimuli from a fixed location in the median plane. When the source location changed randomly in subsequent tests, the identification of low-frequency noise bands remained normal, but the identification of high-frequency noise bands fell to chance levels. These errors suggest that the listeners could not dissociate the source spectrum from directional filtering effects of the outer ear. Interestingly, the subjects retained the ability to localize the stimuli despite their inability to identify the source spectrum. These results support the existence of an independent localization process that does not require direct access to knowledge of the source spectrum.

There are various algorithms by which the auditory system may estimate the spectrum of a free-field sound from acoustic energy in the ear canal. Natural sounds are characterized by spectral shapes that change slowly in frequency and therefore are able to communicate the sharp discontinuities of the HRTF (Zakarauskas and Cynader, 1993). Binaural comparisons of HRTF-filtering effects may allow the listener to derive the spectrum of a free-field sound or perhaps compute its location without explicit knowledge of the emitted spectrum. These calculations are possible because each ear exerts a unique filtering effect when sounds reach the head from locations outside the median plane and physical disparities between the two ears yield similar differences when sound sources are located within the median plane (Searle *et al.*, 1975). Regardless of the mechanism, it is clear that the auditory system resolves these ambiguities under all but the most extreme conditions.

The consistency of spectral illusions across observers implies that spatial hearing is based on a common set of species-specific cues. This interpretation is supported by principal component analyses of human HRTFs, which indicate that individual variance may be explained by the linear summation of a surprisingly small number of basis vectors (Kistler and Wightman, 1992; Middlebrooks and Green, 1992). Despite these general properties, best virtual localization is achieved when sounds are shaped by a listener's own HRTFs (Butler and Belendiuk, 1977; Morimoto and Ando, 1982; Wenzel *et al.*, 1993). The errors experienced with non-individualized transfer functions tend to involve poor elevation accuracy and front–back confusions, where monaural spectral cues are particularly important (Wightman and Kistler, 1992).

Inter-subject differences in the HRTF are highly correlated with the physical dimensions of the listener (i.e., interaural delays, size of the external ear, and head width) (Xu and Middlebrooks, 2000). The disparities may be reduced by compressing or expanding the frequency axis of directional transfer functions. This linear relationship suggests that virtual sound localization may be enhanced by scaling procedures that align synthetic spectral shapes to a listener's natural cues (Middlebrooks, 1999a,b). Such findings have important implications for improving the directional qualities of recreational headphones and assistive listening devices.

13.4 The auditory nerve

The energy spectrum of a complex sound is distributed along the cochlear partition in a frequency-dependent or tonotopic manner (Narayan *et al.*, 1998; Ruggero *et al.*, 2000). Because the auditory nerve makes punctate synaptic contacts along the cochlear axis (Kim and Molnar, 1979), each fiber responds best to a select frequency range within the disassembled spectrum. The complete representation of a complex sound, therefore, requires a population of fibers with complementary tuning properties. Within the population, fibers show high discharge rates if they are tuned to energy peaks, or low rates if they are tuned to spectral nulls (Sachs and Young, 1979).

13.4.1 Coding of HRTF shapes by the discharge rates of auditory nerve fibers

The representation of HRTF shapes by auditory nerve fibers has been described in domestic cats (Poon and Brugge, 1993; Rice *et al.*, 1995). Potential rate coding mechanisms are suggested by a simple linear relationship between spectrum level at the fiber's best frequency and the magnitude of the neural response (May and Huang, 1997). Fibers with high spontaneous rates produce a robust representation in which spectral peaks and nulls are encoded by high and low rates, respectively. Fibers with low spontaneous rates are less sensitive to changes in spectrum level and exhibit a more constrained range of rate changes. These fibers play a critical role in the coding of spectral information at high sound levels and in background noise (Le Prell *et al.*, 1996).

A signal detection analysis of the auditory nerve representation of the cat's HRTF reveals an important role for mid-frequency spectral notches (May and Huang, 1997). They produce the most salient discharge rate information at central locations in the horizontal and median planes, where cats show their most accurate localization behaviors (May and Huang, 1996; Populin and Yin, 1998a, b).

The functional significance of directional information in the mid-frequency HRTF spectrum has been verified by measuring the cat's ability to orient to brief sound presentations (May and Huang, 1996). This natural reflex can be adapted to behavioral testing with very little training investment (Sutherland et al., 1998b). If the bandwidth of the stimulus is modified in a manner that conserves its mid-frequency spectral information, accurate behavior is maintained. Limiting the sound spectrum to high frequencies, where large cues lack statistical distinction, elicits poorly directed head movements (Huang and May, 1996).

13.4.2 Effects of cochlear deficits on spectral coding

Auditory structures may be silenced by design in experimental animals to reveal their role in directional hearing. Although physiological mechanisms cannot be tied to perceptual performance with planned lesions in humans, damage to the human cochlea by disease, acoustic overexposure, or aging is no less profound and offers equally enlightening insights into the auditory processes that govern sound localization.

Age-related degeneration of cochlear hair cells (i.e., presbycusis) is a pervasive form of sensorineural hearing loss (SNHL) with significant consequences for sound detection, discrimination, and localization. The disorder is marked by a progressive base-to-apex hair cell loss that usually involves both ears (Rokay and Penzes, 1988; Soucek et al., 1987). Localization in the horizontal plane is relatively resistant to SNHL, but a significant disturbance of vertical plane discrimination is observed (Noble et al., 1994), presumably reflecting the encoding of high-frequency spectral cues in the basal cochlea. When hair cell loss progresses to mid frequencies, the added degradation of spectral coding leads to increased front–back confusions. High-frequency amplification may significantly improve performance (Rakerd et al., 1998).

Cochlear outer hair cells (OHCs) are the target of descending projections from the olivocochlear efferent system (Kimura and Wersall, 1962). Electrical stimulation of the olivocochlear bundle can expand the dynamic range properties of auditory nerve fibers, particularly when transient signals are embedded in continuous background noise (Guinan and Gifford, 1988; Wiederhold, 1970; Winslow and Sachs, 1987). In cats, these adjustments are strongest at frequencies between 5 and 20 kHz (Wiederhold, 1970) because efferent innervation is most profuse in the middle turns of the cochlea (Liberman et al., 1990). This frequency bias is ideal for enhancing the coding of spectral cues for sound localization. Severe deficits in vertical localization are observed when the pathway is lesioned (May et al., 2004).

The following material describes how the distributed auditory nerve representation of spectral cues for sound localization is transformed by spectrally selective neurons in the central auditory system. These descriptions focus on the dorsal cochlear nucleus and inferior colliculus where neural subpopulations establish an ascending auditory pathway that is exquisitely sensitive to monaural directional information.

13.5 The dorsal cochlear nucleus

When the discharge rates of auditory nerve fibers reach the dorsal cochlear nucleus (DCN), linear coding properties give way to central representations that are broadband, convergent, and non-linear. The transformation is achieved by merging auditory nerve inputs with spectrally sensitive inhibition and proprioceptive feedback. This multisensory integration creates a neuron that responds to spectral features, and not simply spectral energy (Oertel and Young, 2004).

13.5.1 **Anatomy**

The projections of spiral ganglion neurons bifurcate upon entering the cochlear nucleus. The ascending branch recapitulates the cochlear frequency map in the anteroventral subdivision of the nucleus. The descending branch innervates the posteroventral subdivision and the dorsal cochlear nucleus (Lorente de Nó, 1933; Ryugo and Parks, 2003). The tonotopic organization of the cochlea is not simply transferred to the brainstem. In keeping with the nucleus' central role in HRTF coding, the frequency map of the cat's DCN is skewed toward mid-frequency sounds where spectral notches provide important monaural localization cues (Spirou *et al.*, 1993). It is common for auditory nuclei to show an exaggerated representation of functionally relevant frequencies. For example, the medial superior olive is specialized for coding low-frequency ITDs (Tsuchitani, 1977) while the lateral superior olive is biased toward processing high-frequency ILDs.

13.5.2 **Physiological response types and spectral coding**

The major cell types of the dorsal cochlear nucleus and their topographical distribution within the laminar structure of the nucleus are illustrated in Fig. 13.6A. In anatomical parlance, projection neurons of the DCN are known as pyramidal cells or giant cells. Their physiological counterpart is designated the type IV neuron. Type IV response patterns are sculpted by multiple sources of

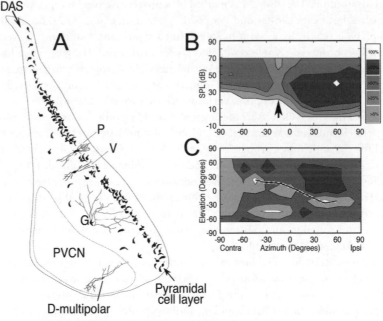

Fig. 13.6 Functional anatomy of the DCN. **A** Topographical organization of major cell types. Pyramidal (P) and giant cells (G) project to the inferior colliculus by way of the dorsal acoustic stria (DAS). These outputs are shaped by excitation from the auditory nerve (not shown) and inhibition from vertical cells (V) in the deep layer of the nucleus and D-multipolar cells in the posteroventral cochlear nucleus (PVCN). **B** Effects of level and azimuth on the discharge rates of a DCN type IV neuron (BF = 10 kHz). It is assumed that these responses are recorded from pyramidal and giant cells. Response magnitude is expressed as a percentage of maximum. A spectral notch produces the rate decrease at −15° azimuth (*arrow*). **C** Effects of azimuth and elevation on the responses of a second neuron (BF = 11 kHz). The trajectory of a spectral notch (*line*) coincides with rate decreases. (Adapted from Imig *et al.*, 2000; Young and Davis, 2002.)

inhibition (Nelken and Young, 1994). Vertical cells are inhibitory interneurons with narrowband tuning. D-multipolar cells provide broadband inhibitory inputs from outside the DCN.

The directional coding properties of the DCN's complex inhibitory circuitry have been demonstrated by recording from type IV neurons under free-field conditions (Imig *et al.*, 2000). Figure 13.6B plots representative responses in the DCN of an anesthetized cat. As the stimulus moves in the horizontal plane, the neuron's discharge rates recapitulate the essential coding properties of the auditory nerve. Higher discharge rates are observed at positive (ipsilateral) azimuths, and lower discharge rates at negative (contralateral) azimuths. Minimum rates signal locations where spectral notches impinge upon the neuron's best frequency (BF: the frequency evoking sound-driven activity at the lowest sound pressure level).

A more complete picture of directional coding in the DCN is obtained by examining discharge rates as a function of both azimuth and elevation. Figure 13.6C plots the responses of a second type IV neuron in this format. A consistent rate decrease follows the trajectory of a spectral notch that falls near the neuron's BF (line). Because this notch exists at multiple locations, rate decreases define a spatial contour and not a single point in space (Rice *et al.*, 1992). The representation of a specific location along the iso-notch contour requires additional spectral processing in the inferior colliculus, which will be described later (Davis, 2005; May *et al.*, 2008).

The circuit model in Fig. 13.7A summarizes the hypothesized interactions between DCN cell types. Here, the neurons are identified using physiological nomenclature since these results were obtained with recording techniques that do not reveal the anatomical properties of the neuron being studied. The frequency tuning of each neuron is indicated by the distribution of connections on the best frequency axis of the model. The type II inhibitory input to the type IV unit (pyramidal cell) is sharply tuned in frequency and tends to have a BF that is slightly lower in frequency (Hancock *et al.*, 1997). This source of inhibition is attributed to vertical cells in the deep layers of the DCN (Young and Voigt, 1982; Spirou *et al.*, 1999). A second inhibitory input is weaker and broadly tuned (Nelken and Young, 1994; Hancock and Voigt, 1999). Wide-band inhibition (WBI) is assumed to arise from multipolar cells in the posteroventral cochlear nucleus (Oertel *et al.*, 1990; Nelken and Young, 1996; Doucet *et al.*, 1999; Hancock and Voigt, 1999; Arnott *et al.*, 2004).

The ability of the DCN circuit model to predict the spectral integration properties of type II and type IV units has been confirmed under a variety of stimulus conditions. Type IV units are weakly driven by broadband noise because excitatory inputs from the auditory nerve are offset by the combined inhibition of type II and WBI neurons.

As illustrated in Fig. 13.7B, shaping the noise spectrum with directional features of the HRTF may potentiate or reduce the response of a type IV neuron. Panel 1 shows three spectra that were produced by shifting a generic HRTF in the frequency domain. Panel 2 describes the largely inhibitory frequency response map (FRM) of a type IV unit. Letters on the FRM mark the frequency location of the prominent mid-frequency notch for five spectra that were created by shifting the prototypes in panel 1. Panel 3 plots the rate-level functions for the five spectra.

If a spectral notch removes energy from frequencies that excite the type II neuron, the type IV unit will be less inhibited. If energy is removed from frequencies that excite the type IV unit, the balance of inputs will shift toward stronger inhibition. Inhibitory responses are noted across most levels of the rate-level function for HRTF-a because the spectral notch falls on excitatory frequencies near BF. The remaining HRTFs elicit excitatory responses because their spectral notches correspond to inhibitory sidebands.

13.5.3 Lesion effects

The role of the dorsal cochlear nucleus in auditory perception has been explored by assessing the behavioral deficits that follow surgical lesions of the dorsal acoustic stria (DAS) (Sutherland *et al.*,

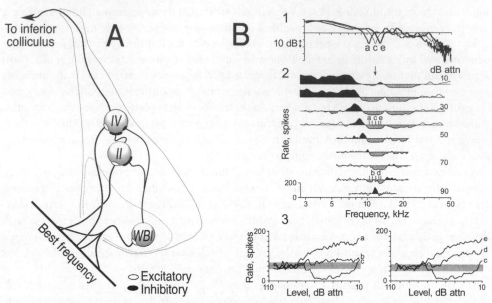

Fig. 13.7 A Neural circuit model of the DCN. The type IV response pattern is assumed to reflect the discharge rates of pyramidal or giant cells. Type II inhibition is likely to arise from vertical cells. Wide-band inhibition (WBI) is associated with inputs from D-multipolar cells. The relative frequency tuning of the multiple input sources is indicated by location along the best frequency axis. **B** Spectral coding properties of a type IV neuron. *1* The spectral notch of a generic HRTF shape is shifted in frequency by changing the sampling rate of a digitized sound file. *2* The frequency response map of a type IV neuron. Most combinations of tone frequency and level elicit inhibitory responses (*gray fill*). At threshold, frequencies near best frequency (12 kHz) excite the neuron (*black fill*). *3* Rate-level functions obtained from the type IV neuron in *2* using generic HRTFs, like those shown in *1*. The frequency of the spectral notch is indicated by *letters* in *2*. The maximum variation of spontaneous rates is bracketed by the *shaded region*. (Adapted from Young and Davis, 2002.)

1998a, b; May, 2000). The ascending axons of type IV principal cells exit the nucleus via the DAS, cross the midline, and terminate in the central nucleus of the inferior colliculus (ICC). If the axons are cut near their point of exit from the DCN, hearing sensitivity in quiet and background noise is not affected (Masterton and Granger, 1988; Masterton *et al.*, 1994). These functions are presumably mediated by the more generalized output pathways of the ventral cochlear nucleus (i.e., the trapezoid body).

Based on the physiological evidence for non-linear processing of spectral information in the DCN, subsequent studies have hypothesized that DAS lesions may influence sound localization in the median vertical plane because this form of directional hearing depends on monaural spectral cues. Various behavioral tests have been used to test this prediction. Without any behavioral training, cats will orient their head reflexively to a sudden burst of noise. The accuracy of head orientations to sound sources in the median plane decreases after DAS lesions (Sutherland *et al.*, 1998b). Cats can also be trained to respond on a lever when a sound changes from one location to another in the median plane. The magnitude of the just detectable change is not affected by DAS lesions (Sutherland *et al.*, 1998a). One explanation for the specificity of the deficit is that an accurate head orientation demands absolute localization competency, while the discrimination of a positional change does not. In other words, the former requires the subject to point to the sound source, while the latter only requires an indication that the source has changed.

The effects of DAS lesions on a cat's sound-directed head movements are summarized in Fig. 13.8, using data taken from May (2000). The cat was trained by positive reinforcement to orient to a brief noise burst and then hold its head at the perceived location until a cue light signaled the availability of a food reward. For these trials, the noise burst was band-pass filtered at 5–20 kHz to restrict monaural localization cues to mid-frequency notches. The scored orientation response was based on the subject's stable position at the conclusion of the head movement. Line segments indicate the error between source locations and average responses. The ellipses show the horizontal and vertical variability of responses (±1 SD).

Prior to lesioning, the cat displayed orientation behaviors that were well directed in azimuth and elevation (Fig. 13.8A). These results have been shown in previous studies of binaurally intact cats (Huang and May, 1996). Monaural localization was investigated by eliminating spectral processing in the right DCN with a unilateral DAS lesion. After the surgical manipulation, the cat continued to identify the elevation and azimuth of most test locations (Fig. 13.8B). The error and variability of responses were slightly magnified, but remained localized to the same eccentric locations that proved problematic prior to the lesion. The near-normal localization performance of unilaterally lesioned cats is reminiscent of the accurate localization behaviors of unilaterally deaf humans (Angell and Fite, 1901a; Slattery and Middlebrooks, 1994), which suggests that both may rely on the monaural processing of spectral cues.

A second surgery disrupted spectral processing bilaterally (Fig. 13.8C). The resulting localization deficits were statistically significant only in terms of response elevation. Regardless of the

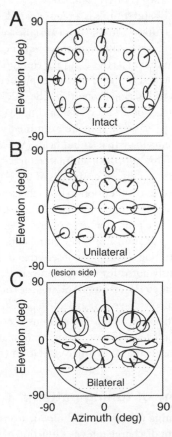

Fig. 13.8 Effects of DCN lesions on orientation behavior. Localization accuracy is shown before the lesion (**A**), after a unilateral lesion (**B**), and after bilateral lesions (**C**). Line segments join orientation responses to stimulus locations. *Ellipses* indicate the standard deviation of responses to each location. (Adapted from May, 2000.)

actual location of the sound source, the subject's orientation responses were seldom directed toward elevations that deviated more than 20 degrees from the interaural horizontal plane. The systematic underestimation of source location exceeded 60 degrees for extreme elevations. It is likely that DAS lesioned cats maintained accurate horizontal localization by relying on ITD and ILD cues (Batteau, 1967; Musicant and Butler, 1984a).

13.6 The inferior colliculus

The central nucleus of the inferior colliculus (ICC) receives direct projections from multiple subdivisions of the cochlear nucleus and superior olivary complex (Aitkin et al., 1984). These parallel inputs combine within the ICC to enhance the selective representation of monaural spectral cues that is created in the DCN (May et al., 2008). Directional tuning is dictated by the bandwidth and timing of inhibition at frequencies that are critical for monaural localization, elevation sensitivity, and the resolution of front–back confusions.

13.6.1 Basic patterns of spatial tuning

A number of studies have characterized the spatial tuning of inferior colliculus neurons with free-field stimuli (Leiman and Hafter, 1972; Bock and Webster, 1974; Semple et al., 1983; Aitkin et al., 1984; Moore et al., 1984). Much of this work has emphasized the binaural processing of ITDs and ILDs by measuring the localization of pure tones in the horizontal plane (Aitkin et al., 1985; Aitkin and Martin, 1987). These measures tend to underestimate the directional acuity that is achieved with spectrally rich sounds (Poirier et al., 2003).

The spectral processing of broadband sounds is a requisite underlying mechanism for localization in the median vertical plane (Aitkin and Martin, 1990). Best elevation sensitivity is observed for ICC neurons with BFs above 6 kHz. Although this frequency tuning conforms well to the domain of spectral information in the cat's HRTF, similar elevation tuning may be demonstrated with tonal stimuli. These unexpected findings may be explained by simple changes in sound pressure level that are introduced by filtering properties of the HRTF. Thus, directionally sensitive responses may be evoked by veritical localization cues or context-dependent loudness cues.

The acoustic basis of spatial processing may be examined with more precise control by conducting localization experiments in virtual sound fields (VSFs) (Delgutte et al., 1999; Davis, 2005; Chase and Young, 2006). This approach simulates a free-field environment by shaping closed-field sounds with computer-generated properties of the HRTF. Localization cues may be eliminated, transformed, or placed in competition to evaluate their functional significance.

The azimuth tuning that is evoked by VSF stimuli may encompass large regions of the contralateral hemifield (Fig. 13.9A) or rise to a peak at a best azimuth (Fig. 13.9B). These spatial receptive fields reflect the degree to which excitation from the contralateral ear is constrained by binaural inhibitory interactions. Azimuth tuning also may be observed in the absence of binaural sensitivity (Delgutte et al., 1999). As previously noted for free-field measures, monaural neurons may attain similar directionality by responding to HRTF-based spectral cues or simple changes in sound level.

Approximately half of ICC neurons have VSF receptive fields that are tuned to vertical locations in the median plane (Delgutte et al., 1999). The neurons may display elevation-sensitive rate peaks (Fig. 13.9C) or troughs (Fig. 13.9D). These strongly modulated responses imply a sensitivity to HRTF-based spectral patterns that maximize excitation (peak responses) or inhibition (trough responses) at BF.

13.6.2 Functional anatomy of tuning patterns

The excitatory and inhibitory tuning patterns of auditory neurons are demarcated by frequency response maps (FRMs), which plot discharge rates as a function of pure tone frequency and level.

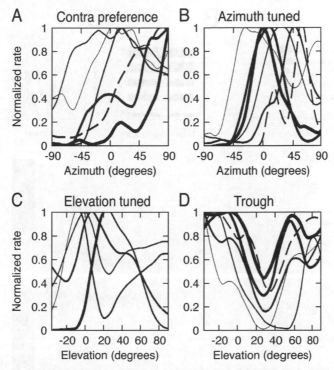

Fig. 13.9 Responses of inferior colliculus neurons to virtual sound field stimuli. **A** Examples of neurons that are broadly tuned to azimuths in the contralateral hemifield. **B** Neurons with sharp tuning. **C** and **D** Peak (excitatory) and trough (inhibitory) elevation tuning. (Adapted from Delgutte *et al.*, 1999.)

The inhibitory receptive field is revealed by frequency-dependent rate decreases relative to spontaneous activity. Excitatory tuning is indicated by rate increases.

When measured in domestic cats, the FRMs of spectrally sensitive inferior colliculus neurons display two general patterns of inhibition (Davis *et al.*, 1999; Ramachandran *et al.*, 1999). Type I neurons (as in the letter *i*) are distinguished by an I-shaped excitatory region that is bounded at higher and lower frequencies by lateral inhibitory areas (Fig. 13.10A). When spectral notches remove energy from the narrowly tuned excitatory field, the neurons are strongly inhibited (Fig. 13.10B). The projection neurons of the lateral superior olive (LSO) show similar FRM shapes and therefore are assumed to be an important source of input to type I units (Ramachandran *et al.*, 1999).

Type I units also share patterns of binaural sensitivity with the LSO (Davis *et al.*, 1999; Ramachandran *et al.*, 1999; Ramachandran and May, 2002). They are excited by contralateral sounds and inhibited by ipsilateral sounds. Maximum inhibition requires coincident arrival of contralateral and ipsilateral stimulation (Batra *et al.*, 1997). Consequently, a limited range of sound locations will create the ITD that optimizes the inhibitory interaction. When tested with different tone frequencies, the type I neuron is consistently inhibited by the 'characteristic delay' (CD) that compensates for conduction time inequalities between the two ears (Fig. 13.10C). The negative CD observed for this example predicts azimuth tuning in the contralateral hemifield (Fig. 13.10D).

Type O neurons (as in the letter *o*) take their name from the O-shaped island of near-threshold excitation that is a stable feature of a largely inhibitory FRM (Fig. 13.11A). Several lines of evidence

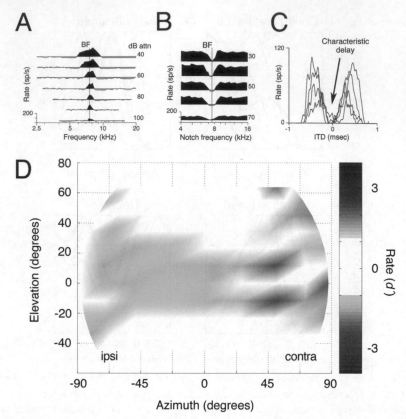

Fig. 13.10 Physiological characteristics of an ICC type I neuron (BF = 7 kHz). **A** Frequency response map showing narrowly tuned excitation (*black fill*) and lateral inhibition (*gray fill*). *Horizontal lines* represent spontaneous activity. *Numerical labels* state presentation levels in decibel attenuation (0 dB attenuation is approximately 100 dB SPL). **B** Responses to a spectral notch that is swept in frequency across the neuron's receptive field. **C** ITD sensitivity measured with a pure-tone binaural beat paradigm. The functions were obtained at different frequencies but yielded a consistent characteristic delay. **D** The spatial receptive field determined by closed-field presentations of virtual sound field stimuli. Statistically significant rate increases are indicated in *red*. Rate decreases are shown in *blue*. The neuron was excited by most locations in the contralateral hemifield. (Adapted from May *et al.*, 2008.)

link this response type to ascending projections from the DCN; consequently, this response type plays an important role in the coding of monaural localization cues that are passed to the midbrain from the cochlear nucleus. In addition to sharing strong inhibitory effects at BF, type O neurons and their DCN counterparts are largely monaural. Consequently, most type O neurons are insensitive to ITD cues even when timing information is conveyed by the low-frequency envelopment modulations of high-frequency stimuli (Fig. 13.11C). Type O neurons are silenced when pharmacological manipulations block conduction in the output pathways of the DCN (Davis *et al.*, 2003).

Type O neurons also display the wideband spectral integration properties of DCN projection neurons. Like their hypothesized inputs, they respond selectively to spectral notches that simulate HRTF-based directional features (Fig. 13.11B). The sharp frequency tuning of this notch sensitivity

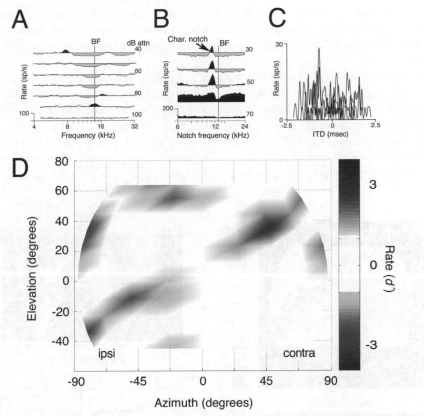

Fig. 13.11 Physiological characteristics of an ICC type O neuron (BF = 14 kHz). **A** The neuron produced a frequency response map with near-threshold excitation and large regions of inhibition. **B** Discharge rates were strongly modulated by changes in the frequency of a spectral notch. **C** The neuron was insensitive to ITD cues. **D** Responses to virtual sound field stimuli were tuned in azimuth and elevation. Plotting conventions are described in Fig. 13.9. (Adapted from May *et al.*, 2008.)

suggests that type O neurons encode changes in sound source elevation (Fig. 13.11D), whereas type I neurons are better suited for coding changes in azimuth.

13.6.3 Spectral template matching

Despite the diverse nature of localization cues for azimuth and elevation, most ICC neurons react to multiple forms of directional information (Chase and Young, 2005). When the information is arranged to complement individualized receptive field properties, type I neurons provide a more sensitive representation than type O units under a variety of testing conditions. These characteristics reflect the narrowband versus wideband integration properties of the unit types. The narrowly tuned type I neurons encode slight variations in the magnitude of local HRTF features, but ignore the broader context in which they occur. As a result, the neurons show strongly modulated responses, but little directional selectivity (Fig. 13.10D). By contrast, the wideband integration properties of type O neurons diminish their generalized spectral sensitivity, but maximize their selectivity for HRTF shapes (Fig. 13.11D).

Spectral selectivity is achieved by matching specific HRTF shapes to a neuron's broadband inhibitory patterns (May *et al.*, 2008). Discharge rates are increased when spectral peaks coincide with ON-BF excitatory inputs and spectral notches fall within OFF-BF inhibitory regions. The process of spectral template matching is not a unique property of type O units. Some type I neurons also display broadband inhibitory sidebands that tune their responses to particular HRTF shapes.

The VSF receptive field of a spatially tuned type I neuron is shown in Fig. 13.12A. The plot shows the neuron's discharge rates for diotic stimuli that simulate binaural HRTF effects at 99 locations in the frontal sound field. The rates are plotted in spatial coordinates that refer to the free-field locations of the HRTF filter shapes. Maximum rates (red) are elicited by a narrow contour of sound locations that fall from high ipsilateral elevations in the vertical plane to eccentric contralateral azimuths in the horizontal plane (diagonal line). These preferred locations are not predicted by the topography of sound energy in the contralateral ear. To illustrate these differences,

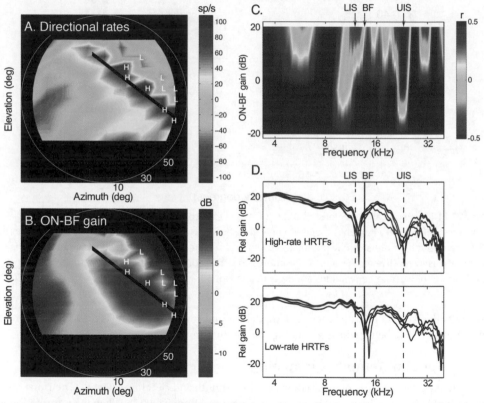

Fig. 13.12 Role of spectral templates in spatial selectivity. **A** Responses of a type I neuron (BF = 13.6 kHz) to virtual sound field stimuli. Maximum discharge rates (*red*) are aligned with a contour in the contralateral hemifield (*diagonal line*). **B** Spatial distribution of ON-BF gains for the VSF stimuli. Locations that produced maximum discharge rates (*diagonal line*) are more restricted than areas with maximum gains (*red*). **C** Correlation map showing the strength of association between discharge rates and OFF-BF spectral energy (see text for details). The *x-axis* indicates the frequency bin of the correlation. The *y-axis* is presentation level, which is plotted in terms of ON-BF gain. Positive correlations (*red*) indicate excitatory influences. Negative correlations (*blue*) indicate inhibition. **D** HRTF shapes that evoke relatively high (*upper panel*) or low (*lower panel*) discharge rates. The spatial locations of the five high-rate HRTFs are indicated by the *letter H* in **A** and **B**. The locations of the low-rate HRTFs are indicated by the *letter L*. (Adapted from May *et al.*, 2008.)

the gain of the HRTF at the best frequency of the neuron is shown in Fig.13.12B. Locations where the HRTF transmits high levels of sound energy (red) are broadly distributed and do not conform to the locations where highest discharge rates are observed in Fig 13.12A. The mismatch between discharge rates and ON-BF spectrum levels is observed because the neuron's responses to VSF stimuli are modified by sound energy at frequencies remote to BF.

The frequency domain of the neuron's excitatory and inhibitory inputs is revealed by correlating discharge rates with directional changes in discrete frequency bands of the HRTF (Fig. 13.12C). First, the spectral energy in the frequency band is calculated for each of the 99 HRTF pairs. Then, the HRTF-driven rates are sorted by order of spectrum level. Finally, the rate-level function is searched for its region of maximum correlation. Excitatory interactions produce positive correlations (red), whereas inhibitory interactions generate negative correlations (blue). The correlation map of the type I neuron in this example is dominated by lower (LIS) and upper inhibitory sidebands (UIS) that persist across presentation levels.

The critical role of OFF-BF inhibition in spatial tuning is summarized in Fig. 13.12D. Five HRTFs (upper panel) have been selected from the spatially tuned region of the neuron's maximum discharge rates. The locations of these high-rate HRTFs are indicated by the letter H in Fig. 13.12A and B. Although the HRTFs vary in azimuth by as much as 45° and in elevation by as much as 37.5°, their common regions of maximum and minimum gain correspond favorably to the neuron's integration properties. Energy is present in the narrowly tuned ON-BF excitatory region, but it is removed from the lower (LIS) and upper (UIS) inhibitory sidebands by deep spectral notches. Consequently, the balance of excitatory and inhibitory inputs shifts toward maximum excitation.

Five HRTFs (lower panel) with the opposite combination of spectral features evoked low discharge rates. Their locations are indicated by the letter L in Fig. 13.12A and B. Although ON-BF gain is closely matched to the high-rate HRTFs, the balance of converging inputs is tipped toward inhibition by high levels of energy within inhibitory sidebands.

OFF-BF inhibition must be powerful, tuned in frequency, and broadly distributed to produce the spectral template that is displayed by type O neurons and a subset of directionally selective type I neurons. In the case of type O neurons, ascending inputs from the DCN may convey the basic characteristics of these patterns of inhibition. Additional sources of inhibition must be invoked to explain broadband inhibition among type I neurons. Direct projections from the ventral cochlear nucleus (Blackburn and Sachs, 1992) and lateral superior olive (Sanes and Rubel, 1988) appear to lack sufficient bandwidth and complexity. Binaural inhibitory interactions also are unlikely because discharge rates are poorly correlated with directional features of the ipsilateral HRTF. One possibility is that the inhibition arises from potential GABAergic sources in the lateral lemniscus, which may explain the powerful effects of bicuculline on inhibitory tuning in the inferior colliculus. Regardless of the source, these inputs endow the inferior colliculus with spectral templates that are dominated by the contralateral ear, level tolerant, and tuned in both azimuth and elevation (May et al., 2008).

13.6.4 Lesion effects

The role of the inferior colliculus in sound localization has been investigated by evaluating the behavioral deficits that follow surgical lesions (Aitkin, 1986). When unilateral lesions are applied to lower commissural pathways, their effects on sound localization are pervasive and complete (Masterton et al., 1967; Moore et al., 1974; Casseday and Neff, 1975; Jenkins and Masterton, 1982). The magnitude of the deficits suggests that the surgical manipulation disrupts binaural processes that are critical for localization in both hemifields. Unilateral lesions of the higher commissural pathways produce localization errors that are limited to the contralateral hemifield. The spatial organization of lesion effects led Masterton and colleagues (Glendenning and Masterton, 1983; Masterton, 1997) to propose a two-stage localization process that creates a bias toward contralateral representations in the higher auditory nuclei. The binaural stage of the process involves the integration of activity from the two ears in the brainstem. The distributive stage makes the system functionally contralateral as it converges on the inferior colliculus. By analogy with visual pathways, this selective decussation is termed the 'acoustic chiasm.'

Early behavior-ablation studies relied heavily on domestic cats as experimental subjects and used free-field testing arenas to characterize the accuracy of directional hearing. In the two-alternative forced-choice paradigm, one of two goal boxes was temporarily unlocked to allow access to a food reward. The location of the randomly selected food receptacle was signaled by the presentation of sounds from a nearby speaker. Directional thresholds were determined by measuring how the probability of correct responding related to the physical separation between the two goal boxes.

An advantage of the goal-box paradigm is that it is a true localization task. The subject must identify and approach a sound source. A disadvantage, at least when testing terrestrial animals, is that the auditory targets are arranged along the floor of the arena and therefore do not assess performance in the vertical plane where monaural spectral cues are an essential component of the localization process. Nevertheless, variations in performance after central auditory lesions suggest that monaural localization does play a role in compensation for binaural deficits.

Moore *et al.* (1974) used the goal-box paradigm to investigate the effects of commissural lesions on directional hearing. Their results suggest an absence of localization deficits after destruction of the commissures of the inferior colliculus or cerebral cortex. Lesions of the trapezoid body produced more striking effects, but only in some subjects. The larger, persistent deficits may be explained by collateral damage to the dorsal and intermediate acoustic striae. Therefore, the lesions abolished not only binaural interactions that act on the outputs of the ventral cochlear nucleus, but also the monaural ascending projections of the dorsal cochlear nucleus. More focused lesions spared spatial discrimination, presumably because cats were able to rely on alternative directional cues in the intact spectral processing pathways.

Casseday and Neff (1975) also lesioned the trapezoid body, lateral lemniscus, and brachium of the inferior colliculus. Significant localization deficits were only observed after trapezoid body lesions, and, as noted in their previous study (Moore *et al.*, 1974), the loss of function was complete and permanent in a limited number of subjects. An interesting distinction between this study and their previous surgical procedure is that the trapezoid body incisions were placed in the midline of the brainstem and therefore did not directly involve the cochlear nuclei. Under these conditions, the magnitude of the impairment was predicted not by the laterality of the lesion site, but by its depth. Large localization errors were associated with deep cuts that not only severed the trapezoid body, but also were likely to involve the crossing fibers of both dorsal cochlear nuclei *en route* to the contralateral inferior colliculus. The loss of spatial acuity in these subjects was even more pronounced than deficits that were observed after unilateral cochlear ablation. Destruction of one cochlea completely disrupts binaural processing, but spares monaural localization in the opposite ear.

Subsequent investigations by Jenkins and Masterton (1982) have revealed potentially confounding listening strategies in the classic goal-box task. When two sound sources are located in the left and right hemifield of the testing arena, the subject may identify the active speaker by detecting binaural cues for stimulus azimuth (that is, *left* versus *right*). This is the anticipated decision criterion for localization testing. When directional processing has been compromised, for example by lesioning the left lateral lemniscus, the subject may continue to respond correctly by adopting a strategy that is based on *left* versus *not-left*. If the localization deficit is accompanied by hearing loss, *loud* versus *quiet* is an effective strategy. These undesirable modes of compensation must be carefully avoided when impaired subjects are repetitively tested under stable listening conditions (May *et al.*, 2004).

Jenkins and Masterton (1982) corrected the ambiguities of the goal-box task by adding multiple sound sources to the left and right hemifield of the testing arena. Although these more complex stimulus conditions did not alter the robust effects of trapezoid body lesions, results for higher-order lesions differed significantly from the transient impairments that were previously observed with the two-choice paradigm (Casseday and Neff, 1975). Without the aid of alternative listening strategies, unilateral damage to the lateral lemniscus, inferior colliculus, and brachium produced permanent deficits throughout the contralateral sound field. These findings support the utility of the 'acoustic chiasm,' as a theoretical construct for interpreting the functional consequences of higher-order lesions.

A coherent view of sound localization anatomy has emerged from the behavioral outcomes of lesioning studies. At processing levels below and including the superior olive, the pathways for binaural and monaural processing appear to be discrete. When spectrally sensitive projections of the dorsal cochlear nucleus are unilaterally interrupted *en route* to the inferior colliculus, vertical localization is compromised in the contralateral hemifield, but horizontal localization is spared (May, 2000). Bilateral lesions produce a complete loss of elevation sensitivity. In both cases, the deficits are permanent because reliable elevation cues cannot be synthesized by the intact binaural pathways. By contrast, losing one source of input extinguishes the brain's capacity for binaural processing. Consequently, unilateral ablations of the cochlea, ventral cochlear nucleus, trapezoid body, or superior olive produce pervasive disruptions of horizontal localization. The impairments may appear transitory because subjects may be inadvertently trained by the contingencies of the testing procedure to make better use of monaural cues for azimuth or alternative listening strategies. Severe and persistent deficits are only noted when lower-level lesions involve both pathways and both ears (e.g., a deep cut on the midline of the ventral medulla), and the localization task provides a valid assessment of directional acuity.

Processing levels beyond the superior olive receive ascending projections from the auditory brainstem that are sensitive to the azimuth and elevation of sound source locations. The convergence of this pre-processed spatial information creates a representation that is largely self contained. The spatial deficits produced by unilateral damage to the lateral lemniscus, inferior colliculus, or auditory cortex are restricted to the contralateral hemifield. Spatial tuning within the preferred hemifield may be dictated by binaural or monaural localization cues, which operate discretely or in combination. Consequently, the deficits are observed in the vertical and horizontal dimensions of auditory space (Beitel and Kaas, 1993).

13.7 Conclusions

Ablation studies are designed to isolate the functional significance of directionally sensitive neurons in the central auditory system by comparing localization accuracy before and after surgical manipulations. Although there is sufficient corroborative evidence from decades of research to integrate these findings into cohesive models of monaural and binaural localization, ambiguities arise from the imprecise nature of surgical procedures. Actual processing deficits may be obscured by small lesions that spare too much of the structure of interest. Spurious deficits may be generated by large or misplaced lesions that damage nearby structures or fibers of passage. Surgical approaches also are limited in their ability to resolve the discrete processing role of a particular morphology or response type that lies scattered in a complex neuropil such as the central nucleus of the inferior colliculus. For these reasons, ablation paradigms have been supplanted by pharmacological and genetic approaches that are able to manipulate specific components of processing pathways, often in a reversible manner.

As hearing scientists look forward to newer and better genetic tools, excellent animal models of the mechanisms of sound localization also may be found by looking backward. The cumulative effects of generations of evolution have yielded unique solutions to the biological problems that are endemic to a species-specific lifestyle.

An appreciation of evolutionary biology and its influence on the nervous system has been particularly enlightening in studies of binaural hearing. Masterton et al. (1975) referred to this neuroethological perspective as a study of 'natural ablation.' Structure–function relationships in the medial superior olive (MSO) provide a prime example of the approach. Mammalian species (hedgehogs, rats, tree shrews, cats, and dogs) may be ordered along a continuum of increasing MSO size and cell number (additional species were later added to the analysis by Heffner and Masterton, 1990). These naturally occurring variations in brainstem anatomy reflect the common or unusual lifestyle of the comparison species. When testing conditions demand the accurate processing of ITD information, behavioral performance is correlated with anatomical diversification.

The inferior colliculus plays a central role in multiple modes of directional coding. Natural ablations of this essential nucleus do not occur among mammalian species. In lieu of overt anatomical diversification, structure–function relationships may be inferred by examining perceptual performance in the context of more subtle physiological dichotomies. The analysis is made possible by species-specific variations of the neural response types that populate the midbrain.

Although the mouse shows the same ICC response types as the cat, the distribution of neurons is markedly different. Spectrally sensitive type O neurons dominate the population of IC neurons in cats (53%) (Ramachandran et al., 1999; Davis, 2005). They are rarely observed in mice (4%) (Ehret and Dreyer, 1984; Egorova et al., 2001; Ma et al., 2006). A similar underrepresentation of O-like neurons has been noted in guinea pigs (LeBeau et al., 2001), rats (Malmierca et al., 2003), and gerbils (Gdowski and Voigt, 1997).

The behavior consequences of DCN lesions (Sutherland et al., 1998a, b; May, 2000) predict poor monaural sound localization in species lacking a dedicated spectral processing pathway. Although existing cross-species comparisons have neglected this dimension of localization, directional acuity in the horizontal plane appears to correlate well with predatory versus prey lifestyles (Fay, 1988). In situations where an evolutionary premium is placed on accurate localization, the central auditory system manifests physiological specializations to enhance the auditory processing of spectral information. Consequently, exquisite thresholds for spatial discrimination are observed among predatory species such as the cat, bat, and barn owl. Prey species like the mouse or gerbil exhibit poor localization and appear to lack specialized spectral processing pathways.

An alternative explanation for the inferior localization abilities of the mouse is its small head size. As a result, the same angle of incidence will produce binaural cues that are of smaller magnitude in the mouse than in the cat. This argument is challenged by psychophysical measures in the least weasel (Heffner and Heffner, 1987) and grasshopper mouse (Heffner and Heffner, 1988), which are predators with physical dimensions that are comparable to small rodents. Sound localization thresholds in these animals suggest that the predators make more efficient use of localization cues than size-matched prey. The underlying mechanisms for this advantage have not been explored, but it is intriguing to speculate that the refinements for monaural localization first described in the cat may generalize to other predatory species.

The spectral processing pathway is a useful concept for exploring the fundamental principles of monaural sound localization. Like the brain's binaural pathways, the existence of this hypothetical construct is inferred from its unique physiological characteristics. Although the mechanisms for directional hearing have long been the subject of intense scientific interest, the computational nature of the spectral pathway continues to offer a unique foundation for future studies of how neural responses to biological signals are transformed into a coherent spatial identity by the convergence of ascending auditory representations, descending feedback systems, and contextual cues from other sensory modalities.

Acknowledgements

The author acknowledges the colleagues and students who have contributed ideas and experimental observations that are presented in this chapter. Sound localization research in the laboratory of B.J. May was sponsored by NIDCD grant R01 DC000954.

References

Aitkin L (1986) The Auditory Midbrain: Structure and Function in the Central Auditory Pathway. Humana Press, Clifton, New Jersey.

Aitkin LM, Martin RL (1987) The representation of stimulus azimuth by high best-frequency azimuth-selective neurons in the central nucleus of the inferior colliculus of the cat. *J Neurophysiol* 57: 1185–200.

Aitkin L, Martin R (1990) Neurons in the inferior colliculus of cats sensitive to sound-source elevation. *Hear Res* 50: 97–105.

Aitkin LM, Gates GR, Phillips SC (1984) Responses of neurons in inferior colliculus to variations in sound-source azimuth. *J Neurophysiol* 52: 1–17.

Aitkin LM, Pettigrew JD, Calford MB, Phillips SC, Wise LZ (1985) Representation of stimulus azimuth by low-frequency neurons in inferior colliculus of the cat. *J Neurophysiol* 53: 43–59.

Angell JR, Fite W (1901a) Further observations on the monaural localization of sound. *Psychol Rev* 8: 449–58.

Angell JR, Fite W (1901b) The monaural localization of sound. *Psychol Rev* 8, 225–46.

Arnott RH, Wallace MN, Shackleton TM, Palmer AR (2004) Onset neurones in the anteroventral cochlear nucleus project to the dorsal cochlear nucleus. *J Assoc Res Otolaryngol* 5: 153–70.

Batra R, Kuwada S, Fitzpatrick DC (1997) Sensitivity to interaural temporal disparities of low-and high-frequency neurons in the superior olivary complex. II. Coincidence detection. *J Neurophysiol* 78: 1237–47.

Batteau DW (1967) The role of the pinna in human localization. *Proc R Soc Lond B Biol Sci* 168: 158–80.

Beitel RE, Kaas JH (1993) Effects of bilateral and unilateral ablation of auditory cortex in cats on the unconditioned head orienting response to acoustic stimuli. *J Neurophysiol* 70: 351–69.

Blackburn CC, Sachs MB (1992) Effects of OFF-BF tones on responses of chopper units in ventral cochlear nucleus. I. Regularity and temporal adaptation patterns. *J Neurophysiol* 68: 124–43.

Blauert J (1969/1970) Sound localization in the median plane. *Acustica* 22: 205–13.

Blauert J (1997) *Spatial Hearing: The Psychophysics of Human Sound Localization.* The MIT Press, Cambridge, Massachusetts.

Bloom PJ (1977) Creating source elevation illusions by spectral manipulation. *J Audio Eng Soc* 25: 560–65.

Bock GR, Webster WR (1974) Coding of spatial location by single units in the inferior colliculus of the alert cat. *Exp Brain Res* 21: 387–98.

Butler RA, Belendiuk K (1977) Spectral cues utilized in the localization of sound in the median sagittal plane. *J Acoust Soc Am* 61: 1264–9.

Butler RA, Flannery R (1980) The spatial attributes of stimulus frequency and their role in monaural localization of sound in the horizontal plane. *Percept Psychophys* 28: 449–57.

Casseday JH, Neff WD (1975) Auditory localization: role of auditory pathways in brain stem of the cat. *J Neurophysiol* 38: 842–58.

Chase SM, Young ED (2005) Limited segregation of different types of sound localization information among classes of units in the inferior colliculus. *J Neurosci* 25: 7575–85.

Chase SM, Young ED (2006) Spike-timing codes enhance the representation of multiple simultaneous sound-localization cues in the inferior colliculus. *J Neurosci* **26**: 3889–98.

Davis KA (2005) Spectral processing in the inferior colliculus. *Int Rev Neurobiol* **70**: 169–205.

Davis KA, Ramachandran R, May BJ (1999) Single-unit responses in the inferior colliculus of decerebrate cats. II. Sensitivity to interaural level differences. *J Neurophysiol* **82**: 164–75.

Davis KA, Ramachandran R, May BJ (2003) Auditory processing of spectral cues for sound localization in the inferior colliculus. *J Assoc Res Otolaryngol* **4**: 148–63.

Delgutte B, Joris PX, Litovsky RY, Yin TC (1999) Receptive fields and binaural interactions for virtual-space stimuli in the cat inferior colliculus. *J Neurophysiol* **81**: 2833–51.

Doucet JR, Ross AT, Gillespie MB, Ryugo DK (1999) Glycine immunoreactivity of multipolar neurons in the ventral cochlear nucleus which project to the dorsal cochlear nucleus. *J Comp Neurol* **408**: 515–31.

Egorova M, Ehret G, Vartanian I, Esser KH (2001) Frequency response areas of neurons in the mouse inferior colliculus. I. Threshold and tuning characteristics. *Exp Brain Res* **140**: 145–61.

Ehret G, Dreyer A (1984) Localization of tones and noise in the horizontal plane by unrestrained house mice (*Mus musculus*). *J Exp Biol* **109**: 163–74.

Fay RR (1988) *Hearing in Vertebrates: a Psychophysics Databook*. Hill-Fay Associates, Winnetka, Illinois.

Flannery R, Butler RA (1981) Spectral cues provided by the pinna for monaural localization in the horizontal plane. *Percept Psychophys* **29**: 438–44.

Gatehouse RW (1976) Further research in localization of sound by completely monaural subjects. *J Aud Res* **16**: 263–73.

Gdowski GT, Voigt HF (1997) Response map properties of units in the dorsal cochlear nucleus of barbiturate-anesthetized gerbil (*Meriones unguiculatus*) *Hear Res* **105**: 85–104.

Glendenning KK, Masterton RB (1983) Acoustic chiasm: efferent projections of the lateral superior olive. *J Neurosci* **3**: 1521–37.

Guinan JJ Jr, Gifford ML (1988) Effects of electrical stimulation of efferent olivocochlear neurons on cat auditory-nerve fibers. III. Tuning curves and thresholds at CF. *Hear Res* **37**: 29–45.

Hancock KE, Voigt HF (1999) Wideband inhibition of dorsal cochlear nucleus type IV units in cat: a computational model. *Ann Biomed Eng* **27**: 73–87.

Hancock KE, Davis KA, Voigt HF (1997) Modeling inhibition of type II units in the dorsal cochlear nucleus. *Biol Cybern* **76**: 419–28.

Hebrank J, Wright D (1974) Spectral cues used in the localization of sound sources on the median plane. *J Acoust Soc Am* **56**: 1829–34.

Heffner RS, Heffner HE (1987) Localization of noise, use of binaural cues, and a description of the superior olivary complex in the smallest carnivore, the least weasel (*Mustela nivalis*). *Behav Neurosci* **101**: 701–8, 44–5.

Heffner RS, Heffner HE (1988) Sound localization in a predatory rodent, the northern grasshopper mouse (*Onychomys leucogaster*). *J Comp Psychol* **102**: 66–71.

Heffner RS, Masterton RB (1990) Sound localization in mammals: brain-stem mechanisms. In: *Comparative Perception* (eds Berkley MA, Stebbins WC), pp. 285–314. John Wiley, New York.

Hofman PM, Van Riswick JG, Van Opstal AJ (1998) Relearning sound localization with new ears. *Nat Neurosci* **1**: 417–21.

Huang AY, May BJ (1996) Sound orientation behavior in cats. II. Mid-frequency spectral cues for sound localization. *J Acoust Soc Am* **100**: 1070–80.

Imig TJ, Bibikov NG, Poirier P, Samson FK (2000) Directionality derived from pinna-cue spectral notches in cat dorsal cochlear nucleus. *J Neurophysiol* **83**: 907–25.

Jenkins WM, Masterton RB (1982) Sound localization: effects of unilateral lesions in central auditory system. *J Neurophysiol* **47**: 987–1016.

Kawase T, Koiwa T, Yuasa R, *et al.* (1999) Sound localization for a virtual sound source in cases of chronic otitis media. *Audiology* **38**: 83–90.

Kim DO, Molnar CE (1979) A population study of cochlear nerve fibers: comparison of spatial distributions of average-rate and phase-locking measures of responses to single tones. *J Neurophysiol* **42**: 16–30.

Kimura R, Wersall J (1962) Termination of the olivo-cochlear bundle in relation to the outer hair cells of the organ of Corti in guinea pig. *Acta Otolaryngol* **55**: 11–32.

Kistler DJ, Wightman FL (1992) A model of head-related transfer functions based on principal components analysis and minimum-phase reconstruction. *J Acoust Soc Am* **91**: 1637–47.

Kuhn GF (1987) Physical acoustics and measurements pertaining to directional hearing. In: *Directional Hearing* (eds Yost WA, Gourevitch G). Springer, New York.

Le Prell GS, Sachs MB, May BJ (1996) Representation of vowel-like spectra by discharge rate responses of individual auditory-nerve fibers. *Aud Neurosci* **2**: 275–88.

LeBeau FE, Malmierca MS, Rees A (2001) Iontophoresis in vivo demonstrates a key role for GABA(A) and glycinergic inhibition in shaping frequency response areas in the inferior colliculus of guinea pig. *J Neurosci* **21**: 7303–12.

Leiman AL, Hafter ER (1972) Responses of inferior colliculus neurons to free field auditory stimuli. *Exp Neurol* **35**: 431–49.

Liberman MC, Dodds LW, Pierce S (1990) Afferent and efferent innervation of the cat cochlea: quantitative analysis with light and electron microscopy. *J Comp Neurol* **301**: 443–60.

Lorente de Nó R (1933) Anatomy of the eighth nerve. III. General plan of structure of the primary cochlear nuclei. *Laryngoscope* **43**: 327–50.

Ma WL, Hidaka H, May BJ (2006) Spontaneous activity in the inferior colliculus of CBA/J mice after manipulations that induce tinnitus. *Hear Res* **212**: 9–21.

Malmierca MS, Hernandez O, Falconi A, Lopez-Poveda EA, Merchan M, Rees A (2003) The commissure of the inferior colliculus shapes frequency response areas in rat: an in vivo study using reversible blockade with microinjection of kynurenic acid. *Exp Brain Res* **153**: 522–9.

Masterton B, Thompson GC, Bechtold JK, RoBards MJ (1975) Neuroanatomical basis of binaural phase-difference analysis for sound localization: a comparative study. *J Comp Physiol Psychol* **89**: 379–86.

Masterton RB (1997) Neurobehavioral studies of the central auditory system. *Ann Otol Rhinol Laryngol Suppl* **168**: 31–4.

Masterton RB, Granger EM (1988) Role of the acoustic striae in hearing: contribution of dorsal and intermediate striae to detection of noises and tones. *J Neurophysiol* **60**: 1841–60.

Masterton RB, Jane JA, Diamond IT (1967) Role of brainstem auditory structures in sound localization. I. Trapezoid body, superior olive, and lateral lemniscus. *J Neurophysiol* **30**: 341–59.

Masterton RB, Granger EM, Glendenning KK (1994) Role of acoustic striae in hearing: mechanism for enhancement of sound detection in cats. *Hear Res* **73**: 209–22.

May BJ (2000) Role of the dorsal cochlear nucleus in the sound localization behavior of cats. *Hear Res* **148**: 74–87.

May BJ, Huang AY (1996) Sound orientation behavior in cats. I. Localization of broadband noise. *J Acoust Soc Am* **100**: 1059–69.

May BJ, Huang AY (1997) Spectral cues for sound localization in cats: a model for discharge rate representations in the auditory nerve. *J Acoust Soc Am* **101**: 2705–19.

May BJ, Budelis J, Niparko JK (2004) Behavioral studies of the olivocochlear efferent system: learning to listen in noise. *Arch Otolaryngol Head Neck Surg* **130**: 660–64.

May BJ, Anderson M, Roos M (2008) The role of broadband inhibition in the rate representation of spectral cues for sound localization in the inferior colliculus. *Hear Res* **238**: 77–93.

McPartland JL, Culling JF, Moore DR (1997) Changes in lateralization and loudness judgements during one week of unilateral ear plugging. *Hear Res* **113**: 165–72.

Middlebrooks JC (1992) Narrow-band sound localization related to external ear acoustics. *J Acoust Soc Am* **92**: 2607–24.

Middlebrooks JC (1999a) Virtual localization improved by scaling nonindividualized external-ear transfer functions in frequency. *J Acoust Soc Am* **106**: 1493–510.

Middlebrooks JC (1999b) Individual differences in external-ear transfer functions reduced by scaling in frequency. *J Acoust Soc Am* **106**: 1480–92.

Middlebrooks JC, Green DM (1990) Directional dependence of interaural envelope delays. *J Acoust Soc Am* **87**: 2149–62.

Middlebrooks JC, Green DM (1992) Observations on a principal components analysis of head-related transfer functions. *J Acoust Soc Am* **92**: 597–9.

Moore CN, Casseday JH, Neff WD (1974) Sound localization: the role of the commissural pathways of the auditory system of the cat. *Brain Res* **82**: 13–26.

Moore DR, Semple MN, Addison PD, Aitkin LM (1984) Properties of spatial receptive fields in the central nucleus of the cat inferior colliculus. I. Responses to tones of low intensity. *Hear Res* **13**: 159–74.

Morimoto M, Ando Y (1982) On the simulation of sound localization. In: *Localization of Sound: Theory and Applications* (ed. Gatehouse RW), pp. 85–9. Amphora Press, Groton Connecticut.

Musicant AD, Butler RA (1980) Monaural localization: an analysis of practice effects. *Percept Psychophys* **28**: 236–40.

Musicant AD, Butler RA (1984a) The influence of pinnae-based spectral cues on sound localization. *J Acoust Soc Am* **75**: 1195–200.

Musicant AD, Butler RA (1984b) The psychophysical basis of monaural localization. *Hear Res* **14**: 185–90.

Narayan SS, Temchin AN, Recio A, Ruggero MA (1998) Frequency tuning of basilar membrane and auditory nerve fibers in the same cochleae. *Science* **282**: 1882–4.

Nelken I, Young ED (1994) Two separate inhibitory mechanisms shape the responses of dorsal cochlear nucleus type IV units to narrowband and wideband stimuli. *J Neurophysiol* **71**: 2446–62.

Nelken I, Young ED (1996) Why do cats need a dorsal cochlear nucleus? *J Basic Clin Physiol Pharmacol* **7**: 199–220.

Noble W, Byrne D, Lepage B (1994) Effects on sound localization of configuration and type of hearing impairment. *J Acoust Soc Am* **95**: 992–1005.

Oertel D, Young ED (2004) What's a cerebellar circuit doing in the auditory system? *Trends Neurosci* **27**: 104–10.

Oertel D, Wu SH, Garb MW, Dizack C (1990) Morphology and physiology of cells in slice preparations of the posteroventral cochlear nucleus of mice. *J Comp Neurol* **295**: 136–54.

Oldfield SR, Parker SP (1986) Acuity of sound localisation: a topography of auditory space. III. Monaural hearing conditions. *Perception* **15**: 67–81.

Poirier P, Samson FK, Imig TJ (2003) Spectral shape sensitivity contributes to the azimuth tuning of neurons in the cat's inferior colliculus. *J Neurophysiol* **89**: 2760–77.

Poon PW, Brugge JF (1993) Virtual-space receptive fields of single auditory nerve fibers. *J Neurophysiol* **70**: 667–76.

Populin LC, Yin TC (1998a) Behavioral studies of sound localization in the cat. *J Neurosci* **18**: 2147–60.

Populin LC, Yin TC (1998b) Pinna movements of the cat during sound localization. *J Neurosci* **18**: 4233–43.

Pratt CC (1930) The spatial character of high and low tones. *J Exp Psychol* **13**: 278–85.

Rakerd B, Vander Velde TJ, Hartmann WM (1998) Sound localization in the median sagittal plane by listeners with presbyacusis. *J Am Acad Audiol* **9**: 466–79.

Rakerd B, Hartmann WM, McCaskey TL (1999) Identification and localization of sound sources in the median sagittal plane. *J Acoust Soc Am* **106**: 2812–20.

Ramachandran R, May BJ (2002) Functional segregation of ITD sensitivity in the inferior colliculus of decerebrate cats. *J Neurophysiol* **88**: 2251–61.

Ramachandran R, Davis KA, May BJ (1999) Single-unit responses in the inferior colliculus of decerebrate cats. I. Classification based on frequency response maps. *J Neurophysiol* **82**: 152–63.

Rice JJ, May BJ, Spirou GA, Young ED (1992) Pinna-based spectral cues for sound localization in cat. *Hear Res* **58**: 132–52.

Rice JJ, Young ED, Spirou GA (1995) Auditory-nerve encoding of pinna-based spectral cues: rate representation of high-frequency stimuli. *J Acoust Soc Am* **97**: 1764–76.

Rokay E, Penzes L (1988) Pathophysiological changes of the cochlea during ageing – a review. *ZFA* **43**: 185–9.

Ruggero MA, Narayan SS, Temchin AN, Recio A (2000) Mechanical bases of frequency tuning and neural excitation at the base of the cochlea: comparison of basilar-membrane vibrations and auditory-nerve-fiber responses in chinchilla. *Proc Natl Acad Sci USA* **97**: 11744–50.

Ryugo DK, Parks TN (2003) Primary innervation of the avian and mammalian cochlear nucleus. *Brain Res Bull* **60**: 435–56.

Sachs MB, Young ED (1979) Encoding of steady-state vowels in the auditory nerve: representation in terms of discharge rate. *J Acoust Soc Am* **66**: 470–9.

Sanes DH, Rubel EW (1988) The ontogeny of inhibition and excitation in the gerbil lateral superior olive. *J Neurosci* **8**: 682–700.

Searle CL, Braida LD, Cuddy DR, Davis MF (1975) Binaural pinna disparity: another auditory localization cue. *J Acoust Soc Am* **57**: 448–55.

Semple MN, Aitkin LM, Calford MB, Pettigrew JD, Phillips DP (1983) Spatial receptive fields in the cat inferior colliculus. *Hear Res* **10**: 203–15.

Shaw EAG (1974) The external ear. In: *Handbook of Sensory Physiology*, (eds Keidel WD, Neff WD), pp. 455–90. Springer, New York.

Shinn-Cunningham BG, Durlach NI, Held RM (1998) Adapting to supernormal auditory localization cues. I. Bias and resolution. *J Acoust Soc Am* **103**: 3656–66.

Slattery WH 3rd, Middlebrooks JC (1994) Monaural sound localization: acute versus chronic unilateral impairment. *Hear Res* **75**: 38–46.

Soucek S, Michaels L, Frohlich A (1987) Pathological changes in the organ of Corti in presbyacusis as revealed by microslicing and staining. *Acta Otolaryngol Suppl* **436**: 93–102.

Spirou GA, May BJ, Wright DD, Ryugo DK (1993) Frequency organization of the dorsal cochlear nucleus in cats. *J Comp Neurol* **329**: 36–52.

Spirou GA, Davis KA, Nelken I, Young ED (1999) Spectral integration by type II interneurons in dorsal cochlear nucleus. *J Neurophysiol* **82**: 648–63.

Starch D (1908) The perimetry of the localization of sound. *Psychol Rev Mon* **38**(Suppl 9): 1–55.

Sutherland DP, Glendenning KK, Masterton RB (1998a) Role of acoustic striae in hearing: discrimination of sound-source elevation. *Hear Res* **120**: 86–108.

Sutherland DP, Masterton RB, Glendenning KK (1998b) Role of acoustic striae in hearing: reflexive responses to elevated sound-sources. *Behav Brain Res* **97**: 1–12.

Tollin DJ, Yin TC (2003) Spectral cues explain illusory elevation effects with stereo sounds in cats. *J Neurophysiol* **90**: 525–30.

Tsuchitani C (1977) Functional organization of lateral cell groups of cat superior olivary complex. *J Neurophysiol* **40**: 296–318.

Van Wanrooij MM, Van Opstal AJ (2004) Contribution of head shadow and pinna cues to chronic monaural sound localization. *J Neurosci* **24**: 4163–71.

Van Wanrooij MM, Van Opstal AJ (2005) Relearning sound localization with a new ear. *J Neurosci* **25**: 5413–24.

Viehweg R, Campbell RA (1960) Localization difficulty in monaurally impaired listeners. *Ann Rhino Laryngol* **69**: 622–34.

Wenzel EM, Arruda M, Kistler DJ, Wightman FL (1993) Localization using nonindividualized head-related transfer functions. *J Acoust Soc Am* **94**: 111–23.

Wiederhold ML (1970) Variations in the effects of electric stimulation of the crossed olivocochlear bundle on cat single auditory-nerve-fiber responses to tone bursts. *J Acoust Soc Am* **48**: 966–77.

Wiener FM, Ross DA (1946) The pressure distribution in the auditory canal in a progressive sound field. *J Acoust Soc Am* 18: 401–8.

Wightman FL, Kistler DJ (1989a) Headphone simulation of free-field listening. II: Psychophysical validation. *J Acoust Soc Am* 85: 868–78.

Wightman FL, Kistler DJ (1989b) Headphone simulation of free-field listening. I: Stimulus synthesis. *J Acoust Soc Am* 85: 858–67.

Wightman FL, Kistler DJ (1992) The dominant role of low-frequency interaural time differences in sound localization. *J Acoust Soc Am* 91: 1648–61.

Wightman FL, Kistler DJ (1997) Monaural sound localization revisited. *J Acoust Soc Am* 101: 1050–63.

Wightman FL, Kistler DJ, Perkins ME (1987) A new approach to the study of human sound localization. In: *Directional Hearing* (eds Yost WA, Gourevitch G), pp. 26–48. Springer New York.

Winslow RL, Sachs MB (1987) Effect of electrical stimulation of the crossed olivocochlear bundle on auditory nerve response to tones in noise. *J Neurophysiol* 57: 1002–21.

Xu L, Middlebrooks JC (2000) Individual differences in external-ear transfer functions of cats. *J Acoust Soc Am* 107: 1451–9.

Young ED, Davis, KA (2002) Circuitry and function of the dorsal cochlear nucleus. In: *Integrative Functions in the Mammalian Auditory Pathway* (eds Oertel D, Fay RR, Popper AN), pp. 160–206. Springer, New York.

Young ED, Voigt HF (1982) Response properties of type II and type III units in dorsal cochlear nucleus. *Hear Res* 6: 153–69.

Zakarauskas P, Cynader M (1993) A computational theory of spectral cue localization. *J Acoust Soc Am* 94: 1323–31.

Chapter 14

Physiological correlates of the precedence effect and binaural masking level differences

Ruth Y. Litovsky and David McAlpine

14.1 Introduction

Humans spend much of their time in complex acoustic environments, where multiple sounds arise from many locations simultaneously. These sounds often interact with physical objects to create reverberations. Under such conditions, significant implications for functional and communication abilities can arise, including reduced ability to localize the source of a sound and problems in understanding speech. For adult listeners, examples of such environments include restaurants, meeting rooms, and places of entertainment. For children, one should consider classrooms, play-spaces, gymnasiums, and the like. However, despite the apparent 'clutter' of acoustic signals that exist in complex environments, most normal-hearing listeners show remarkable abilities in hearing and understanding speech, and in making themselves understood. Decades of research in human and animal auditory psychophysics have provided a theoretical framework for understanding brain mechanisms responsible for mediating these functional abilities.

Parallel to this, research aimed at uncovering the anatomical and physiological substrates of behavioral and perceptual effects has suggested a range of neural mechanisms underlying our ability to perform complex listening tasks. Two of the effects that have been widely studied, and that are the topic of this chapter, are the precedence effect and binaural unmasking. As we elaborate below, these perceptual phenomena are thought to reflect basic auditory mechanisms that enhance localization, detection, and perception of signals under complex listening situations. Briefly, the precedence effect occurs when two sounds arrive at the ears in close succession and from different locations, as might occur in an idealized space containing a single reflective surface. Humans, and several other mammalian species, are known to fuse the two sounds into a single auditory event whose perceived location is dominated by the leading sound. This effect is akin to an auditory illusion, and is especially compelling when one considers the fact that the effect is observed even when the delayed signal is presented with equal intensity. For delayed signals of lower-intensity, the effect is particularly strong, and is thus thought to account for our ability to suppress localization information from reflections, facilitating the communication of sounds under naturally reverberant environments.

Binaural unmasking is a related phenomenon that is most pronounced when listening over headphones where signals – often tones – presented in a background of masking noise are made more audible when the signal (or masking noise) is inverted at one ear relative to the other. This specific case, referred to as the binaural masking level difference (BMLD), has been the subject of intensive psychophysical investigation for over 60 years. The more recent physiological investigation of binaural masking has built upon research examining basic aspects of binaural processing in the auditory brain, and potentially provides an opportunity for exploring brain mechanisms involved in perceptual segregation of sound sources in the environment. The precedence effect and binaural unmasking constitute those relatively rare occasions where physiological correlates of human and, in some cases, animal, perceptual measures have been investigated in the auditory pathway. In this chapter we examine the neural basis of these effects in greater detail, and provide an overview of recent studies in the field of electrophysiology that potentially illuminate those processes by which perceptual effects are achieved.

14.2 The precedence effect

14.2.1 Background on psychophysical phenomena

A fundamental feature of acoustic environments is the presence of barrage of echoes. When a sound is emitted in a reverberant setting it arrives at the listener's ears through a direct path, which is the most rapid and least disturbed path. In addition, reflections of the sound from nearby surfaces, including walls and various objects, reach the ears, subsequently creating a cacophony of stimuli, each with their own set of localization cues. A simplified version of this scenario is depicted in Fig. 14.1. The potential for listeners to experience chaos and confusion with respect to the source of the sound is thus tremendous. However, the auditory system of mammals appears to be remarkably adept at sorting and prioritizing amongst potentially competing signals. In reverberant rooms, the listener is keenly aware of the presence of echoes; in fact, echoes enrich the quality of the first-arriving sound. However, localization cues carried by the echoes are de-emphasized relative to the cues carried by the leading sound, such that localization errors are minimized. This phenomenon is commonly known as the *precedence effect* (PE) since the auditory system assigns greater weight to the localization cues belonging to the preceding, or first-arriving, sound.

Studies of the PE actually utilize stimuli that represent a stripped-down, simplified version of sounds that occur in the real world, as shown in Fig. 14.2A. Typically, the first-arriving sound and a single reflection (hereby referred to as the 'lead' and 'lag', respectively) are simulated as a pair of identical stimuli, with the onset of the lag delayed relative to that of the lead. Figure 14.2B shows

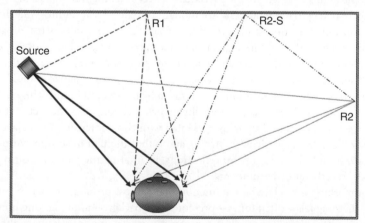

Fig. 14.1 A simplified version of sound source propagation in a reverberant environment. A source emits signals that reach the ears via direct paths, as well as via indirect paths that reflect from nearby walls (reflections R1 and R2) prior to reaching the ears. Additional reflections of reflections may also occur (R2-S). The indirect paths have longer propagation time.

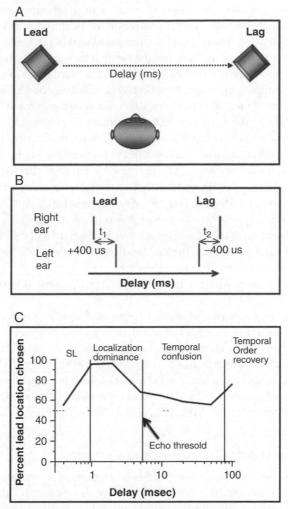

Fig. 14.2 Stimulus configurations and schematics of data. **A** Studies on the PE typically utilize stimuli that represent simplified features of real-world acoustic scenarios. Here, in an anechoic chamber, a source (lead) occurs from the *left*, and a single echo (lag) occurs from the *right*. **B** The interaural timing differences arising from the stimulus configuration in **A** can be simulated using headphones. The lead and lag are each represented by click pairs whose perceived locations are simulated with ITDs (t1, t2) favoring the left and right ears, respectively. Onset delays due to sound propagation differences are simulated using the delay (in milliseconds). **C** Schematic of results obtained using the stimuli shown in **A** and **B**. SL (summing localization) occurs at delays of 0–1 ms. Localization dominance is an aspect of the PE that begins at 1 ms and persists until the PE breaks down. As part of the breakdown, temporal order confusion occurs, whereby listeners hear two sounds but cannot identify which is the lead and lag. As delays increase further, the PE is no longer operative, and temporal order is restored as well.

a schematic of another common stimulus configuration in which interaural timing difference (ITD) cues are manipulated to simulate the relative timing of stimuli with dichotic headphone stimulation. A conspicuous feature of these stimulus paradigms is a lack of attenuation of the lag source intensity relative to that of the lead, and the fact that they are typically identical in spectral content, which is not a natural representation of echoes that might occur in a room with absorbent materials. These stimulus parameters have been deliberately selected by investigators because of the dominant interest in the role of temporal delays between the lead and lag. When the onset of the lag relative to the lead is varied, several perceptual phenomena can be measured. A full review of these can be found elsewhere (Blauert, 1997; Litovsky et al., 1999).

When there is a brief delay between the onset of the lead and lag (<5 ms for clicks), listeners perceive a single, fused auditory event. The perceived location of that event depends on the weighting of localization cues that the auditory system attributes to each source. The weighting is distributed equally amongst the lead and lag for a delay of 0 ms; hence the fused image is heard at a phantom location midway between the two locations (see Fig. 14.2C). As the delay increases from 0 to 1 ms, the lead gains a disproportional amount of weight and the perceived location of the fused auditory image shifts towards the lead location, hence the phenomenon of 'localization dominance'. As delays continue to increase, the lag becomes increasingly more audible; in fact, listeners are unable to judge whether the lead or lag was presented first, hence 'temporal confusion'.

'Echo threshold' is the delay at which fusion of the lead and lag as well as localization dominance become weak. The concept of an echo threshold was invoked as a means of quantifying the temporal window over which localization cues carried by the lag are not accessible to the listener. Psychophysical studies have also utilized a paradigm whereby the ability of a listener to discriminate between two locations from which the lag might occur is measured as a function of delay. Another aspect of the PE, known as 'discrimination suppression' is thus characterized by chance performance for discrimination at brief delays, with increasing ease of the task as delays are increased.

14.2.2 Behavioral studies in non-human species

In the section that follows we review recent studies on physiological correlates of the PE. Prior to that, there is value in knowing the extent to which there is evidence for the PE in behavioral studies with non-human animals. Physiological studies have been undertaken in areas of the brain that are known to mediate mechanisms responsible for sound localization abilities. As they relate to the PE, physiological studies were initiated in the same anatomical regions, with the justification that correlates of the PE should be found in the same neural populations.

Beginning in the 1970s there was interest in studying sound localization and the PE in animals such as cats. Studies by Whitfield and colleagues (e.g., Whitfield et al., 1972) used ablation paradigms, whereby regions of primary auditory cortex were removed to study the functional importance of the auditory cortex for localization of lead–lag sounds in a PE paradigm. These studies suggested that the auditory cortex is necessary for the perception of the lead as the dominant source in the localization process, and were perhaps an impetus for studies in which the role of the immature auditory cortex was implicated in the developmental progression seen in the PE in young infants and children (for review see Litovsky and Ashmead, 1997). As reviewed by Litovsky et al. (1999), using simple discrimination paradigms several researchers succeeded in demonstrating that cats, rats, and crickets orient towards a leading sound source rather than the lagging source at about the same lead–lag delay as that seen in human listeners. More recent experiments, using more sophisticated methodological approaches, demonstrated that cross-species similarities in the PE are indeed remarkably high.

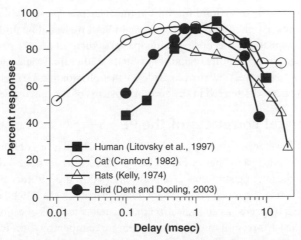

Fig. 14.3 Measures of the PE in humans and other animals. Each data set shows the percentage of trials in which the listener was able to correctly identify the location of the leading source. At short delays, performance is near 50% (chance); as delays increase to the range of localization dominance, performance rises, and a drop is observed at longer delays when the PE breaks down, and temporal order confusion occurs.

Yin and colleagues implemented a magnetic search coil method to measure eye and ear movements in cats that are behaviorally trained to look at a small light source and in the direction of sounds. Cats tested with this method show remarkable accuracy for sound localization of noise, bursts, and clicks. When presented with lead–lag pairs of clicks using delays of up to 300 μs in the azimuthal plane, the cats exhibited summing localization by looking in the direction of phantom source locations that are predicted by the lead–lag delay (Populin and Yin, 1998). Tollin and Yin (2003a) confirmed that summing localization occurs for noise stimuli as well; in addition, at delays of between 1 and 10 ms cats looked towards the leading source position with little evidence that they also localize the lagging source, suggesting that they exhibit localization dominance. This study further showed that delays at which the PE breaks down, i.e., at which behavioral echo thresholds are reached, range from 10–15 ms, which is remarkably similar to thresholds reported in human listeners (see Litovsky *et al.*, 1999).

Takahashi and colleagues (e.g., Spitzer *et al.*, 2003; Spitzer and Takahashi, 2006) showed similar effects in the barn owl, by employing infrared methods to measure changes in dilation of the pupil that occur when the animal detects a salient, novel stimulus, in a habituation and recovery paradigm. This powerful approach enabled measurement of the relative weighting attributed by the auditory system to the lead and lag sounds to generate a model of localization dominance for the owl (Spitzer and Takahashi, 2006). The delays at which the perceptual illusion of localization dominance was strongest were in the range of 3–5 ms, indicating remarkable similarity between owls and humans. Using operant conditioning methods, similar measures of performance were discovered between the aforementioned species and several other species of birds, such as budgerigars (Dent and Dooling, 2003), canaries, and zebra finches (Dent and Dolling, 2004).

Overall, the range of delays for which behavioral manifestation of the PE occurs is similar across several species, although not identical. The variation is more likely a function of the stimuli and behavioral paradigms than species differences. While inter-species differences merit consideration, there are remarkable ways in which the phenomenon holds up for animals that have different communication needs and that evolved to exist in different environmental habitats.

Figure 14.3 summarizes the behavioral findings in these various species, which suggests that, in general, the PE is a robust phenomenon that exists in both mammalian and non-mammalian species. Heuristically speaking, it is unsurprising that placement of greater perceptual weighting on leading sources is a general feature of auditory systems, rather than a specialized aspect unique to human perception. Thus, we now turn to evidence that physiological correlates of the PE, and its phenomena, have been discovered in the auditory systems of various species.

14.2.3 Physiological correlates of the PE

Correlates of the PE have been studied physiologically at nearly all levels of the auditory pathway. At early stages in the pathway, where monaural stimulation drives neural discharge, reduced neural responses to the lagging stimulus have been reported in the auditory nerve (e.g., Parham *et al.*, 1996) and cochlear nucleus (e.g., Wickesberg, 1996; Fitzpatrick *et al.*, 1999) at delays of 1–2 ms. These findings were interpreted as an indication that neural correlates of echo suppression exist. While monaural echo suppression might be important for dampening the audibility of the lag as a separate auditory event, the time window in which the physiological responses occur cannot account for longer-lasting (up to tens of milliseconds) effects that are measured behaviorally (see Litovsky *et al.*, 1999). At more central levels of the auditory pathway there have been extensive studies demonstrating correlates of the PE at much longer delay ranges. Of particular importance is the evidence for the existence of neural mechanisms that impact spatial hearing under conditions of the PE, which cannot be accounted for by the responses observed at monaural levels.

Although sounds originate from locations that vary in both azimuth and elevation, much of the work on the PE has been done using stimuli whose locations vary primarily in the horizontal plane, for which spatial information is encoded using interaural differences in timing and level. The auditory system is well known for having neural circuits that code for interaural differences, also known as *binaural* cues, at the level of the brainstem (see Chapter 12) and in cortical areas A1 (e.g., Middlebrooks and Pettigrew, 1981; Brugge *et al.*, 1996) and A2 (Middlebrooks, 1998). Binaural coding for timing and level are first measured at the level of the medial and lateral superior olives (MSO and LSO), respectively. However, the inferior colliculus (IC) has been the target of studies on physiological correlates of the PE, since it is there that information regarding both binaural timing and level converge are subsequently transmitted to higher brain centers.

Correlates of the PE in the responses of single neurons in the IC were first described in detail by Yin (1994). Responses of IC neurons to lead–lag click pairs with delays in the range of summing localization (0–1 ms) reflected the responses of those neurons to single sounds presented from the location at which the phantom image would be perceptually localized. By studying neural responses at longer delays, Yin and colleagues (Yin, 1994; Litovsky and Yin, 1998a, b; Tollin *et al.*, 2004) observed correlates of echo suppression at delays that overlap with the behavioral data. A characteristic response, reported by now in hundreds of IC neurons, is a delay-dependent spike rate. When lead–lag stimulus pairs such as clicks are presented with brief delays, the response resembles that of each neuron's response to the leading sound alone, in other words, a form of suppressed response to the lagging stimulus. A common metric used to quantify recovery from suppression has been the half-maximal delay or the lead–lag delay at which the lagging response recovered to 50% of its response in absence of the leading stimulus.

The early work of Yin and Litovsky was conducted in the barbiturate anesthetized cat, where neural echo threshold ranged from 2–100 ms (mean 34.8 ±8.5 ms). Although those delays certainly overlap with the psychophysical echo thresholds measured in humans and other animals, they are at the high end of the distribution. After Fitzpatrick *et al.*'s (1995) finding that recovery functions in similar structures in the awake rabbit were shifted towards smaller delays (mean 11.9

±3.3 ms), it was suspected that the additional inhibitory effects induced by barbiturates may have shifted the echo thresholds upwards, although the potential effect of species differences could not be discounted. The contribution of anesthesia was verified when Tollin and Yin (2003a) recorded in the IC of awake, behaving cats using stimuli that were known to evoke behavioral PE. Recovery functions were in delay ranges (mean 9.8 ±2.3 ms) similar to those of Fitzpatrick *et al.* and comparable to psychophysically measured echo thresholds in cats. Thus it appears that anesthesia, and not species differences, accounts for the different neural correlates of echo threshold (half-maximal delay) reported in the earlier studies.

Increased neural echo thresholds occur not only when inhibition is increased in the presence of barbiturates, but also at more central regions of the auditory pathway. In the auditory cortex, single-neuron studies to date have focused on species such as rabbit and cat (see below). In field A1 of awake rabbits, Fitzpatrick *et al.* (1999) found that half-maximal thresholds were overall approximately 20 ms, twice those in the brainstem of the awake rabbit. Reale and Brugge (2000) reported that in area A1 of the anesthetized cat, half-maximal delays ranged from 50–200 ms (median 94.7 ms); these values, again, were significantly larger than the ones reported in lower brainstem structures of the same species using similar stimuli and anesthesia. A third representative study by Mickey and Middlebrooks (2005) examined responses in three cortical fields of the anesthetized cat, including A1, A2, and posterior auditory field (PAF), and in A1 of awake cats. The median half-maximum delay was longer in this study than in Reale and Brugge's (>300 ms in A1 and PAF; 259 ms in A2).

Differences across studies in the delays at which recovery from suppression is observed may be accounted for by stimulus presentation mode (free field in Mickey and Middlebrooks' study; virtual space simulation of free field in Reale and Brugge's research). In addition, variants in anesthesia may have contributed to these differences (see discussion in Mickey and Middlebrooks). In fact, in a small number of animals, Mickey and Middlebrooks found that the proportion of units with a lagging response at a given delay was greater in the awake than in the anesthetized animal. Consistent with the rabbit data, it appears that in the cat barbiturates also increase inhibition and are likely to cause stronger measures of physiological correlates of the PE in anesthetized animals. Using an information transmission approach, these authors considered the extent to which information about the locations of the leading and lagging signals is preserved and extractable from single neuron responses. It appears that although neural responses to lagging stimuli appear, and are used to quantify echo thresholds, information regarding the locations of the delayed signals is not well coded until much longer delay ranges are used. This parallels psychophysical findings whereby the delays at which listeners hear the echo are typically shorter than the delays at which they are able to identify its location.

14.2.4 Spatial cue sensitivity

One of the hallmarks of IC neurons is that the vast majority are tuned to binaural difference cues; hence the original interest in understanding the extent to which spatial hearing phenomena are captured by the responses of these neurons. Neural recordings show there are robust effects of varying lead and lag spatial position on physiological correlates of PE in the IC. Reduced neural spike rate, i.e., suppression of the lag response, has been found to vary with the locations of both the lead and lag stimuli. In the anesthetized cat, Litovsky and Yin (1998b) used a free-field setup to vary the lead location along the azimuth while positioning the lag at a location to which the neuron responded vigorously, i.e., at the neuron's 'best' location. For most IC neurons, suppression was strongest when the lead was also at the 'best' location, and weakest when the lead was in the 'worst' location. Using dichotic stimulation with ITDs in the awake rabbit, Fitzpatrick *et al.* (1995)

found that about 50% of neurons showed greater suppression with the lead in the neuron's 'best' ITD (best-best) and 50% with the lead in the neuron's 'worst' ITD. This work suggested that there is some relationship between the suppression seen under conditions of the PE and the neuron's spatially dependent excitation pattern. Recall that the work was conducted under conditions in which only ITDs were present, or in which the full set of localization cues that are available in the free field co-varied; thus the extent to which suppression was linked to specific localization cues was not established.

Litovsky and Delgutte (2002) examined in more detail how the directionality of neural suppression is related to the directionally dependent excitability of the neuron, i.e., the neuron's preference regarding the lead location. Using virtual space stimuli obtained by digitally filtering sound waveforms through head-related transfer functions (HRTFs) of cats, partial-cue stimuli were synthesized in which one or two of the cues were held constant regardless of azimuth while the remaining cue(s) varied (Fig. 14.4A). This method had been used by this group in previous studies to investigate the processing of directional cues in the IC with single stimuli.

By applying this approach to the PE paradigm, it was possible to have the directional cues in the lead and lag either co-varied or dissociated, providing the opportunity to tease apart generally suppressive mechanisms (such as forward masking) from suppression that is specifically dependent on directional cues. Results from 63 neurons taken from 10 cats suggested that both the excitation produced by the lead and suppression of the lag responses were highly directional (Fig. 14.4). For some neurons, the degree of inhibition of the lag response was a mirror-image of the excitation that produced the lead response, suggesting that similar networks of neural inputs were engaged in mediating the responses of those neurons. In other neurons, there appeared to be no relationship between the excitation and inhibition. Furthermore, manipulation of the directional cues revealed interesting dissociations between the mechanisms that presumably mediate excitation and inhibition of IC neurons. The authors suggested that in neuron types for which there are dissociations, inhibitory inputs causing suppression may originate from subcollicular or other auditory nuclei that process different directional cues than the inputs that determine the pattern of directionally dependent excitation. It is these neurons in particular that may play the most important role, not just in fusion and echo suppression, but also in directionally dependent aspects of the PE, such as localization dominance, and discrimination suppression (see Litovsky et al., 1999).

The neural circuitry that mediates these complex spatio-temporal interactions is far from understood. There are species in which, although neural responses to delayed signals can be suppressed in the order of tens of milliseconds, the behavioral (perceptual) outcome can be quite different. Differences in outcomes between behavior and physiology have been seen when recordings were made from the dorsal nucleus of the lateral lemniscus (DNLL) in the bat (e.g., Yang and Pollak, 1994) and gerbil (Pecka et al., 2007). It appears that long-lasting inhibition for delayed signals is observed in the physiology, although behavioral correlates of spatial echo suppression are not found in bats in the same way as observed in humans and other animals (Saitoh and Suga, 1995; Schuchmann et al., 2006). From an evolutionary perspective this is perhaps not surprising since bats emit signals whose echoes are used to judge location and the distance of objects. This apparently adaptive mechanism may well have evolved in these animals in particular since they localize primarily in the dark and while in flight. In the bat, there appears to be a mechanism in which long-lasting inhibition such as that seen with PE stimuli, referred to as 'persistent inhibition' (PI), might actually enable the organism to utilize some cues that are available in the lagging sound.

More recently, the existence of PI was demonstrated in the mongolian gerbil (Pecka et al., 2007), suggesting that the PI mechanism is not limited to the bat, but is found in other mammals

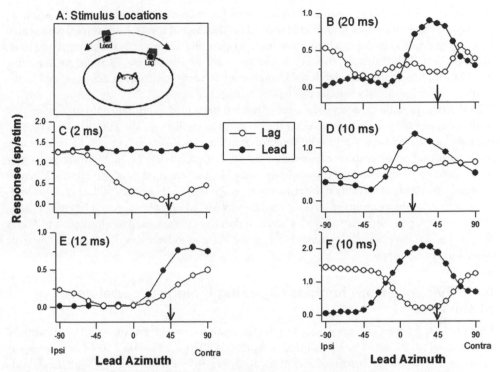

Fig. 14.4 Examples of responses from single IC neurons in the anesthetized cat, in which HRTF stimuli were used to manipulate lead and lag locations in a 'virtual space'. Each of the neurons shown here is representative of a different class of neurons. **A** Stimulus configuration; the lead stimulus varies in azimuth from *left* to *right*, while the lag stimulus is fixed at a location that produces a robust response. **B** Responses of both the lead and lag vary with source direction in azimuth, but there appears to be little relationship between the excitation produced by the lead and suppression of the lag. **C** Response to the lead does not vary with source direction, but the suppression of the lag is modulated nonetheless. **D** Opposite to **C**: response to the lead varies with source direction, but the suppression of the lag remains unmodulated. **E** Responses of both the lead and lag vary with source direction in azimuth, and the lag is well-predicted from the lead; unlike the neuron in **B**, when the lead produces strong excitation, the lag is weakly suppressed. **F** Responses of both the lead and lag vary with source direction in azimuth, and the lag is well-predicted from the lead such that when the lead produces strong excitation the lag is strongly suppressed. *Numbers in parentheses* indicate the delay between the lead and lag at which the measurements were obtained for each neuron. *Arrows* show the position of the lag stimulus. (After Litovsky and Delgutte, 2002.)

as well. Pollak and colleagues, as well as Pecka *et al.*, suggest that the PI is derived from the contralateral DNLL, and that its potential utility lies in the extraction of important usable information from echoes. One well-known example is the buildup and breakdown of echo suppression (the Clifton effect (Clifton and Freyman, 1997)) which is thought to involve higher-order processes that enable a listener to build dynamic internal models of auditory spaces, whereby echoes are initially heard and utilized, and subsequently suppressed when the auditory system has acquired sufficient information regarding their location.

This review of physiological studies on the PE has so far focused on paradigms in which the stimuli remained in the horizontal (azimuthal) plane, where interaural difference cues are primarily used for sound localization. Sound sources of course vary not only in location along the azimuth, but also in elevation, where sounds are localized on the basis of spectral shape cues, represented by peaks and valleys in the spectrum introduced by directionally dependent filtering of the head, torso, and ears (see Blauert, 1997). Psychophysical studies on the PE have shown that summing localization, fusion, and localization dominance also occur when sounds are presented in the midline vertical plane, where binaural cues are minimal or absent.

In the first investigation on correlates of human perception and neurophysiology in cats, Litovsky *et al.* (1997) demonstrated that the PE operates similarly in the azimuthal and median sagittal planes. Tollin and Yin (2003a) demonstrated that cats also experience the PE behaviorally for sounds that occur in the median sagittal plane. The occurrence of the PE in elevation is of particular note here because it cannot be explained by current models of the PE which invoke binaural processing of directional information to assign weighted averages to the perceived locations of fused auditory events (for review see Litovsky *et al.*, 1999). As suggested by Litovsky *et al.* (1997), in order to fully account for localization dominance, summing localization, and fusion that are known to occur in elevation, models of the PE need to be revised to include monaurally based directional inputs.

14.2.5 Evidence from humans regarding biological correlates of the PE

This final section on the PE is devoted to the few studies in which physiological or anatomical substrates of the PE could be investigated in humans. Litovsky *et al.* (2002) had a unique opportunity to investigate the functional role of the IC in the PE by conducting psychophysical measures in a subject who had suffered a unilateral small traumatic hemorrhage of the right brainstem involving the IC. The subject had normal pure-tone audiometric measures, but complained of difficulty localizing sounds. In addition, this individual's brainstem auditory evoked potentials showed abnormally small wave V amplitude following stimulation to the ear contralateral to the lesion. Perceptually, the strength of echo suppression was substantially weaker when the leading sound was on the side contralateral to the site of lesion than when it was ipsilateral to the lesion. A fascinating finding was that discrimination suppression, i.e., the extent to which changes in the ITD of the lagging sound can be discriminated (see Litovsky *et al.*, 1999), was abnormal: the subject's performance was excellent, whereas it should have been poor owing to suppression of the directional information carried by the lagging sound.

These findings suggest that the IC on the side of the brainstem contralateral to the leading sound plays an important role in activating or sustaining suppressive processes that are important for a PE that operates with fidelity. A lesion of the IC appears to be associated with atypical responses to tasks that measure the strength of echo suppression. Similar studies in which the IC is deliberately lesioned in other species have not been conducted, possibly because of the difficult nature of such experiments. Several studies have approached the role of the human auditory system in the PE using evoked potentials with stimuli that are known to evoke the PE perceptually. Correlates of the PE appear to be fairly robust at the level of the brainstem (Damaschke *et al.*, 2005) as well as the auditory cortex (Pratt *et al.*, 2001; Damaschke *et al.*, 2005). In general, the extent of suppression is much weaker at the level of the brainstem compared with the auditory cortex, in a way that is much more pronounced than the differences observed in physiology studies in non-human animals. This difference might be due to the fact that the human studies used field potentials as opposed to measuring single-neuron responses, and that the mechanisms underlying the PE are perhaps not as readily apparent in the gross potential measures that have been used.

14.2.6 Modeling studies

The PE has captured the interest and attention of numerous investigators, and has been the focus of several compelling models whose authors attempted to account for perceptual phenomena and/or related physiological findings. Existing models are either descriptive in that they account for particular perceptual effects, or physiologically based in that they feature known neural responses and anatomical pathways. For their inputs, the models primarily rely on binaural cues which are interpreted by the auditory system to code for source locations in the azimuth (horizontal plane). As was described earlier in the chapter, several studies have shown that the PE also operates in elevation (median plane), where spectral cues provide information about sound location, although these results have not yet been accounted for by existing models of the PE. These models are rooted in bottom-up approaches that focus on brainstem processes, and appear to account for many of the phenomena that have been described in this chapter.

The success of these models depended on their use of parameters such as interaural timing, level, and phase to code for relative source locations, and by invoking weighting schemes and inhibitory circuits that are akin to those found in the mammalian auditory system. These models were reviewed in detail by Litovsky *et al.* (1999), who noted that inhibition is a key factor in representing the processes engaged by the auditory system when greater weighting of location information is assigned to the first-arriving wave-front.

An alternative approach may be preferred for its simplicity, since it invokes solely peripheral auditory processing to account for some of the same phenomena that are related to the PE. Specifically, Hartung and Trahiotis (2001) showed that an internal representation of a fused auditory image can be accounted for without invoking binaural or central models. One drawback to this approach, noted by the authors, is the limitation of the model to transient stimuli separated by brief delays (~ 1 ms), and the lack of its extension to complex stimuli.

Finally, a limitation that is common to all existing models is their inability to account for phenomena related to the PE that are thought to involve higher-order processes such as attention, cognition, and memory.

14.2.7 Summary

Every-day acoustic environments are filled with multitudes of echoes whose presence is clearly noticed by the listener, but whose directional information is buried, perhaps suppressed, by the auditory system. Studies that address this issue have utilized a simplified set of stimuli to simulate aspects of source locations and delays in arrival times that mimic realistic propagation of sounds in rooms. The precedence effect (PE) refers to the auditory illusion which arises when two similar sounds are presented from different locations, but with a delay between their onsets, whereby listeners perceive a single fused auditory image whose perceived location is dominated by the first-arriving wave-front.

In the past few decades physiological investigations have uncovered the underlying mechanisms involved in mediating the PE. Overall, results from this work suggest that neurons at various levels in the auditory pathway respond to pairs of sounds that produce the PE perceptually in a delay-dependent manner. That is, responses to the first (leading) stimulus are generally robust, whereas responses to the second (lagging) stimulus are smaller or absent, suggesting the existence of forward-masking or suppressive mechanisms. The extent to which the lagging response is suppressed depends on a number of variables. These include the level within the auditory pathway, the relative locations of the leading and lagging stimuli, and whether the animal is awake or anesthetized. Overall, studies on physiological correlates of the PE suggest that the mechanisms involved in mediating the PE include monaural as well as binaural centers. What differentiates the binaural centers, where directional information is coded and transmitted to higher centers, is the location-dependent suppression.

14.3 Binaural masking level differences

This section examines a phenomenon that is thought to lie at the heart of the detection and perception of signals under complex listening situations. The ability to understand speech in noisy listening conditions is at least partly dependent on binaural hearing and the ability to perform binaural unmasking, a phenomenon first described independently, for speech and tones respectively, by J.C.R. Licklider and Ira Hirsh in 1948. In its most common form, the binaural masking level difference, or BMLD, is considered to be the difference in masked threshold for an *in-phase* signal (zero interaural phase difference between the ears) and an *anti-phase* signal (180°, or π, interaural phase difference between the ears) when the masker consists of identical noise tokens at the two ears. This configuration, referred to as N_0S_0 *vs* N_0S_π, is just one of a range of different signal and masker configurations that have been employed in the investigation of binaural unmasking in the 60 years since its discovery.

An extensive body of literature now exists reporting the influence on binaural unmasking of factors such as the relative interaural configurations of signal and masker, the frequency existence region over which unmasking is observed, the spectral composition of maskers and signals, and, where more behaviorally relevant signals are of interest, the use of speech-on-speech masking (for a review of the psychophysical literature see Durlach and Colburn, 1978). BMLD experiments have also been employed to address fundamental questions concerning the nature of binaural processing *per se*, including the existence of brain mechanisms that process interaural time differences (ITDs) by means of internal delay mechanisms, and the range of ITDs encoded by these internal delays (van der Heijden and Trahiotis, 1999).

Modern instantiations of psychophysically inspired models of binaural unmasking propose neural elements that bear striking resemblance to patterns of neural activation known to exist in the auditory brain. Generally, these models posit exclusively one of the two forms of known binaural interaction. Models based on Durlach's equalization-cancellation (E-C) hypothesis, which suggests that binaural unmasking arises by means of a differencing operation on the signal at each ear, include neural elements excited by one ear and inhibited by the other (in a manner dependent on the ITD of the stimulus). In contrast, modern correlation-based models employ purely excitatory neural elements that accord with Jeffress' (1948) model of coincidence detection. These models comprise arrays of binaural neurons that are maximally responsive when inputs from the two ears are timed so as to offset interaural differences in axonal conduction delay. In both cases, a wide range of internal delays is usually considered necessary to account for the data; internal delays corresponding to multiple cycles of the stimulus centre frequency are not uncommon in these models. Note, however, that Durlach's E-C hypothesis did not specify neural elements responsible for the model's required differencing function, whilst the vector model proposed by Webster (1951), to which later correlation-based models can be sourced, has no requirement for internal delays, necessitating only brain mechanisms sensitive to interaural correlation *per se*.

14.3.1 Neural elements contributing to binaural unmasking

Despite the apparent mutual exclusivity of the competing models of BMLD, electrophysiological studies suggest that neural elements corresponding to certain features of both models co-exist in the mammalian brain. A basic requirement of neurons underpinning binaural unmasking is that they exhibit sensitivity to ITDs in the fine-structure of the stimulus waveform. Such neurons are now well described throughout the ascending auditory pathway, including at the level of the brainstem, where it is now established that the MSO and LSO nuclei constitute the primary sites of binaural integration. Neurons in these nuclei, as well as in the IC of the midbrain, the thalamus, and the auditory cortex, respond to interaurally delayed sounds with discharge patterns that depend on the precise value of the ITD, the extent to which the sounds presented to the two ears are correlated, the bandwidth of the stimulus, and differences in the intensity of the sound presented to the two ears.

Neurons of the MSO, in accordance with the general principles of Jeffress' (1948) model, appear to act as binaural coincidence detectors, responding maximally when the externally applied acoustic delay offsets an internal, transmission delay (Fig. 14.5A). Such neurons provide a plausible physiological basis for the neural elements required in correlation-based models of binaural unmasking. In contrast to the MSO, ITD-sensitive neurons of the LSO, including those sensitive to low-frequency sounds, appear to act as *anti*-coincidence detectors, showing a response minimum when the externally applied ITD offsets the transmission delay (Fig. 14.5B).

The basis for this form of response appears to be the convergence of timed excitatory and inhibitory inputs such that, for appropriately delayed sounds, neural activity generated by one ear is essentially abolished by inhibition generated from the other. Such neurons potentially function as the elements described in the E-C hypothesis, and are explicitly implemented in recent implementations of the model (e.g., Breebaart *et al.*, 2001). Although the MSO and LSO represent the primary stages of binaural integration, the majority of studies examining sensitivity of auditory neurons to ITDs in mammals have, in fact, been investigated in the IC. From these studies it is not clear that the neural elements themselves represent distinct classes rather than a continuum (see Fig. 14.5C) between responses based largely on excitation from both ears, through to those based largely on excitation from one ear and inhibition from the other. The possibility of 'mixed' binaural excitatory and inhibitory processes is supported by recent evidence indicating that neural tuning for ITD in MSO neurons is at least partly determined by inhibitory mechanisms (Brand *et al.*, 2002).

14.3.2 Basic physiological investigations using single-neuron electrophysiology

Initial investigations of the neural basis of binaural unmasking failed to demonstrate any convincing explanation for the psychophysically observed results in the responses of single neurons. Recordings from the MSO of the chinchilla and the IC of the cat, respectively, Langford (1984) and Caird *et al.* (1989) were unable to provide evidence for a neural substrate of binaural unmasking, the latter concluding that '. . . it seems that single cells in the central nucleus of the inferior colliculus cannot code BMLDs'. In both studies, responses of single neurons were obtained to tones at a neuron's characteristic frequency (CF) in noise, when either the phase of both signal and noise were identical at the two ears or the phase of either the tone or noise at one ear was inverted. Although neither study was able to demonstrate sufficient differences in response patterns between the different stimulus configurations to provide a basis for the psychophysically observed BMLDs, Langford (1984) made the observation that the addition of a π-phase signal to a zero-phase noise masker produced a reduction in the discharge rate of single neurons in the MSO.

The failure to observe a neural substrate for the BMLD when the standard BMLD configurations were employed (i.e., those generating the greatest degree of psychophysical unmasking) led to a change in the strategy used to assess the capacity of single neurons to perform binaural unmasking. This culminated in a series of reports, spanning a decade, in which Palmer and colleagues demonstrated neural responses of binaural neurons in the IC consistent with at least some of the elements in the existing models of BMLD.

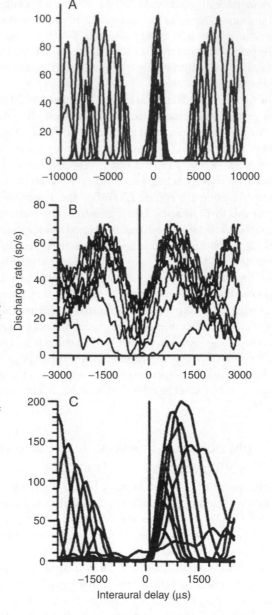

Fig. 14.5 Examples of ITD functions for three IC neurons. **A** Response of a 'peak-type' neuron, in which the response maxima of rate-vs-ITD functions for interaurally delayed tones of different frequencies are aligned at a common ITD. **B** Response of a 'trough-type' neuron, in which the response minima of rate-vs-ITD functions for interaurally delayed tones of different frequencies are aligned at a common ITD. **C** Response of a neuron in which the ITD functions are aligned at neither a common peak nor a trough in the response, but at an intermediate location (the ITD at which the functions align is indicated by the *vertical lines*). (Modified from McAlpine *et al.*, 1998.)

In the first of these studies (Caird *et al.*, 1991), and in a later study by McAlpine *et al.* (1996), an apparently critical factor was the use of signals in which the frequency, intensity, and interaural configurations were optimized for each neuron's sensitivity to these stimulus parameters. In both studies, neural correlates of binaural unmasking were observed. Caird *et al.* (1991) examined the effects of masking noise on the responses of single neurons in the guinea pig IC to 50-ms tone bursts at neural CF, or to 50-ms segments of a synthetic vowel, presented at a neuron's best ITD. Broadband noise maskers were presented at a range of ITDs, and the level of the noise was adjusted using an adaptive tracking paradigm to obtain a criterion spike difference. This method compared the discharge rate in a noise-alone interval with that in an interval containing both the noise and the signal, increasing or decreasing the intensity of the noise until a step of less than 1 dB was required for a difference in spike count in the two intervals to occur on 75% of trials. For most neurons, the level of noise required to elicit an increase in discharge rate was lowest at its best ITD to interaurally delayed noise. Similarly, desynchronization (to the fundamental frequency) of the temporal response to longer (500-ms) segments of the synthetic vowel by masking noise was most apparent when the noise was presented at each neuron's best ITD. Masked threshold differences across the population of neurons were reported as being very similar to the BMLD measured for human listeners using the same signal and masker conditions.

McAlpine *et al.*'s (1996) study extended the observations of Caird *et al.* (1991), confirming that when signals are optimized for the delay sensitivities of IC neurons, binaural unmasking is observed in the same direction as, and of a magnitude consistent with, human psychophysical observations. This study introduced a modified nomenclature for the binaural configurations employed that was suited to single-neuron studies, but which nevertheless followed the traditional subscripting employed to denote the binaural configuration of the stimulus (e.g., N_0 for diotically presented noise). By this nomenclature, signal and masker conditions were individualized for each neuron such that, for example, $N_{WD}S_{BD}$ was used to denote noise presented with an interaural delay equivalent to a neuron's least-preferred ITD (worst delay, WD: that evoking the response minimum) with the signal presented at the preferred ITD or best delay (BD).

In McAlpine *et al.*'s study, the magnitude of binaural unmasking was also compared across a range of non-optimized (for single-neuron unmasking) interaural configurations, including the configurations employed in the standard comparisons N_0S_0 vs N_0S_π and N_0S_0 vs $N_\pi S_0$, giving a total of eight binaural configurations, four in which the signal was presented at best ITD (S_{BD}) with the noise in one of four configurations N_{BD}, N_{WD}, N_0, and N_π, and the four standard configurations generated from S_0, S_π, N_0, and N_π. This included standard configurations in which the signal was a 500-Hz tone, independent of the neuron's frequency tuning. In general, masked thresholds were lowest for signals in the S_{BD} and S_0 configurations and highest for S_{WD} and S_π. The largest BMLDs were obtained for the comparison $N_{WD}S_{BD}$ vs $N_{BD}S_{BD}$, followed by N_0S_{BD} vs $N_\pi S_{BD}$. Again, however, both the sign and the magnitude of BMLDs for the standard configurations were opposite to those observed psychophysically; the comparison N_0S_0 vs N_0S_π producing largely negative BMLDs (signals more detectable in the S_0 than in the S_π configuration). Positive BMLDs of 3 dB or more were obtained for the comparison $N_\pi S_0$ vs N_0S_0 for 11/18 neurons, but only one neuron showed a positive BMLD for the comparison N_0S_0 vs N_0S_π.

For all binaural comparisons, both positive (π-phase signals more detectable, as is observed in the psychophysics) and negative BMLDs were obtained, often in the same neuron, a result entirely consistent with each neuron's sensitivities to the interaural delay of the noise and tone signals. Indeed, the dependence of binaural unmasking on the delay sensitivities of individual IC neurons, with maskers presented at either best or worst ITD, or in the N_0 or N_π configurations, highlighted the strong relationship between the noise-evoked discharge rate and the magnitude of binaural unmasking, with the major determinant of the masked threshold being the activity evoked in the neuron by the masking noise.

Despite the continued failure to replicate the psychophysical unmasking properties for the standard configurations, other features of the neural responses were consistent with behavioral data. For example, a common observation in human psychophysics is that the magnitude of the BMLD increases as the masker level is increased. This arises as a result of thresholds for out-of-phase signals increasing more slowly with increasing masker level compared with in-phase signals. Consistent with this, the magnitude of binaural unmasking for signals optimized for neural sensitivities in McAlpine *et al.* (1996) also increased with the level of the noise, by 5 dB over a 40-dB range of noise levels. As in the psychophysics, this arose because, as noise level was increased, masked threshold for optimized tones increased more slowly in N_π noise than in N_0 noise.

14.3.3 **Neural metrics of signal detection in binaural unmasking**

The importance of Langford's (1984) and McAlpine *et al.*'s (1996) findings is that they seem to suggest that increases in spike rate may not be an appropriate cue for masked threshold under these conditions. Nevertheless, the methods employed allowed only for the presence of a signal in background noise being rendered detectable by virtue of it evoking an *increase* in discharge rate above that evoked by the masker alone. Indeed, the threshold-tracking procedure employed by both Caird *et al.* (1991) and McAlpine *et al.* (1996) in determining single-neuron masked thresholds depended on such an outcome. This assumption is not necessarily a valid one, particularly with respect to correlation models of BMLD that posit reductions in neural activity upon the introduction of π-phase signals to diotic noise as being the basis for their enhanced detectability compared with zero-phase signals.

Jiang *et al.* (1997a) addressed this issue directly, employing the methodology of signal detection theory to demonstrate that reductions in discharge rate upon the introduction of a tone to masking noise were more detectable than increases. This study also employed, for the first time since Langford's (1984) study, a fixed level of masker noise for each neuron upon which signal level was varied. Thresholds for different signal and masker conditions were then assessed for single IC neurons by fixing the level of a supra-threshold noise masker (arbitrarily 7–15 dB above threshold for diotic noise) and measuring masked rate-vs-level functions over a range of signal levels. By calculating the mean and standard deviation of spikes evoked, it was possible to determine when the response first increased significantly above (or decreased below) that of the noise masker. Threshold was taken to be the signal level at which the standard separation 'D' first reached 1.0, either in the positive or the negative direction, when compared with the mean and standard deviation of the responses evoked by the lowest (subthreshold) 10-dB range of tone levels. In another significant change to previous studies, all neurons were assessed with respect to their ability to perform binaural unmasking using 500-Hz tones rather than their CF. The rationale for the choice of a fixed signal frequency was based on the nature of a standard psychophysical experiment in which the tone frequency is fixed; presumably the contribution of neurons with a range of CFs (here, in the range 168 Hz to 2.09 kHz) varies according to their frequency tuning characteristics.

Under these stimulus conditions – non-optimized for neural delay sensitivity – the noise-evoked response predictably dominated the masked rate-vs-level function at low signal levels. However, as the signal level was increased, its impact on the noise-evoked response became apparent. This effect was most likely a result of the specific binaural configuration of the signal. With some variation across neurons, and dependent largely on a neuron's ITD sensitivity, discharge rates either increased or decreased in response to increasing signal level. Neurons in which a 'D' of 1 (threshold) was reached with an increase in spike rate were labeled type-P (for Positive change) and those in which a 'D' of 1 was reached with a reduction in spike rate were labeled type-N (for Negative change) (see Fig. 14.6). Note that the BMLD responses (Fig. 14.6C) are in accordance with the delay functions to tones and noise in Fig 14.6A and B.

In half the neurons, increasing levels of either S_0 or S_π signals produced an increase in discharge rate above that evoked by the noise alone (thus P-P corresponding to an increase in spike rate for both binaural configurations at D = 1), with approximately one third showing positive BMLDs > 3 dB, one third showing negative BMLDs > 3 dB, and the remaining third showing no effect of signal configuration on masked threshold. In a third of neurons, however, increasing the signal level produced an increase in discharge rate for S_0 signals, but a reduction for S_π signals (N-P). Of these neurons, the vast majority (73%) showed positive BMLDs > 3 dB, i.e., in the direction consistent with psychophysics, with fewer than 5% showing negative BMLDs of similar magnitude.

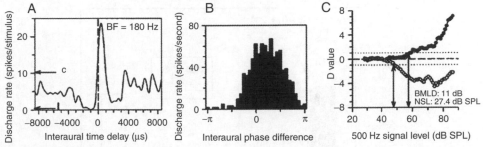

Fig. 14.6 Response of an IC neuron with CF of 180 Hz to **A** interaurally delayed noise, **B** binaural beats, where the signal in the left ear (contralateral to the recording site) was a 500-Hz tone and the signal in the right ear a 499-Hz tone, and **C** increasing levels of binaural 500-Hz tones in the S_0 (*closed symbols*) or S_π (*open symbols*) configurations. Note that the threshold value of the standard separation 'D' (where the spike rate increased significantly above the average rate for the lowest 10 dB of tone levels, i.e., below tone threshold) is positive for the S_0 signal (a type-P response) and negative for S_π (a type-N response). The magnitude of binaural unmasking for this neuron was +11 dB. (Modified from Jiang *et al.*, 1997a.)

Few neurons (<7%) showed a reduction in discharge rate for both signal configurations (N-N), and fewer still (<2%) a reduction in discharge rate in response to increasing levels of S_0 tones and an increase of S_π (N-P).

This study demonstrated two important points. First, that it is possible to identify a neural substrate of the BMLD using the standard psychophysical configurations, including a fixed signal frequency. Second, that binaural unmasking observed in single neurons supports a specific psychophysical model of the BMLD, in which S_π signals are rendered more detectable by virtue of a reduction and S_0 signals by virtue of an increase in the activity evoked by a N_0 masker alone. It was also noted that neurons contributing to the psychophysical BMLD for a 500-Hz tone are, perhaps unsurprisingly, those with CFs close to 500 Hz, and that the detection of S_0 and S_π signals may depend on different populations of neurons. The rationale for this statement relates to the fact that detection threshold is likely based on those neurons in which threshold occurs at the lowest signal-to-noise ratio.

This notion was explored further by Jiang *et al.* (1997b), who took the return to psychophysical parameters to its logical conclusion by examining the responses of a large population of IC neurons ($n = 121$) in a small number of animals ($n = 5$) for the N_0S_0 and N_0S_π configurations for a fixed level of noise across all neurons. Across all neurons (with CFs in the range 100 Hz to 2.33 kHz), the BMLD for the standard comparison N_0S_0 vs N_0S_π was 5.5 dB and 6.6 dB for those neurons with CFs in the range 300–800 Hz. As Fig. 14.7 indicates, the lowest thresholds to S_0 signals were obtained for neurons in which this configuration produced a type-P response (i.e., discharge rates increased with increasing signal level and D was positive at threshold – see Fig. 14.6C). Conversely, the lowest thresholds for S_π signals were obtained in neurons in which a type-N response was evoked (discharge rates fell with increasing signal level and D at threshold was negative – see Fig. 14.6C). The highest thresholds were obtained for those neurons in which adding an S_0 signal reduced the discharge rate to noise alone. Based purely on neurons in which introducing an S_0 signal led to an increase in discharge rate (type-P responses), the BMLD across the population of neurons was less than 2 dB (for a noise with a fixed spectrum level of 23 dB SPL). Thus, it appears that different neuronal populations are required to account for the BMLD, responding differently to the different signal and masker configurations.

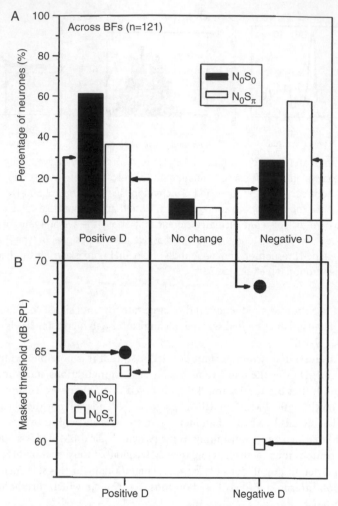

Fig. 14.7 A Proportions of IC neurons with type-P or type-N responses (increases or decreases in discharge rate at masked threshold compared with noise-evoked responses) and their average masked thresholds. *Across BFs* indicates that neurons of all BF sampled were included. **B** Average masked thresholds for S_0 (*filled circles*) and S_π (*open squares*) tones computed separately for neurons yielding positive and negative D values, as indicated by the *arrows* from the histogram bars to the corresponding masked thresholds. (From Jiang *et al.*, 1997b.)

From the same data set, Palmer *et al.* (2000) reported binaural unmasking for another comparison of the standard configurations, N_0S_0 vs $N_\pi S_0$. Psychophysically, this comparison provides for a smaller BMLD (6–12 dB) than N_0S_0 vs N_0S_π, which can be as high as 15 dB. Consistent with this, the single-neuron BMLD for the N_0S_0 vs $N_\pi S_0$ comparison was just 3.6 dB, compared with 6.6 dB for N_0S_0 vs N_0S_π. In this case, however, because noise presented in the N_π configuration evokes little activity in most neurons, due to the least favourable ITD of most neurons corresponding to roughly half a cycle of their CF, the predominant response to an S_0 signal was an increase in discharge rate. Thus, for this comparison, signal detection was largely mediated by neurons increasing their response above the (low) background level of activity generated by the N_π noise.

14.3.4 Signal-to-noise ratios and neural unmasking

An important consideration in psychophysical studies of binaural unmasking is the signal-to-noise (S/N) ratio at which unmasking occurs. The advantages in detection gained by having masker and signal in opposite phase relationships occur when the S/N ratio at masked threshold is negative for S_π signals in N_0 noise. Thus, for at least some neurons, it is likely to be the case that they indicate the presence of a tone at negative S/N ratios. This was examined directly in a study by Jiang *et al.* (1997b) in which the effect of increasing masker level was assessed for several different S/N ratios, where the S/N ratio within the auditory channel (i.e., the ratio of the signal to the noise within the neural filter) was calculated according to the effective bandwidth of 200 Hz for center frequencies of 500 Hz (data for the guinea pig; Evans *et al.*, 1992). From this calculation, and for a fixed signal level of 50 dB SPL, the S/N ratio within the 500-Hz frequency channel was estimated to be 0 dB.

Taking the view that across the population detection of the tone will be mediated by those neurons with the lowest masked thresholds, Jiang *et al.* (1997b) determined which neurons would be responsible for tone detection (based on an arbitrary requirement of 5–8% of neurons necessary for detection to occur) at different S/N ratios. At 0 dB S/N ratio, and in response to S_π tones, 17/121 neurons showed significant changes in discharge rate – either an increase or a reduction – compared with the N_0-evoked response alone. A smaller number of neurons showed increases in discharge rate when S_0 signals were introduced at this S/N ratio. These neurons tended not to be the same as those that responded to S_π signals with a reduction in discharge rate at this S/N ratio. Reducing the S/N ratio further to –5 dB (i.e., by examining those neurons contributing to detection when the tone level was 45 dB SPL) revealed fewer neurons in which either signal configuration evoked sufficient change in spike rate to distinguish the response from that to noise alone, and, in response to S_π signals, only those neurons that responded with a reduction in discharge rate contributed to detection. From this it can be concluded that different populations of neurons potentially contribute to detection of S_0 and S_π signals, but that detection at the lowest S/N ratios is largely mediated by neurons responding to S_π signals with a reduction in discharge rate.

14.3.5 Support for specific models of BMLD

The cross-correlation model of binaural detection suggests that adding an S_π signal to N_0 noise desynchronizes the response to N_0 noise alone, the consequence of within-channel disruption of the interaural phase. Palmer *et al.* (1999) examined this proposition directly by recording responses of IC neurons to interaurally delayed noise with various levels of interaural correlation (between 1.0 – fully correlated at the two ears – and 0.0 – independent noises at the two ears), and then comparing the responses evoked to adding a 500-Hz tone in either 0 or π interaural phase to the interaurally delayed noise.

Generally, the effect of adding S_0 tones was to saturate a neuron's noise delay function, raising discharge rates at all ITDs to those corresponding to the peak rate (Fig. 14.8). Adding S_π tones had the opposite effect: as tone level was increased, discharge rates at response peaks decreased, and those at troughs increased, reducing the modulation of the noise delay function until discharge rates at all ITDs lay midway between those of the original response peaks and troughs. The effect was largely consistent with that produced by reducing the interaural correlation of the noise, suggesting support for cross-correlation models of BMLD, although some evidence of inhibitory influences was also observed in that discharge rates sometimes fell below those evoked by the uncorrelated noise. Note, however, that it is not strictly necessary to invoke inhibitory mechanisms to explain these data; since S_π signals are anti-correlated, not simply de-correlated, the discharge rate will tend to reflect that evoked by the worst ITD when the signal overwhelms completely the noise-evoked response.

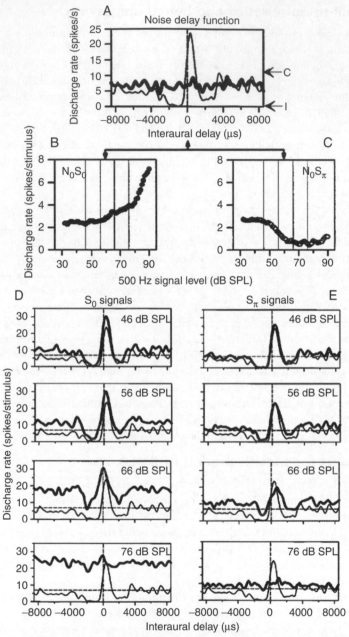

Fig. 14.8 Responses of an IC neuron with CF of 300 Hz. **A** Response to interaurally delayed noise with interaural correlation of 1.0 (*fine line*) and 0.0 (*heavy line*). **B** and **C** Masked rate-level functions to 500-Hz tones in the presence of identical noise at a spectral level of 31 dB SPL at the two ears, with tones presented in either zero (**B**) or π (**C**) interaural phase difference. *Thin vertical lines* in **B** and **C** show the tone levels in **D** and **E** at which noise-vs-ITD functions were obtained. **D** and **E** Responses to interaurally delayed noise with increasing levels of 500-Hz tones in S_0 (**D**) and S_π (**E**). (Modified from Palmer *et al.*, 1999.)

One general caveat for the apparent support these data provide for cross-correlation models of BMLD is that such models do not necessarily include internal delay mechanisms, but, rather, neural mechanisms by which changes in interaural correlation are rendered detectable. Nevertheless, the fact that ITD-sensitive neurons show such sensitivity is at least consistent with the contribution of internal delays to binaural unmasking.

Since, in Jiang et al.'s (1997a) study, the lowest thresholds occurred for those neurons in which discharge rates fell with increasing levels of an S_π signal, minimum detection thresholds appear to be associated with those neurons in which a reduction in interaural correlation leads to a reduction in neural activity. Nevertheless, the extent to which a reduction in neural activity constitutes, per se, the neural marker for detecting a signal in masking noise is moot. A second possibility, also consistent with the physiological data, is that the reduction in activity in response to S_π signals in the majority of neurons, and the increase in activity in the minority, act in concert to enhance signal detection. As Jiang et al. (1997b) comment 'the effective contrast in neural activation between these two populations contributes to the S_π signal audibility'.

Such physiological data do not sit easily with current psychophysically inspired models of BMLD. However, it should be remembered that the stimulus configurations used in BMLD studies are largely physiologically implausible, in that they employ a constant phase shift at all frequencies. The BMLD is a consequence of mechanisms that evolved to enhance signal detection in noisy environments. To this end it would be important to assess binaural unmasking in the wider context of spatial release from masking, the ability to hear out signals in background noise under more natural listening conditions, where cues other than ITD contribute: for example, release from masking by the monaural mechanism of listening through the ear with the most advantageous signal-to-noise ratio – the 'better ear effect'.

In a recent study by Lane and Delgutte (2005) spatial release from masking was examined using more realistic signal and masker conditions. Targeting low-CF neurons in the cat IC and employing virtual acoustic space (VAS) stimuli (broadband chirp trains presented at 40 Hz with a continuous broadband masker), these authors confirmed the basic findings of Palmer and colleagues. Single-neuron unmasking abilities reflected more the azimuthal tuning properties of individual neurons than the relative (virtual) location of signal and masker. These authors found the best neural thresholds to correspond to human psychophysical performance. In addition, although many of the data could be accounted for in terms of a binaural cross-correlation model, indicating ITD to be a major contributor to unmasking effects, the responses of at least some neurons appeared to be influenced by further processing. In particular, an enhanced response to the chirp stimuli employed was observed, suggesting that although both signal and masker may have similar spectra, the tuning of IC neurons to stimulus 'features' such as amplitude modulation likely also plays a role in signal detection in noise.

14.3.6 Human physiological studies of binaural unmasking

Although studies of binaural unmasking in humans with disorders of central auditory processing suggest that the BMLD reflects brainstem processing of sound, direct electrophysiological investigations measuring auditory brainstem and middle latency responses (ABRs and MLRs) or the auditory steady-state response (ASSR) (e.g., Wong and Stapells, 2004) have failed to demonstrate evidence for the involvement of brainstem mechanisms in generating binaural unmasking. Responses to BMLD stimuli have reliably been measured in cortical potentials. For example, using magneto-encephalography (MEG), Sasaki et al. (2005) demonstrated cortical responses consistent with many of the psychophysical findings, including the dependence of binaural unmasking on the overall signal level – unmasking is greater for signal levels close to threshold and disappears altogether some 15–20 dB above this. Nevertheless, the failure to observe brainstem markers for binaural unmasking is, at first glance, surprising, given the likely location of neural elements sensitive to interaurally delayed sounds.

Explanations for the failure to observe neural markers for the BMLD below the cortical level include the possibility that interaural phase information underpinning binaural unmasking is not extracted until this level of processing, a highly unlikely scenario given its dependence on neural phase-locking, which is known to degrade substantially in transmission to the level of primary cortex. A more compelling explanation for the failure of non-invasive measures of neural activity to reveal BMLD-like responses lies in the possibility, supported by the findings of Jiang *et al.* (1997b), that binaural unmasking may be the product of both increases and decreases in the activity of small populations of neurons, with different neurons contributing to signal detection for different signal or masker conditions. Transformation or amplification of these small neural signals at the cortical level might be necessary for their capture by the relatively insensitive techniques employed in whole-brain measures of neural activity.

14.3.7 Summary

Clear evidence exists, from single-neuron studies in the auditory midbrain at least, of a neural substrate of binaural unmasking and the psychophysically determined BMLD in particular. A synopsis of the physiological studies would conclude that having initially abandoned, or down-played, the standard binaural configurations in favour of optimizing signals for individual neurons' proclivities, the subsequent extension of possible neural metrics for detecting tones in noise to include reductions in discharge rate proved decisive. However, the extent to which any particular brain mechanism might be thought both necessary and sufficient to account for the psychophysical data remains to be determined. The failure to demonstrate neural markers for the BMLD below the cortical level using non-invasive techniques may be the result of the diverse neural responses to BMLD signals suggested by single-neuron studies.

14.4 Conclusions

The precedence effect (PE) and binaural masking level difference (BMLD) are two effects that have been studied in depth in order to understand auditory mechanisms that enhance localization, detection, and perception of signals under complex listening situations. These two phenomena are notable in that correlates of both have been found in responses of single neurons in the auditory pathway. The work on the PE suggests that, while suppression of echoes occurs at low-level, monaurally driven levels in the auditory pathway, the extent of the suppression increases at higher levels. The best characterization of differences between the binaural and monaural auditory centers is that directionally dependent suppression is coded and transmitted to higher centers in the binaural pathway, i.e., the midbrain. It is at this same level of auditory processing that clear evidence for a neural substrate of BMLD is found. In both cases, the underlying neural mechanisms involved remain to be fully understood. Methods that involve multi-unit recordings and non-invasive brain function measures, in both human and non-human species, are shedding light on these issues.

References

Blauert J (1997) *Spatial Hearing: The Psychophysics of Human Sound Localization*, revised edition. MIT Press, Cambridge, Massachusetts.

Brand A, Behrend O, Marquardt T, McAlpine D, Grothe B (2002) Precise inhibition is essential for microsecond interaural time difference coding. *Nature* 417: 543–47.

Breebaart J, van de Par S, Kohlrausch A (2001) Binaural processing model based on contralateral inhibition. I. Model structure. *J Acoust Soc Am* **110**: 1074–88.

Brugge JF, Reale RA, Hind JE (1996) The structure of spatial receptive fields of neurons in primary auditory cortex of the cat. *J Neurosci* **15,16**(14): 4420–37.

Caird D, Pillmann F, Klinke R (1989) Responses of single cells in the cat inferior colliculus to binaural masking level difference signals. *Hear Res* **43**: 1–23.

Caird DM, Palmer AR, Rees A (1991). Binaural masking level difference effects in single units of the guinea pig inferior colliculus. *Hear Res* **57**: 91–106.

Clifton RK, Freyman RL (1997) The precedence effect: beyond echo suppression. In: Binaural and Spatial Hearing in Real and Virtual Environments (eds Gilkey RH, Anderson TR), pp. 233–55. Lawrence Earlbaum, Mahwah, New Jersey.

Cranford JL (1982) Localization of paired sound sources in cats: effects of variable arrival times. *J Acoust Soc Am* **72**(4): 1309–11.

Damaschke J, Riedel H, Kollmeier B (2005). Neural correlates of the precedence effect in auditory evoked potentials. *Hear Res* **205**: 157–71.

Dent ML, Dooling RJ (2003) Investigations of the precedence effect in budgerigars: the perceived location of auditory images. *J Acoust Soc Am* **113**: 2159–69.

Dent ML, Dooling RJ (2004) The precedence effect in three species of birds (*Melopsittacus undulatus*, *Serinus canaria*, and *Taeniopygia guttata*). *J Comp Psychol* **118**(3): 325–31.

Durlach N, Colburn H (1978) Binaural phenomena. In: Handbook of Perception. Volume IV: Hearing (eds Carterette E, Friedman M), pp. 365–466. Academic Press, New York.

Evans EF, Pratt SR, Spencer H, Cooper NP (1992) Comparisons of physiological and behavioural properties: auditory frequency selectivity. *Adv Biosci* **83**: 159–69.

Fitzpatrick DC, Kuwada S, Batra R, Trahiotis C (1995) Neural responses to simple, simulated echoes in the auditory brainstem of the unanesthetized rabbit. *J Neurophysiol* **74**: 2469–86.

Fitzpatrick DC, Kuwada S, Kim DO, Parham K, Batra R (1999) Responses of neurons to click-pairs as simulated echoes: auditory nerve to auditory cortex. *J Acoust Soc Am* **106**: 3460–72.

Hartung K, Trahiotis C (2001) Peripheral auditory processing and investigations of the "precedence effect" which utilize successive transient stimuli. *J Acoust Soc Am* **110**: 1505–13.

Hirsch IJ (1948) Binaural summation and interaural inhibition as a function of the noise level of the masking noise. *Am J Psychol* **56**: 205–13.

Jeffress LA (1948) A place theory of sound localization. *J Comp Physiol Psychol* **61**: 468–86.

Jiang D, McAlpine D, Palmer AR (1997a) Responses of neurons in the inferior colliculus to binaural masking level difference stimuli measured by rate-versus-level functions. *J. Neurophysiol* **77**: 3085–106.

Jiang D, McAlpine D, Palmer AR (1997b) Detectability index measures of binaural masking level difference across populations of inferior colliculus neurons. *J. Neurosci* **17**: 9331–9.

Kelly JB (1974) Localization of paired sound sources in the rat: small time differences. *J Acoust Soc Am* **55**: 1277–84.

Lane CC, Delgutte B (2005) Neural correlates and mechanisms of spatial release from masking: single-unit and population responses in the inferior colliculus. *J. Neurophysiol* **94**: 1180–98.

Langford TL (1984) Responses elicited from medial superior olivary neurons by stimuli associated with binaural masking and unmasking. *Hear Res* **15**: 39–50.

Licklider JCR (1948) The influence of interaural phase relations upon the masking of speech by white noise. *J Acoust Soc Am* **20**: 150–9.

Litovsky R, Ashmead D (1997) Developmental aspects of binaural and spatial hearing. In: Binaural and Spatial Hearing (eds Gilkey RH, Anderson TR), pp. 571–92. Earlbaum, Hillsdale, New Jersey.

Litovsky RY, Delgutte B (2002) Neural correlates of the precedence effect in the inferior colliculus: effect of localization cues. *J Neurophysiol* **87**: 976–94.

Litovsky RY, Yin TC (1998a) Physiological studies of the precedence effect in the inferior colliculus of the cat. I. Correlates of psychophysics. *J Neurophysiol* 80(3): 1285–301.

Litovsky RY, Yin TC (1998b) Physiological studies of the precedence effect in the inferior colliculus of the cat. II. Neural mechanisms. *J Neurophysiol* 80: 1302–16.

Litovsky RY, Rakerd B, Yin TC, Hartmann WM (1997) Psychophysical and physiological evidence for a precedence effect in the median sagittal plane. *J Neurophysiol* 77(4): 2223–6.

Litovsky RY, Colburn HS, Yost WA, Guzman SJ (1999) The precedence effect. *J Acoust Soc Am* 106: 1633–54.

Litovsky RY, Fligor BJ, Tramo MJ (2002) Functional role of the human inferior colliculus in binaural hearing. *Hear Res* 165: 177–88.

McAlpine D, Jiang D, Palmer AR (1996) Binaural masking level differences in the inferior colliculus of the guinea pig. *J Acoust Soc Am* 100: 490–503.

McAlpine D, Jiang D, Shackleton TM, Palmer AR (1998) Convergent input from brainstem coincidence detectors onto delay-sensitive neurons in the inferior colliculus. *J Neurosci* 18: 6026–39.

Mickey BJ, Middlebrooks JC (2005) Sensitivity of auditory cortical neurons to the locations of leading and lagging sounds. *J Neurophysiol* 94(2): 979–89.

Middlebrooks JC, Pettigrew JD (1981) Functional classes of neurons in primary auditory cortex of the cat distinguished by sensitivity to sound location. *J Neurosci* 1(1): 107–20.

Middlebrooks JC, Xu L, Eddins AC, Green DM (1998) Codes for sound source location in non-tonotopic auditory cortex. *J Neurophysiol* 80: 863–81.

Palmer AR, Jiang D, McAlpine D (1999) Desynchronizing responses to correlated noise: a mechanism for binaural masking level differences at the inferior colliculus. *J Neurophysiol* 81: 722–34.

Palmer AR, Jiang D, McAlpine D (2000) Neural responses in the inferior colliculus to binaural masking level differences created by inverting the noise in one ear. *J Neurophysiol* 84: 844–52.

Parham K, Zhao HB, Kim DO (1996) Responses of auditory nerve fibers of the unanesthetized decerebrate cat to click pairs as simulated echoes. *J Neurophysiol* 76(1): 17–29.

Pecka M, Zahn TP, Saunier-Rebori B, *et al.* (2007) Inhibiting the inhibition: a neuronal network for sound localization in reverberant environments. *J Neurosci* 27(7): 1782–90.

Populin LC, Yin TCT (1998) Behavioral studies of sound localization in the cat. *J Neurosci* 18: 2147–60.

Pratt H, Bleich N, Mittelman N (2001) Echo suppression in the human cortex is affected by the spatial and temporal proximity of the primary sound and echo. *J Basic Clin Physiol Pharmacol* 12: 109–23.

Reale RA, Brugge JF (2000) Directional sensitivity of neurons in the primary auditory (AI) cortex of the cat to successive sounds ordered in time and space. *J Neurophysiol* 84: 435–50.

Saitoh I, Suga N (1995) Long delay lines for ranging are created by inhibition in the inferior colliculus of the mustached bat. *J Neurophysiol* 74(1): 1–11.

Sasaki T, Kawase T, Nakasato N, *et al.* (2005) Neuromagnetic evaluation of binaural unmasking. *Neuroimage* 25: 684–9.

Schuchmann M, Hubner M, Wiegrebe L (2006) The absence of spatial echo suppression in the echolocating bats *Megaderma lyra* and *Phyllostomus discolor*. *J Exp Biol* 209: 152–7.

Spitzer MW, Takahashi TT (2006) Sound localization by barn owls in a simulated echoic environment. *J Neurophysiol* 95: 3571–84.

Spitzer MW, Bala AD, Takahashi TT (2003) Auditory spatial discrimination by barn owls in simulated echoic conditions. *J Acoust Soc Am* 113: 1631–45.

Tollin DJ, Yin TCT (2003a) Psychophysical investigation of an auditory spatial illusion in cats: the precedence effect. *J Neurophysiol* 90: 2149–62.

Tollin DJ, Yin TC (2003b) Spectral cues explain illusory elevation effects with stereo sounds in cats. *J Neurophysiol* 90: 525–30.

Tollin DJ, Populin LC, Yin TCT (2004) Neural correlates of the precedence effect in the inferior colliculus of behaving cats. *J Neurophysiol* 92: 3286–97.

van der Heijden M, Trahiotis C (1999) Masking with interaurally delayed stimuli: the use of "internal" delays in binaural detection. *J Acoust Soc Am* **105**: 388–99.

Webster FA (1951) The influence of interaural phase on masked thresholds. I. The role of interaural time deviation. *J Acoust Soc Am* **23**: 452–62.

Whitfield IC, Cranford J, Ravizza R, Diamond IT (1972) Effects of unilateral ablation of auditory cortex in cat on complex sound localization. *J Neurophysiol* **35**: 718–31.

Wickesberg RE (1996) Rapid inhibition in the cochlear nuclear complex of the chinchilla. *J Acoust Soc Am* **100**: 1691–702.

Wong YS, Stapells DR (2004) Brain stem and cortical mechanisms underlying the binaural masking level difference in humans: an auditory steady-state response study. *Ear Hear* **25**: 57–67.

Yang L, Pollak GD (1994) The roles of GABAergic and glycinergic inhibition on binaural processing in the dorsal nucleus of the lateral lemniscus of the mustache bat. *J Neurophysiol* **71**: 1999–2013.

Yin TCT (1994) Physiological correlates of the precedence effect and summing localization in the inferior colliculus of the cat. *J Neurosci* **14**: 5170–86.

Section 4

Development, aging, and plasticity of the auditory brain

Chapter 15

Development of the auditory pathway

Douglas E.H. Hartley and Andrew J. King

15.1 The importance of studying auditory development

Over the past few decades, the study of auditory development has added significantly to our understanding not only of the processes that underlie auditory function in adulthood, but also of the effects of hearing loss on the developing brain. Although the auditory system is by no means mature in young animals, much of the rudimentary structure of the auditory pathways from the cochlea to cortex is in place at birth. After birth, the individual components of these pathways and the perceptual abilities to which they contribute develop with different time-constants. With this in mind, we can utilize ontogenesis as a research tool to dissect some of the critical components of hearing. In so doing, we can identify how different elements interact to form the mature auditory system, be it at a genetic, molecular, cellular, neuronal, network, or behavioral level.

Some components of the immature and, to a lesser extent, the mature auditory system are shaped by experience to fit their acoustic environment. Studies of visual perception have shown that abnormal visual input in young animals causes significantly greater and more lasting deficits in visual perception than in older animals (Wiesel and Hubel, 1965). This leads us to a crucial question in auditory research, namely, to what extent is the influence of experience restricted to a 'sensitive' or 'critical period' of development? Recent experimental evidence has shown that extensive plasticity is possible in adulthood (see Chapter 16). Subsequently, it has been necessary to modify our concept of a 'sensitive period'. Nevertheless, it does appear that neural circuitry emerging during development can, to a large degree, constrain the plasticity seen later in life.

Ultimately, the evolution of the auditory system has helped many species adapt to their surroundings. Hearing has aided their survival through both the search for food and avoidance of prey. Many animals have also utilized their hearing abilities to facilitate communication between con-specific individuals, a capacity that reaches its zenith in humans. Thus, in our communication-based societies, it is arguable that hearing loss impacts upon one of our most distinguishing characteristics. Indeed, the very plasticity that allows the auditory system to become tuned to a rich acoustic environment can also result in it being corrupted by auditory deprivation. However, provided normal sensation is restored at a sufficiently early stage, normal function can eventually be recovered. Optimistically, it is through the study of auditory development that we can aspire to discover treatments for deafness that are directed at specific processes and at appropriate times, whist improving our understanding of the biological mechanisms of hearing.

15.2 When does hearing start?

It is tempting to think that the auditory system simply blossoms into being: we are born and we begin to hear. Instead, it is during embryology that the development of the auditory system begins, including, at least in humans and certain other precocial species, the appearance of the first sensory responses to sound. Although much of the structure of the auditory system is in place at birth (Moore and Linthicum, 2007), an infant still has to learn how to make sense of sounds from the world around it, which is a skill that must be mastered in stages. This section reviews some of the key embryological and perinatal milestones that contribute to the formation of the adult auditory system. Indeed, the identification of milestones in auditory development provides us with potential insights into processes of rapid development that might be vulnerable to the effects of hearing loss, compared with more robust systems that have already reached a more advanced stage of maturity (Moore and Linthicum, 2007).

The early development of the peripheral auditory system is extremely complex, with the external, middle, and inner ear structures having different embryological origins (Fritzsch *et al.*, 1998). A consequence of this developmental complexity is that hearing impairments could potentially result from any one of a myriad of possible errors. Moreover, the maturation of certain parts of the auditory periphery is a lengthy process that extends from early embryonic life until well into the postnatal period. For instance, although the pinna and external auditory canal are formed during the 4 and 5th fetal weeks, they do not reach adult-like proportions for another decade (Wright, 1997). As we shall see, this can help to explain some of the postnatal changes in neuronal response properties that take place within the brain.

The initial stage in the development of the human inner ear is marked by a thickening of the ectoderm in the region of the hindbrain, called the otic placode. Subsequently, the otic placode develops into the otocyst, which contributes to the formation of the auditory nerve and hair cells through the development of the otic ganglion and the cochlear duct, from which the cochlea is formed. By extending processes in two directions, the cochlear ganglion cells provide a link between the cochlea and the central nervous system (Rubel and Fritzsch, 2002). The ganglion cell fibers reach the cochlear hair cells and their targets in the brainstem very early in development and well before the onset of hearing (Rubel and Fritzsch, 2002). Central auditory nuclei appear in a specific order (Cant, 1998) and, by the 8th fetal week in humans, the cochlear nuclei, trapezoid body, superior olivary complex, lateral lemniscus, inferior colliculus (IC), and medial geniculate nucleus are all evident (Cooper, 1948; Dekaban, 1954). These structures subsequently increase in size while retaining the same basic configuration.

The development of the inner ear and the cochlear nerve is rapid. For example, by the 14th fetal week, cochlear ganglion cells form robust synaptic connections with the rows of inner and outer hair cells. By the 26th fetal week cochlear structure is almost mature, apart from smaller and fewer afferent terminals (Lavigne-Rebillard and Pujol, 1988). In terms of function, evidence from distortion product otoacoustic emissions (DPOAE) and cochlear traveling wave delay measurements implies that the human cochlea is largely adult-like a few weeks before birth (Eggermont, 1996a). Furthermore, both morphological and DPOAE studies suggest that the olivocochlear system and efferent function reach maturity around the time of birth (Moore *et al.*, 1997, 1999; Abdala *et al.*, 1999). Myelination of neurons, which is critical for rapid and synchronized neuronal conduction, occurs relatively late in development, first appearing within the human central auditory system at around the 27th week of gestation and continuing well into postnatal life (Moore *et al.*, 1995; Moore and Linthicum, 2001, 2007). It is only by the 22nd fetal week that afferent axons from the thalamus begin to connect with the cortical plate (Krmpotic-Nemanic *et al.*, 1983) and, by the 27th week, the temporal lobe can be identified as a distinct structure in the forebrain (Moore and Linthicum, 2007).

It seems little short of miraculous that the complex fusion of these developmental processes results in hearing. Notwithstanding, in the majority of human pregnancies, this does occur and, by the end of the second trimester, there are sufficient neural connections for sounds to elicit responses throughout the auditory pathway. The onset of myelination in central auditory structures seems to coincide with the first electrophysiological and behavioral responses to sound.

Both auditory brainstem responses (ABRs) and cortical auditory evoked potentials (CAEPs) recorded from premature infants born between 27 and 29 weeks suggest that a large proportion of the auditory system is responsive to sound *in utero* (Krumholz *et al.*, 1985; Ponton *et al.*, 1993). However, in general, high stimulus levels are required in order to elicit a response and the morphology of the evoked potential waveforms differs from those seen in later life. Indeed, ABR latency continues to decrease throughout the first few postnatal months (Ponton *et al.*, 1993). This maturation is paralleled by increased myelination of the cochlear nerve and brainstem pathways, which becomes adult-like around a year after birth. From as early as the 25th fetal week, ultrasound scans show that fetal movement occurs in response to vibroacoustic stimulation across the maternal abdomen (Birnholz and Benacerraf, 1983; Kuhlman *et al.*, 1988). Together, this suggests that, in humans, there is a synchronous onset of both physiological and behavioral responses to sound close to the end of the second trimester of pregnancy.

Throughout the perinatal period, the temporal lobe expands in size and a period of rapid cortical maturation ensues, particularly within the marginal layer. Indeed, by 5 months after birth, the marginal layer consists of a dense lower tier and a more lightly labeled upper tier of axons, which coincides with a period of neuronal differentiation and cortical lamination (Moore and Guan, 2001). Evidence from electrophysiological studies in animals and functional magnetic resonance imaging studies in human infants (Dehaene-Lambertz *et al.*, 2002) suggests that cortical activity is driven by marginal layer axons. Furthermore, long-latency evoked potentials (Pasman *et al.*, 1991) and mismatch negativity signals (Cheour *et al.*, 1998) recorded in human infants may reflect the slow conduction velocities of sparsely myelinated neurons within the marginal layer. Other, shorter-latency cortical-evoked responses emerge during the next 10 years, most likely as a result of the maturation of thalamocortical circuits (Kraus *et al.*, 1993). Thus, while newborn babies can certainly engage with their acoustic environment and can even discriminate between different speech sounds (Ramus *et al.*, 2000; Dehaene-Lambertz *et al.*, 2002; Pena *et al.*, 2003; Winkler *et al.*, 2003), these and other perceptual abilities show marked improvements throughout childhood as higher levels of the auditory pathway continue to develop.

15.3 Behavioral development of hearing capabilities

In comparison to adults, newborns seem to respond to sounds in the world around them in a very different way. Over the first decade of life, human performance improves in almost every aspect of hearing, ranging from pure-tone detection thresholds to the perception of complex sounds such as vocalizations. When interpreting behavioral maturation, it is important to recognize that a perceptual improvement with age could reflect development of (1) the auditory periphery (external, middle, or inner ear), (2) neural circuits at different levels of the auditory pathway, or (3) 'non-sensory' factors, namely variables, such as attention or memory, that influence auditory processing and which are not directly related to the physical characteristics of the stimulus. Here we focus on developmental trends in pure-tone sensitivity, frequency selectivity, and temporal resolution, all of which play a pivotal role in speech perception and the ability to localize sound. However, for more general reviews of developmental psychoacoustics, readers are referred to Werner and Rubel (1992) and Werner and Gray (1998).

Behavioral studies of pure-tone sensitivity in humans have shown that infants have much higher thresholds than adults and a relatively flat audiogram (Werner, 1996). Thresholds improve progressively during infancy, particularly, at least to begin with, for high-frequency sounds. Indeed, it seems that thresholds for low frequencies mature as late as 10 years of age (Trehub *et al.*, 1988), whereas thresholds for higher frequencies are adult-like much earlier (~2 years old) (Schneider *et al.*, 1980). Because 2-year-old listeners can master detection tasks, it has been argued that the parametric differences in performance between children and adults, namely higher thresholds for low- but not high-frequency signals, likely reflect immaturity of the auditory system (Olsho *et al.*, 1987), rather than non-sensory factors. Compared with humans, audiometric thresholds mature over a shorter period in other mammals. However, as in humans, sensitivity to higher frequencies appears to mature before lower frequencies in both cats and mice. Based on studies in animals, the range of audible sound frequencies is thought to expand upwards with increasing age (Rubel, 1978). This expansion of bandwidth during development has not been observed in humans, but could potentially occur *in utero*.

Age-related improvements in auditory sensitivity appear to depend, at least in large part, on the maturation of the conductive properties of the ear. Thus, the resonant frequencies of the external ear become adult-like after about 2 months of age in ferrets (Carlile, 1991) and 9 years in humans (Keefe *et al.*, 1994), while the power transfer of the middle ear is lower in infant humans (Keefe *et al.*, 1993) and gerbils (Cohen *et al.*, 1993) than in adults. Another key factor in the maturation of the audiogram in mammals is likely to be cochlear development. Although the basal, high-frequency end of the cochlea develops first, this initially responds best to lower frequencies. During early postnatal life, a systematic shift occurs in the spatial encoding of sound frequency along the cochlea, introducing sensitivity to progressively higher-frequency sounds (Echteler *et al.*, 1989; Rübsamen and Lippe, 1998). However, behavioral improvements in pure-tone sensitivity persist beyond the time that the cochlea is thought to have matured. For example, although cochlear mechanics appear to be mature at around postnatal day 18 (P18) in mice, pure-tone sensitivity has still not reached adult values by 2–3 months of age (Ehret, 1976). Because the time course over which neuronal thresholds in kitten auditory cortex improve resembles that of the auditory nerve (Brugge *et al.*, 1988), it seems likely that improvements in pure-tone sensitivity occurring beyond the age of cochlear maturation primarily reflect the development of the external and middle ear rather than changes within the central auditory pathway.

Behavioral measures of frequency selectivity, defined as the ability to detect a signal of one frequency in the presence of masking energy at other frequencies, also improve with age. Frequency selectivity can be assessed by the notched-noise method (Patterson, 1976), which tests a listener's ability to detect a tone in the presence of a noise with variable bandwidth deletions ('notches') around the tone frequency. This allows sensory cues to be varied as the notch width is changed, while non-sensory factors, which can influence the estimate of threshold, remain constant. Most studies carried out using this method (Allen *et al.*, 1989; Veloso *et al.*, 1990; Hall and Grose, 1991) have found that frequency resolution reaches adult levels before 6 years of age. Hall and Grose (1991) noted that detection by young children seems to require higher signal levels, regardless of the notch width. This suggests that although young listeners may possess adult-like frequency resolution, their performance is more affected by non-sensory factors.

Several lines of evidence suggest that frequency selectivity is determined in the cochlea (for review see Ruggero, 1992), implying that the limiting factor in the emergence of psychophysical auditory filters is the maturity of the auditory periphery. However, developmental changes in frequency tuning have been reported in the auditory cortex of different species (Zhang *et al.*, 2001; Bonham *et al.*, 2004; Pienkowski and Harrison, 2005; Razak and Fuzessery, 2007), which presumably contribute to behavioral measures of frequency selectivity. The ability to detect a change in the frequency of a sound relies more on the slope of the frequency-tuning curves or on the neural coding of temporal cues to sound frequency, which is provided by the phase-locked responses of auditory nerve fibers. Frequency discrimination of brief-duration tones matures by 7 years of age in humans (Thompson *et al.*, 1999), which may, at least in part, reflect developmental changes in neuronal phase locking (Kettner *et al.*, 1985).

The time scale for the development of temporal resolution is more uncertain. Temporal resolution has been defined as the minimum time interval within which different acoustic events can be distinguished. Development of temporal resolution has been measured using a number of different methods, including gap detection, amplitude modulation (AM) detection, and tone-in-noise masking. Gap detection, measured by the smallest detectable silent interval in a stimulus, has been reported to reach adult levels at different ages depending upon the type of sound used (Irwin *et al.*, 1985; Wightman *et al.*, 1989; Trehub *et al.*, 1995). Trehub and colleagues (1995) suggested that this variability with stimulus parameters might reflect an increased sensitivity to the effects of adaptation amongst younger listeners.

Other studies have investigated the development of temporal resolution using the detection of sinusoidal AM in noise as a function of depth and frequency of modulation (Hall and Grose, 1994; Hartley and Moore, 2005). Hall and Grose (1994) found that sensitivity to the depth of modulation improves until 9–10 years of age, whereas the effects of modulation frequency were the same for all ages tested (4 years of age to adult; Fig. 15.1A). This implies that while temporal information is adequately represented in the auditory periphery in younger children, the central auditory system may not process that information efficiently.

Development of temporal resolution has also been examined using non-simultaneous masking. In this paradigm, thresholds are measured for a signal that is presented just after (forward masking) or before (backward masking) a masking sound. Werner (1999) found that, compared to adults, 6-month-old infants showed more masking for tones presented at 5 ms after a broadband

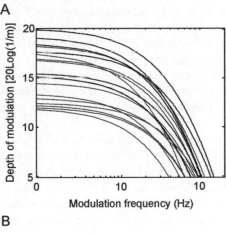

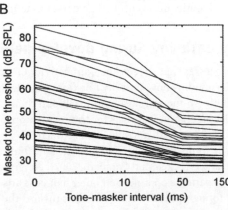

Fig. 15.1 Development of temporal resolution. **A** Sinusoidal amplitude modulation detection thresholds for school-age children (*n* = 9; *red lines*) and adults (*n* = 9; *black lines*) as a function of depth and frequency of modulation. (Adapted from Hall and Grose, 1994.) **B** Backward masking thresholds for school-age children (*n* = 12; *red lines*) and adults (*n* = 12; *black lines*) as a function of signal-masker interval. (Adapted from Hill *et al.*, 2004.)

noise masker, but not at longer delays. Similarly, Hartley *et al.* (2000) found that children perform poorly relative to adults on a backward masking task. Indeed, adult-like performance is not reached on this task until about 15 years of age. Modeling and analysis of these (Hartley and Moore, 2002) and similar data (Hill *et al.*, 2004) suggest that developmental differences in backward masking thresholds could be explained by poor processing efficiency, rather than immaturity of temporal resolution (Fig. 15.1B). Processing efficiency refers to all the factors, aside from temporal resolution, that influence the ability to detect acoustic signals in noise. This includes neural events intrinsic to the auditory system, as well as cognitive factors such as attention and memory.

Another important aspect of auditory processing that matures over a protracted period of post-natal development is spatial hearing. Newborn infants can turn to face a sound source, but the accuracy with which they do improves during the first 18 months of life (Morrongiello and Rocca, 1987). Measurements of minimum audible angles have shown that the ability of humans to detect a change in sound-source location steadily improves after birth, reaching adult values at about 5 years of age (Clifton, 1992; Litovsky, 1997). This is also the age at which adult-like binaural masking-level differences (BMLDs) have been recorded (Hall and Grose, 1990), although more recent studies with different stimulus parameters have reported reduced BMLDs at 5–10 years of age (Grose *et al.*, 1997; Hall *et al.*, 2007). Similarly, the precedence effect seems to develop beyond 5 years old (Litovsky, 1997), suggesting that the capacity to perceive sounds within more realistic, reverberant environments emerges gradually as the auditory system matures.

As with other aspects of auditory perception, the development of spatial hearing is influenced by the maturation of both the peripheral and central auditory system. Because sound-source direction is computed from a combination of monaural spectral cues produced by the filter properties of the head and external ears and differences between the ears in the level and time of arrival of the sound, growth of these structures will change the cue values associated with each direction in space (Clifton *et al.*, 1988; Carlile, 1991; Mrsic-Flogel *et al.*, 2003; Campbell *et al.*, 2008). Consequently, a major challenge in the study of spatial hearing development is to unravel the relative contributions of age-related changes at the periphery and in the neural circuits that process auditory localization cues.

In summary, a wide variation in the time scale of development of different perceptual abilities has been reported. In addition to peripheral and central auditory maturation, cognitive factors, such as attention and memory, have to be considered, which likely account for some of the conflicting results that have been reported in different studies even when similar techniques have been used. Nevertheless, a major goal in the study of auditory development, and which will be the focus of the rest of this chapter, is to identify the events that give rise to mature neural circuits.

15.4 Wiring the auditory pathway during development

Unraveling the developmental processes that specify the connectivity of neurons within the auditory pathway is critical to understanding how auditory functions are established. The precise organization of the connections between the spiral ganglion cells and their targets in both the cochlea and the brainstem provides an anatomical basis for the cochleotopic representation of sound frequency within the central auditory system (Rubel and Fritzsch, 2002). The ganglion cell fibers reach the hair cells very early in development, and various pathfinding cues have been implicated in guiding them to their targets (Fekete and Campero, 2007). Nevertheless, it is presently unclear how the specific innervation patterns on inner and outer hair cells arise.

Cochlear ganglion cells extend topographically ordered axons toward the cochlear nucleus (CN) before their postsynaptic targets have matured. Neurons from the basal end of the cochlea reach their targets before those from the apical end, but very little is known about the molecular guidance cues responsible for the formation of this pathway (Rubel and Fritzsch, 2002; Cramer, 2005). Neural activity appears to play little, if any, role in establishing the initial topographic order, but may contribute to the selection of synaptic targets, once morphogenesis within the CN is complete. In the adult auditory system, neurons in both the mammalian anteroventral CN (AVCN) and the avian nucleus magnocellularis (NM) are innervated by large, calyceal endbulbs of Held, which are important for conveying temporal information with high fidelity. Initially, these endings are much simpler, but, under the influence of afferent activity, become larger and more complex over a protracted period of postnatal development (Limb and Ryugo, 2000; Rubel and Fritzsch, 2002; Fig. 15.2).

The normal development of CN neurons relies on activity-dependent interactions with the auditory nerve. Removal of afferent input by cochlear ablation in embryonic or young animals results in the rapid death of a substantial number of CN neurons and atrophy of the surviving neurons (Rubel and Fritzsch, 2002). Because pharmacological blockade of auditory nerve fiber activity also produces atrophy of CN neurons, which can be reversed by restoring presynaptic activity (Pasic and Rubel, 1991), it seems likely that neurotransmission at the auditory-nerve-CN synapse is accompanied by the release of neurotrophic factors that are critical for the survival of those neurons. Spontaneous activity in the auditory nerve, which occurs in bursts before the onset of hearing, rather than acoustically evoked activity (Tucci et al., 1987), is likely to be responsible for maintaining the target neurons in the CN. Afferent deprivation appears to result in an apoptotic-like process in the CN neurons that gives rise to toxic levels of intracellular calcium (Harris and Rubel, 2006). This dependence on trophic support provided by the auditory nerve declines with age and, at least in mammals, ceases at around the time when hearing begins (Tierney et al., 1997; Fig. 15.3A). The molecular basis for the age-dependent regulation of CN neurons by their afferent inputs is not presently well understood, but is likely to involve an upregulation of genes that promote the stability of neurons in the face of changes in afferent input (Harris and Rubel, 2006).

Projections from the CN to their targets are established before or around birth (Kubke and Carr, 2005). Although these projections are topographically organized from the outset, substantial rearrangements take place during normal maturation, particularly where inhibitory synapses are present. In some mammals that can localize low-frequency sounds using interaural time differences (ITDs), there is good evidence that precisely timed glycinergic inputs to the soma and proximal dendrites of neurons in the medial superior olive (MSO) are responsible for adjusting their sensitivity to the physiological range of ITDs (Grothe, 2003). It has been shown in gerbils

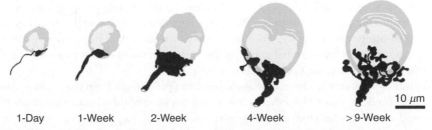

1-Day   1-Week   2-Week   4-Week   > 9-Week

Fig. 15.2 Developmental changes in the mouse endbulb of Held (shown in *black*), the large synaptic ending formed by auditory nerve fibers on neurons in the anteroventral cochlear nucleus. The structural complexity of the endbulb increases from the 2nd to the 8th postnatal weeks and is mature by 9 weeks after birth. (From Limb and Ryugo, 2000.)

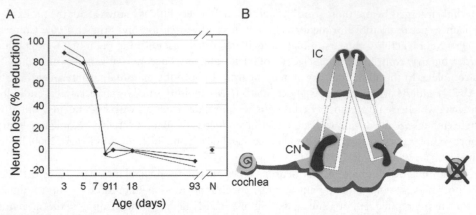

Fig. 15.3 Anatomical reorganization within the central auditory pathway following unilateral cochlear ablation. **A** Age at cochlear removal versus the mean (±1 standard deviation) neuronal loss within the cochlear nucleus (CN) ipsilateral to the ablated cochlea relative to the CN on the non-operated side. (Adapted from Tierney *et al.*, 1997.) **B** Schematic representation of the remodeled projections from the CN to the inferior colliculus (IC) following early cochlear removal. These comprise both crossed (contralateral IC) and uncrossed (ipsilateral IC) components. In normally hearing animals, the contralateral projection is much larger (e.g., in the ferret, contralateral:ipsilateral ratio = 50:1). After unilateral cochlear removal, the number of neurons projecting from the CN on the non-operated side to the ipsilateral IC may be twice that in controls.

that, before hearing onset, these glycinergic synapses are distributed uniformly along the dendrites of MSO neurons, and are subsequently selectively lost, leaving only the inhibitory synapses on the soma (Fig. 15.4). This reorganization of inhibitory inputs requires auditory experience, as the infant distribution persists if binaural localization cues are eliminated by ablating the cochlea on one side or by raising gerbils in omnidirectional noise (Kapfer *et al.*, 2002).

The inhibitory projection from the medial nucleus of the trapezoid body (MNTB) to the lateral superior olive (LSO), which is critical for conferring sensitivity to interaural level differences (ILDs), the other major binaural localization cue, is also reorganized during the course of normal development. Most of the synaptic inputs from the MNTB to the LSO are lost during the first postnatal week and those remaining become more effective, after which these connections switch from being excitatory to inhibitory (Kim and Kandler, 2003; Kandler, 2004). This is followed, once hearing begins, by a refinement of axonal and dendritic arbors, which results in more precise topography within this pathway (Sanes and Siverls, 1991; Sanes *et al.*, 1992b). The early functional refinement of the MNTB-LSO connections is thought to rely on spontaneous activity generated within the cochlear hair cells, whereas the later phase of structural remodeling may be influenced by auditory experience. Thus, unilateral cochlear ablation results in more widely spread axon terminals and dendritic arbors that resemble those found in younger animals (Sanes *et al.*, 1992a; Sanes and Takacs, 1993).

These studies show that the tonotopic organization of projections from the cochlear ganglion cells to the CN and from the CN to other auditory structures is established at an early stage of development and certainly before the onset of hearing. Nevertheless, morphological and biochemical changes take place at both pre- and postsynaptic sites at multiple levels of the pathway, which have important implications for the emergence of the coding properties of auditory neurons. Unilateral deafferentation can disrupt the structural refinements that normally take place during development (Cant, 1998; Kandler, 2004) and even results in abnormal, but tonotopically

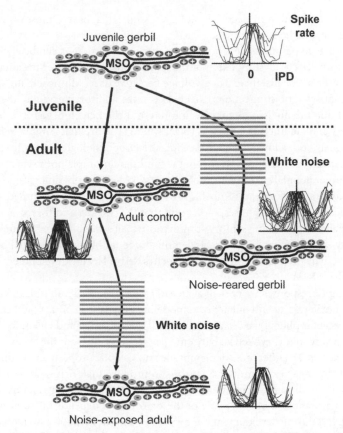

Fig. 15.4 Maturation of brainstem circuits for processing interaural time differences. In juvenile gerbils at around the time of hearing onset, excitatory and inhibitory inputs are distributed on the dendrites and somata of neurons in the medial superior olive (MSO). At this age, neurons prefer interaural phase differences (IPD) of around 0. In adult gerbils, glycinergic inhibition is restricted to the cell somata and is absent from the dendrites, and IPD response curves are shifted away from 0, so that the maximal slope lies within the physiological range. This developmental refinement depends on acoustic experience, as demonstrated by the effects of raising gerbils in omnidirectional white noise, which preserves the juvenile state. Exposing adults to noise has no effect on the distribution of glycinergic synapses on the MSO neurons or on the IPD functions. (From Seidl and Grothe, 2005, with permission from the American Physiological Society.)

appropriate, projections from the contralateral CN to other structures within the central auditory pathway (Lippe *et al.*, 1992; Kitzes *et al.*, 1995; Russell and Moore, 1995; Fig. 15.3B). Some of these effects are also observed with conductive hearing loss or other experimental manipulations, highlighting the role that patterned activity can play in adjusting neural circuitry once hearing begins.

15.5 **Maturation of neuronal response properties**

Methods that sample activity throughout one or more regions of the brain, such as 2-deoxyglucose expression (Ryan *et al.*, 1982), immediate-early gene expression (Friauf, 1992), and optical imaging (Momose-Sato *et al.*, 2006; Mrsic-Flogel *et al.*, 2006), have been applied to the developing auditory system. However, most of what we know about the maturation of neuronal response properties has been derived from electrophysiological studies that have, almost without exception, been carried out in anesthetized animals.

Using brain-slice preparations, it is possible to show that responses can be elicited in central auditory neurons by electrical stimulation of the auditory nerve soon after the afferent terminals arrive at their targets. For instance, using voltage-sensitive dyes, Momose-Sato and colleagues (2006) found that synaptic connections exist between the auditory nerve and the two cochlear nuclei, the NM and the nucleus angularis, in 6-day-old chicken embryos and, by 1 day later, between the NM and the nucleus laminaris (NL), where ITDs are first computed. This is earlier than had previously been shown using extracellular electrophysiological recordings, presumably reflecting the capacity of the optical recording techniques to sample both synaptic and spiking events from a larger population of neurons. Sound-evoked electrophysiological (Saunders *et al.*, 1973) and behavioral (Jackson and Rubel, 1978) responses have been recorded soon after the onset of electrically evoked responses, indicating that the chicken auditory system is relatively mature and capable of processing sensory stimuli more than a week before hatching. By contrast, in mammals, synaptic transmission can be demonstrated in the brainstem well before the first sound-evoked activity (Wu and Oertel, 1987), which is delayed by the development of the cochlea (Sanes and Walsh, 1998).

Although synaptic responses are present at an early stage, the efficacy of transmission continues to mature, presumably as a consequence of remodeling of synaptic contacts and changes in neurotransmitter-receptor phenotype (Sanes and Walsh, 1998; Kandler and Gillespie, 2005). Indeed, this may explain why sound-evoked activity emerges sequentially from the brainstem to the thalamus (Ryan *et al.*, 1982). Differences in membrane and synaptic properties in young animals also appear to limit the capacity of auditory neurons to produce high firing rates or to respond to rapidly changing stimuli, and give rise to more variable and longer latency responses than are seen in adults. The maturation of at least some of these properties depends on auditory experience. Thus, a hearing loss during development has been shown to alter synaptic strength and plasticity, as well as the excitability and temporal characteristics of neurons at different levels of the auditory pathway (Vale and Sanes, 2002; Francis and Manis, 2000; Kotak *et al.*, 2007; Xu *et al.*, 2007). In conjunction with the anatomical changes described in the previous section, such abnormal neuronal physiology presumably contributes to the various perceptual deficits associated with impaired hearing.

The earliest sound-evoked responses elicited in central auditory neurons are immature in various ways. During the course of postnatal development, improvements are seen in neuronal thresholds, in the capacity to follow rapidly changing stimuli, and in phase locking, while maximum discharge rates increase and response latencies decrease. The age at which they attain adult values depends on the response property in question, the level in the auditory pathway, and the species in which it is being studied. For instance, electrophysiological recordings in cats have revealed that phase locking matures more rapidly in the auditory nerve than in the AVCN (Kettner *et al.*, 1985), while in the primary auditory cortex (A1) thresholds for pure tones mature first, followed by frequency resolution, and then various measures of temporal processing (Eggermont, 1996b).

Because the tonotopic organization of the central auditory pathway has its origin in the properties of the hair cells, the maturation of the cochlea would be expected to constrain the emergence of the frequency maps found in adult animals. While this seems to be the case in mammals (for a review see King and Moore, 1991), recent studies indicate that developmental changes take place at higher levels of the auditory system, which shape the cortical representation of sound frequency. In infant rats, electrophysiological recordings have shown that tone-evoked cortical responses first appear in A1 during the second postnatal week and are initially both more broadly tuned and cover a smaller range of best frequencies – the sound frequencies to which the neurons are most sensitive – than those found in adult animals (Zhang *et al.*, 2001). The tonotopic representation is adult-like by about 4 weeks after birth (Zhang *et al.*, 2001; Chang *et al.*, 2005), with sideband inhibition maturing 2–3 weeks later (Chang *et al.*, 2005). Tonotopy has been observed at the youngest ages examined in other species, with frequency tuning sharpening with age in pallid bats (Razak and Fuzessery, 2007), whereas it remains unchanged in chinchillas (Pienkowski and Harrison, 2005) and becomes broader in cats (Bonham *et al.*, 2004). The significance of these species-specific differences in the ontogeny of cortical frequency selectivity is unclear, but, in cats, this results in segregated regions of narrow or broad tuning within the isofrequency dimension of A1 (Bonham *et al.*, 2004).

While the frequency selectivity of central auditory neurons will be influenced by the development of the cochlea, Bonham *et al.* (2004) suggested that changes in cortical bandwidths with age might be due to pruning or selection of thalamic inputs, perhaps under the influence of the animal's acoustic environment. The postnatal development of tonotopy in the auditory cortex does indeed appear to be dependent upon the acoustic environment experienced during early life (Fig. 15.5). For example, rat pups exposed to pulsed single-tone stimuli develop an over-representation of that sound frequency at the expense of other frequencies (Zhang *et al.*, 2001). Han and colleagues (2007) showed that rat pups are impaired in their ability to discriminate the over-represented frequencies, whereas discrimination of the neighboring under-represented frequencies is substantially improved. Furthermore, they suggested that reorganization of the frequency representation in A1 could fully account for these altered perceptual abilities. Rearing rats in continuous noise, in order to remove patterned acoustic inputs, seems to maintain the cortex in its immature state, with subsequent exposure to either normal conditions or pulsed tone stimuli leading to a rapid reorganization of A1 frequency selectivity (Chang *et al.*, 2005).

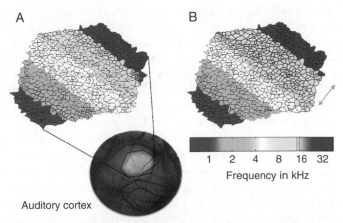

Fig. 15.5 The tonotopic map in the primary auditory cortex (A1) becomes reorganized after presenting rats with continuous pure-tone stimulation during infancy. **A** Schematic representation of a normal frequency map in adult A1. Neurons with the highest 'best frequencies' (BFs) are positioned in the *upper right-hand corner* while neurons with progressively lower BFs follow in the opposite direction. The area occupied by each frequency band is roughly equal. **B** Schematic of a frequency map in which there is an expansion of the region occupied by neurons with BFs of about 15 kHz following exposure to pure tones at this frequency during infancy, while frequency regions adjacent to 15 kHz are underrepresented. (Based on Zhang *et al.*, 2001.)

Plasticity of the frequency representation in A1 can also be induced in adulthood (see Chapter 16). Nevertheless, in terms of the changes elicited by placing animals in an artificial acoustic environment, it does seem as though the capacity for reorganization is restricted to a sensitive period of development. De Villers-Sidani *et al.* (2007) reported that exposure to pulsed single-tone stimuli results in an expansion of the region of A1 tuned to that frequency only if these sounds are presented within a short 3-day window during the second postnatal week, the age at which various A1 response properties are maturing. This sensitive period of cortical development can, however, be extended by raising animals in the presence of environmental noise in an attempt to eliminate patterned acoustic input (Chang and Merzenich, 2003; Chang *et al.*, 2005).

While these studies illustrate the importance of experience in shaping cortical response properties during development, it remains to be seen where and how the underlying changes are brought about. Plasticity at this level is often thought to originate from modifications of thalamocortical circuitry, but it is has been shown that raising animals in abnormal acoustic environments can also alter frequency tuning in the IC (Sanes and Constantine-Paton, 1985). Recordings in deaf cats in response to unilateral electrical intra-cochlear stimulation also suggest that altered sensory experience can lead to expansion of the 'activated area' in both the auditory cortex (Klinke *et al.*, 1999; Kral *et al.*, 2002; Fig. 15.6A, B) and IC (Snyder *et al.*, 1990, 1991). Moreover, Kral and colleagues (2002) found that the effect on cortical activation of chronic stimulation during development decreased when the cats received a unilateral cochlear implant after the age of 5 months (Fig. 15.6C). Specifically, they observed smaller areas of activation, longer latencies, and smaller long-latency responses in these older implanted animals, providing further evidence for the existence of a sensitive period for cortical plasticity.

15.6 Maturation of auditory spatial response properties

Developmental studies of spatial response properties have concentrated largely on the maturation of sensitivity to binaural cues, with particular attention on ILDs. As discussed above, the synaptic connectivity of the LSO and MSO changes in an activity-dependent fashion during early postnatal life. Nevertheless, neurons in these structures receive inputs from each ear from a very early stage. It is therefore not surprising that sensitivity to ILDs has been demonstrated in the LSO (Sanes and Rubel, 1988), as well as in both the IC (Moore and Irvine, 1981; Blatchley and Brugge, 1990) and A1 (Brugge *et al.*, 1988) at the youngest ages examined. Similarly, ITD sensitivity is found in the MSO (Seidl and Grothe, 2005) and IC (Blatchley and Brugge, 1990) of juvenile mammals and in the young barn owl NL, where it first appears when the delay line axons from the NM have matured (Kubke and Carr, 2005).

Adult-like ILD functions have been described in the auditory cortex of cats (Brugge *et al.*, 1988) and pallid bats (Razak and Fuzessery, 2007) soon after the onset of hearing, implying that these may emerge in the absence of sensory experience. However, other studies indicate that binaural response properties do change with age, as might be expected from the synaptic and structural reorganization that has been observed at the level of the superior olivary complex. For instance, the ITD sensitivity of neurons in the gerbil brainstem is fine-tuned during development by a process that is disrupted by rearing the animals in omnidirectional noise (Seidl and Grothe, 2005; Fig. 15.4). It seems likely that this maturation of ITD sensitivity is a consequence of the experience-dependent rearrangement of glycinergic inputs to MSO neurons described in an earlier section of this chapter, which occurs at around the same stage of postnatal life (Kapfer *et al.*, 2002; Fig. 15.4). At the same time, however, noise-exposure does not impair auditory spatial acuity (Maier *et al.*, 2008), so a behavioral correlate of these structural and functional changes has yet to be identified.

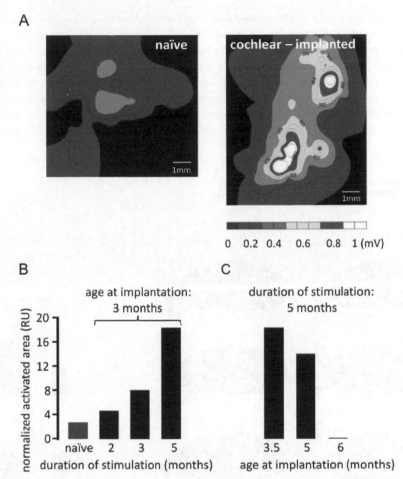

Fig. 15.6 Cortical plasticity in deaf cats following cochlear implantation. **A** Cortical activated areas obtained from approximately 150 recording sites within the primary auditory cortex of congenitally deaf cats in response to intracochlear electrical stimulation. Cortical maps from an unstimulated 'naïve' animal (*left*) and a chronically stimulated 'cochlear-implanted' animal (*right*) are shown **D** Bar chart showing the mean normalized area activated in the cortex for adult naïve animals (*n* = 5), and for cats implanted at 3 months and stimulated for 2 months' (*n* = 1), 3 months' (*n* = 1), and 5 months' duration (*n* = 1). With increasing duration of stimulation, the activated cortical area increases in size, suggesting cortical plasticity. **C** Bar chart showing the mean normalized area activated in the cortex for cats stimulated for 5 months following cochlear implantation at 3.5 months (*n* = 1), 5 months (*n* = 1), and 6 months (*n* = 1) of age. With increasing age at implantation, the activated cortical area decreases in size, which suggests a sensitive period for cortical plasticity. RU Relative units. (Adapted from Kral and Tillein (2006), with permission from S. Karger AG, Basel.)

The spatial receptive fields of auditory neurons are shaped not only by their binaural interactions, but also by the directional properties of the external ear. Investigation of the maturation of auditory *spatial* tuning therefore requires the presentation of sounds either from free-field loudspeakers or in virtual acoustic space (VAS), which is achieved by presenting stimuli over headphones that mimic the directional-specific acoustic filtering of the head and external ears. Using the latter approach, Mrsic-Flogel *et al.* (2003) found that young ferrets have broader spatial response fields (SRFs) that transmit less information about stimulus direction than older animals. In principle, this could reflect the different localization cue values provided by the smaller head and external ears of younger animals, the immaturity of the neural circuits underlying spatial processing in the brain, or a combination of the two. However, VAS stimuli allow an experimenter to separate the contributions of the auditory periphery from more central factors. Presenting infant animals with stimuli through virtual adult ears led to an immediate sharpening of the spatial receptive fields and an increase in the amount of information transmitted by the neurons (Fig. 15.7). Indeed, the

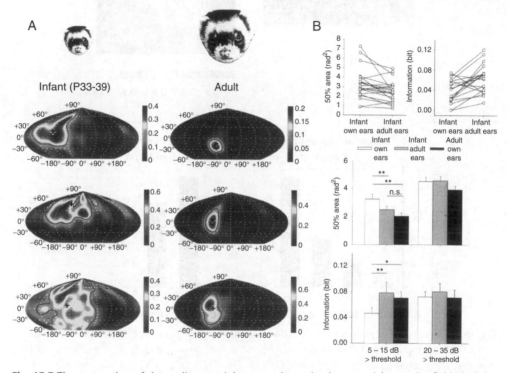

Fig. 15.7 The maturation of the auditory periphery can determine how spatial receptive fields (SRFs) change during development in ferrets. Listening through adult ears reduces the size of, and increases the amount of information transmitted by, near-threshold SRFs in infant animals. **A** Representative examples of SRFs recorded at a sound level of 10 dB above neuronal threshold for different neurons in the auditory cortex of infant and adult ferrets. The SRFs from infant cortex (P33−39; *left column*) are more irregular and larger than those recorded in adults (*right column*). *Crosses* indicate the direction of the SRF centroid vector. The *color bar* denotes the evoked spike count per stimulus presentation, averaged over five repetitions. The *black contour line* runs along the half-maximal response level, demarcating the 50% response area. **B** Pair-wise comparisons of near-threshold 50% area and number of bits of information transmitted between the stimulus location and response for SRFs recorded from infant cortex through the animal's own ears ('infant own ears') and then through virtual adult ears ('infant adult ears'). Note that the 50% areas become smaller and the transmitted information increases when mature localization cue values are provided. The histograms show the mean 50% area and information values derived from infant (own-ear and adult-ear) SRFs and adult (own-ear) SRFs recorded at near threshold (5−15 dB above unit threshold) and at higher sound levels (20−35 dB above threshold; $n = 40$) (n.s., not significant; *$P < 0.05$; **$P < 0.01$). *Error bars* indicate standard error of the mean. (Adapted from Mrsic-Flogel *et al.*, 2003.)

values of these parameters were statistically indistinguishable from those measured in the A1 of adult ferrets. This suggests that the maturation of spatial sensitivity in A1 is governed by peripheral rather than central auditory factors.

Nevertheless, there is considerable evidence that the development of neural mechanisms of sound localization can be shaped by experience, implying plasticity in the way in which neurons at one or more levels of the pathway process spatial cues. This plasticity is necessary so that the neural circuits responsible for auditory localization can be calibrated by experience of the cues available to individual listeners; cues that vary in value according to the size, shape, and separation of the ears. A variety of paradigms have been used to manipulate the sensory cues available to young animals (for a review see Moore and King, 2004). For example, inducing a reversible conductive hearing loss by occluding one ear will alter the auditory cue values corresponding to different directions in space and therefore disrupt both auditory localization accuracy and the spatial tuning of neurons in the brain (Fig. 15.8). However, raising animals with a unilateral earplug results in compensatory changes that allow sounds to be localized with near-normal accuracy (Knudsen *et al.*, 1984; King *et al.*, 2000). A neural correlate of this adaptive plasticity is seen in the superior colliculus (SC), where, despite the continued presence of abnormal cue values, a map of auditory space emerges in register with the maps of other sensory modalities (Knudsen, 1985; King *et al.*, 2000). These studies also suggest that plasticity of auditory spatial tuning in the SC is developmentally regulated, as comparable periods of monaural occlusion in adulthood do not result in adaptive changes in these responses.

Other experiments have shown that vision provides a guiding role in shaping the developing auditory responses. If visual signals are degraded during infancy, then the auditory representation in the SC fails to develop normally. On the other hand, shifting the visual world representation relative to the head by optical or surgical means can produce a corresponding shift in auditory spatial tuning in the SC, even though normal sound localization cues are available (for a review see King, 2002; Moore and King, 2004). Using experience to bring these maps into register is useful as this allows individual neurons to synthesize multisensory cues in ways that can enhance the localization of biologically important objects, such as potential predators or prey. Once again, this experience-mediated plasticity is most pronounced during development. However, studies in barn owls have shown that the sensitive period for visual refinement of both the auditory space map and auditory localization behavior can be extended under certain conditions (Brainard and Knudsen, 1998).

In owls, visual signals also alter auditory spatial tuning in the external nucleus of the IC (ICX), where a map of auditory space is first generated and then relayed to the optic tectum, the avian equivalent of the SC. This appears to be achieved by conveying visual cues via a topographically organized projection from the tectum to the ICX (Hyde and Knudsen, 2002; Fig. 15.9). The shifts in auditory spatial tuning are then brought about by systematic remodeling of the projection from the central nucleus of the IC to the ICX.

15.7 Development of complex vocalizations

Progress in our understanding of the neural processing of species-specific vocalizations has recently been made by recording cortical responses in several species, including mice, echolocating bats, and non-human primates. However, investigation of vocalization learning and its neural underpinnings has focused primarily on songbirds. Although the complexity of meaning in human language is not conveyed by birdsong, birdsong learning may provide a valuable model for examining various aspects of a human's ability to learn to speak and has provided important insights into the neural processing of complex signals that evolve over time (for a review see

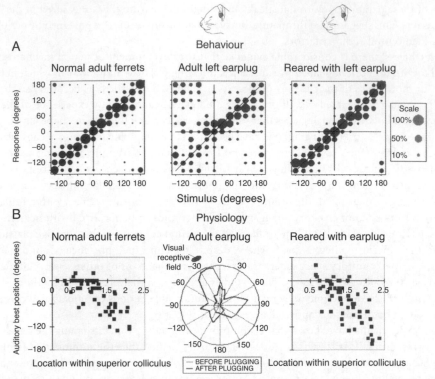

Fig. 15.8 Auditory experience shapes the maturation of sound localization behavior and the map of auditory space in the superior colliculus. **A** Stimulus-response plots showing the combined data of three normally reared ferrets ('Normal adult ferrets'), another three animals just after inserting an earplug into the left ear ('Adult left earplug'), and three ferrets that had been raised and tested with the left ear occluded with a plug that produced 30–40 dB attenuation ('Reared with left earplug'). These plots illustrate the distribution of approach-to-target responses (*ordinate*) as a function of stimulus location (*abscissa*). The stimuli were bursts of broadband noise. The size of the *dots* indicates, for a given speaker angle, the proportion of responses made to different response locations. Correct responses fall on the diagonal (x = y). Occluding one ear disrupts sound localization accuracy, but adaptive changes take place during development that enable the juvenile plugged ferrets to localize sound almost as accurately as the controls. **B** The map of auditory space in the ferret SC, illustrated by plotting the best azimuth of neurons versus their location within the nucleus. Occluding one ear disrupts this spatial tuning, as shown by the shift in the azimuth-response profile of one representative neuron in the middle panel, but, as with the behavioral data, near-normal spatial tuning is present in ferrets that were raised with one ear occluded. (Based on King *et al.*, 2000.)

Doupe and Kuhl, 1999). Songbirds display a predisposition to vocal learning that is guided, through a sensitive period in development, by performance feedback. As with other aspects of auditory development, the timing of this sensitive period is not fixed, but can vary with acoustic experience, hormonal factors, and the species in question.

Certain species of songbird have regional dialects reminiscent of human speech. For recent reviews of how songbirds learn their complex vocalizations see Brainard and Doupe (2002) and Bolhuis and Gahr (2006). If they are moved as an embryo or hatchling, these birds will acquire vocalizations similar to their adopted guardians or 'tutors', rather than their genetic parents. Also, compared with their 'tutored' peers, the birdsong of an 'untutored' songbird (reared in isolation)

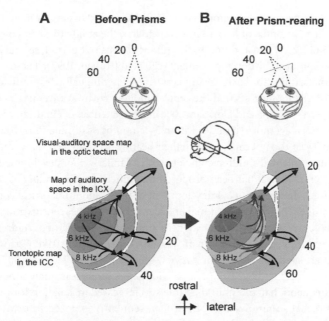

Fig. 15.9 Effects of prism rearing on the midbrain auditory localization pathway of the barn owl. **A** The central nucleus of the inferior colliculus (ICC) is organized tonotopically. In this species, information is combined across different frequency channels in the projection from the ICC to the external nucleus of the inferior colliculus (ICX) to produce a map of auditory space. The map in the ICX is then relayed via a topographic projection to the optic tectum, where it becomes superimposed on a map of visual space. The location of the optic tectum can be seen in the side view of the owl's brain in the *inset* (c, caudal; r, rostral). **B** If owls are raised wearing prisms, a systematic change in the ICC-ICX projection takes place (*red arrows*), which brings the ICX map back into alignment with the optically displaced visual map in the tectum. The instructive signal for this appears to be delivered to the ICX via a topographically organized visual projection from the optic tectum.

is grossly abnormal. Again, abnormal vocalizations are produced if a bird is prevented from hearing its own song through deafening. This occurs even if the bird is exposed to songs made by others before deafening. Together, these results suggest that normal birdsong acquisition is dependent upon an animal hearing (1) sounds from other birds and (2) its own vocal attempts within a sensitive period of development. Likewise, humans need to experience the sounds of other individuals, as suggested by both the diverse cultural languages and dialects that exist and the abnormal vocalizations of children raised without exposure to speech (Kuhl, 2004). Furthermore, the importance of a child hearing its own voice is revealed by the detrimental effect of profound hearing loss on speech production amongst children.

There is evidence to suggest that the neural circuitry for birdsong recognition and learning may, in part, be genetically predetermined. With no previous song exposure, young birds exhibit behavioral and physiological differences in response to playback of songs from their own as opposed to other species. This suggests that they can recognize conspecific song at an early age. Also, despite being able to learn the song of another species, young birds will preferentially learn the songs of their own species. Furthermore, the birdsong of normally hearing, 'untutored' birds contains more species-specific structure compared with birds deafened before they were able to practise their own songs. Together, this evidence suggests that there are innate influences on the development of neural circuitry responsible for birdsong.

Arguably, one of the best known examples of a 'sensitive' period of development involves human speech. After the first 6 months of life, infants start to lose the ability to distinguish phonemes in other languages (Kuhl, 2004). In addition to this phonetic-sensitive period, several other aspects of speech acquisition appear to be developmentally regulated (Ruben, 1997). These sensitive periods have important implications for cochlear implantation of prelingually deaf individuals. Evidence from the latency of CAEPs suggests that the central auditory pathways are maximally plastic for a period of about 4 years (Sharma and Dorman, 2006). CAEP latencies of children who are implanted within that period reach age-normal values within 3–6 months of stimulation. However, individuals implanted after 7 years do not catch up with their hearing peers. Indeed, abnormal CAEP latency development in late-implanted children coincides with a similarly poor development of speech and language skills (Geers, 2006). It has been proposed that functional decoupling of A1 from higher-order auditory cortex, due to restricted development of inter- and intracortical connections (Kral *et al.*, 2006) and/or the reorganization of higher order cortex by other sensory modalities (Sharma and Dorman, 2006), may account for these deficits amongst late-implanted children.

In a similar vein, there are a number of well-documented sensitive periods of birdsong development that are species-specific (for a review see Brainard and Doupe, 2002). For example, white-crowned sparrows that have been reared with tutors rarely learn new songs after 100 days of age. On the other hand, hatchlings of the same species reared in isolation for the first 100 days rarely produce normal songs, even if they are subsequently exposed to tutor vocalizations. However, the closure of this sensitive period relies on experience rather than a strict age limit. Thus, hatchlings tutored by birds from another species can subsequently incorporate new songs from their own species even after other birds exposed only to songs from their own species have stopped learning. Learning from live tutors, rather than taped recordings, and decreased testosterone levels may also increase the duration of the sensitive period. Together this evidence suggests that abnormal experience, together with attentional, motivational and hormonal factors, allows the brain to be shaped by its environment for longer.

In the songbird auditory system, various forebrain areas have been implicated in the recognition of natural sounds, such as conspecific song. These include field L, the equivalent of A1 in mammals, and higher-level areas, such as the caudal mesopallium. Compared to adults, neurons in field L of juvenile zebra finches are both less responsive to acoustic stimuli and less selective for natural calls over statistically equivalent synthetic sounds (Amin *et al.*, 2007). The emergence of neuronal selectivity for conspecific songs coincides with the age at which the animals exhibit a behavioral preference for individual songs (Clayton, 1988), suggesting that the development of these response properties is involved in the maturation of song recognition.

The auditory forebrain areas of songbirds project to the 'song system', a cluster of structures that have been shown to be involved with vocal learning. Electrophysiological studies have shown that certain neurons within the avian song system respond more to the bird's own song or the tutor's song, compared with songs from other species or similar sounds of comparable complexity (Margoliash, 1983; Doupe, 1997; Fig. 15.10). The discovery of these neurons naturally led to the suggestion that their selectivity is shaped by experience during development. Song-selective neurons could be useful to the animals' vocal practice by indicating the degree of success in mimicking the tutor's song. However, this idea has been challenged by developmental studies which show that neuronal song selectivity develops closer to the timing of the birds' own vocal output, rather than the earlier tutored phase of birdsong learning. Evidence for this is provided by the altered song selectivity of neurons in birds that produce abnormal songs following denervation of their vocal apparatus. Therefore, current evidence suggests that the emergence of song-selective neurons depends on exposure to the animal's own vocal attempts, rather than those of its vocal tutors (Solis and Doupe, 1999).

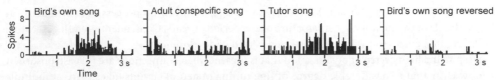

Fig. 15.10 Song-selective neurons are found throughout the song system of adult male songbirds. These neurons respond more strongly to the animal's own song, and in some cases the tutor song, than to equally complex conspecific songs. They also respond more strongly to the natural song than to the same song reversed in time. (Adapted from Brainard and Doupe (2002) with permission from Macmillan Publishers Ltd.)

Attempts have been made to identify the contribution of nuclei within the avian brain to song learning by examining the effects of lesioning particular structures on the ability of birds to discriminate and memorize conspecific songs and other sounds. These studies have pointed to the involvement of the higher vocal centre HVc and the lateral magnocellular nucleus of the anterior neostriatum (LMAN) in these processes. Furthermore, blockade of N-methyl-D-aspartate (NMDA) receptors in LMAN during the tutored phase of learning, but not during vocal practice, reduces song learning in experimental birds compared with controls (Basham *et al.*, 1996), suggesting that this forebrain region is a potential locus of vocal learning.

In zebra finches, the closure of the sensitive period for song learning normally occurs at around 60 days of age. This coincides with the completion of numerous morphological changes that occur in the song system nuclei, including the LMAN (Brainard and Doupe, 2002). For example, in the LMAN, neuron spine density decreases and the terminal arbors of their inputs from the thalamus are pruned during the sensitive period. This is accompanied by changes in the properties of NMDA receptors and a loss of activity-dependent plasticity at synapses within the LMAN. The decrease in LMAN spine density by around 60 days of age is not seen in birds raised without tutors, suggesting that these cellular changes may be a consequence of experience-mediated learning, rather than other developmental factors. Thus, at least some of the structural and functional changes that have been reported in the song system may underlie the decline in the capacity for sensory learning with age.

While the birdsong system has provided the primary animal model for the study of perception and learning, a preference for species-specific vocalizations over those of another species has also been described in mammalian A1 (Wang and Kadia, 2001), implying that experience of complex sounds can shape the response properties of neurons in other species too. Very little work has so far been done on the development of call selectivity in mammals, but a recent study in pallid bats has shown that the maintenance and refinement of cortical selectivity for the frequency-modulated sweeps that characterize their echolocation calls depends on experience (Razak *et al.*, 2008). Interestingly, as in the development of brainstem circuits involved in the processing of binaural spatial cues, the effects on the response properties of these neurons of depriving the animals of normal experience appear to be mediated by plasticity of inhibitory inputs.

15.8 **Conclusions**

The neural complexity of the auditory system arises in a precisely timed and ordered manner through development. The connectivity of the central pathways is largely in place at birth, having been specified by a combination of molecular guidance cues and spontaneous patterns of neuronal activity. At this stage, peripheral auditory function is still changing, a process that appears to last for the first few postnatal months in humans, thereby constraining the range of sounds that can be delivered to the infant brain. Moreover, some aspects of central processing, particularly at higher levels of the auditory system, mature over a period of years. Consequently, adult perceptual abilities often emerge only after a protracted period of development.

Despite the high degree of organization that is present when connections are first established, it is now clear that a considerable degree of fine tuning of neural circuits takes place at multiple stages of the auditory pathway, both before and after the onset of sensory-evoked neuronal activity. This dependence on afferent input makes the maturing auditory system highly susceptible to hearing disorders. Indeed, a desire to characterize – and potentially reverse – the effects of sensorineural or conductive hearing loss at levels ranging from synaptic function to perception is one of the driving forces behind the study of auditory development.

There are numerous instances, from the survival of neurons in the brainstem to the acquisition of language and musical abilities, where the influence of experience or other signals seems to be confined to a sensitive or critical period of development. Despite the considerable evidence for plasticity in adulthood, there is no doubt that variations in the statistics of the acoustic environment can change the response properties of auditory neurons in the developing brain in ways that are not normally possible later in life. Moreover, the neural circuits formed as the auditory system is maturing appear to constrain the plasticity that is possible in later life. Our understanding of what causes these sensitive periods to end is still very limited, although valuable progress in answering this fundamental question is being made by studying the developmental regulation of neuron number in the auditory brainstem.

During the last few years, some advances have been made in unraveling the cellular and molecular mechanisms that underlie the structural and functional changes that take place during development. This progress has, to a large extent, been possible through the use of brain slice preparations, which have provided a window into the maturation of the synaptic and cellular properties of specific neurons. Future progress in this area will require an examination of how isolated neural circuits respond to natural patterns of stimulation. Moreover, if we are to understand the processes that give rise to the auditory perceptual abilities, it will be necessary to combine methods for monitoring neuronal activity and behavior in developing animals, in order to identify the physiological changes responsible for, and not just correlated with, perceptual maturation.

Acknowledgements

The authors' research was supported by the Wellcome Trust through a Clinician Scientist Fellowship to D.E.H.H. and a Principal Research Fellowship to A.J.K.

References

Abdala C, Ma E, Sininger YS (1999) Maturation of medial efferent system function in humans. *J Acoust Soc Am* **105**: 2392–402.

Allen P, Wightman F, Kistler D, Dolan T (1989) Frequency resolution in children. *J Speech Hear Res* **32**: 317–22.

Amin N, Doupe A, Theunissen FE (2007) Development of selectivity for natural sounds in the songbird auditory forebrain. *J Neurophysiol* **97**: 3517–31.

Basham ME, Nordeen EJ, Nordeen KW (1996) Blockade of NMDA receptors in the anterior forebrain impairs sensory acquisition in the zebra finch (*Poephila guttata*). *Neurobiol Learn Mem* **66**: 295–304.

Birnholz JC, Benacerraf BR (1983) The development of human fetal hearing. *Science* **222**: 516–18.

Blatchley BJ, Brugge JF (1990) Sensitivity to binaural intensity and phase difference cues in kitten inferior colliculus. *J Neurophysiol* **64**: 582–97.

Bolhuis JJ, Gahr M (2006) Neural mechanisms of birdsong memory. *Nat Rev Neurosci* **7**: 347–57.

Bonham BH, Cheung SW, Godey B, Schreiner CE (2004) Spatial organization of frequency response areas and rate/level functions in the developing AI. *J Neurophysiol* **91**: 841–54.

Brainard MS, Doupe AJ (2002) What songbirds teach us about learning. *Nature* **417**: 351–8.

Brainard MS, Knudsen EI (1998) Sensitive periods for visual calibration of the auditory space map in the barn owl optic tectum. *J Neurosci* **18**: 3929–42.

Brugge JF, Reale RA, Wilson GF (1988) Sensitivity of auditory cortical neurons of kittens to monaural and binaural high frequency sound. *Hear Res* **34**: 127–40.

Campbell RA, King AJ, Nodal FR, Schnupp JWH, Carlile S, Doubell TP (2008) Virtual adult ears reveal the roles of acoustical factors and experience in auditory space map development. *J Neurosci* **28**: 11557–70.

Cant NB (1998) Structural development of the mammalian auditory pathways. In: *Development of the Auditory System. Springer Handbook of Auditory Research, Vol. 9* (eds Rubel EW, Popper AN, Fay RR), pp. 315–413. Springer, New York.

Carlile S (1991) The auditory periphery of the ferret: postnatal development of acoustic properties. *Hear Res* **51**: 265–77.

Chang EF, Merzenich MM (2003) Environmental noise retards auditory cortical development. *Science* **300**: 498–502.

Chang EF, Bao S, Imaizumi K, Schreiner CE, Merzenich MM (2005) Development of spectral and temporal response selectivity in the auditory cortex. *Proc Natl Acad Sci USA* **102**: 16460–5.

Cheour M, Alho K, Ceponiene R, *et al.* (1998) Maturation of mismatch negativity in infants. *Int J Psychophysiol* **29**: 217–26.

Clayton NS (1988) Song discrimination learning in zebra finches. *Anim Behav* **36**: 1016–24.

Clifton RK (1992) The development of spatial hearing in human infants. In: *Developmental Psychophysics* (eds Werner LA, Rubel EW), pp. 135–57. American Psychological Association, Washington DC.

Clifton RK, Gwiazda J, Bauer JA, Clarkson MG, Held RM (1988) Growth in head size during infancy: implications for sound localization. *Dev Psychol* **24**: 477 83.

Cohen YE, Doan DE, Rubin DM, Saunders JC (1993) Middle-ear development. V: Development of umbo sensitivity in the gerbil. *Am J Otolaryngol* **14**: 191–8.

Cooper ERA (1948) The development of the human auditory pathway from the cochlear ganglion to the medial geniculate body. *Acta Anat* **5**: 99–122.

Cramer KS (2005) Eph proteins and the assembly of auditory circuits. *Hear Res* **206**: 42–51.

De Villers-Sidani E, Chang EF, Bao S, Merzenich MM (2007) Critical period window for spectral tuning defined in the primary auditory cortex (A1) in the rat. *J Neurosci* **27**: 180–9.

Dehaene-Lambertz G, Dehaene S, Hertz-Pannier L (2002) Functional neuroimaging of speech perception in infants. *Science* **298**: 2013–15.

Dekaban A (1954) Human thalamus; an anatomical, developmental and pathological study. II. Development of the human thalamic nuclei. *J Comp Neurol* **100**: 63–97.

Doupe AJ (1997) Song- and order-selective neurons in the songbird anterior forebrain and their emergence during vocal development. *J Neurosci* **17**: 1147–67.

Doupe AJ, Kuhl PK (1999) Birdsong and human speech: common themes and mechanisms. *Annu Rev Neurosci* **22**: 567–631.

Echteler SM, Arjmand E, Dallos P (1989) Developmental alterations in the frequency map of the mammalian cochlea. *Nature* **341**: 147–9.

Eggermont JJ (1996b) Differential maturation rates for response parameters in cat primary auditory cortex. *Aud Neurosci* **2**: 309–27.

Eggermont JJ, Brown DK, Ponton CW, Kimberley BP (1996a) Comparison of distortion product otoacoustic emission (DPOAE) and auditory brain stem response (ABR) traveling wave delay measurements suggests frequency-specific synapse maturation. *Ear Hear* **17**: 386–94.

Ehret G (1976) Development of absolute auditory thresholds in the house mouse (*Mus musculus*). *J Am Audiol Soc* **1**: 179–84.

Fekete DM, Campero AM (2007) Axon guidance in the inner ear. *Int J Dev Biol* **51**: 549–56.

Francis HW, Manis PB (2000) Effects of deafferentation on the electrophysiology of ventral cochlear nucleus neurons. *Hear Res* **149**: 91–105.

Friauf E (1992) Tonotopic order in the adult and developing auditory system of the rat as shown by c-fos immunocytochemistry. *Eur J Neurosci* **4**: 798–812.

Fritzsch B, Barald KF, Lomax MI (1998) Early embrology of the vertibrate ear. In: *Development of the Auditory System. Springer Handbook of Auditory Research, Vol. 9* (eds Rubel EW, Popper AN, Fay RR), pp. 80–145. Springer, New York.

Geers AE (2006) Factors influencing spoken language outcomes in children following early cochlear implantation. *Adv Otorhinolaryngol* **64**: 50–65.

Grose JH, Hall JW 3rd, Dev MB (1997) MLD in children: effects of signal and masker bandwidths. *J Speech Lang Hear Res* **40**: 955–9.

Grothe B (2003) New roles for synaptic inhibition in sound localization. *Nat Rev Neurosci* **4**: 540–50.

Hall JW 3rd, Grose JH (1990) The masking-level difference in children. *J Am Acad Audiol* **1**: 81–8.

Hall JW 3rd, Grose JH (1991) Notched-noise measures of frequency selectivity in adults and children using fixed-masker-level and fixed-signal-level presentation. *J Speech Hear Res* **34**: 651–60.

Hall JW 3rd, Grose JH (1994) Development of temporal resolution in children as measured by the temporal modulation transfer function. *J Acoust Soc Am* **96**: 150–4.

Hall JW 3rd, Buss E, Grose JH (2007) The binaural temporal window in adults and children. *J Acoust Soc Am* **121**: 401–10.

Han YK, Kover H, Insanally MN, Semerdjian JH, Bao S (2007) Early experience impairs perceptual discrimination. *Nat Neurosci* **10**: 1191–7.

Harris JA, Rubel EW (2006) Afferent regulation of neuron number in the cochlear nucleus: cellular and molecular analyses of a critical period. *Hear Res* **216–217**: 127–37.

Hartley DE, Moore DR (2002) Auditory processing efficiency deficits in children with developmental language impairments. *J Acoust Soc Am* **112**: 2962–6.

Hartley DE, Moore DR (2005) Effects of otitis media with effusion on auditory temporal resolution. *Int J Pediatr Otorhinolaryngol* **69**: 757–69.

Hartley DE, Wright BA, Hogan SC, Moore DR (2000) Age-related improvements in auditory backward and simultaneous masking in 6- to 10-year-old children. *J Speech Lang Hear Res* **43**: 1402–15.

Hill PR, Hartley DE, Glasberg BR, Moore BCJ, Moore DR (2004) Auditory processing efficiency and temporal resolution in children and adults. *J Speech Lang Hear Res* **47**: 1022–9.

Hyde PS, Knudsen EI (2002) The optic tectum controls visually guided adaptive plasticity in the owl's auditory space map. *Nature* **415**: 73–6.

Irwin RJ, Ball AK, Kay N, Stillman JA, Rosser J (1985) The development of auditory temporal acuity in children. *Child Dev* **56**: 614–20.

Jackson H, Rubel EW (1978) Ontogeny of behavioral responsiveness to sound in the chick embryo as indicated by electrical recordings of motility. *J Comp Physiol Psychol* **92**: 682–96.

Kandler K (2004) Activity-dependent organization of inhibitory circuits: lessons from the auditory system. *Curr Opin Neurobiol* **14**: 96–104.

Kandler K, Gillespie DC (2005) Developmental refinement of inhibitory sound-localization circuits. *Trends Neurosci* **28**: 290–6.

Kapfer C, Seidl AH, Schweizer H, Grothe B (2002) Experience-dependent refinement of inhibitory inputs to auditory coincidence-detector neurons. *Nat Neurosci* **5**: 247–53.

Keefe DH, Bulen JC, Arehart KH, Burns EM (1993) Ear-canal impedance and reflection coefficient in human infants and adults. *J Acoust Soc Am* **94**(5): 2617–38.

Keefe DH, Bulen JC, Campbell SL, Burns EM (1994) Pressure transfer function and absorption cross section from the diffuse field to the human infant ear canal. *J Acoust Soc Am* **95**: 355–71.

Kettner RE, Feng JZ, Brugge JF (1985) Postnatal development of the phase-locked response to low frequency tones of auditory nerve fibers in the cat. *J Neurosci* 5: 275–83.

Kim G, Kandler K (2003) Elimination and strengthening of glycinergic/GABAergic connections during tonotopic map formation. *Nat Neurosci* 6: 282–90.

King AJ (2002) Neural plasticity: how the eye tells the brain about sound location. *Curr Biol* 12: R393–R395.

King AJ, Moore DR (1991) Plasticity of auditory maps in the brain. *Trends Neurosci* 14: 31–7.

King AJ, Parsons CH, Moore DR (2000) Plasticity in the neural coding of auditory space in the mammalian brain. *Proc Natl Acad Sci USA* 97: 11821–8.

Kitzes LM, Kageyama GH, Semple MN, Kil J (1995) Development of ectopic projections from the ventral cochlear nucleus to the superior olivary complex induced by neonatal ablation of the contralateral cochlea. *J Comp Neurol* 353: 341–63.

Klinke R, Kral A, Heid S, Tillein J, Hartmann R (1999) Recruitment of the auditory cortex in congenitally deaf cats by long-term cochlear electrostimulation. *Science* 285: 1729–33.

Knudsen EI (1985) Experience alters the spatial tuning of auditory units in the optic tectum during a sensitive period in the barn owl. *J Neurosci* 5: 3094–109.

Knudsen EI, Esterly SD, Knudsen PF (1984) Monaural occlusion alters sound localization during a sensitive period in the barn owl. *J Neurosci* 4: 1001–11.

Kotak VC, Breithaupt AD, Sanes DH (2007) Developmental hearing loss eliminates long-term potentiation in the auditory cortex. *Proc Natl Acad Sci USA* 104: 3550–5.

Kral A, Hartmann R, Tillein J, Heid S, Klinke R (2002) Hearing after congenital deafness: central auditory plasticity and sensory deprivation. *Cereb Cortex* 12: 797–807.

Kral A, Tillein J (2006) Brain plasticity under cochlear implant stimulation. *Adv Otorhinolaryngol* 64: 89–108.

Kral A, Tillein J, Heid S, Klinke R, Hartmann R (2006) Cochlear implants: cortical plasticity in congenital deprivation. *Prog Brain Res* 157: 283–313.

Kraus N, Mcgee T, Carrell T, Sharma A, Micco A, Nicol T (1993) Speech-evoked cortical potentials in children. *J Am Acad Audiol* 4: 238–48.

Krmpotic-Nemanic J, Kostovic I, Kelovic Z, Nemanic D, Mrzljak L (1983) Development of the human fetal auditory cortex: growth of afferent fibres. *Acta Anat (Basel)* 116: 69–73.

Krumholz A, Felix JK, Goldstein PJ, Mckenzie E (1985) Maturation of the brain-stem auditory evoked potential in premature infants. *Electroencephalogr Clin Neurophysiol* 62: 124–34.

Kubke MF, Carr CE (2005) Development of the auditory centres responsible for sound localization. In: *Sound Source Localization. Springer Handbook of Auditory Research Vol. 25* (eds Popper AN, Fay RR), pp. 179–237. Springer, New York.

Kuhl PK (2004) Early language acquisition: cracking the speech code. *Nat Rev Neurosci* 5: 831–43.

Kuhlman KA, Burns KA, Depp R, Sabbagha RE (1988) Ultrasonic imaging of normal fetal response to external vibratory acoustic stimulation. *Am J Obstet Gynecol* 158: 47–51.

Lavigne-Rebillard M, Pujol R (1988) Hair cell innervation in the fetal human cochlea. *Acta Otolaryngol* 105: 398–402.

Limb CJ, Ryugo DK (2000) Development of primary axosomatic endings in the anteroventral cochlear nucleus of mice. *J Assoc Res Otolaryngol* 1: 103–19.

Lippe WR, Fuhrmann DS, Yang W, Rubel EW (1992) Aberrant projection induced by otocyst removal maintains normal tonotopic organization in the chick cochlear nucleus. *J Neurosci* 12: 962–9.

Litovsky RY (1997) Developmental changes in the precedence effect: estimates of minimum audible angle. *J Acoust Soc Am* 102: 1739–45.

Maier JK, Kindermann T, Grothe B, Klump GM (2008) Effects of omni-directional noise-exposure during hearing onset and age on auditory spatial resolution in the Mongolian gerbil (*Meriones unguiculatus*) – a behavioral approach. *Brain Res* 1220: 47–57.

Margoliash D (1983) Acoustic parameters underlying the responses of song-specific neurons in the white-crowned sparrow. *J Neurosci* **3**: 1039–57.

Momose-Sato Y, Glover JC, Sato K (2006) Development of functional synaptic connections in the auditory system visualized with optical recording: afferent-evoked activity is present from early stages. *J Neurophysiol* **96**: 1949–62.

Moore DR, Irvine DR (1981) Development of responses to acoustic interaural intensity differences in the car inferior colliculus. *Exp Brain Res* **41**: 301–9.

Moore DR, King AJ (2004) Plasticity of binaural systems. In: *Plasticity of the Auditory System* (eds Parks TN, Rubel EW, Popper AN, Fay RR), Springer Handbook of Auditory Research, Vol. 23, pp. 96–172. Springer, New York.

Moore JK, Guan YL (2001) Cytoarchitectural and axonal maturation in human auditory cortex. *J Assoc Res Otolaryngol* **2**: 297–311.

Moore JK, Linthicum FH Jr (2001) Myelination of the human auditory nerve: different time courses for Schwann cell and glial myelin. *Ann Otol Rhinol Laryngol* **110**: 655–61.

Moore JK, Linthicum FH Jr (2007) The human auditory system: a timeline of development. *Int J Audiol* **46**: 460–78.

Moore JK, Perazzo LM, Braun A (1995) Time course of axonal myelination in the human brainstem auditory pathway. *Hear Res* **87**: 21–31.

Moore JK, Guan YL, Shi SR (1997) Axogenesis in the human fetal auditory system, demonstrated by neurofilament immunohistochemistry. *Anat Embryol (Berl)* **195**: 15–30.

Moore JK, Simmons DD, Guan Y (1999) The human olivocochlear system: organization and development. *Audiol Neurootol* **4**: 311–25.

Morrongiello BA, Rocca PT (1987) Infants' localization of sounds in the horizontal plane: effects of auditory and visual cues. *Child Dev* **58**: 918–27.

Mrsic-Flogel TD, Schnupp JW, King AJ (2003) Acoustic factors govern developmental sharpening of spatial tuning in the auditory cortex. *Nat Neurosci* **6**: 981–8.

Mrsic-Flogel TD, Versnel H, King AJ (2006) Development of contralateral and ipsilateral frequency representations in ferret primary auditory cortex. *Eur J Neurosci* **23**: 780–92.

Olsho LW, Koch EG, Halpin CF (1987) Level and age effects in infant frequency discrimination. *J Acoust Soc Am* **82**: 454–64.

Pasic TR, Rubel EW (1991) Cochlear nucleus cell size is regulated by auditory nerve electrical activity. *Otolaryngol Head Neck Surg* **104**: 6–13.

Pasman JW, Rotteveel JJ, de Graaf R, Maassen B, Notermans SL (1991) Detectability of auditory evoked response components in preterm infants. *Early Hum Dev* **26**: 129–41.

Patterson RD (1976) Auditory filter shapes derived with noise stimuli. *J Acoust Soc Am* **59**: 640–54.

Pena M, Maki A, Kovacic D, *et al.* (2003) Sounds and silence: an optical topography study of language recognition at birth. *Proc Natl Acad Sci USA* **100**: 11702–5.

Pienkowski M, Harrison RV (2005) Tone frequency maps and receptive fields in the developing chinchilla auditory cortex. *J Neurophysiol* **93**: 454–66.

Ponton CW, Eggermont JJ, Coupland SG, Winkelaar R (1993) The relation between head size and auditory brain-stem response interpeak latency maturation. *J Acoust Soc Am* **94**: 2149–58.

Ramus F, Hauser MD, Miller C, Morris D, Mehler J (2000) Language discrimination by human newborns and by cotton-top tamarin monkeys. *Science* **288**: 349–51.

Razak KA, Fuzessery ZM (2007) Development of functional organization of the pallid bat auditory cortex. *Hear Res* **228**: 69–81.

Razak KA, Richardson MD, Fuzessery ZM (2008) Experience is required for the maintenance and refinement of FM sweep selectivity in the developing auditory cortex. *Proc Natl Acad Sci USA* **105**: 4465–70.

Rubel EW (1978) Ontogeny of structure and function in the vertebrate auditory system. In: *Handbook of Sensory Physiology. Vol. 9. Development of Sensory Systems* (ed. Jacobson M), pp. 135–237. Springer, New York.

Rubel EW, Fritzsch B (2002) Auditory system development: primary auditory neurons and their targets. *Annu Rev Neurosci* **25**: 51–101.

Ruben RJ (1997) A time frame of critical/sensitive periods of language development. *Acta Otolaryngol* **117**: 202–5.

Rübsamen R, Lippe WR (1998) The development of cochlear function. In: *Development of the Auditory System. Springer Handbook of Auditory Research, Vol. 9* (eds Rubel EW, Popper AN, Fay RR), pp. 193–270. Springer, New York.

Ruggero MA (1992) Responses to sound of the basilar membrane of the mammalian cochlea. *Curr Opin Neurobiol* **2**: 449–56.

Russell FA, Moore DR (1995) Afferent reorganisation within the superior olivary complex of the gerbil: development and induction by neonatal, unilateral cochlear removal. *J Comp Neurol* **352**: 607–25.

Ryan AF, Woolf NK, Sharp FR (1982) Functional ontogeny in the central auditory pathway of the Mongolian gerbil. A 2-deoxyglucose study. *Exp Brain Res* **47**: 428–36.

Sanes DH, Constantine-Paton M (1985) The sharpening of frequency tuning curves requires patterned activity during development in the mouse, *Mus musculus. J Neurosci* **5**: 1152–66.

Sanes DH, Rubel EW (1988) The ontogeny of inhibition and excitation in the gerbil lateral superior olive. *J Neurosci* **8**: 682–700.

Sanes DH, Siverls V (1991) Development and specificity of inhibitory terminal arborizations in the central nervous system. *J Neurobiol* **22**: 837–54.

Sanes DH, Takacs C (1993) Activity-dependent refinement of inhibitory connections. *Eur J Neurosci* **5**: 570–4.

Sanes DH, Walsh EJ (1998) The development of central auditory processing. In: *Development of the Auditory System. Springer Handbook of Auditory Research, Vol. 9* (eds Rubel EW, Popper AN, Fay RR), pp. 271–314. Springer, New York.

Sanes DH, Markowitz S, Bernstein J, Wardlow J (1992a) The influence of inhibitory afferents on the development of postsynaptic dendritic arbors. *J Comp Neurol* **321**: 637–44.

Sanes DH, Song J, Tyson J (1992b) Refinement of dendritic arbors along the tonotopic axis of the gerbil lateral superior olive. *Brain Res Dev Brain Res* **67**: 47–55.

Saunders JC, Coles RB, Gates GR (1973) The development of auditory evoked responses in the cochlea and cochlear nuclei of the chick. *Brain Res* **63**: 59–74.

Schneider B, Trehub SE, Bull D (1980) High-frequency sensitivity in infants. *Science* **207**: 1003–4.

Seidl AH, Grothe B (2005) Development of sound localization mechanisms in the mongolian gerbil is shaped by early acoustic experience. *J Neurophysiol* **94**: 1028–36.

Sharma A, Dorman MF (2006) Central auditory development in children with cochlear implants: clinical implications. *Adv Otorhinolaryngol* **64**: 66–88.

Snyder R L, Rebscher SJ, Cao KL, Leake PA, Kelly K (1990) Chronic intracochlear electrical stimulation in the neonatally deafened cat. I: Expansion of central representation. *Hear Res* **50**: 7–33.

Snyder RL, Rebscher SJ, Leake PA, Kelly K, Cao K (1991) Chronic intracochlear electrical stimulation in the neonatally deafened cat. II. Temporal properties of neurons in the inferior colliculus. *Hear Res* **56**: 246–64.

Solis MM, Doupe AJ (1999) Contributions of tutor and bird's own song experience to neural selectivity in the songbird anterior forebrain. *J Neurosci* **19**: 4559–84.

Thompson NC, Cranford JL, Hoyer E (1999) Brief-tone frequency discrimination by children. *J Speech Lang Hear Res* **42**: 1061–8.

Tierney TS, Russell FA, Moore DR (1997) Susceptibility of developing cochlear nucleus neurons to deafferentation-induced death abruptly ends just before the onset of hearing. *J Comp Neurol* **378**: 295–306.

Trehub SE, Schneider BA, Morrongiello BA Thorpe LA (1988) Auditory sensitivity in school-age children. *J Exp Child Psychol* **46**: 273–85.

Trehub SE, Schneider BA, Henderson JL (1995) Gap detection in infants, children, and adults. *J Acoust Soc Am* **98**: 2532–41.

Tucci DL, Born DE, Rubel EW (1987) Changes in spontaneous activity and CNS morphology associated with conductive and sensorineural hearing loss in chickens. *Ann Otol Rhinol Laryngol* **96**: 343–50.

Vale C, Sanes DH (2002) The effect of bilateral deafness on excitatory and inhibitory synaptic strength in the inferior colliculus. *Eur J Neurosci* **16**: 2394–404.

Veloso K, Hall JW 3rd, Grose JH (1990) Frequency selectivity and comodulation masking release in adults and in 6-year-old children. *J Speech Hear Res* **33**: 96–102.

Wang X, Kadia SC (2001) Differential representation of species-specific primate vocalizations in the auditory cortices of marmoset and cat. *J Neurophysiol* **86**: 2616–20.

Werner LA (1996) The development of auditory behavior (or what the anatomists and physiologists have to explain). *Ear Hear* **17**: 438–46.

Werner LA (1999) Forward masking among infant and adult listeners. *J Acoust Soc Am* **105**: 2445–53.

Werner LA, Gray L (1998) Behavioural studies of hearing development. In: *Development of the Auditory System. Springer Handbook of Auditory Research, Vol. 9* (eds Rubel EW, Popper AN, Fay RR), pp 12–79. Springer, New York.

Werner LA, Rubel EW (1992) *Developmental Psychophysics*. American Psychological Association, Washington, DC.

Wiesel TN, Hubel DH (1965) Comparison of the effects of unilateral and bilateral eye closure on cortical unit responses in kittens. *J Neurophysiol* **28**: 1029–40.

Wightman F, Allen P, Dolan T, Kistler D, Jamieson D (1989) Temporal resolution in children. *Child Dev* **60**: 611–24.

Winkler I, Kushnerenko E, Horvath J, *et al.* (2003) Newborn infants can organize the auditory world. *Proc Natl Acad Sci USA* **100**: 11812–15.

Wright CG (1997) Development of the human external ear. *J Am Acad Audiol* **8**: 379–82.

Wu SH, Oertel D (1987) Maturation of synapses and electrical properties of cells in the cochlear nuclei. *Hear Res* **30**: 99–110.

Xu H, Kotak VC, Sanes DH (2007) Conductive hearing loss disrupts synaptic and spike adaptation in developing auditory cortex. *J Neurosci* **27**: 9417–26.

Zhang LI, Bao S, Merzenich MM (2001) Persistent and specific influences of early acoustic environments on primary auditory cortex. *Nat Neurosci* **4**: 1123–30.

Chapter 16

Plasticity in the auditory pathway

Dexter R.F. Irvine

16.1 Summary

In the last 20 years, evidence from human and animal studies has revealed that the adult auditory system exhibits a remarkable degree of plasticity. Such plasticity has been demonstrated using a wide range of experimental paradigms in which auditory input or the behavioural significance of particular inputs is manipulated. Changes over the same time period in the way in which the receptive fields (RFs) of sensory neurons are conceptualized, and well-established mechanisms for use-related changes in synaptic function, provide at least a framework for understanding the mechanisms of auditory system plasticity. The evidence for plasticity in auditory cortex and, to a lesser extent, auditory subcortical structures, indicates that central auditory processing mechanisms are dynamic and are constantly modified to optimize processing of salient events in the organism's acoustic environment.

16.2 Introduction

One of the seminal discoveries of sensory neuroscience in the last 40 years has been the important role of sensory experience during development in establishing the response characteristics of sensory neurons and the functional organization of sensory systems. The classic exemplars of this *developmental* plasticity, the massive changes produced by altered sensory input in the ocular dominance organization of visual cortex and in the representation of the vibrissae in the rodent somatosensory cortex, and analogous changes in the auditory system, were reported to occur only in restricted 'critical' or 'sensitive' periods during development (for reviews see Keuroghlian and Knudsen, 2007; Chapter 15). As a consequence, and despite the fact that the life-long capacity of humans and other animals for new learning and memory formation is *prima facie* evidence that many brain areas are plastic throughout the life span, it was widely believed that adult sensory systems were not plastic. This assumption is intuitively plausible, in that stability of the neural mechanisms responsible for processing sensory input would seem to be a necessary condition of reliable perception.

In the last two decades, however, a number of lines of evidence have required revision of this view. The strongest impetus to recognition that sensory system plasticity is not restricted to critical developmental periods was provided by evidence for reorganization of the topographic representations ('maps') of receptor surfaces in primary sensory cortices as a consequence of elimination of input from a restricted region of the receptor epithelium. Such reorganization was first demonstrated in somatosensory cortex, but was subsequently described in both auditory and visual cortices after analogous lesions (for review see Kaas and Florence, 2001). The impact of these demonstrations of injury-induced plasticity derived from the fact that cortical topographic maps had long been thought of as simple reflections of orderly projections from receptor surfaces to target structures in the brain, established early in development.

In the auditory system, earlier evidence of adult plasticity had been provided by studies of changes in cortical and subcortical responses as a result of various forms of behavioural conditioning, in which the significance of specific acoustic stimuli for the organism was modified. This evidence had initially struggled to achieve acceptance within auditory neuroscience, at least partly because of the entrenched view that primary sensory cortical processing areas were not subject to such change (Weinberger, 2004a, b; Chapter 18). More recently, another type of learning that is characteristic of all perceptual systems, the improvement in discriminative ability with practice (termed 'perceptual learning'), has provided further evidence that adult sensory systems are modifiable by experience. The evidence for these different forms of plasticity, given the need alluded to above to maintain a degree of stability of perceptual systems, creates a problem which is directly analogous to the 'stability/plasticity dilemma' that has long been recognized in neural network and other models of learning and memory (e.g., Seitz and Watanabe, 2005). Stated in general terms, the nub of this problem (which is considered in greater detail in a later section) is how a neural system can be endowed with the plasticity that allows it to be modified by experience without compromising the stability necessary to execute its previously established functions.

As illustrated by the examples presented above, some of the interventions that have been used to demonstrate adult auditory system plasticity involve the production of changes in auditory input by modifying receptor function or the transmission of information from the receptors to the central nervous system (CNS), while others involve manipulation of the organism's sensory environment or of the significance for the organism of particular stimuli in that environment. The various lines of evidence for such plasticity will be reviewed in this chapter, and evidence bearing on the mechanisms and functional significance of this plasticity will be examined. Before doing so, however, it is necessary to consider briefly some of the issues related to identifying plasticity.

16.3 The definition and locus of plasticity

Neural plasticity can be broadly defined as dynamic changes in the structural and functional characteristics of neurons that occur in response to changes in the nature or significance of their input. This definition is intended to distinguish plasticity from changes that occur as *passive* consequences of the altered input or as a direct consequence of changes in the organism's state (e.g., arousal state and age). In the auditory system, for example, changes in the frequency tuning of auditory nerve fibres and central neurons occur as an immediate and direct consequence of destruction of the outer hair cells (e.g., Dallos and Harris, 1978). These changes are passive consequences of the elimination of the cochlear amplifier rather than instances of plasticity, which involves some form of dynamic change in neural properties as a consequence of the altered input. This distinction between passive and plastic changes is superficially straightforward, and is indeed usually made quite easily, but as will be shown in later sections, there are borderline cases where the distinction is difficult (see Calford, 2002).

Multiple forms of auditory learning are manifest in everyday life, and many have been investigated in psychological and psychophysical studies. All learning undoubtedly involves plasticity in some part of the CNS. In many cases it is unclear, however, whether the neural changes underlying learning have taken place in the auditory system itself or in 'higher-order' attentional or cognitive processing areas. Although some uncertain cases of this sort will be considered in this chapter, the emphasis will be on plasticity within the classically defined auditory system. It must also be acknowledged, however, that the definition of this system itself presents challenges, and has exhibited fluidity (if not plasticity) in recent years, as has the distinction between sensory and cognitive areas of the cortex (for discussion see Näätänen et al., 2001; Irvine, 2007; Chapter 18).

16.4 Forms of adult plasticity

16.4.1 Plasticity induced by restricted cochlear lesions

Damage to a restricted region of the cochlea results in a hearing loss over the frequency range represented in that region of the cochlea (Fig. 16.1A). A mechanical lesion producing a cochlear 'dead region' (Thai-Van et al., 2007) of this sort in one ear of adult guinea pigs (Robertson and Irvine, 1989) or cats (Rajan et al., 1993) results in a reorganization of the frequency map in primary auditory cortex (field AI) contralateral to the lesioned cochlea. The general form of this reorganization is that the neurons in the region of cortex in which the lesioned section of the cochlea would normally be represented, which for convenience will be termed the lesion projection zone (LPZ), have a new characteristic frequency (CF: the frequency at which the threshold is lowest) at frequencies represented at the edge(s) of the cochlear lesion (Fig. 16.1B). As a consequence of this change in frequency tuning, the LPZ is wholly or partly occupied by an expanded representation of the lesion-edge frequency or frequencies (Fig. 16.1D). Analogous changes in frequency organization have been described in AI of adult animals of a variety of species, including non-human primates, and as a consequence of different forms of cochlear insult (e.g., ototoxic lesions and noise trauma) and of congenital sensori-neural hearing losses (for reviews see Seki and Eggermont, 2002; Irvine and Wright, 2005). That such changes also occur in auditory cortex of adult humans as a consequence of cochlear lesions is indicated by magneto-encephalographic (MEG) evidence for an expanded representation of lesion-edge frequencies in humans with steeply sloping hearing losses of the sort that produce reorganization in animals (Dietrich et al., 2001).

As discussed in detail elsewhere (e.g., Rajan et al., 1993), changes in frequency organization of the type seen in these studies do not in themselves constitute evidence for plasticity, because they could also occur as a passive consequence of cochlear lesions. Most neurons at all levels of the auditory system respond over a relatively wide frequency range at suprathreshold sound pressure levels (SPLs). At levels above the auditory nerve, these responses at higher SPLs reflect convergent input derived from regions of the cochlea other than that from which the neurons' CF input is derived (e.g., Snyder and Sinex, 2002). For neurons with CF at and above the lesion-edge frequencies, elimination of input over the frequency range affected by the cochlear lesion would therefore be expected to leave intact input derived from lower-frequency channels. If the changed frequency organization observed in the studies cited above reflected a passive process of this sort, it would be associated with a progressive increase in threshold at CF across the LPZ (for detailed discussion see Rajan et al., 1993). In Robertson and Irvine's (1989) and Rajan et al.'s (1993) studies, however, the thresholds of neurons in the LPZ at their new CFs (and their other response characteristics) were normal or near-normal, indicating that the changes were not simply passive consequences of the cochlear lesion but reflected a dynamic process of reorganization.

A fundamental issue raised by cortical reorganization of this sort concerns the extent to which it is the consequence of processes intrinsic to the cortex or reflects changes at subcortical levels. Similar changes in frequency organization after mechanical cochlear lesions in adult cats have been shown to occur in the dorsal cochlear nucleus (DCN) (Rajan and Irvine, 1998), the central nucleus of the inferior colliculus (ICC) (Irvine et al., 2003), and the ventral division of the medial geniculate nucleus (MGv) (Kamke et al., 2003). However, the thresholds of neurons in the LPZ in DCN, and in the majority of penetrations through that in ICC, indicate that the changes in these structures are explicable as passive consequences of the lesion. In contrast, thresholds in MGv indicate that reorganization in this structure is attributable to a dynamic process of plasticity. This finding does not necessarily mean that the thalamus is the primary site of plasticity, because – as discussed below in the context of the mechanisms of plasticity – the changes in MGv might reflect

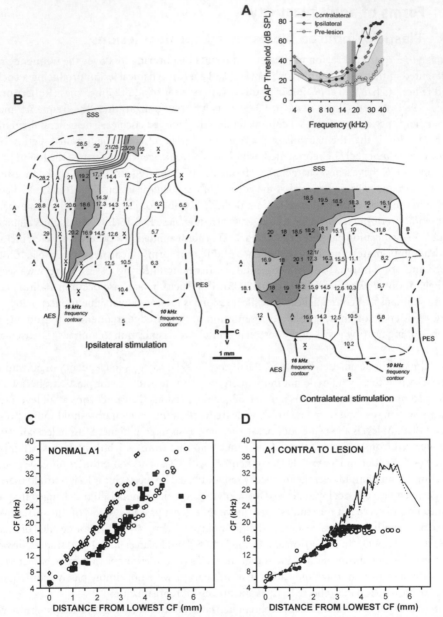

Fig. 16.1 Reorganization of AI produced by restricted cochlear lesions in adult cats. **A** Compound action potential (CAP) audiograms for a chronically lesioned cat. CAP thresholds prior to cochlear lesioning in the to-be-lesioned ear ('pre-lesion'; *open circles*), and at the time of cortical mapping for both the lesioned ('contralateral'; *filled circles*) and the normal ('ipsilateral'; *diamonds*) ears. The *grey shaded area* gives mean normal ± 1 SD CAP thresholds from a large pool of cats (*n* > 50). The lesion produced a steeply sloping hearing loss with edge-frequency in the region of 18 kHz. The normal ear has a mild high-frequency loss at the time of cortical recording, but all thresholds are close to 1 SD above the mean. The *vertical coloured bars* indicate the frequency bands at the edge of the lesion for which the cortical representations (in **B**) are enlarged. **B** Frequency maps of AI in the hemisphere contralateral to the (unilateral) cochlear lesion for monaural stimulation of the ipsilateral (normal) ear and of the contralateral (lesioned) ear in the cat for which the CAP audiogram is shown in **A**.

Fig. 16.1 (*continued*) *Dots* indicate sites at which microelectrode penetrations were made, and *solid black lines* indicate the physiological boundary of AI as defined from the data shown in the map. The characteristic frequency (CF) of the neuron cluster recorded in each penetration is indicated above the *dot* marking the penetration site; other penetrations are labeled *X* (no response to acoustic stimulation), *A* (acoustically responsive, but CF could not be determined), *B* (broadly tuned), and *I* (inhibitory response). The *line* defining the physiological boundary of AI is broken where this boundary was not determined unequivocally. *Thin lines* indicate iso-CF contours fitted to the data at 2-kHz intervals using an inverse-distance smoothing function, and the 10- and 16-kHz contours are identified (*arrows*). *Blue and purple bands* indicate the area of cortex containing neurons with CFs in the range 16–18 and 18–20 kHz, respectively, which are greatly enlarged in the map for stimulation of the lesioned (contralateral) ear relative to the map for stimulation of the normal (ipsilateral) ear. AES Anterior ectosylvian sulcus; PES posterior ectosylvian sulcus; SSS suprasylvian sulcus; R, C, D, and V rostral, caudal, dorsal, and ventral directions, respectively. **C** and **D** Plots of CF against cortical distance (as measured from the position of the lowest CF along an axis orthogonal to the predominant orientation of iso-frequency contours) for AI in three normal animals (**C**) and two unilaterally lesioned cats (**D**) with high-frequency losses similar to those shown in A. In each case, the plots are for the hemisphere contralateral to the stimulated ear, which was the lesioned ear in the case of the lesioned cats. The frequency reversal at the largest distances in **C** marks the border between AI and the anterior auditory field. In **D**, the plots for the lesioned animals are shown relative to a smoothed function fitted to the normal data. (**A** and **B** are modified with permission from Kamke *et al.* (2003); **C** and **D** are modified with permission from Rajan and Irvine (1996).)

centrifugal influences from the cortex. These data do, however, establish that this form of auditory plasticity in adults is a characteristic of the thalamo-cortico-thalamic system.

As with mechanical lesions, plastic reorganization of the frequency map is not seen in the ICC after restricted ototoxic lesions in adult chinchillas (Harrison, 2001). However, ototoxic lesions in neonatal cats result in plastic reorganization in ICC (Harrison *et al.*, 1996), suggesting that *developmental* lesion-induced plasticity is not restricted to the thalamo-cortical system.

16.4.2 Plasticity associated with behavioural conditioning tasks

As noted above, the first reports of auditory system plasticity were provided by studies of the effects of behavioural conditioning procedures on auditory responses. However, many of the early studies did not include the control procedures necessary to establish that the observed changes were associative in nature, rather than reflecting changes in state variables. The pioneering studies of Weinberger and colleagues were the first to use appropriate controls for the general activating properties of the commonly used aversive unconditioned stimulus (UCS) (e.g., foot shock) and to establish the specificity of the effects to the characteristics of the acoustic conditioned stimulus (CS) (for reviews see Weinberger, 2004a, b; Chapter 18). In subsequent studies, a wider range of learning tasks have been employed, and it has become clear that the effects of conditioning procedures depend critically on the nature of the task requirements presented by the particular learning situation, rather than on the mere occurrence of learning (e.g., Ohl and Scheich, 2005).

The most commonly reported effect of classical conditioning with a tonal CS is an increase in the response at the CS frequency and a decrease in response at the pre-training best frequency (BF; that evoking maximum response), such that the BF shifts towards, or becomes the same as, the CS frequency (for reviews see Suga and Ma, 2003; Weinberger, 2004a, b). Weinberger and colleagues have typically investigated these effects by examining changes in iso-level functions (i.e., the response profile across frequency at a fixed SPL). The characteristic stimulus-specific effect of conditioning in these studies is illustrated in Fig. 16.2a and b, and the non-specific effects of state factors are illustrated by the overall increase in auditory responses produced by either auditory or visual sensitization (unpaired presentation of the CS and UCS) in Fig. 16.2b.

A similar pattern of stimulus-specific change has been described by Fritz *et al.* (2003, 2005) in the spectro-temporal RFs (STRFs) of neurons in AI of unanaesthetized ferrets during training on a conditioned avoidance task in which the discriminative stimulus (S^D) signaling shock presentation was a pure tone presented in a background of broadband reference stimuli. Their data are illustrated in Fig. 16.3, and the population pattern of enhancement of the response to the target tone and suppression at adjacent frequencies (Fig. 16.3f) is remarkably similar to that shown in Fig. 16.2a (inset). In a subsequent study using a frequency discrimination task, Fritz *et al.* (2005) reported that the responses of individual neurons varied, but population responses showed a potentiation of response at the S^D ('target') frequency and a depression of response at the background ('reference') frequency. On both tasks, the STRF returned to its pre-training form within a relatively short time in some neurons, while in others the changes persisted for some time after training.

In most conditioning studies, the measured changes in neuronal responses are associated with the (animal or human) subject's learning the task, i.e., moving from the naïve to the trained state. An interesting feature of the behavioural procedures used by Fritz and colleagues is that the ferrets were initially trained in a test box on the avoidance (conditioned suppression of drinking) task for a number of weeks until they reached the criterion. Neurophysiological recordings were subsequently made in repeated test sessions in which the animal was restrained (in a different apparatus), and in which the particular tone frequency used as S^D (and/or as the reference frequency in the discrimination task) was selected on the basis of the STRF of the neuron(s) isolated in a given test session, and thus changed from day to day. In this situation, it seems likely that the change in neural spectral sensitivity is not associated with learning *per se*, but with attention to the particular tonal stimulus that is salient in that test session. Attention alone cannot account for the effects, however, as the different changes in response to the target (S^D) and reference frequencies in the frequency discrimination task, both of which are behaviourally salient, indicate that the nature of the information conveyed by the stimulus (viz. whether or not it signals the occurrence of the aversive stimulus) is also a critical factor.

In contrast to these reports of enhanced responsiveness, some early studies reported either no change or decreases in the response to the CS in classical conditioning tasks, or to the S^D in operant tasks, and these patterns of results have also been observed in recent, carefully controlled studies. A notable example is a study by Ohl and Scheich (1996), who studied the effects of discrimination training on the responses of AI neurons in anaesthetized gerbils. They used a procedure in which all the frequencies that were presented in determining the preconditioning frequency receptive field (FRF), other than that used as CS^+ (i.e., paired with the UCS), were used as unpaired stimuli (CS^-) during training. Although individual neurons showed either increases or decreases in spike rate at CS^+ at different times during the response, the pooled data from the entire sample of neurons showed a decrease in the early (onset) part of the response at the CS^+ frequency, whereas increases in response at this time were greatest at frequencies above and below the CS^+ frequency, such that the latter came to lie at a local minimum. In what appears to be the only study of frequency-specific changes in human auditory cortex associated with behavioural conditioning, Morris *et al.* (1998) used positron emission topography (PET) to investigate the effects of discriminatory classical conditioning using a noxious intense noise as the unconditioned stimulus (UCS) and tones of different frequencies as CS^+ and CS^-. They reported that behavioural conditioning of the skin conductance response was associated with a decrease in the response to the CS^+ frequency, a finding similar to that reported by Ohl and Scheich (1996).

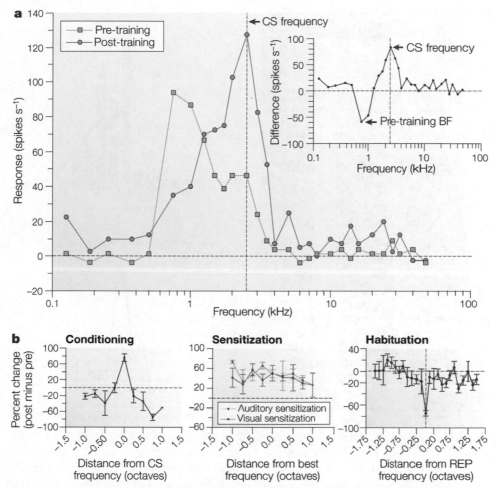

Fig. 16.2 Enhancement of responses to the conditioned stimulus (CS) frequency as a result of classical conditioning procedures. **a** Receptive field plasticity of a single AI neuron is manifested in iso-level functions obtained (at 70 dB SPL) before and after tone-shock conditioning ('pre-training' and 'post-training', respectively). The best frequency (that evoking the maximum response) shifts from below 1 kHz to the frequency of the CS. The *inset* shows the difference in frequency selectivity (post-training minus pre-training), with the maximum increase in response at the frequency of the CS. **b** Normalized group difference functions (post-training minus pre-training), showing change in response to a probe frequency as a function of distance from the frequency used in behavioural training in conditioning (*left*), sensitization (*middle*), and habituation (*right*) conditions. Conditioning (*left*) produces a selective increase in response at the CS frequency, with reduced responses at most other frequencies. Sensitization training produces a non-selective increase in response at all frequencies both for auditory sensitization (tone–shock unpaired) and visual sensitization (light–shock unpaired), showing that this non-associative effect occurs across modalities. Habituation (repeated presentation of the same tone ('REP frequency') alone) produces a selective decrease in response at that frequency. (Reproduced with permission from Weinberger, 2004.)

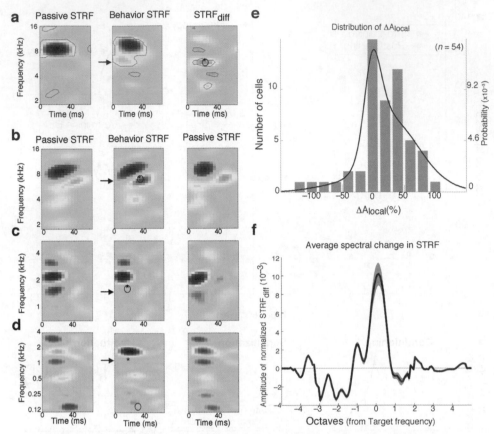

Fig. 16.3 Plasticity of spectrotemporal receptive fields (STRFs) of neurons in AI of the ferret.
a–d STRFs of four single neurons showing changes typical of those observed during performance of the detection task. For each neuron, the *left column* shows a pre-behaviour 'passive STRF', and the *middle column* shows a 'behaviour STRF' recorded when the animal's task was to detect a target tone at the frequency indicated by the *black arrow*. The STRF in each panel was normalized, and all STRFs were then depicted using the same color scale. The contours in **a** demarcate the excitatory (*red*) and inhibitory (*blue*) regions with statistically significant fluctuations (±3 SD) from the mean (for details see 'Methods' in Fritz *et al.*, 2003). These contours are not drawn on the *panels* in **b**, **c**, and **d** to avoid cluttering the figures. **a** In the *right column*, the difference between the normalized passive and behaviour STRFS ('STRF$_{diff}$') is shown. An *asterisk* marks the location of maximum change in the region of the target frequency (local change; ΔA_{local}), and a *circle* marks the location of the maximum change over the entire frequency range spanned by the STRF (global change; ΔA_{global}) (defined in Fritz *et al.*, 2003). In this case the local and global maximal changes were both at the target frequency, as in about half of all neurons. **b–d** The *right column* shows a repeat passive RTF obtained after the behavioural STRF, and the locations of the local and global maximum changes are shown on the behaviour STRF (*middle column*). **b** Localized enhancement of an excitatory region in the STRF during behaviour (*left* and *middle columns*). The two maxima were nearly coincident at the target frequency. The post-behaviour passive STRF (*right column*) reverted immediately to its original shape. **c** Local decrease or elimination of inhibitory sidebands in the behaviour STRF (coincident maxima at target frequency). The inhibition recovered quickly afterwards, but the overall STRF shape was different.

Fig. 16.3 (*continued*) **d** A global weakening of inhibitory fields during behaviour. In this example the local maximum difference occurred at the target tone frequency, whereas the global maximum was located over a low-frequency inhibitory field (which was also knocked out during behaviour). Immediately following behaviour the STRF recovered its pre-behaviour shape. **e** Summary histogram and smoothed distribution of ΔA_{local} (local STRF changes) from all STRFs in the study. The histogram (*left ordinate*) and distribution (*right ordinate*) are significantly skewed toward positive changes (overall mean = +20.2%). **f** Average spectral change in the STRF at all frequencies relative to the target frequency. The *curve* shows the average plastic change in STRF amplitude as a function of octave distance from the target frequency (centered at 0). The *shaded region* around the curve represents the variance around the mean. There was facilitation for about one octave around the target (half-width of ± 0.56 octave) and asymmetric suppressive sidebands outside of this range. (Modified with permission from Fritz *et al.*, 2003.)

Recent evidence for a lack of change in frequency tuning under some conditions is provided by Rutkowski and Weinberger's (2005) report of no change in the number of neurons tuned to the frequency of a tone used as S^D in an operant task. These authors did, however, report that the overall size of AI in trained animals was reduced, such that a larger proportion of AI was devoted to the representation of the training frequency (for a discussion of this puzzling result see Irvine, 2007).

The different patterns of results reported in various studies of the effects of behavioural conditioning on the frequency selectivity of auditory cortical neurons undoubtedly reflect a range of methodological, contextual, and task-related factors. The way in which the observed pattern of changes depends on specific task requirements is a major focus of current research (e.g., Ohl and Scheich, 2005) and is likely to be an area of substantial progress in the next few years. The precise nature of the task determines, amongst other things, the particular features of the presented stimuli to which the subject must attend, and – as will be seen in later sections – attention is an important determinant of many forms of plasticity. Despite these unresolved issues, the data from the various conditioning studies constitute one of the strongest lines of evidence that the frequency selectivity of individual neurons, and hence the way in which spectral information is represented by populations of neurons, exhibits a high degree of plasticity in adult animals.

It should also be emphasized that the changes in frequency selectivity produced by behavioural conditioning procedures can emerge very rapidly, after as few as five training trials (over a period of approximately 10 min) (e.g., Edeline *et al.*, 1993; Fritz *et al.*, 2003, 2005). The rapidity of these changes imposes restraints on the nature of the mechanisms involved, as will be discussed below.

A final point is that the overwhelming majority of behavioural conditioning studies have used tonal stimuli, and have therefore concentrated on plasticity in the spectral processing domain (viz. in frequency tuning and tonotopicity), but it is likely that other features of auditory responses and functional organization will also exhibit plasticity as a consequence of behavioural training. The auditory system is specialized for the processing of time-varying stimuli, and temporal processing mechanisms would therefore be expected to be modifiable by experience. This expectation is supported by the results of Bao *et al.* (2004), who trained rats on an operant task in which the repetition rate of noise pulses increased as the distance between the rat and a target location associated with reward presentation decreased. After training, AI neurons in trained rats exhibited stronger responses, and stronger phase locking, to high-rate noise pulses than neurons in control rats. Evidence for plasticity of temporal processing mechanisms has also been found using other plasticity paradigms (see sections 16.4.4, 16.4.5, and 16.4.8 below).

16.4.3 Plasticity associated with auditory perceptual learning

Another form of auditory learning that has been postulated to involve auditory cortical plasticity is perceptual learning, the improvement in discriminative capacity with training that is a common observation in all sensory modalities, both in psychophysical experiments and in everyday life (see Chapter 13 in Hearing, Volume 3 of this Handbook). The possibility that such learning might reflect plastic changes at early stages of cortical processing was initially suggested by psychophysical evidence that many forms of visual perceptual learning exhibited a remarkable specificity to the region of the receptor surface to which the training stimuli were presented, or to particular parameters of the stimuli (for review see Karni and Bertini, 1997). However, direct evidence from studies of the response characteristics of neurons in primary visual cortex (V1) of monkeys exhibiting perceptual learning on various discrimination tasks have not shown dramatic changes in V1 response characteristics or topography, and indicate that the changes underlying perceptual learning are more likely to occur in higher-order visual areas (for review see Ghose, 2004).

In the auditory system, the evidence is more limited and is also equivocal (for reviews see Irvine and Wright, 2005; Irvine, 2007). Animal studies of auditory perceptual learning in frequency discrimination tasks, in which auditory cortex was mapped in detail in acute experiments at the completion of training, have yielded conflicting results. Recanzone *et al.* (1993) reported that in owl monkeys the area of representation in AI of the frequencies used in training was enlarged (by a factor of ~7 to ~9, depending on frequency) relative to untrained (control) monkeys, and that larger areas of representation were associated with superior discrimination performance. In contrast to these results, Brown *et al.* (2004) found no change in the frequency organization of AI in cats that were trained and showed perceptual learning on a somewhat different frequency discrimination task. The only change in neural response characteristics was a tendency for neurons with CF immediately above the training frequency to have slightly broader tuning in the trained cats than in controls. More recently, Witte and Kipke (2005) reported decreases in the summed response of auditory cortical neurons in AI and the anterior auditory field to the training frequencies, and in the number of neurons with CF in that range, in cats in which chronic recordings were made during the course of frequency discrimination training. The summed response at frequencies below the training frequencies increased, such that there was a local minimum in the response at the training frequencies, a result reminiscent of those obtained in the classical conditioning study by Ohl and Scheich (1996) described above.

Further evidence for increased representational areas in AI has been provided by a recent study, which also provides compelling evidence for top-down influences on the neural changes associated with perceptual learning. Polley *et al.* (2006) trained rats on an operant task to identify a target tonal stimulus (the S^D; defined by either a particular frequency or a particular SPL) from a set of distracter stimuli varying in frequency and SPL. The difference between the S^D (5 kHz in the frequency discrimination task; 35 dB SPL in the level discrimination task) and the distracter stimuli was progressively reduced, and task difficulty was therefore increased, in the course of training. On both tasks the rats showed perceptual learning, in that they exhibited asymptotic performance with smaller S^D – distracter stimulus differences as training progressed. An ingenious feature of this study was that the groups of rats trained on the frequency and level discrimination tasks received the same distracter stimuli and therefore had almost identical stimulus exposure, but were required to learn discriminations based on different stimulus characteristics. In rats trained on the frequency discrimination task, the area of representation of frequencies around the S^D frequency (viz. 5 kHz) in AI was found to be enlarged, but there was no change in responses to SPL, whereas in rats trained in the level discrimination task the relative area containing neurons with best level (viz. the level eliciting the maximum response) close to the level S^D (viz. 35 dB) was enlarged, but there was no change in frequency representation.

A puzzling feature of the level data, however, is that while the animals were trained with pure tones, the rate-level functions were obtained with broad-band noise stimuli. Given the sharp tuning of AI neurons, only a small proportion of the energy of a broad-band noise stimulus falls within the frequency response range of a given cortical neuron. Thus, if neurons had come to respond best to 35-dB tones as a consequence of training, they would be expected to have best SPLs for the broad-band noise stimulus that were substantially higher than 35 dB. Putting this concern aside, an important aspect of Polley *et al.*'s results is that different effects were seen in animals trained on different tasks, despite their receiving basically the same stimulus sets, strongly supporting the importance of attention to a particular stimulus attribute (that made salient by the task) in producing the changes in the neural mechanisms involved in processing that attribute.

A different pattern of effects was reported by Blake *et al.* (2002), who studied the effects of frequency discrimination training in two owl monkeys in which chronic recordings were made from neurons at the same AI loci throughout the course of training. These experiments were directed at elucidating the neural correlates of reinforcement, rather than those of perceptual learning *per se*, but nevertheless bear on the latter issue. In both animals, the summed responses of all neurons sampled by the electrode array decreased during training, but the decrease was non-monotonic: at the time at which the monkey's performance began to improve, responses to both the S^D ('target') frequency and control frequencies transiently increased, with a greater increase in the response to the target frequency. The method of data summation leaves it unclear whether this increase reflected a change in the frequency selectivity of some or all of the neurons, or simply a greater increase in responsiveness of those neurons tuned to the target frequency. Response strength declined over further training trials, while behavioural discrimination continued to improve, suggesting that the period of increased responsiveness was not the substrate of the improved discrimination but was a correlate of the behaviour coming under the control of the reinforcement contingency.

Numerous procedural differences between the studies described above might explain their different results (see Brown *et al.* (2004) and Irvine *et al.* (2005) for discussion of differences between their and Recanzone *et al.*'s studies), and it is likely that the nature of the task and other related variables determine both the nature of the associated neural changes and the site at which they occur However, it should also be noted that the massive increase in the representation of the training frequencies reported by Recanzone *et al.* (1993) and Polley *et al.* (2006) raises in an explicit fashion the stability/plasticity dilemma referred to earlier. Any such increase must occur at the expense of the representation of other frequencies, and thus implies the loss of discriminative ability at those other frequencies. As discussed by Irvine *et al.* (2005) such a loss in discriminative ability has not been reported in studies of frequency discrimination in either human or animal research. In fact, there is a high degree of generalization from trained to untrained frequencies, even to immediately adjacent frequency ranges, the representation of which would be expected to be supplanted by an expanded representation of the training frequencies. It has long been recognized that neural network models (or any other learning algorithm) in which new learning results in catastrophic forgetting of old memories do not match the performance of biological learning systems. Proposed mechanisms of perceptual learning that imply that improvement on one task necessarily involves a loss of ability on other tasks are similarly implausible (for discussion see Seitz and Watanabe, 2005).

A number of studies in humans have demonstrated that extensive training and perceptual learning on a range of auditory discrimination tasks are correlated with changes in a variety of characteristics of cortical activity recorded using electro- or magneto-encephalographic methods

(EEG or MEG, respectively) or imaging techniques (positron emission tomography (PET) or functional magnetic resonance imaging (fMRI)). The most commonly reported effect of training in EEG and MEG studies is an increase in the amplitude of event-related potentials (ERPs) with latencies in the 100- to 200-ms range, although decreased responses have also been reported, and increases in the amplitude of some ERP components have been reported in untrained control groups (for recent reviews see Sheehan *et al.*, 2005; Alain *et al.*, 2007). Larger ERPs could reflect either an increase in the number of responsive neurons or increased synchrony in the discharge of the responding population. The ERP components investigated in these studies have multiple generators, including (but not restricted to) primary and belt areas of auditory cortex, so the cortical fields in which the changes occur cannot be specified with certainty.

There is also a large body of human data indicating differences between musicians and non-musicians in auditory cortical responses, which could reflect perceptual learning by the former. Although the correlations reported in some of these studies could indicate either that musical training had produced plastic changes in auditory cortical responses or that individuals with these traits are more likely to pursue musical careers, a number of lines of evidence indicate that the changes are likely to be the product of training (for review see Irvine and Wright, 2005).

As with the conditioning data reviewed in the previous section, the perceptual learning data provide compelling evidence for plasticity in the adult auditory system, although the different patterns of effects in different studies indicate that much further work is required to determine the precise nature and locus of the changes associated with particular task characteristics and requirements.

Although the term 'perceptual learning' is commonly used with the specific meaning of improved discriminative capacity with practice that has been given here, there are other forms of learning on auditory perceptual tasks that also appear to involve changes in auditory cortical processing mechanisms. One of these is category learning, in which observers learn to discriminate not between two specific stimuli, but between stimuli in different categories (e.g., rising and falling frequency modulated (FM) tones, independent of the particular frequency ranges traversed by the sweeps). In a study of category learning with such stimuli in gerbils, Ohl *et al.* (2001) found that category learning was associated with a change in the spatial distribution of electrical activity in AI.

Finally, two forms of auditory perceptual learning that are of great practical significance relate to speech perception. The first is the effect of language experience on the perception of speech sounds, and thus on language acquisition, during a critical period of development (e.g., Kuhl, 2004). There is a growing body of imaging evidence indicating language-specific modification of the responses of belt and parabelt areas of human auditory cortex to speech sounds (e.g., Näätänen *et al.*, 1997; Jacquemot *et al.*, 2003). The second is the improvement in speech perception shown by cochlear implantees over the post-implantation period (e.g., McKay, 2005). Although there is evidence of post-implantation changes in auditory cortical responsiveness (for review see Green *et al.*, 2005), the extent to which plasticity in auditory cortex itself and/or in higher-level language-related areas contributes to this form of learning remains unclear.

16.4.4 Plasticity in sound localization mechanisms

As described in Chapter 15, some of the most compelling evidence for developmental plasticity in the auditory system has been provided by changes in the neural mechanisms by which sound localization cues are processed and maps of auditory space are generated in the midbrain (viz. in the IC and the superior colliculus (SC) or optic tectum (OT)). In both barn owls and mammals, interventions during 'sensitive' periods in development that alter the relationship between binaural cues and spatial location, or that between visual and auditory space, result in profound changes in these mechanisms. Although the same interventions have little or no effect in adult animals, there is nevertheless evidence for more limited, and in some cases qualitatively different, forms of plasticity of sound localization mechanisms in adults.

In juvenile barn owls, exposure to a chronic horizontal displacement of the visual field produced by distorting prisms results in a shift in the tuning of neurons in the OT to interaural time differences (ITDs), which is reversed when the prisms are removed. Although normal adult owls exposed to such prismatic displacement show little or no change in ITD tuning, Bergan *et al.* (2005) found that owls exposed as adults that hunted live prey (rather than being fed dead food, as was the case in previous studies of prism effects in juveniles and adults) showed shifts in ITD tuning approximately five times greater than those observed in non-hunting owls (Fig. 16.4), albeit of approximately half the magnitude of the shifts seen with juvenile prism experience. The shifts in ITD tuning in the OT were highly correlated with the success rate of the hunting owls in striking their prey. A number of factors could have contributed to this enhanced adult plasticity (Bergan *et al.*, 2005), but it is likely that the increased attention and arousal associated with hunting was at least one of the factors.

Another, more subtle, form of plasticity in adult owls is indicated by the finding that when prisms were fitted to adults that had experienced displacement as juveniles, a change in ITD tuning comparable to that shown as juveniles occurred (Knudsen, 1998; Linkenhoker *et al.*, 2005). This change in adults occurred only for the specific displacement that had been experienced during development, and depended on the survival of an aberrant projection from the external nucleus of the IC to the OT formed in response to the juvenile exposure. The plasticity exhibited by these adult owls therefore depends on the underlying developmental plastic change (viz. the formation of a new pathway), but involves the reactivation of this pathway, which had been non-functional in the absence of disturbed input. The mechanisms by which this acquired projection is made ineffective and then reactivated remain to be determined.

A similar behavioural adaptation has been reported in adult ferrets in which the normal relationship between spatial locations and binaural cues was modified by occlusion of one ear. When the ferrets were trained on a behaviourally relevant task, they relearned accurate sound localization. In this case, however, the plasticity does not seem to involve changes in neural sensitivity to binaural cues. Rather, the animals apparently learn to ignore the altered binaural cues and to attend to those cues that are less affected by the earplug (Kacelnik *et al.*, 2006). Whether this learning involves changes in the auditory system itself or in higher-order attentional structures is not clear.

A final intriguing form of adult plasticity in sound localization is provided by studies in which the spectral shape cues to sound source elevation (see Chapter 13) are modified in adult human subjects by the insertion of ear moulds. In Hofman *et al.*'s (1998) study using this procedure, vertical localization was massively disrupted immediately after insertion of bilateral moulds, but improved greatly over 3–6 weeks' experience with the moulds. Most surprisingly, when the moulds were removed, participants were immediately able to perform at the levels exhibited prior to the experiment. The plasticity demonstrated in this study therefore seems to have involved the acquisition of a new representation of the pinna transfer function without disruption of the original representation. However, the location of these representations in the CNS is not known, and the site of this plasticity is consequently uncertain.

16.4.5 Plastic effects of cochlear electrical stimulation in profoundly deaf animals

The occurrence of plastic changes in the central auditory system of profoundly deaf animals (or humans) obviously cannot be investigated using acoustic stimuli. However, the responsiveness of

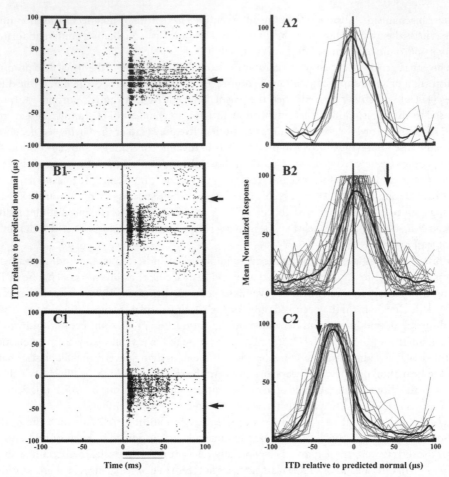

Fig. 16.4 Effect of prism experience with and without hunting on ITD tuning in the optic tectum of an individual adult barn owl. **A1**, **B1** and **C1** are raster displays of multiunit responses to a range of ITD values for single recording sites. **A2**, **B2**, and **C2** are ITD tuning curves derived from data such as those shown on the *left* for all of the sites sampled in this owl. The ITD axes in both columns are in microseconds relative to the ITD to which neurons at that recording site would be tuned in normal animals, based on the previously established relationship between the location of the visual receptive field and ITD tuning (for details see Bergan *et al.*, 2005). Negative ITDs designate left-ear leading ITDs. In **A1**, **B1**, and **C1**, time is measured relative to stimulus onset, and the duration of the stimulus is indicated by the *bar* at the bottom. In **A2**, **B2**, and **C2**, the *thin lines* are curves from individual sites, and the *thick lines* are population averages. In both columns, *arrows* indicate the ITD value that was instructed by prism experience. Prior to prism experience ('initial'; **A1** and **A2**), the individual and group data indicate tuning to the normal ITD for the site. After prism experience without hunting ('no hunting'; **B1** and **B2**) there was a small (~5 µs) shift in ITD tuning. In contrast, prism experience while hunting live prey ('hunting'; **C1** and **C2**) resulted in a much larger (~25 µs) shift in tuning. (Reproduced with permission from Bergan *et al.*, 2005.)

the central auditory pathways in such cases can be assessed by direct electrical stimulation of surviving spiral ganglion neurons via intracochlear electrodes. This stimulation is directly comparable to that provided by cochlear implants, which have been used to restore functional hearing to many thousands of profoundly deaf humans. Plasticity in the auditory system of congenitally deaf or neonatally deafened animals has generally been demonstrated by comparing responses to cochlear electrical stimulation in adult animals that have received chronic electrical stimulation for some specified period with those in unstimulated controls. In the majority of studies, the stimulation is initiated at an early stage of development (as soon as implant surgery can be carried out), but continues during adulthood, so it is unclear to what extent the plastic changes occur during development or adulthood. Kral and colleagues (2006) made observations on animals that were implanted as young adults, and reported that the effects of chronic stimulation on the response parameters they measured were much smaller in these cases, indicating a sensitive period during development for such plasticity.

The temporal pattern of AERs to cochlear electrical stimulation, and a number of the response characteristics of single AI neurons, are modified by chronic stimulation (for reviews see Kral *et al.*, 2006; Fallon *et al.*, 2008). AERs in congenitally deaf adult animals are characterized by small middle-latency responses and the complete absence of long-latency responses. Chronic cochlear electrical stimulation (initiated early in development) results in increased amplitude and a broader spatial distribution of middle-latency responses, and the appearance of long-latency responses (Kral *et al.*, 2006). Single- and multi-unit responses in chronically stimulated animals show more sustained responses and an increase in the maximum following rate for pulse trains compared to deaf controls (Fallon *et al.*, 2009).

When chronic electrical stimulation is restricted to a single intracochlear location, the area of AI activated by stimulation of that location increases greatly and as a function of the duration of stimulation during the sensitive period, but is only slightly increased by stimulation in adults (Kral *et al.*, 2006). In contrast, expansion of the representation of the stimulated cochlear region has been reported to occur in ICC in both neonatally deafened cats and cats deafened as adults (Moore *et al.*, 2002). The different cortical and midbrain effects in adults reported in these studies are puzzling, given that the injury-induced reorganization results reviewed in section 16.4.1 indicate greater adult plasticity in AI than in ICC.

Cochleotopic organization of AI is rudimentary or absent in congenitally deaf or neonatally deafened adult cats, although that in ICC is near-normal. Chronic stimulation via a multichannel cochlear electrode in neonatally deafened cats, initiated as soon as implantation is possible (at around 2 months of age), results in the maintenance (or restoration) of basic cochleotopy in the adult AI (Fallon *et al.*, 2009). As noted above, it is unclear to what extent this effect is attributable to developmental or adult plasticity.

These effects have obvious parallels in the way in which the performance of cochlear implantees improves with experience. The remarkable expressive and receptive language performance of children given cochlear implants at an early age is testimony to the existence of greater plasticity during sensitive periods in development, although these sensitive periods undoubtedly include those for language acquisition as well as for auditory processing. Also, as noted above, the improvement in speech discrimination shown by adult cochlear implantees over the months and years following implantation (e.g., McKay, 2005) is undoubtedly a manifestation of plasticity at one or more CNS locations. In both cases, the extent to which the improved performance involves plasticity in the auditory system *per se*, or in specialized speech processing and/or language areas, is not yet known.

16.4.6 **Plasticity associated with environmental enrichment**

One of the most intensively studied aspects of structural brain plasticity over the last 60 years has been the effects of so-called environmental enrichment. The brains of rats raised in enriched environments show a wide range of cellular and molecular changes relative to those of littermates raised in (admittedly often impoverished) standard conditions (e.g., Nithianantharajah and Hannan, 2006). There has been only limited investigation of the effects of environmental enrichment on the response characteristics of auditory cortical neurons, but Kilgard and colleagues (e.g., Engineer *et al.*, 2004) have reported that a combination of generalized and specifically acoustic enrichment results in changes in the response strength, RF characteristics, and temporal processing characteristics of AI neurons in rats. In a recent intriguing study of the effects of an enhanced acoustic environment in adult cats, Noreña *et al.* (2006) reported that an environment consisting of tone pips of 32 different frequencies in the range 5–20 kHz resulted in a reduction in the strength of short-latency neuronal responses to, and in the area of representation of, those frequencies, and to over-representation of frequencies neighbouring those in the enhanced acoustic environment. This result was unexpected, but might indicate that adaptation to the exposure stimuli resulted in reduced input to the area in which they were represented (which could be regarded as a functional lesion), and thus in changes similar to those produced by cochlear lesions.

A more general point relating to environmental enrichment is suggested by Bergan *et al.*'s (2005) finding that adult owls that hunted live prey showed much greater plasticity of ITD tuning in response to prism displacement than owls fed dead mice (see section 16.4.4 above). As Keuroghlian and Knudsen (2007) pointed out, it is not unlikely that the plasticity demonstrated in many experiments using laboratory animals is limited by the impoverished conditions under which the animals are maintained.

16.4.7 **Plasticity induced by cortical microstimulation**

Changes in the frequency selectivity of AI neurons (and consequently in the cortical frequency map) as a consequence of focal electrical stimulation of the cortex have been observed in a number of studies. Gerstein and colleagues reported that in both anaesthetized and awake rats, stimulation at a specific AI location changed the FRFs of nearby neurons (within ~300 µm) such that they became more responsive to the BF of the cells at the stimulation site and (in some cases) their BF shifted towards that at the stimulation site (e.g., Talwar and Gerstein, 2001). This response enhancement occurred rapidly (in the course of a few hours of stimulation) and lasted for a period of some hours. Some rats were tested within that period on a frequency discrimination task at the BF of neurons at the stimulation site, but the enlarged area of strong responses at that frequency did not result in better discrimination (Talwar and Gerstein, 2001).

More dramatic effects of microstimulation in AI of gerbils and echolocating bats have been reported by Suga and colleagues, who reported that the BF of neurons surrounding the stimulation site shifted towards that of the neurons at the stimulation site, resulting in an enlarged representation of that frequency (Suga and Ma, 2003). In a smaller area surrounding the region in which BF shifted toward that at the stimulating site, smaller shifts in BF away from that at the stimulating site were observed. In experiments on both echolocating bats (e.g., Suga and Ma, 2003) and mice (e.g., Yan *et al.*, 2005), the frequency selectivity (and other tuning characteristics) of neurons in the tonotopically corresponding area of the ICC were also found to change as a consequence of cortical microstimulation, presumably as a consequence of the activation of corticofugal fibres.

16.4.8 **Plasticity induced by direct activation of neuromodulatory systems**

The neocortex receives diffuse extrathalamic projections from five different subcortical cell groups, which act to modulate cortical sensitivity and have been implicated in cortical plasticity (e.g., Gu, 2002). The most extensively studied of these systems is the system of cholinergic fibres originating in the basal forebrain. A number of lines of evidence indicate that acetylcholine (ACh) and the cholinergic basal forebrain are involved in at least some forms of auditory cortical plasticity.

Pairing a tonal stimulus of a particular frequency with direct application to the cortex of either cholinergic agents or acetylcholinesterase inhibitors alters the FRFs of a large proportion of auditory cortical neurons by selectively modifying the response to tones at or near the paired frequency (for review see Weinberger, 2003). These observations imply that endogenous ACh has a role in modulating the frequency selectivity of auditory cortical neurons, and this role is supported by data obtained under more physiological conditions by pairing electrical stimulation of the basal forebrain with tonal stimulation. Such pairing has been shown to result in frequency-selective changes in FRFs in a number of species (for reviews see Suga and Ma, 2003; Weinberger, 2003) and in an enlarged representation of the paired frequency in AI of the rat (Fig. 16.5; for review see Kilgard *et al.*, 2002).

When paired with tone-pip stimulation at particular rates, basal forebrain stimulation can also modify the temporal information processing characteristics of auditory cortical neurons (Fig. 16.6; Kilgard *et al.*, 2002). Such stimulation also activates non-cholinergic basal forebrain neurons (notably the large population of GABAergic neurons that also project to the cortex), but in a number of cases these effects were shown to be blocked by application of ACh antagonists to the cortex, indicating that they were mediated by activation of cholinergic neurons. These effects of direct electrical activation of the basal forebrain suggest that it might be involved in the range of injury- and use-related plasticity in auditory cortex described in previous sections. This possibility is examined in the following section.

16.5 **Mechanisms of auditory system plasticity**

Almost all of the various forms of plasticity described in animal studies and reviewed in the previous sections involve changes in the efficacy of particular stimuli in 'driving' (i.e., producing action potentials in) auditory system neurons. In the human studies, the nature of the changes is less clear for a number of reasons: changes in AER amplitude could reflect changes in the synchrony rather than the amount of neural activity; synaptic potentials as well as action potentials contribute to the recorded response; and the relationship between the haemodynamic changes measured using some imaging techniques and the associated neural changes is complex. For these reasons, the following consideration of the mechanisms of auditory system plasticity will largely be restricted to evidence from animal studies.

In some cases the change in stimulus efficacy involves stimuli that are normally ineffective in driving the neuron becoming effective; in others the relative efficacy of different stimuli is altered. An explanation of the former cases requires an account of the source of the apparently 'new' input, and of the mechanisms by which it becomes effective. Explanation of the latter cases requires an account of the change in the relative efficacy of the inputs. Evidence that has required substantial revision of classical ideas about neuronal RFs provides at least part of the answer (and perhaps the entire answer) to the question concerning the source of new inputs. Evidence regarding

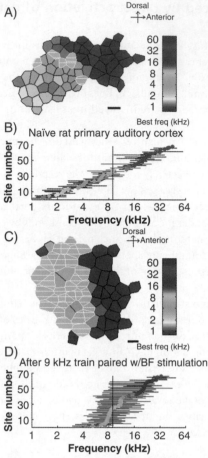

Fig. 16.5 Effect on tonotopic organization of AI in the rat of pairing electrical activation of the basal forebrain with tonal stimulation. **A** Frequency organization of AI in a representative, experimentally naïve rat, demonstrating the normal orderly progression of characteristic frequency (CF). Each *polygon* represents one microelectrode penetration (scale bar = 0.25 mm), and its *colour* indicates the CF (here designated best frequency (BF)) of the neurons at that site. Sites with a CF within a third of an octave of 9 kHz are indicated by *white hatching*. **B** Every AI receptive field for the naïve control rat in **A** is shown to illustrate the systematic progression of tone frequency and typical receptive-field sizes. *Coloured dots* represent the CF at each site, and *horizontal lines* indicate the width of each receptive field 10 dB above threshold. Lines for tuning curves that include 9 kHz are *coloured red*. **C** Map from a representative experimental rat following 4 weeks of sensory experience with 9-kHz tone trains modulated at 15 Hz paired with basal forebrain stimulation. Conventions as in **A**. The area with sites close to 9 kHz (*white hatching*) is greatly expanded relative to that in the naïve animal in **A**. Note that this expansion has resulted in the elimination of sites with CF below about 3 kHz. **D** CFs and breadth of tuning for every recording site in the experimental rat in **C**, illustrating the increase in the number of sites with CF near 9 kHz and the broader tuning of neurons at those sites. (Reproduced with permission from Kilgard *et al.*, 2002.)

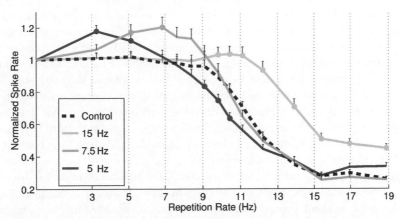

Fig. 16.6 Effect on rate sensitivity of neurons in AI of the rat of pairing electrical activation of the basal forebrain with stimulation at specific rates. Stimuli in each case were trains of tone pulses, the carrier frequencies of which varied from train to train, at repetition rates from 1–19 Hz. The experimental groups received identical basal forebrain stimulation paired with trains at repetition rates of 5, 7.5, or 15 Hz (see *key*). The data were collected from a total of 15 rats and over 500 cortical recording sites, and the repetition-rate transfer function for each site was normalized using the number of spikes evoked by the first tone in each train. *Error bars* indicate standard error, and the rates that were significantly different from controls are marked with *dots* (one-way ANOVA, Fischer's projected least-significant difference, $p < 0.05$). Relative to controls, stimulation at 5 Hz resulted in stronger responses at rates near the paired rate, and decreased sensitivity at higher rates; stimulation at 7.5 and 15 Hz resulted in stronger responses at rates around the paired rate. (Reproduced with permission from Kilgard *et al.*, 2002.)

this issue, and the mechanisms by which new inputs become effective or the efficacy of existing inputs is modified, will be reviewed in the following sections.

16.5.1 Sources of 'new' input: changes in the conceptualization of receptive fields

In the early period of sensory neuroscience, RFs were described simply in terms of the range of the given stimulus parameter(s) that evoked an increase in action potential frequency above the background resting activity. In the visual cortex literature, the 'classical' RF so defined has been referred to as the 'minimum discharge field' (MDF) (e.g., Bringuier *et al.*, 1999). An auditory neuron's MDF in the frequency domain comprises the range of frequencies and SPLs that evoke an increased discharge (i.e., the area delimited by its tuning curve). In the absence of spontaneous activity, these studies could not identify inhibitory components of RFs, but studies using various masking paradigms, or the iontophoretic application of inhibitory transmitter antagonists, revealed that many neurons at all levels of the central auditory system receive excitatory and/or inhibitory input at a range of frequencies and SPLs outside the MDF, the latter often manifested as flanking or 'side-band' inhibition. The immediate expansion of the RFs of some auditory cortical neurons following iontophoretic application of the GABA-A receptor antagonist bicuculline indicates that in these neurons suprathreshold excitatory input outside the MDF is masked by inhibition (for review see Irvine, 2007). The complex combinations of excitatory and inhibitory regions comprising the suprathreshold RFs of auditory cortical neurons, and the way in which these components vary over time, are particularly clearly illustrated in STRFs (e.g., Fritz *et al.*, 2003, 2005; Fig. 16.3).

Excitatory and inhibitory components of auditory RFs were defined in these studies in terms of the spiking activity of the neurons, but the most dramatic changes in our conceptualization of RFs have undoubtedly been those produced by *in vivo* intracellular recordings. In visual cortex, such recordings have revealed that many neurons receive *subthreshold* excitatory and inhibitory input over an area (the 'synaptic integration field') many times larger than the MDF (e.g., Bringuier *et al.*, 1999). Similarly, intracellular data indicate that the RFs of AI neurons defined in terms of subthreshold excitatory post-synaptic potentials (EPSPs) are much broader than those defined in terms of spike responses, and can extend over 5 octaves or more at moderate SPLs (Fig. 16.7). As in the visual system, this synaptic integration field reflects input derived from intrinsic cortico-cortical connections over horizontal fibres (for review see Metherate *et al.*, 2005). Finally, there is compelling evidence for the existence of 'silent' synapses which can be rapidly activated by patterns of stimulation that evoke long-term potentiation (LTP). It is possible that such silent inputs could be derived from points beyond the synaptic integration field of AI neurons, thus increasing even further the range of locations within the cortical tonotopic map from which input can be derived.

16.5.2 Mechanisms by which the efficacy of particular inputs is modified

The supra- and sub-threshold inputs outside the classic RF revealed by the studies reviewed in the previous section provide a broad matrix from which the short- and long-term RF changes observed in various plasticity paradigms could potentially be sculpted. Given this broad range of potential inputs, the major question raised by the various forms of plasticity concerns the nature of the 'sculpting' processes involved: what are the mechanisms by which the efficacy of various inputs is modified (i.e., by which excitatory and inhibitory synaptic weights are changed)? It must be acknowledged that direct evidence bearing on this question in the case of auditory plasticity is limited, and the following account is therefore based partly on evidence from other sensory systems and is leavened by a fair measure of speculation. It should also be noted that different forms of plasticity are likely to involve different mechanisms or combinations of mechanisms with different time courses.

Undoubtedly the best established mechanism for the strengthening of synaptic connections is correlated pre- and post-synaptic activity, as originally postulated by Hebb, and realized in the phenomenon of LTP or, more specifically, in spike-timing dependent plasticity (for review see Dan and Poo, 2006). Auditory cortical plasticity produced by cortical micro-stimulation would appear to be readily explicable in terms of this mechanism, as would the preservation/restoration of cochleotopicity by electrical stimulation at discrete cochlear places. In the former case, cortical microstimulation would be expected to activate nearby neurons via intrinsic intracortical connections, such that these inputs to those neurons would be strengthened. In the latter case, the pathways projecting from the cochlear regions activated by intracochlear stimulation to (more or less) discrete cortical regions would also be selectively strengthened. It must be acknowledged, however, that although this mechanism is intuitively plausible there is currently no direct evidence for its involvement in these forms of plasticity.

Synaptic LTP and long-term depression (LTD) would also appear to be strong candidates for the processes involved in changes in synaptic weights in injury-induced reorganization. Evidence from the somatosensory system indicates that the first stage of reorganization after digit amputation is an immediate expansion onto peri-lesion skin areas of the RFs of neurons in the LPZ (for review see Calford, 2002). The immediacy of this expansion can only be explained in terms of the 'unmasking' (presumably, the release from inhibition) of pre-existing suprathreshold excitatory

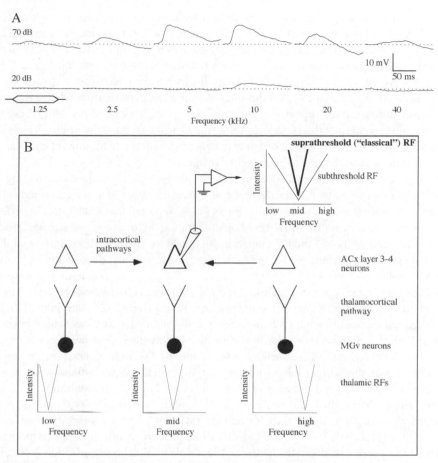

Fig. 16.7 The synaptic integration field (the combination of supra- and sub-threshold RFs) of an AI neuron, and a schematic illustration of the derivation of the classical and subthreshold RFs.
A Intracellular synaptic potentials evoked in response to a 5-octave range of frequencies at 20 and 70 dB SPL. Tone duration was 100 ms, beginning at trace onset (10-ms rise times). Synaptic potentials were obtained using whole-cell recording from a layer 3 neuron in AI of a urethane anaesthetized rat; resting potential ~ –60 mV. At 20 dB, near threshold, an EPSP is evoked only at 10 kHz (the neuron's CF). At 70 dB, however, EPSPs are recorded at all frequencies from 1.25 to 40 kHz. **B** Schematic illustration of the hypothesis that direct thalamo-cortical inputs to auditory cortical neurons convey information about stimuli within the classical RF and intracortical horizontal projections carry information mostly about spectrally distant non-CF stimuli. ACx Auditory cortex. (Reproduced with permission from Metherate *et al.*, 2005.)

inputs, and down-regulation of inhibition is known to be associated with cortical plasticity (for review see Rajan, 2001). Over a period of weeks after digit amputation, the expanded RFs gradually reduced in size, a process that Calford and colleagues (Calford, 2002) attributed to a re-establishment of excitatory–inhibitory balance. LTP and LTD are likely to be involved in this second phase of plastic change, and there is evidence for the involvement of NMDA receptor-mediated LTP in lesion-induced (and other forms of) somatosensory cortical plasticity (for review see Calford, 2002).

The role of unmasking of previously inhibited excitatory inputs in auditory cortical lesion-induced plasticity has not been established with certainty. Such unmasking as a consequence of loud-sound-induced hearing losses has been demonstrated in the immediate expansion of the frequency-SPL response areas of some AI neurons and associated changes in CF (e.g., Calford *et al.*, 1993; Noreña *et al.*, 2003). In the only study of the acute effects of mechanical cochlear lesions, Robertson and Irvine (1989) did not see an immediate expansion of RFs. Rather, the post-lesion tuning curves appeared to be explicable as the residue of pre-lesion responses. However, interpretation of this observation is qualified by the fact that the mechanical lesioning technique used in that study almost certainly produced short-term disruptions of cochlear processes at regions around the area of permanent damage.

Although unmasking of normally inhibited inputs almost certainly contributes to reorganization of frequency maps after restricted peripheral lesions, a number of observations indicate that it is not sufficient for such reorganization. Rajan (1998) reported that small losses in peripheral auditory sensitivity, associated with either idiopathic or noise-induced cochlear damage, produced a loss of surround inhibition and the unmasking of excitatory inputs in AI neurons in adult cats, but did not result in reorganization of the AI frequency map. A similar dissociation is apparent in the ICC. Snyder and Sinex (2002) reported that restricted spiral ganglion lesions resulted in the immediate post-lesion appearance of low-threshold excitation at frequencies below (or, in fewer cases, above) the borders of the pre-lesion frequency tuning curve in neurons in the LPZ in the ICC. Although this suggests that such unmasking would also occur after mechanical or ototoxic cochlear lesions, long-term reorganization after such lesions either does not occur in or occurs only in restricted regions of ICC (for review see Irvine, 2007). These observations indicate that unmasking is not sufficient for injury-induced auditory system reorganization, but it might well be a necessary first stage in the cascade of processes involved in such reorganization.

In the visual system, there is direct evidence that input derived over long-range horizontal intracortical connections is necessary for reorganization in V1 after restricted retinal lesion in adults (Calford *et al.*, 2003). The conclusion that visual cortex reorganization reflects mechanisms intrinsic to the cortex is supported by the fact that only minimal reorganization is seen in the visual thalamus after such lesions (for review see Calford, 2002). In the auditory system, however, cochlear lesions in adult cats result in reorganization in the MG_V that is indistinguishable from that in AI (Kamke *et al.*, 2003). If the reorganization in cortex partially or wholly reflects that in MG_V, it would indicate that reorganization in AI involves mechanisms other than changes in intracortical circuitry. However, it could be that the cortical changes are primary and are transferred to the thalamus via corticofugal projections. The possible importance of corticofugal projections in subcortical plasticity is indicated by the demonstration by Suga and colleagues that changes in the frequency organization of ICC induced by conditioning and by cortical microstimulation depend on corticofugal projections from AI (for review see Suga and Ma, 2003). In the somatosensory system, there is extensive reorganization in the thalamus after peripheral lesions, and corticofugal projections contribute substantially to thalamic plasticity (for review see Calford, 2002). Despite the similarities between lesion-induced reorganization in the major sensory systems, that in the auditory and somatosensory systems seems to be a characteristic of the entire thalamo-cortico-thalamic system, while that in the visual system seems to depend more on intrinsically cortical mechanisms.

In both microstimulation- and injury-induced plasticity, the nature of the intervention is such as to result in substantial changes in the relative frequency with which different inputs activate a given AI neuron, and thus in changes in synaptic strength. In the case of conditioning and other forms of behavioural and perceptual training, however, the training procedure itself would be expected to involve only a slight increase in the frequency of activation of inputs associated with the training or discrimination frequency, and little or no change in the wide range of other inputs activated in the course of the animal's interaction with its environment. In these forms of plasticity, the critical point seems to be that the training stimuli have increased salience for the organism (because of their association with reinforcement in the case of animal studies, or because of task demands in human perceptual learning) and therefore become the focus of attention. Under these conditions, it is widely held that the modulating influence of the cholinergic projections to AI is the critical factor in modifying the strength of inputs associated with that stimulus.

This view is supported by the evidence reviewed above for the effects of cholinergic agents and of stimulation of the basal forebrain on the response characteristics of auditory cortical neurons. ACh antagonists have also been shown to block the BF changes in auditory cortical neurons in bats (Ji et al., 2001) and the changes in auditory cortical fMRI responses in humans (Thiel et al., 2002), that are produced by classical conditioning procedures. However, although these studies establish that cortical ACh is necessary to produce those changes, they do not directly establish that the cholinergic projections from the basal forebrain are involved. In what appears to be the only study of the effects of inactivation of this system on auditory learning, Kudoh et al. (2004) found that immunotoxic injections into the auditory cortex in rats disrupted the learning of a sound-sequence discrimination, but in that study no evidence on plasticity of neuronal response characteristics was presented. Thus, although there is a substantial body of indirect evidence pointing to the role of the cholinergic basal forebrain in learning-induced auditory cortical neural plasticity, it has not been directly established that it is necessary for such changes. What is required is a study in which the effects of appropriate training procedures on auditory cortical neurons are determined in animals in which the cholinergic projections from the basal forebrain (but not cholinergic neurons intrinsic to the cortex) have been eliminated.

In the only study of the role of the basal forebrain in injury-induced auditory cortical plasticity, Kamke et al. (2005) found that immunotoxic lesions of the cholinergic basal forebrain regions projecting to AI did not prevent cochlear-lesion-induced reorganization in AI of adult cats. If one assumes that injury-induced reorganization in different sensory cortices involves the same mechanisms, this result is apparently at variance with evidence from the somatosensory system that injury-induced reorganization is blocked by lesions of the basal forebrain (for review see Irvine, 2007). The latter effect cannot unequivocally be attributed to destruction of the cholinergic system, however, as the neurotoxic lesions used in these somatosensory studies would also have destroyed non-cholinergic neurons in the basal forebrain. The finding that the cholinergic basal forebrain is not involved in cochlear-lesion-induced plasticity in AI is perhaps not surprising, given the evidence that cholinergic input to the cortex is critically associated with attentional processes (e.g., Sarter et al., 2003). As emphasized in previous sections, attention is critical to many forms of auditory system plasticity, but it is unlikely that it is important for injury-induced reorganization. Animals with restricted cochlear lesions obviously attend to their acoustic environment, but there is no reason to suppose that they attend specifically to lesion-edge frequencies, or that such attention is required for those frequencies to gain an enlarged representation in the thalamo-cortical system.

Finally, on a longer time scale, a number of studies of injury-induced plasticity in other modalities have found evidence of structural changes associated with cortical reorganization. Reorganization of the retinotopic map in VI after restricted retinal lesions in adult cats is associated with axonal sprouting of horizontal fibres in the superficial layers (for review see Calford, 2002). More recently, analogous reorganization in VI of adult mice has been shown by in vivo two-photon imaging to be associated with a massive increase in the turnover of dendritic spines in the superficial layers in the LPZ (Keck et al., 2008). In that study, the increased spine turnover was not associated with changes in the dendrites themselves, but changes in dendrites have been observed in association with reorganization in somatosensory cortex. Vibrissal deafferentation in adult rats results in an expansion of the influence of intact vibrissae into the area of the barrel cortex in which the deafferented vibrissae were represented. This change was found to be associated with a shift in the orientation of the dendrites of neurons in the LPZ toward the sources of this new input (Tailby et al., 2005). Structural changes of this sort have not yet been shown in injury-induced auditory plasticity, but the similarity of many forms of adult plasticity in different sensory systems suggests that such changes could well be involved.

16.6 Functional significance of central auditory system plasticity

As noted previously, a number of the forms of adult auditory system plasticity reviewed here have also been shown to occur in the visual and somatosensory systems of adults (for review see Kaas and Florence, 2001). This evidence has established that the properties of single neurons, and the functional organization of ensembles of neurons, in adult sensory systems are dynamic, and are constantly modified in ways that, in most cases, serve to optimize processing of salient stimuli in the organism's environment. The adaptive nature of adult plasticity in auditory processing mechanisms is most clearly indicated by the changes in the frequency selectivity of auditory cortical neurons that have been described in association with various forms of auditory learning. These changes result in a stronger response to, or better discrimination of, acoustic stimulus characteristics that are salient for the organism. Some other forms of plasticity (e.g., those produced by microstimulation or by direct activation of neuromodulatory systems) are not in themselves adaptive, but reveal the operation of mechanisms that are likely to be involved in adaptive forms of plasticity.

Injury-induced reorganization does not seem to fit into either of these categories. Although it is tempting to think of the central reorganization consequent on a cochlear lesion as a central compensation for the peripheral loss, this form of plasticity does not in fact seem to be adaptive. Central reorganization does nothing to ameliorate profound deafness in the frequency range corresponding to the damaged region of the cochlea, just as visual cortical reorganization does not eliminate the blind spot in the part of the visual field corresponding to the retinal lesion. This type of injury-induced reorganization should probably be thought of as an extreme manifestation of the processes that normally result in adaptive forms of plasticity.

In the case of injury-induced reorganization in the auditory cortex, however, the marked changes in the pattern of cortical activation produced by peri-lesion frequencies would be expected to have perceptual consequences, even if they are not compensatory. A number of studies in humans with steeply sloping hearing losses of the type that would be expected to result in auditory cortical reorganization have found that listeners with such losses exhibited improved frequency difference limens (DLFs) in the region of the cut-off (edge) frequency of their hearing loss (for review see Thai-Van et al., 2007). The improved DLFs are not attributable to loudness cues, and do not reflect spontaneous otoacoustic emissions at or near the edge frequency, which might interact with external tones in that frequency range and provide additional discrimination cues. These observations strengthen the possibility that the enhanced DLFs might reflect cortical reorganization, but it must be emphasized that there is no *direct* evidence of such reorganization having occurred in the participants in these studies.

It is also possible that some forms of cortical plasticity might have pathological consequences. In the somatosensory system, there is evidence that cortical reorganization might be responsible for some features of phantom limb experiences in amputees (e.g., Flor et al., 2006). It has similarly been suggested that tinnitus might be a consequence of cortical reorganization consequent on a cochlear lesion (for review see Irvine et al., 2000).

Finally, it has been argued that some forms of learning impairment might involve deficiencies in aspects of auditory processing that exhibit plasticity, and that could therefore be modified by training. These considerations have resulted in the recent development of a number of auditory training software packages (for review see Hayes *et al.*, 2003).

16.7 Conclusions

The evidence reviewed in this chapter for the various forms of plasticity exhibited by the adult auditory system, particularly at the thalamo-cortical level, establishes unequivocally that the neural systems by which information about the acoustic environment is processed are highly adaptive. However, although the phenomenon of adult auditory system plasticity is well established, very different patterns of change have been observed in different studies of the effects of, for example, conditioning and perceptual learning. These diverse and apparently contradictory results reflect the fact that we are far from a complete understanding of the particular auditory processing or perceptual demands that produce particular patterns of neural change.

One aspect of this concerns the role of attention. Although it has been argued that attention to salient events in the environment is a critical factor in many forms of sensory system plasticity, and thus that top-down processes play a major role, there is also evidence from the perceptual learning literature that discrimination of unattended stimuli can improve (e.g., Seitz and Watanabe, 2005). There is similar uncertainty concerning the mechanisms involved in adult auditory system plasticity; although we have evidence on a number of potential mechanisms, we are far from understanding the cascade of events that give rise to plastic changes, and the extent to which different forms of plasticity might involve different mechanisms. Finally, the implications of this plasticity for the development of remedial procedures, not only for the hearing impaired but also for those with other disabilities that might reflect auditory processing disorders, are only beginning to be explored.

Acknowledgements

The research by the author and colleagues cited in this chapter was supported by grants from the National Health and Medical Research Council of Australia and by a contract from the National Institute of Deafness and Communication Disorders (NIH-N01-DC-3-1005).

References

Alain C, Snyder JS, He Y, Reinke KS (2007) Changes in auditory cortex parallel rapid perceptual learning. *Cereb Cortex* 17: 1074–84.

Bao S, Chang EF, Woods J, Merzenich MM (2004) Temporal plasticity in the primary auditory cortex induced by operant perceptual learning. *Nat Neurosci* 7: 974–81.

Bergan JF, Ro P, Ro D, Knudsen EI (2005) Hunting increases adaptive auditory map plasticity in adult barn owls. *J Neurosci* 25: 9816–20.

Blake DT, Strata F, Churchland AK, Merzenich MM (2002) Neural correlates of instrumental learning in primary auditory cortex. *Proc Natl Acad Sci USA* 99: 10114–19.

Bringuier V, Chavane F, Glaeser L, Fregnac Y (1999) Horizontal propagation of visual activity in the synaptic integration field of area 17 neurons. *Science* 283: 695–9.

Brown M, Irvine DRF, Park VN (2004) Perceptual learning on an auditory frequency discrimination task by cats: association with changes in primary auditory cortex. *Cereb Cortex* 14: 952–65.

Calford MB (2002) Dynamic representational plasticity in sensory cortex. *Neuroscience* 111: 709–38.

Calford MB, Rajan R, Irvine DRF (1993) Rapid changes in the frequency tuning of neurons in cat auditory cortex resulting from pure-tone-induced temporary threshold shift. *Neuroscience* 55: 953–64.

Calford MB, Wright LL, Metha AB, Taglianetti V (2003) Topographic plasticity in primary visual cortex is mediated by local corticocortical connections. *J Neurosci* 23: 6434–42.

Dallos P, Harris D (1978) Properties of auditory nerve responses in absence of outer hair cells. *J Neurophysiol* 41: 365–83.

Dan Y, Poo M-M. (2006) Spike timing-dependent plasticity: from synapse to perception. *Physiol Rev* 86: 1033–48.

Dietrich V, Nieschalk M, Stoll W, Rajan R, Pantev C (2001) Cortical reorganization in patients with high frequency cochlear hearing loss. *Hear Res* 158: 1–7.

Edeline J-M, Pham P, Weinberger NM (1993) Rapid development of learning-induced receptive field plasticity in the auditory cortex. *Behav Neurosci* 107: 539–51.

Engineer ND, Percaccio CR, Pandya PK, Moucha R, Rathbun DL, Kilgard MP (2004) Environmental enrichment improves response strength, threshold, selectivity, and latency of auditory cortex neurons. *J Neurophysiol* 92: 73–82.

Fallon JB, Irvine DRF, Shepherd RK (2008) Cochlear implants and brain plasticity. *Hear Res* 238: 110–17.

Fallon JB, Irvine DRF, Shepherd RK (2009) Cochlear implant use following neonatal deafness influences the cochleotopic organization of the primary auditory cortex in cats. *J Comp Neurol* 512: 101–14.

Flor H, Nikolajsen L, Jensen TS (2006) Phantom limb pain: a case of maladaptive CNS plasticity? *Nat Rev Neurosci* 7: 873–81.

Fritz J, Shamma S, Elhilali M, Klein D (2003) Rapid task-related plasticity of spectrotemporal receptive fields in primary auditory cortex. *Nat Neurosci* 6: 1216–23.

Fritz JB, Elhilali M, Shamma SA (2005) Differential dynamic plasticity of A1 receptive fields during multiple spectral tasks. *J Neurosci* 25: 7623–35.

Ghose GM (2004) Learning in mammalian sensory cortex. *Curr Opin Neurobiol* 14: 513–18.

Green KMJ, Julyan PJ, Hastings DL, Ramsden RT (2005) Auditory cortical activation and speech perception in cochlear implant users: effects of implant experience and duration of deafness. *Hear Res* 205: 184–92.

Gu Q (2002) Neuromodulatory transmitter systems in the cortex and their role in cortical plasticity. *Neuroscience* 111: 815–35.

Harrison RV (2001) Age-related tonotopic map plasticity in the central auditory pathways. *Scand Audiol* 30: 8–14.

Harrison RV, Ibrahim D, Stanton SG, Mount RJ (1996) Reorganization of frequency maps in chinchilla auditory midbrain after long-term basal cochlear lesions induced at birth. In: *Auditory System Plasticity and Regeneration* (eds Salvi RJ, Henderson D, Fiorino F, Colletti V), pp 238–55. Thieme Medical, New York.

Hayes EA, Warrier CM, Nicol TG, Zecker SG, Kraus N (2003) Neural plasticity following auditory training in children with learning problems. *Clin Neurophysiol* 114: 673–84.

Hofman PM, Van Riswick JGA, Van Opstal AJ (1998) Relearning sound localization with new ears. *Nat Neurosci* 1: 417–21.

Irvine D, Brown M, Martin R, Park V (2005) Auditory perceptual learning and cortical plasticity. In: *Auditory Cortex: Towards a Synthesis of Human and Animal Research* (eds Koenig R, Heil P, Budinger E, Scheich H), pp 409–28. Lawrence Erlbaum, Mahwah, New Jersey.

Irvine DRF (2007) Auditory cortical plasticity: does it provide evidence for cognitive processing in the auditory cortex? *Hear Res* 229: 158–70.

Irvine DRF, Wright BA (2005) Plasticity in spectral processing. In: *Auditory Spectral Processing* (eds Malmierca M, Irvine DRF), pp 435–72. Elsevier, San Diego.

Irvine DRF, Rajan R, McDermott HJ (2000) Injury-induced reorganization in adult auditory cortex and its perceptual consequences. *Hear Res* 147: 188–99.

Irvine DRF, Rajan R, Smith S (2003) Effects of restricted cochlear lesions in adult cats on the frequency organization of the inferior colliculus. *J Comp Neurol* 467: 354–74.

Jacquemot C, Pallier C, LeBihan D, Dehaene S, Dupoux E (2003) Phonological grammar shapes the auditory cortex: a functional magnetic resonance imaging study. *J Neurosci* **23**: 9541–6.

Ji WQ, Gao EQ, Suga NB (2001) Effects of acetylcholine and atropine on plasticity of central auditory neurons caused by conditioning in bats. *J Neurophysiol* **86**: 211–25.

Kaas JH, Florence SL (2001) Reorganization of sensory and motor systems in adult mammals after injury. In: *The Mutable Brain* (ed. Kaas JH), pp 165–242. Harwood, Amsterdam.

Kacelnik O, Nodal FR, Parsons CH, King AJ (2006) Training-induced plasticity of auditory localization in adult mammals. *PLoS Biol* **4**: 627–38.

Kamke MR, Brown M, Irvine DRF (2003) Plasticity in the tonotopic organization of the medial geniculate body in adult cats following restricted unilateral cochlear lesions. *J Comp Neurol* **459**: 355–67.

Kamke MR, Brown M, Irvine DRF (2005) Basal forebrain cholinergic input is not essential for lesion-induced plasticity in mature auditory cortex. *Neuron* **48**: 675–86.

Karni A, Bertini G (1997) Learning perceptual skills: behavioral probes into adult cortical plasticity. *Curr Opin Neurobiol* **7**: 530–5.

Keck T, Mrsic-Flogel TD, Vaz Afonso M, Eysel UT, Bonhoeffer T, Hubener M (2008) Massive restructuring of neuronal circuits during functional reorganization of adult visual cortex. *Nat Neurosci* **11**: 1162–7.

Keuroghlian AS, Knudsen EI (2007) Adaptive auditory plasticity in developing and adult animals. *Progr Neurobiol* **82**: 109–21.

Kilgard MP, Pandya PK, Engineer ND, Moucha R (2002) Cortical network reorganization guided by sensory input features. *Biol Cyber* **87**: 333–43.

Knudsen EI (1998) Capacity for plasticity in the adult owl auditory system expanded by juvenile experience. *Science* **279**: 1531–3.

Kral A, Tillein J, Heid S, Klinke R, Hartmann R (2006) Cochlear implants: cortical plasticity in congenital deprivation. *Progr Brain Res* **157**: 283–313.

Kudoh M, Seki K, Shibuki K (2004) Sound-sequence discrimination learning is dependent on cholinergic inputs to the rat auditory cortex. *Neurosci Res* **50**: 113–23.

Kuhl PK (2004) Early language acquisition: cracking the speech code. *Nat Rev Neurosci* **5**: 831–43.

Linkenhoker BA, von der Ohe CG, Knudsen EI (2005) Anatomical traces of juvenile learning in the auditory system of adult barn owls. *Nat Neurosci* **8**: 93–8.

McKay CM (2005) Spectral processing in cochlear implants. In: *Auditory Spectral Processing* (eds Malmierca M, Irvine DRF), pp 473–509. Elsevier, San Diego.

Metherate R, Kaur S, Kawai H, Lazar R, Liang K, Rose HJ (2005) Spectral integration in auditory cortex: mechanisms and modulation. *Hear Res* **206**: 146–58.

Moore CM, Vollmer M, Leake PA, Snyder RL, Rebscher SJ (2002) The effects of chronic intracochlear electrical stimulation on inferior colliculus spatial representation in adult deafened cats. *Hear Res* **164**: 82–96.

Morris JS, Friston KJ, Dolan RJ (1998) Experience-dependent modulation of tonotopic neural responses in human auditory cortex. *Proc R Soc Lond Ser B* **265**: 649–57.

Näätänen R, Lehtokoski A, Lennes M, *et al.* (1997) Language-specific phoneme representations revealed by electric and magnetic brain responses. *Nature* **385**: 432–4.

Näätänen R, Tervaniemi M, Sussman E, Paavilainen P, Winkler I (2001) 'Primitive intelligence' in the auditory cortex. *Trend Neurosci* **24**: 283–8.

Nithianantharajah J, Hannan AJ (2006) Enriched environments, experience-dependent plasticity and disorders of the nervous system. *Nat Rev Neurosci* **7**: 697–709.

Noreña A, Tomita M, Eggermont JJ (2003) Neural changes in cat auditory cortex after a transient pure-tone trauma. *J Neurophysiol* **90**: 2387–401.

Noreña AJ, Gourevich B, Aizawa N, Eggermont JJ (2006) Spectrally enhanced acoustic environment disrupts frequency representation in cat auditory cortex. *Nat Neurosci* **9**: 932–9.

Ohl FW, Scheich H (1996) Differential frequency conditioning enhances spectral contrast sensitivity of units in auditory cortex (field Al) of the alert Mongolian gerbil. *Eur J Neurosci* 8: 1001–17.

Ohl FW, Scheich H (2005) Learning-induced plasticity in animal and human auditory cortex. *Curr Opin Neurobiol* 15: 470–7.

Ohl FW, Scheich H, Freeman WJ (2001) Change in pattern of ongoing cortical activity with auditory category learning. *Nature* 412: 733–6.

Polley DB, Steinberg EE, Merzenich MM (2006) Perceptual learning directs auditory cortical map reorganization through top-down influences. *J Neurosci* 26: 4970–82.

Rajan R (1998) Receptor organ damage causes loss of cortical surround inhibition without topographic map plasticity. *Nat Neurosci* 1: 138–43.

Rajan R (2001) Plasticity of excitation and inhibition in the receptive field of primary auditory cortical neurons after limited receptor organ damage. *Cereb Cortex* 11: 171–82.

Rajan R, Irvine DRF (1996) Features of and boundary conditions for lesion-induced reorganization of adult auditory cortical maps. In: *Auditory System Plasticity and Regeneration* (eds Salvi RJ, Henderson D, Fiorino F, Colletti V), pp 224–37. Thieme Medical, New York.

Rajan R, Irvine DRF (1998) Absence of plasticity of the frequency map in dorsal cochlear nucleus of adult cats after unilateral partial cochlear lesions. *J Comp Neurol* 399: 35–46.

Rajan R, Irvine DRF, Wise LZ, Heil P (1993) Effect of unilateral partial cochlear lesions in adult cats on the representation of lesioned and unlesioned cochleas in primary auditory cortex. *J Comp Neurol* 338: 17–49.

Recanzone GH, Schreiner CE, Merzenich MM (1993) Plasticity in the frequency representation of primary auditory cortex following discrimination training in adult owl monkeys. *J Neurosci* 13: 87–103.

Robertson D, Irvine DRF (1989) Plasticity of frequency organization in auditory cortex of guinea pigs with partial unilateral deafness. *J Comp Neurol* 282: 456–71.

Rutkowski RG, Weinberger NM (2005) Encoding of learned importance of sound by magnitude of representational area in primary auditory cortex. *Proc Natl Acad Sci USA* 102: 13664–9.

Sarter M, Bruno JP, Givens B (2003) Attentional functions of cortical cholinergic inputs: what does it mean for learning and memory. *Neurobiol Learn Mem* 80: 245–56.

Seitz A, Watanabe T (2005) A unified model for perceptual learning. *Trend Cognit Sci* 9: 329–34.

Seki S, Eggermont JJ (2002) Changes in cat primary auditory cortex after minor-to-moderate pure-tone induced hearing loss. *Hear Res* 173: 172–86.

Sheehan KA, McArthur GM, Bishop DVM (2005) Is discrimination training necessary to cause changes in the P2 auditory event-related brain potential to speech sounds? *Cognit Brain Res* 25: 547–53.

Snyder RL, Sinex DG (2002) Immediate changes in tuning of inferior colliculus neurons following acute lesions of cat spiral ganglion. *J Neurophysiol* 87: 434–52.

Suga N, Ma X (2003) Multiparametric corticofugal modulation and plasticity in the auditory system. *Nat Rev Neurosci* 4: 783–94.

Tailby C, Wright LL, Metha AB, Calford MB (2005) Activity-dependent maintenance and growth of dendrites in adult cortex. *Proc Natl Acad Sci USA* 102: 4631–6.

Talwar SK, Gerstein GL (2001) Reorganization in awake rat auditory cortex by local microstimulation and its effect on frequency-discrimination behavior. *J Neurophysiol* 86: 1555–72.

Thai-Van H, Micheyl C, Noreña A, Veuillet E, Gabriel D, Collet L. (2007) Enhanced frequency discrimination in hearing-impaired individuals: a review of perceptual correlates of central neural plasticity induced by cochlear damage. *Hear Res* 233: 14–22.

Thiel CM, Friston KJ, Dolan RJ (2002) Cholinergic modulation of experience-dependent plasticity in human auditory cortex. *Neuron* 35: 567–74.

Weinberger NM (2003) The nucleus basalis and memory codes: auditory cortical plasticity and the induction of specific, associative behavioral memory. *Neurobiol Learn Mem* 80: 268–84.

Weinberger NM (2004a) Experience-dependent response plasticity in the auditory cortex: issues, characteristics, mechanisms, and functions. In: *Plasticity of the Auditory System* (eds Parks TN, Rubel EW, Popper AN, Fay RR), pp 173–227. Springer, New York.

Weinberger NM (2004b) Specific long-term memory traces in primary auditory cortex. *Nat Rev Neurosci* **5**: 279–90.

Witte RS, Kipke DR (2005) Enhanced contrast sensitivity in auditory cortex as cats learn to discriminate sound frequencies. *Cognit Brain Res* **23**: 171–84.

Yan J, Zhang Y, Ehret G (2005) Corticofugal shaping of frequency tuning curves in the central nucleus of the inferior colliculus of mice. *J Neurophysiol* **93**: 71–83.

Chapter 17

Aging changes in the central auditory system

Robert D. Frisina

17.1 Introduction

The neural processing capabilities of the central auditory system tend to decline with age. However, perhaps counterintuitively, the central auditory system can also show signs of plasticity in response to changing inputs from the aging cochlea, which can sometimes be beneficial. Alterations, which take place in the parts of the brain used for hearing, which are somewhat independent of aging changes in the cochlea, may be related to age-linked neurodegenerative changes in the brain itself. In contrast, age-related reorganizations or plasticity in the central auditory system that take place in response to age-dependent losses of inputs from the cochlea are sometimes referred to as 'hearing-loss induced plasticity' (Carlson and Willott, 1996), or 'peripherally induced central effects' (Frisina *et al.*, 2001). Interestingly, these plastic changes sometimes occur well into a human's or animal's oldest ages, as has been observed in central visual and somatosensory systems (Syka, 2002). In this chapter age-related changes in the central auditory system are examined first from anatomical and neurochemical vantage points, and then the functional consequences of these structural changes are presented in the context of human perception and the underlying physiology of animal model systems.

17.2 Structural changes in the central auditory system

17.2.1 Cochleotopic or tonotopic plasticity with age

Illustrative cases of peripherally induced central effects reside in the brainstem and auditory cortex of aging mice, particularly the C57Bl/6J (C57, B6) and DBA mouse strains. These strains possess recessive alleles for the *ahl* gene, inducing age-related conformational abnormalities in cadherin 23, a protein critical for the proper development and functionality of inner ear hair cell stereocilia. The auditory phenotypes of C57 and DBA mice manifest a rapid, age-dependent high-frequency hearing loss, where, at 1 year of age, these mice have a severe-to-profound sensorineural loss, due to massive hair cell atrophy starting with outer hair cells in the cochlear base. In some sense, at 1 year of age, these mouse models have an 'old' cochlea, but still a relatively young brain, allowing for meaningful studies of reorganizational changes in the central auditory system that are primarily due to deafferentation (loss of cochlear outputs), rather than to aging of the brain itself.

Willott and colleagues provided convincing evidence of age-related alterations in the tonotopic map in the C57 and DBA strains, at the level of the inferior colliculus and auditory cortex (Willott, 1991). By recording from single neurons or multi-unit clusters, they discovered that middle and old age C57 mice had a paucity of neurons with high best frequencies (BF: the sound frequency to which a single neuron is most sensitive). However, in the regions of the inferior colliculus (in the ventral part of the central nucleus) and auditory cortex that normally would code for high frequencies, they recorded a preponderance of neurons with lower BFs (Willott *et al.*, 1988a, 1991; Willott and Turner, 2000). They observed that these lower-frequency neurons often had good sensitivity to sounds, indicating that they were not simply the low frequency 'tails' of the high-frequency response areas of neurons that are normally found in these regions in younger mice. No such age-related tonotopic reorganizations were seen in the inferior colliculus of CBA mice (Willott *et al.*, 1988b). Walton and colleagues recently verified the tonotopic reorganization of C57s with age, by comparing recordings of single units in the inferior colliculus of unanesthetized 1- to 2-month and 6- to 10-month-old C57s (Barsz *et al.*, 2007). In addition, they observed changes in the coding of wideband noise that were consistent with a loss of lateral inhibition with age and peripheral hearing loss.

The reorganization in C57s and DBAs was further substantiated by observations that startle responses for middle- and low-frequency sounds are *potentiated* in middle-age C57 and DBA mice, but not in middle-age CBAs (Willott *et al.*, 1994; Carlson and Willott, 1996; Ison *et al.*, 2007). A consequence of this over-representation is given in Fig. 17.1 for behavioral measures of prepulse inhibition in 1- and 6-month-old C57s. This over-representation of middle and lower frequencies in the central auditory system of aging C57 mice was also observed physiologically in a brainstem region that receives projections from the auditory system: the caudal pontine reticular formation (Carlson and Willott, 1998). So, Willott and colleagues' body of anatomical, behavioral, and neurophysiological evidence suggests that between the lower brainstem auditory centers, such as the cochlear nucleus, and the higher centers, including the inferior colliculus, some rewiring or plasticity occurs. In terms of pathways or local circuitry within these auditory brainstem centers, novel lower-frequency inputs are re-routed to principal neurons that normally receive inputs predominantly from high-BF cochlear output pathways in young adult mice.

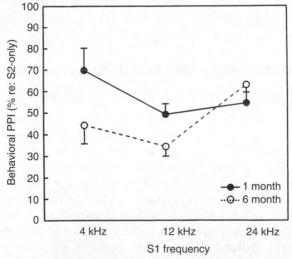

Fig. 17.1 Behavioral prepulse inhibition (PPI) in 1- and 6-month-old C57 mice indicates enhancement of the behavioral response in the older mice at frequencies below the hearing loss, i.e., 4 and 12 kHz. For 6-month-old mice, PPI was significantly better (lower percentage) when the S1 was 4 or 12 kHz, whereas PPI was the same at 24 kHz for the two age groups. The *abscissa* gives the frequency of the prepulse. The *ordinate* gives the magnitude of the startle response, as a percentage of the startle response with no prepulse. *Error bars* indicate means ± SE. (From Carlson and Willott (1998), with permission.)

17.2.2 Reductions in neuron size, morphology, and number

Willott and co-workers also discovered, using the C57 and DBA strains, that brainstem regions that receive heavy inputs from the cochlea, such as the cochlear nucleus, will show declines in volume and neuron size and number, which follow the decline in high-frequency cochlear outputs (from the cochlear base) that occur during the first year of life. In contrast, auditory brainstem regions in CBA mice, which lose their hearing slowly with age, like most humans after correcting for the absolute lifespan differences of mice and men, are more stable with age compared to C57s. For example, at the level of the anteroventral cochlear nucleus (AVCN), Willott's team observed that in C57s and DBAs overall volume declines, and packing density and cell number decreased between 1 and 7 months, but remained stable thereafter, despite chronic severe hearing impairment. In contrast, CBA mice displayed a modest reduction in AVCN cell number and packing density only during the second year of life (Willott et al., 1987; Willott and Bross, 1996). The C57 changes were most pronounced in the dorsal, high-frequency regions of AVCN.

Helfert and colleagues looked for age-related changes by studying the ultrastructure of the AVCN in Fischer 344 rats, which lose their hearing slowly with age like most humans and CBA mice (Helfert et al., 2003). Electron microscopy revealed decreases with age in the size of synaptic terminals contacting small-caliber ($< 2 \mu m$) dendrites. Dendrites of this size comprised the largest percentage of dendrites in the AVCN. On these dendrites, round and pleomorphic-vesicle presynaptic terminals were reduced in volume by 44% and 24%, respectively, in old rats compared to the young adults. This decline in presynaptic inputs, particularly the pleomorphic vesicles that are associated with inhibitory neurotransmitters, may be linked to the age-related loss of glycinergic inhibitory transmission (described later in this chapter).

Willott and co-workers examined age-linked structural changes of the posteroventral cochlear nucleus (PVCN) in the C57 and CBA mouse strains (Willott and Bross, 1990). A light microscopy investigation of the octopus cell area, in the caudal PVCN, yielded the following changes with age: a decrease in overall volume of this region, neuron loss, slight decrease in neuron size, increased glial cell packing density, and degradations of dendrites ranging from minor to total loss of primary branches. The greatest changes occurred in extreme old age, beyond the mouse median lifespan. Age-related changes were not exacerbated by sensorineural hearing loss in aging C57s, and there was a great deal of individual variation between octopus cells in the degree of age-related pathology.

For the dorsal cochlear nucleus (DCN), Willott's group discovered that in C57s, DCN overall volume declined with age, as did the mean number and size of neurons, most notably in DCN layer III which is the primary DCN target zone for auditory nerve fiber inputs (Willott et al., 1992). These striking cochlear nucleus aging changes did not occur in the DCN of CBA mice.

At the level of the central nucleus of the inferior colliculus, Kazee and colleagues, using electron microscopy, found similar results in the sense that C57s showed significant age degradations at the synaptic level, as well as shrinkage of principal neurons, especially in ventral regions of the central nucleus (Kazee et al., 1995). Synaptic changes with age included reduction of the number of synapses on principal neuron somata and reductions of up to 67% of the somatic area contacted by synapses. In contrast, a similar investigation in CBA mice showed very little change with age over a similar time course (Kazee and West, 1999).

Helfert and co-workers performed immunohistochemical ultrastructural studies of the aging Fischer 344 rat inferior colliculus (Helfert et al.1999). They observed losses of both excitatory and inhibitory synapses in the central nucleus of the inferior colliculus. Specifically, there were significant reductions in the densities of gamma-aminobutyric acid (GABA)+ and GABA– synaptic terminals (~ 30% and 24%, respectively) and synapses (~ 33% and 26%, respectively) for

28-month-old rats relative to 3-month-olds. They did not observe any reductions in neuron density with age. They concluded that the age-related decrease in GABA identified in previous investigations (described later in this chapter) may be attributable to synaptic and dendritic loss, rather than neuron loss.

Spatial localization of sound sources is one of the neural mechanisms in the central auditory system by which the detection of an acoustic signal is improved in the presence of a masking noise, and which can improve speech perception in noisy situations. Different rat strains have been utilized to elucidate some of the aging changes in this circuitry. To begin to understand some of its neural underpinnings, Casey and Feldman (1985a, 1988) examined the ultrastructure of the synaptic organization of the medial nucleus of the trapezoid body (MNTB), a key nucleus in the pathway providing contralateral inhibition to the lateral superior olive for binaural processing of sounds in space. They discovered, using electron microscopy, that there is a significant amount of neuropil degeneration with age, including declines in axons, dendrites, and nerve endings in the MNTB. For example, the mean percentage of the surface area of principal cells covered by synaptic terminals is 61.7% (SEM = 4.1) in young adults, while in aged animals (27–33 months of age) the coverage is only 43.7% (SEM = 3.3). Similarly, the average number of synaptic terminals present along a 100-μm length of principal cell surface decreases significantly in the old rats. They concluded that because of the significant loss of calycine synaptic specializations with advancing age, the structure of calyces of Held (large synapses found in the sound localization pathways of the auditory brainstem) becomes less complex, resulting in partial deafferentation of principal cells, compromising auditory information processing in the MNTB with age. Consistent with these neural changes, Casey and Feldman (1985b) also uncovered damage to the microvasculature in the MNTB, including large cavitations or spaces, and membranous debris, indicative of cellular degeneration, within leaflets of capillary basal lamina.

Later, Casey (1990) performed cell counts in the three major nuclei of the Fischer 344 rat superior olivary complex, which subserve auditory spatial processing. He found relative stability in the lateral and medial superior olive, but a significant decline in neuron number in the MNTB by 24–30 months of age (8%), although not as quite as dramatic as occurs in the Sprague-Dawley rat strain (34% decline; Casey and Feldman, 1982).

17.2.3 Auditory brainstem pathways degrade with age

Frisina and colleagues examined age-related changes in auditory brainstem pathways that provide inputs to the central nucleus of the inferior colliculus in the CBA mouse. Walton and co-workers physiologically characterized the dorsomedial central nucleus in CBAs of different ages, and then made injections of a retrograde label (horseradish peroxidase – HRP) to examine the inputs as a function of age (Walton et al., 1998). They found that input pathways from all three major divisions of the contralateral cochlear nucleus showed statistically significant declines with age, whereas other prominent input regions, such as the superior olivary complex and nuclei of the lateral lemniscus, were stable with age (Frisina and Walton, 2001a, b).

17.2.4 Intracellular calcium regulation modulates with age

A major theory of age-related central nervous system neurodegenerative diseases focuses upon calcium excitotoxicity. Proper levels of calcium ions are critical for many cellular functions in neurons, including the magnitude and timing of synaptic release of neurotransmitter. The latter requires rapid, specific binding of calcium ions to presynaptic neurotransmitter packets to facilitate movement along presynaptic ribbons, membrane binding, blebbing, and release into the synaptic cleft. Owing to the importance of these calcium-related processes for multiple aspects of neuronal function, proper regulation of calcium concentration by intracellular calcium-binding proteins throughout the life of a neuron is critical. Too little calcium can impair many neuronal functions; too much calcium can become toxic, sometimes inducing excitotoxicity, necrosis, or apoptosis in a central auditory neuron. Three of the most prominent calcium-binding proteins in the central auditory system are calbindin, calretinin, and parvalbumin.

Canlon and colleagues investigated age-related changes in these intracellular calcium regulators in the mouse cochlear nucleus. To examine peripherally induced central effects in the cochlear nucleus, they employed the C57 strain and quantitative stereology (Idrizbegovic *et al.*, 2003, 2004). Comparing young adults with 2.5-year-old mice they found, in both the PVCN and DCN of old C57s, a statistically significant *decrease* in the total number of neurons and *increases* in the proportion of neurons staining positive for parvalbumin, calbindin, and calretinin, which were correlated to peripheral pathologies such as loss of spiral ganglion neurons (SGNs), inner hair cells, and outer hair cells.

In other investigations, Canlon's group studied changes in calcium binding proteins in another mouse strain, BALB/C, with accelerated age-related hearing loss linked to the *ahl* gene. One interesting characteristic of this strain is that, in addition to losing its hearing at a faster rate than C57s (Willott *et al.*, 1998) and displaying severe hair cell losses in old age, there is an 80% loss of SGNs in the cochlear basal turn in 2-year-old mice (Idrizbegovic *et al.*, 2006). Consequences of this severe peripheral loss in the PVCN and DCN of old BALB/Cs were similar to the C57s, including: a statistically significant *decrease* in the density of neurons (25%) and *increases* in the proportion of calretinin+ and parvalbumin+ neurons. The increase of parvalbumin and calretinin neurons was correlated to the loss of SGNs, inner hair cells, and outer hair cells with age.

In a similar study in the CBA mouse cochlear nucleus the results were qualitatively similar to the C57s and BALB/Cs, in that for the PVCN and DCN, there were modest *increases* in the total number of neurons staining for the calcium-binding proteins (except calretinin which remained stable with age), but since the overall number of neurons declined in the DCN and remained stable in the PVCN, there was a *proportionate increase* in the number of neurons staining for calbindin, calretinin, and parvalbumin in the old CBAs, and in the DCN these changes were correlated with loss of SGNs, inner hair cells, and outer hair cells (Idrizbegovic *et al.*, 2001a, b). Canlon and colleagues interpret these age-related upregulations of calcium-binding proteins in the PVCN and DCN of BALB/C, C57, and CBA mice as *compensatory responses* to counterbalance aging neurodegenerative changes in the brain, including excitotoxicity.

These immunocytochemical investigations of the aging cochlear nucleus were taken one step further by Zettel and colleagues, who looked at aging changes in CBAs that were bilaterally deafened with cochlear ablations as young adults, and then allowed to survive to old age (Zettel *et al.*, 2003). They discovered that old deafened CBAs showed a decline of 47% in the mean density of calretinin+ cells in layer III of the DCN compared to old control CBAs, thus supporting the hypothesis that continued auditory neural activity in old age enhances the *upregulation* of calcium-binding proteins, possibly providing neuroprotection and facilitating increased neuron survival in the elderly.

Zettel and co-workers have performed extensive studies at higher brainstem levels as well, including the superior olivary complex and inferior colliculus. Examining immunocytochemical labeling in the inferior colliculus of CBA and C57 mice of different ages, they discovered that calbindin declined with age in both strains, but calretinin was *upregulated* in old CBA mice with good hearing, but not in aged C57s (that are deaf) (Zettel *et al.*, 1997). They interpreted this as, perhaps, a compensatory aging mechanism to combat possible calcium excitotoxicity in auditory midbrain neurons of old CBA mice that are still hearing, and where preserving neural function is a key issue. To start to test this hypothesis, Zettel and co-workers deafened young adult, normal hearing CBAs with cochlear ablation, allowed the mice to survive to old age, and then examined the calretinin immunolabeling. Supporting the activity-dependency hypothesis, the old deafened CBAs *failed to show* the age-dependent upregulation, displaying calretinin levels similar to the old deaf C57s (Zettel *et al.*, 2001). An additional immunohistochemical study revealed declines in calbindin labeling in the medial nucleus of the trapezoid body in C57 mice with age, but not in CBA mice (O'Neill *et al.*, 1997), suggesting that the declines in the C57 mice are a peripherally induced central effect.

17.2.5 Neurotransmitter system modifications – age reduces inhibition

Neural processing in the central auditory system is dependent on the magnitude and timing of excitatory and inhibitory inputs to auditory neurons. Caspary and colleagues carried out an extensive investigation of age changes in the two most prominent inhibitory neurotransmitter systems of the auditory system: glycine and GABA. Glycine is the predominant inhibitory transmitter at the lower levels of the auditory brainstem, such as at the cochlear nucleus. It gives way to GABA as one ascends the auditory brainstem. Both GABA and glycine are critically involved in temporal coding and spatial processing in the auditory brainstem, for neural circuitry from the cochlear nucleus through the inferior colliculus (Pollak and Park, 1993; Park and Pollak, 1993, 1994; Le Beau *et al.*, 1996; Caspary *et al.*, 2002; Frisina and Walton, 2006).

Willott, Caspary, and colleagues examined aging changes in glycine receptor binding and immunoreactivity in the cochlear nucleus of Fischer 344 rat, (Milbrandt and Caspary, 1995), and C57 and CBA mouse (Willott *et al.*, 1997). In old rats and old C57s, an overall decline in the number of glycine-immunoreactive neurons and significant decreases in the number of strychnine-sensitive glycine receptors (GlyR) in the DCN were observed. These deficits were not seen in middle-age C57s or CBAs of any age, suggesting that these changes in glycinergic circuitry are driven by both age and deafferentation associated with peripheral hearing loss. In addition, using *in situ* hybridization techniques (a measure of gene expression) in the cochlear nucleus of the Fischer 344 rat, they observed an age-related alteration in the glycine receptor subunit composition (Krenning *et al.*, 1998). A physiological follow-up experiment by Caspary and colleagues focused upon recording aging changes in DCN cartwheel cells, which are known to provide glycinergic inhibitory inputs onto the apical dendrites of DCN fusiform principal cells (Caspary *et al.*, 2005). Their study revealed that cartwheel cells in old rats displayed higher thresholds, increased spontaneous activity, reduction in off-set suppression, and rate-level functions characterized by hyperexcitability at high intensities, compared to young adults. Their conclusions were that these age changes reflect declines in excitatory inputs from the auditory nerve with age, reducing DCN inhibitory inputs to cartwheel cells, which collectively results in a disruption of tonic or stimulus-driven inhibition that DCN cartwheel neurons would normally provide to fusiform cells in young adults with normal hearing.

To acquire an understanding of the impacts of age and declines in glycinergic circuitry with age in the DCN, Caspary's group recorded from DCN fusiform cells extracellularly in the rat (Caspary *et al.*, 2005). They discovered that aged fusiform neurons exhibited higher maximum discharge rates and fewer non-monotonic rate-intensity functions and disruptions in temporal processing relative to young adults. Although not a complete explanation, these results are consistent with the hypothesized age-related decline in glycinergic, inhibitory inputs from cartwheel cells to these DCN principal neurons with age.

Caspary and colleagues performed an extensive series of investigations demonstrating, in a multidisciplinary manner, that there are age-related declines in the GABA inhibitory neurotransmitter systems of the rat auditory midbrain (Caspary *et al.*, 1995). Specifically, using immunocytochemical and neurochemical techniques, they demonstrated that the number of GABA-positive neurons was reduced by 36% in the ventrolateral portion of the central nucleus of the inferior colliculus in old animals relative to young adults (Caspary *et al.*, 1990). Additionally, they found that in neurochemical experiments, there are significant reductions in GABA transmitter release in the central nucleus of aged rats (−30%, $p < 0.05$), whereas, in contrast, tissue GABA content, basal and evoked release of glutamate and aspartate (the two main excitatory neurotransmitters of the auditory system), and acetylcholine were similar between the young and old age groups. Consistent with these investigations, they uncovered age-related decreases in $GABA_B$ receptor binding utilizing quantitative autoradiography assays (Milbrandt *et al.*, 1994). These receptor binding deficits were found in all three major divisions of the inferior colliculus: central nucleus, external nucleus, and dorsomedial cortex, but not in nearby cerebellar tissue. Milbrandt and colleagues also discovered gene expression changes in $GABA_A$ receptor subunit composition with age, using *in situ* hybridization (Milbrandt *et al.*, 1997). The most noticeable age change was an *upregulation* of the gamma-1 subunit, which they interpreted to be a possible compensatory response to the other predominant declines in the GABA inhibitory system of the inferior colliculus.

Recent evidence suggests that there may be aging changes in other neurotransmitters at the level of the inferior colliculus. Tadros *et al.* (2007a) performed an extensive gene array study, involving 40 CBA mice of different ages, obtaining both cochlear and inferior colliculus tissue for the microarrays ($n = 80$, one array for each mouse cochlea and one array for each inferior colliculus). Prior to sacrifice, each mouse had its hearing tested with auditory brainstem responses (ABRs) and distortion-product otoacoustic emissions (DPOAEs). The serotonin family of genes was investigated for any mRNA gene expression changes that might be linked to aging or hearing loss in the auditory midbrain. Serotonin was selected because it is an important neuromodulator of complex sound processing, as demonstrated by Hurley and Pollak (2001, 2005; Hurley, 2006) in recordings from the inferior colliculus of unanesthetized bats. Tadros and colleagues found an age-related upregulation of the serotonin 2B receptor in the inferior colliculus which was confirmed by PCR and, at the protein level, using immunocytochemistry. Across the three age groups of CBA mice (young adult, middle-aged, and old), they observed correlations between serotonin receptor gene expression and hearing loss. Tadros *et al.* (2007a) postulated that serotonin receptors are upregulated with age to counterbalance age-related declines in serotonin, but this creates the possibility that under certain conditions, intracellular calcium ions could build up to toxic levels because of the increased number of serotonin receptors.

Since glutamate is the primary excitatory neurotransmitter of the auditory system, Tadros and co-workers also looked at the glutamate family of genes ($n = 68$ genes) for the same data set as their serotonin study, by comparing microarray gene expression results and hearing measures (Tadros *et al.*, 2007b). Utilizing PCR verification of gene expression changes in the arrays, they discovered significant changes in two glutamate-related genes: Pyrroline-5-carboxylate synthetase enzyme (*Pycs*) was down-regulated with age and hearing loss (Fig. 17.2), while a high-affinity glutamate transporter (*Slc1a3*) showed an upregulation. Additional research will reveal exactly how these changes in gene expression play a role in presbycusis, but since *Pycs* facilitates the conversion of glutamate to proline, its deficiency in old age could result in glutamate elevation, and possibly glutamate excitotoxicity. In addition, since proline has been implicated as a neuroprotective agent, deficiencies in the aging auditory midbrain might be neurotoxic. The observed upregulation of *Slc1a3* might reflect a cellular compensatory mechanism to help protect against age-linked glutamate or calcium excitotoxicity.

17.3 Decline in central auditory processing with age

The molecular, anatomical, and neurochemical changes occurring with age in the auditory system have functional consequences for central auditory sound processing. As suggested above,

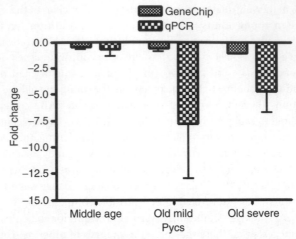

Fig. 17.2 For both GeneChip and real-time PCR, expression of some glutamate-related genes declines significantly with age in the mouse auditory midbrain (inferior colliculus). For example, Pycs enzyme gene expression (fold change) in the inferior colliculus of middle age, old mild hearing loss, and old severe hearing loss groups showed downregulation with age and hearing loss. This enzyme is used to convert glutamate to proline, so a downregulation with age could contribute to glutamate excitotoxicity. (From Tadros *et al.* (2007b), with permission.)

many of these are due to reduced cochlear outputs with age, and others appear to be somewhat independent of these peripheral changes, in line with neurodegenerative deficits of the aging brain.

17.3.1 Decline in temporal processing

It is known with certainty that the temporal resolving capacity of the auditory system degrades with age. Specifically, gap detection at suprathreshold levels becomes more variable and declines with age in human listeners (Schneider and Hamstra, 1999; Snell and Frisina, 2000; Lister *et al.*, 2002; Heinrich and Schneider, 2006). In addition, these investigations found that gap detection thresholds were *uncorrelated* with audiometric thresholds, and therefore unrelated to the most commonly used measure of peripheral, sensorineural hearing loss.

Another approach for gaining insights into the possible contribution of the central auditory system to age-dependent changes in temporal processing in humans is to study two groups of aged subjects, one with the typical, high-frequency sloping sensorineural hearing loss, and another group with audiometric thresholds within the normal range for young adults (sometimes called 'Golden Ears'). The following investigations have utilized this strategy to uncover auditory deficits with age in: gap detection and interaural time-difference thresholds (Strouse *et al.*, 1998); gap discrimination (Lister *et al.*, 2002); discrimination of timing in complex tonal sequences (Fitzgibbons and Gordon-Salant, 2001, 2004); temporal order recognition (Fitzgibbons *et al.*, 2006); and duration coding (Fitzgibbons *et al.*, 2007). In these studies, the differences between the young adults and old listeners with normal audiometric thresholds were significantly greater than those between the old subjects with 'Golden Ears' and those with significant audiometrically defined hearing loss.

In addition, the prevailing evidence links these age-related temporal processing deficits in human listeners to their difficulties with speech understanding, particularly in the presence of background noise. For instance, significant differences in speech perception in background noise exist between young subjects and old subjects with pure-tone thresholds within the normal range (Dubno *et al.*, 1984; Frisina and Frisina, 1997), in part due to *age-related declines* in: identification and discrimination of temporal cues such as temporal gaps in speech segments (Snell, 1997); detection of gaps in speech-like markers, both for within- and between-channel tasks (Mazelova *et al.*, 2003; Pichora-Fuller *et al.*, 2006); and discrimination of silence and transitions important for consonant distinctions (Gordon-Salant *et al.*, 2006). Some of these age-related declines in temporal processing important for speech perception in human listeners, as measured by a variety of gap detection paradigms, are even present in middle-aged subject groups with otherwise normal hearing (Grose *et al.*, 2006). Like most psychoacoustical (e.g., He *et al.*, 1999) or speech perception studies of aging, Grose and colleagues found that the age differences compounded as the listening task complexity was elevated, for example to include greater spectral complexity.

Walton and colleagues investigated aging changes at the auditory midbrain level in CBA mice, which lose their hearing slowly with age. Starting with young adult mice, they noted similarities between the behavioral processing of auditory temporal gaps and the temporal processing abilities of inferior colliculus single neurons (Walton *et al.*, 1997; Ison *et al.*, 1998). Building upon these similarities between auditory behavior and single-neuron processing in the midbrain, they studied changes that occur from young adulthood into old age in recordings from unanesthetized CBA mice (Walton *et al.*, 1998). They found significant declines in temporal processing of gaps in wideband noise. Specifically, the average thresholds for gap detection in the single neurons *increased with age*; gap recovery times were shorter in the young adults; maximal responses to lengthening of gaps *declined with age* across the population of inferior colliculus neurons; and neurons in old mice never showed facilitation in their response to gaps, as often occurs in young adult mice. In addition, most single neurons at the level of the inferior colliculus have a different gap encoding mechanism as compared to auditory nerve fibers. Specifically, auditory nerve fibers have sustained responses and encode gaps with a *decrease* in firing rate during the duration of the gap, whereas most inferior colliculus neurons (in unanesthetized recordings) are transient responders that encode gaps by an *increase* in firing, usually at the termination of the gap. The fact that CBA mice have fairly good hearing in old age, and because of the different neural coding mechanisms for the auditory nerve vs the inferior colliculus, it is likely that some of these age-related temporal processing declines measured at the level of the auditory midbrain are due to disruptions to temporal coding in the brainstem with age, in addition to aging deficits occurring in the cochlea. Furthermore, as presented above, there was an age-related, activity-dependent upregulation of calretinin, and declines in inputs from the contralateral cochlear nucleus in the inferior colliculus region where Walton and colleagues observed the temporal processing deficits at the single neuron level. Lastly, careful comparisons between human gap detection deficits with age and neural and behavioral temporal processing declines in CBA mice revealed some provocative implications for common mammalian aging changes in the central auditory system (Barsz *et al.*, 2002).

Caspary and colleagues investigated age-related temporal processing changes in the auditory midbrain by recording suprathreshold (30 dB above threshold) responses to amplitude modulation (AM) in the Fischer 344 rat (Palombi *et al.*, 2001). They found an age-related shift in the distribution of modulation transfer functions with different shapes in both the central nucleus and external cortex of the inferior colliculus. Old rats showed a lower percentage of bandpass AM transfer functions and a higher percentage of lowpass functions. They surmised that these age-related changes observed in AM coding may be due to an altered balance between excitatory and inhibitory neurotransmitter efficacy in the aged inferior colliculus, consistent with the idea that GABA-ergic inhibition helps shape AM coding in the inferior colliculus (Caspary *et al.*, 2002).

Further, detailed investigations of single neuron temporal processing at the auditory midbrain level in the unanesthetized CBA mouse have uncovered other clues to the possible neural bases of central auditory coding deficits observed in presbycusis. Walton and colleagues recorded responses to suprathreshold AM wideband noise stimuli, and analyzed coding of AM as a function of age (Walton *et al.*, 2002). In unanesthetized mammals, most inferior colliculus neurons respond with some form of an onset response, so their analysis was restricted to phasic responders. The primary result was that there was an overall increase in response rate to AM noise carriers with age, with the greatest differences for the lower AM frequencies, and a decrease in the modulation transfer function's median upper cutoff frequency in neurons from old mice relative to young adults. In addition, onset responses had *shorter* latencies in the old CBA mice relative to young adults, as presented in Fig. 17.3 (Simon *et al.*, 2004). They concluded that these age-related changes in onset response latencies and rate coding of AM are consistent with an age-linked loss of inhibition, or imbalance of excitatory and inhibitory neural mechanisms known to shape encoding of sound envelope periodicities in the inferior colliculus.

These single- and multi-unit studies have been complemented by evoked-potential investigations of changes in temporal processing with age in the auditory brainstem. Boettcher and colleagues investigated brainstem temporal processing using ABR responses in a forward masking paradigm (Boettcher, 2002). They compared responses in young and old gerbils and found significantly greater forward masking in the old animals, even though the old gerbils had fairly good auditory threshold sensitivity (within 15–20 dB of the young gerbils) (Boettcher *et al.*, 1996). Walton and colleagues found similar aging deficits in brainstem temporal processing using ABR forward masking paradigms in humans and mice (CBA and C57 strains) of varying ages (Walton *et al.*, 1995, 1999). In addition, Boettcher and co-workers performed similar ABR experiments in human listeners, with good peripheral hearing across the age-span, and found forward masking temporal processing deficits indicative of auditory brainstem processing problems in the older subjects (Poth *et al.*, 2001).

Age-related declines in frequency and temporal processing have also been observed in the rat auditory cortex. Although unable to localize where in the auditory system the age-related changes in complex sound processing occurred, Mendelson and Ricketts (2001) observed age changes in auditory cortex single neurons in old rats, particularly in response to frequency sweeps that mimic certain aspects of communication sounds, including speech. The age-dependent changes were consistent with declines in auditory temporal processing speed, specifically the ability to follow rapid, neuroethologically relevant frequency glides.

17.3.2 Declines in spatial processing

As presented above, there are age-related structural and neurochemical changes in portions of the central auditory system that mediate different aspects of binaural processing, and these anatomical changes have functional consequences and correlates. For instance, studies of suprathreshold sound localization abilities in humans show declines with age due to loss of both spectral and temporal information, particularly for sounds from the right spatial hemifield (Abel and Hay, 1996; Abel *et al.*, 2000), involving deficits in auditory lateralization (Herman *et al.*, 1977), binaural processing (Strouse *et al.*, 1998), and the precedence effect (Cranford *et al.*, 1990).

17.3.3 An augmented acoustic environment can delay presbycusis

Turner and Willott discovered that raising mice in an acoustically enriched auditory environment can delay the progression of presbycusis for some mouse strains that exhibit rapid age-related hearing loss due to the *ahl* gene. They utilized an augmented acoustic environment (AAE) consisting of

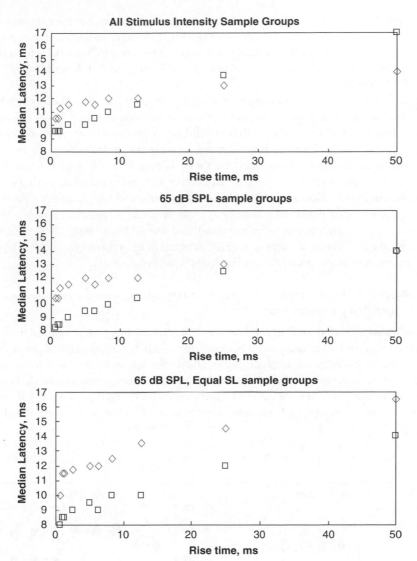

Fig. 17.3 Inferior colliculus single neuron responses to complex sounds show decreased onset latencies with age. Plots showing the relationship between median latency and stimulus rise time for young-adult (*diamonds*) and old (*squares*) CBA mice. *Above* All single units analyzed; *middle* single units stimulated at 65 dB SPL; *below* single units from young-adult and old CBA mice stimulated at 65 dB SPL, which had similar thresholds and equal stimulus sound levels with respect to their single-unit thresholds. Note that latencies *decreased* with age across rise times. (From Simon *et al.* (2004), with permission.)

exposure for 12 hours/night for 10 nights to a 70-dB SPL broadband noise at one of three age periods ranging from the onset of hearing loss (25–35 days of age) to more severe degrees of hearing loss (35–45 days and 45–55 days) (Turner and Willott, 1998). In DBAs they found that the AAE slowed down the accelerated rate of presbycusis normally exhibited by this mouse strain. Specifically, they observed improved auditory processing (only in 35-day and later groups), lower auditory brainstem response (ABR) thresholds (only in 45-day and earlier groups), and bigger startle response amplitudes in the DBAs. However, surprisingly, none of these improvements occurred in the C57s. More recent experiments with DBAs have indicated that exposure to frequency-specific AAEs can enhance ABR thresholds and neuron survivability (neuron size and number) in the regions of the AVCN sensitive to the AAE frequency band, as shown in Fig. 17.4 (Willott *et al.*, 2006).

In a follow-up experiment, Willott and Turner (1999) were also able to delay presbycusis in C57 mice. By significantly increasing the exposure to the AAE, i.e., from 25 days of age to 14 months, improvements in prepulse inhibition, ABR thresholds, and acoustic startle amplitude occurred in the C57 mice. Further experimentation on other mouse strains that lose their hearing at different rates as a function of age revealed that the beneficial effects of AAE take place irrespective of age at the onset of hearing loss, as long as initiation of AAE treatment precedes the occurrence of severe hearing loss (Willott *et al.*, 2000). Delaying AAE treatment beyond such a point results in the progressive loss of threshold sensitivity as usual, although prepulse inhibition benefits are sometimes apparent. Willott and colleagues concluded that AAE treatment can slow down, but not prevent, the occurrence of severe genetically determined age-related hearing loss, depending on AAE parameters and the mouse strain involved (Willott *et al.*, 2001).

17.3.4 Medical conditions can exacerbate age-related changes in central auditory processing

Some studies of co-morbid medical conditions and presbycusis suggest that some of the sequelae of these medical problems of aging might have negative effects on auditory central processing. For example, metabolic conditions, such as diabetes, could have negative effects not only on cochlear processing, but also on central auditory centers. Frisina *et al.* (2006) gained some insights into this situation by running an extensive battery of audiological and speech perception tasks on aged subjects with and without type II diabetes. Comparison of audiometric thresholds, DPOAE

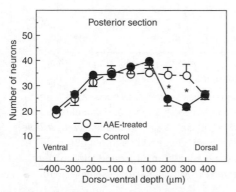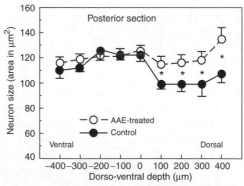

Fig. 17.4 Augmented acoustic environments can affect cochlear nucleus morphology. **A** Number of neurons in the posterior AVCN. The mean number of neurons in the 100- to 200- and, 201- to 300-μm horizontal segments was *significantly greater* in AAE-treated mice compared to controls. **B** Size (area) of AVCN neurons in the posterior AVCN. The mean size of neurons was *significantly larger* in AAE-treated mice in the dorsal four 100-μm horizontal segments compared to controls. *Unfilled circles* are AAE-treated mice; *filled circles* are untreated controls; *error bars* are standard error of the mean; *asterisks* are significant Fisher's LSD tests ($p < 0.05$). AVCN – anteroventral cochlear nucleus. (From Willott *et al.* (2006), with permission.)

amplitudes, wideband noise thresholds, and other peripheral hearing measures showed clear deficits for the type II diabetic group, relative to the age- and sex-matched control subjects, who were otherwise healthy. In addition, some listening measures that involve both peripheral and central auditory processing were utilized. These included the hearing-in-noise-test (HINT), which measures free-field speech perception in background noise, and has a spatial hearing component involving central auditory processing, the results of which are presented in Fig. 17.5. These data show that the diabetics do not benefit as much as the age-matched controls in terms of release-from-masking when the background noise source is moved laterally away from the speech sound source (90 and 270 degrees). Since the HINT is a suprathreshold speech perception task, the impairment in the spatial separation of the background noise from the speech indicates a processing problem in the central auditory system of the diabetics. Frisina and co-workers also measured suprathreshold gap detection and, as with the HINT, the diabetic group showed deficits in this task relative to the controls.

Hormone levels can also affect hearing in aged listeners. More specifically, Tadros *et al.* (2005) conducted a similar battery of audiological and speech perception tasks to those performed in the diabetes study, and correlated them with the levels of aldosterone in the blood. Aldosterone is the main hormone responsible for regulation of sodium and potassium levels, and its concentration tends to decline with age. Tadros and colleagues found a correlation between serum levels of aldosterone and hearing loss: the higher the aldosterone within the normal clinical range, the better the hearing in a group of relatively healthy aged subjects, relative to an age- and sex-matched control group. Significant differences in the peripheral hearing tests were observed, with the low-aldosterone subjects having worse hearing, and low levels of aldosterone were correlated with poor HINT results, the task involving central auditory spatial processing of speech in background noise.

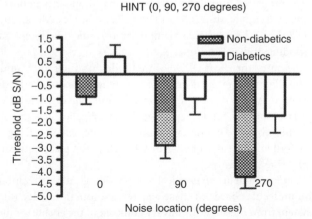

Fig. 17.5 Diabetes-affected speech processing in background noise. Specifically, HINT speech thresholds were lower for non-diabetics than diabetics for all background noise speaker locations. Also, HINT speech recognition in quiet was better for non-diabetics (not shown). ANOVA showed significant main effects of subject group and background noise location. Bonferroni post-hoc tests for subject groups were significant for 90 and 270 degree background noise locations. *Error bars* are SEM. (From Frisina *et al.* (2006), with permission.)

Sex hormones also play a role in the aging of the auditory system. It has been generally observed that women have better hearing than men at most ages, even when correcting for the tendency of men to have greater exposure than women to ototoxic events throughout their lifetimes. The finding that females have better hearing than males at most ages is supported by studies in laboratory animals that have been reared in identical environments, e.g., young adult and middle-age female CBA mice have better hearing than males (Guimaraes *et al.*, 2004).

Guimaraes *et al.* (2006) investigated the effects of hormone replacement therapy on presbycusis in 124 aged women, by comparing hearing test results for those who had taken combination HRT (progestin and estrogen), those who had taken estrogen-alone HRT, and women who had never taken HRT but were otherwise healthy. For the combination HRT group relative to the other two subject groups, they found significant deficits in peripheral hearing measures, such as pure-tone audiograms and DPOAE amplitudes, and in the HINT test, involving brainstem spatial processing. A recent animal model investigation supports the notion that there may be hormone deficits that diminish central auditory processing. Thompson *et al.* (2006) blocked estrogen receptors with tamoxifen, the most common clinically used estrogen receptor blocker, in young adult female CBA mice. Longitudinal measurements of ABRs, DPOAEs, and contralateral suppression (CS) of DPOAEs revealed changes in the medial olivocochlear efferent feedback (MOC) system, prior to any significant changes in the peripheral hearing measures, in experimental mice relative to controls that did not receive estrogen blockers.

17.3.5 Age-related deficits in the auditory efferent feedback system

A major portion of the mammalian auditory efferent feedback system from the brainstem to the cochlea originates in portions of the superior olivary complex, including the dorsomedial periolivary nucleus (DMPO) and the ventral nucleus of the trapezoid body (VNTB), which comprise the medial olivocochlear (MOC) system; and from the lateral periolivary nucleus, which makes up the lateral olivocochlear efferent system. In mammals, the strength of the MOC can be relatively easily measured non-invasively (with or without anesthetics) by measuring the magnitude of contralateral suppression (CS) of DPOAE amplitudes. Measuring the reduction of the amplitudes of DPOAEs is a superlative method for assessing the presence and magnitude of CS in mammals, including humans and mice.

Kim *et al.* (2002) measured the CS of DPOAE amplitudes in young adult, middle-aged, and old human listeners with audiograms in the normal hearing range, and discovered that major declines in the MOC system occur *between young adulthood and middle age*, with further incremental declines into old age. Jacobson *et al.* (2003) replicated this investigation in young adult, middle-aged, and old CBA mice. They observed a similar phenomenon, namely that the greatest age-related declines in the MOC system, measured by CS of DPOAEs, took place between the young adult and middle-aged mice (Fig. 17.6).

Zhu *et al.* (2007) conducted neuroanatomical and physiological investigations to gain insights into the neural and molecular bases of these age-related functional declines in the auditory efferent feedback system from the superior olivary complex to the cochlear outer hair cells. They compared age-related changes in the MOC system in CBA and C57 mice. C57s were found to have much reduced MOC physiological responses at young adult ages. Specifically, most functionality was lost by 8 weeks of age, and C57s showed little increase in CS for increases in the intensity of the contralateral wideband noise (Frisina *et al.*, 2007). Zhu and colleagues then measured neuron density and size in the DMPO and VNTB. Using stereological methods, they

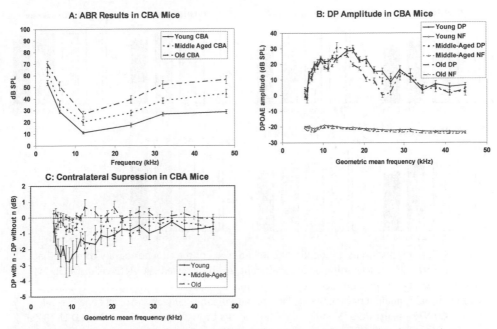

Fig. 17.6 Auditory function of colony-mates of the CBA mice used for age-related expression changes in Kv3.1b. **A** ABR audiograms for young (3–4 months), middle-aged (15 months), and old (24 months) mice (data for mice aged 29–34 months were not available). A flat elevation of threshold with age is evident, but even at 24 months, hearing loss is modest (20–30 dB). **B** DPOAE amplitudes (*upper traces*) and noise floors (*lower traces*) in young, middle-aged, and old CBA mice. DPOAE amplitudes for the oldest group show only a small decline in the mid-frequency range. **C** CS of DPOAEs of young-adult, middle-aged, and old CBA mice show a significant decline in CS by 15 months. (Adapted with permission from Jacobson *et al.* (2003), ©The Triological Society, and Zettel *et al.* (2007), Lippincott Williams and Wilkins, with permission.)

found that C57s had smaller neurons from the outset compared to young adult CBAs, and showed significant neuron shrinkage in both DMPO and VNTB over the same time course that the loss of MOC functionality occurred.

Zettel *et al.* (2007) probed further into the neural bases of this middle-age decline in the MOC efferent feedback system, utilizing physiological and immunocytochemical paradigms. First, they examined the auditory brainstem system of CBA mice with an antibody for the Kv 3.1 voltage-gated K+ channel, a potassium channel which is known to be involved in complex sound processing in the brainstem auditory system. They found that age-related declines in Kv 3.1 channel proteins occurred in the superior olivary complex regions containing the cell bodies of the MOC system, with the biggest differences found between the young adult and middle-age mice, and further declines into the older age groups (Fig. 17.7). To explore further the possible roles of the Kv 3.1 channels in the age-related MOC deficits, Zettel's group measured the CS of DPOAEs in knockout mice for the Kv 3.1 channels. When comparing knockouts with +/+ mice, they discovered that the knockouts had virtually no MOC response, relative to controls (Fig. 17.8). These findings for the MOC efferent feedback system providing inputs to outer hair cells are displayed in Fig. 17.9.

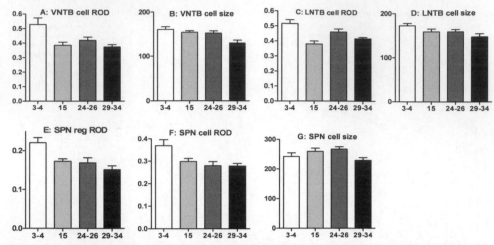

Fig. 17.7 Kv3.1b expression as a function of age in regions of the superior olivary complex that contain neuronal cell bodies of the auditory efferent feedback system. **A** VNTB cellular ROD in neuronal cell bodies. Significant decline occurs by middle age (15 months). **B** VNTB cell area in square microns. A gradual decline takes place with age, particularly by the oldest age (29–34 months). **C** LNTB cellular ROD. Significant decline occurs by middle age (15 months). **D** LNTB cell area in square microns. Decline occurs mostly in the oldest mice (29–34 months). **E** ROD for the entire SPN region. A significant decline occurs by middle age (15 months), with further decreases thereafter. **F** SPN cellular ROD. Significant decline occurs by 15 months. **G** SPN cell body area in square microns. No significant changes with age, except perhaps a trend in the oldest mice. *Error bars* are standard errors of the mean. LNTB Lateral nucleus of the trapezoid body; ROD relative optical density of antibody label; SPN superior paraolivary nucleus; VNTB ventral nucleus of the trapezoid body. (From Zettel *et al.* (2007), with permission.)

17.4 **Summary and conclusions**

It is apparent that there are a number of noteworthy anatomical, molecular genetic, and chemical changes in the aging central auditory system that no doubt play roles in functional declines in sound processing with age. Many changes at lower levels of the auditory pathway, such as the cochlear nucleus, are driven by age-dependent cochlear deafferentation, whereas some changes at higher levels of the system can occur somewhat independently of peripheral changes, such as the noteworthy decline in the auditory efferent feedback system that occurs in mice and humans in middle age, prior to significant decreases in cochlear sensitivity. So, although it is not clear which age-dependent alterations in the auditory central nervous system represent true aging changes in the brain itself, and how many are peripherally induced central effects caused by cochlear deafferentation, the declines are often correlated to age-linked auditory temporal or spatial processing deficits, as determined by psychoacoustic or speech perception tasks in elderly subjects. It is also interesting from the perspectives of both basic neuroscience and future clinical interventions that plasticity in the central auditory system often occurs well into old age. As we continue to uncover alterations of the functional organizational and sound coding properties of central auditory nuclei, we will no doubt move towards more realistic possibilities for clinical interventions that may prevent, slow, or treat age-related sensory processing declines in the brain.

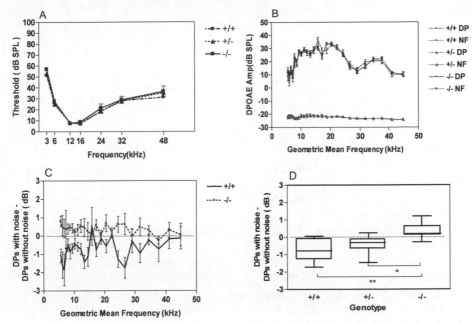

Fig. 17.8 Comparison of auditory function in Kv3.1b –/– (knockouts), +/+, and +/– mice at 6–11 weeks of age. **A** ABR threshold audiograms show no differences among genotypes. **B** DPOAE amplitudes are well above the noise floor (NF, *bottom traces*) for each group at all frequencies tested. No differences in amplitude were found among the three genotypes. **C** Comparison of medial olivocochlear efferent system (CS-DPOAE) function between –/– and +/+ genotypes. The knockout mice have no measurable MOC function and are significantly different from wild-type mice at many frequencies above and at all frequencies below 16 kHz. **D** Box plots (median, interquartile ranges, and total range) summarizing MOC (CS-DPOAEs) activity of the three genotypes. There was a statistically significant difference between the knockout mice compared to both +/– and +/+ mice, *p<0.05; **p<0.01. (From Zettel *et al.* (2007), with permission.)

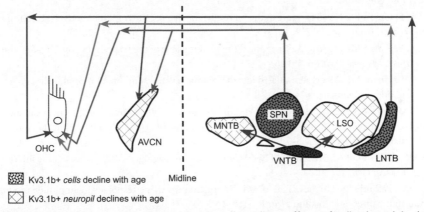

Fig. 17.9 Connections between the olivocochlear bundle auditory efferent feedback nuclei where age-related declines starting in middle age occurred for Kv3.1b antibody labeling of neuronal cell bodies (*stippled*) and nuclei where Kv3.1 antibody is labeled neuropil (*hatched*). Although not stippled here, the MNTB also showed an age-related reduction in neuronal cell body labeling as well. This figure shows primary pathways, but does not show all connections. Notice how the decline in neuropil expression of Kv3.1b in the LSO, MNTB, and AVCN may at least partially result from reduction in expression of Kv3.1b in the MOC neurons that project to them (*red and blue pathways*). AVCN Anteroventral cochlear nucleus; LNTB lateral nucleus of the trapezoid body; LSO lateral superior olive; MNTB medial nucleus of the trapezoid body; MOC medial olivocochlear bundle fiber tract; OHC outer hair cells; SPN superior paraolivary nucleus; VNTB ventral nucleus of the trapezoid body. (From Zettel *et al.* (2007), with permission.)

Acknowledgements

This work was supported by NIH grants P01 AG09524 from the National Institute on Aging, NIDCD P30 DC05409 from the National Institute on Deafness and Communication Disorders, and the International Center for Hearing and Speech Research, Rochester New York, USA.

References

Abel SM, Hay VH (1996) Sound localization: the interaction of HPDs, aging and hearing loss. *Scand Audiol* 25: 3–12.

Abel SM, Giguère C, Consoli A, Papsin BC (2000) The effect of aging on horizontal plane sound localization. *J Acoust Soc Am* 108: 743–52.

Barsz K, Ison JR, Snell KB, Walton JP (2002) Behavioral and neural measures of auditory temporal acuity in aging humans and mice. *Neurobiol Aging* 23: 565–78.

Barsz K, Wilson WW, Walton JP (2007) Reorganization of receptive fields following hearing loss in inferior colliculus neurons. *Neuroscience* 147: 532–45.

Boettcher FA (2002) Presbyacusis and the auditory brainstem response. *J Speech Lang Hear Res* 45: 1249–61.

Boettcher FA, Mills JH, Swerdloff JL, Holley BL (1996) Auditory evoked potentials in aged gerbils: responses elicited by noises separated by a silent gap. *Hear Res* 102: 167–78.

Carlson S, Willott JF (1996) The behavioral salience of tones as indicated by prepulse inhibition of the startle response: relationship to hearing loss and central neural plasticity in C57BL/6J mice. *Hear Res* 99: 168–75.

Carlson S, Willott JF (1998) Caudal pontine reticular formation of C57BL/6J mice: responses to startle stimuli, inhibition by tones, and plasticity. *J Neurophysiol* 79: 2603–14.

Casey MA (1990) The effects of aging on neuron number in the rat superior olivary complex. *Neurobiol Aging* 11: 391–4.

Casey MA, Feldman ML (1982) Aging in the rat medial nucleus of the trapezoid body. I. Light microscopy. *Neurobiol Aging* 3: 187–95.

Casey MA, Feldman ML (1985a) Aging in the rat medial nucleus of the trapezoid body. II. Electron microscopy. *J Comp Neurol* 232: 401–13.

Casey MA, Feldman ML (1985b) Aging in the rat medial nucleus of the trapezoid body. III. Alterations in capillaries. *Neurobiol Aging* 6: 39–46.

Casey MA, Feldman ML (1988) Age-related loss of synaptic terminals in the rat medial nucleus of the trapezoid body. *Neuroscience* 24: 189–94.

Caspary DM, Raza A, Lawhorn Armour BA, Pippin J, Arneric SP (1990) Immunocytochemical and neurochemical evidence for age-related loss of GABA in the inferior colliculus: implications for neural presbycusis. *J Neurosci* 10: 2363–72.

Caspary DM, Milbrandt JC, Helfert RH (1995) Central auditory aging: GABA changes in the inferior colliculus. *Exp Gerontol* 30: 349–60.

Caspary DM, Palombi PS, Hughes LF (2002) GABAergic inputs shape responses to amplitude modulated stimuli in the inferior colliculus. *Hear Res* 168: 163–73.

Caspary DM, Schatteman TA, Hughes LF (2005) Age-related changes in the inhibitory response properties of dorsal cochlear nucleus output neurons: role of inhibitory inputs. *J Neurosci* 25: 10952–9.

Cranford J, Boose M, Moore CA (1990) Effects of aging on the precedence effect in sound localization. *J Speech Hear Res* 33: 654–9.

Dubno JR, Dirks DD, Morgan DE (1984) Effects of age and mild hearing loss on speech recognition in noise. *J Acoust Soc Am* 76: 87–96.

Fitzgibbons PJ, Gordon-Salant S (2001) Aging and temporal discrimination in auditory sequences. *J Acoust Soc Am* 109: 2955–63.

Fitzgibbons PJ, Gordon-Salant S (2004) Age effects on discrimination of timing in auditory sequences. *J Acoust Soc Am* 116: 1126–34.

Fitzgibbons PJ, Gordon-Salant S, Friedman SA (2006) Effects of age and sequence presentation rate on temporal order recognition. *J Acoust Soc Am* 120: 991–9.

Fitzgibbons PJ, Gordon-Salant S, Barrett J (2007) Age-related differences in discrimination of an interval separating onsets of successive tone bursts as a function of interval duration. *J Acoust Soc Am* 122: 458–66.

Frisina DR, Frisina RD (1997) Speech recognition in noise and presbycusis: relations to possible neural sites. *Hear Res* 106: 95–104.

Frisina DR, Frisina RD, Snell KB, Burkard R, Walton JP, Ison JR (2001) Auditory temporal processing during aging. In: Functional Neurobiology of Aging (eds Hof PR, Mobbs CV), pp 565–79. Academic Press, San Diego.

Frisina RD, Walton JP (2001a) Neuroanatomy of the mouse central auditory system. In: Handbook of Mouse Auditory Res: From Behavior to Molecular Biology (ed. Willott JP), pp 243–77. CRC Press, New York.

Frisina RD, Walton JP (2001b) Aging of the mouse central auditory system. In: Handbook of Mouse Auditory Res: From Behavior to Molecular Biology (ed. Willott JP), pp 339–79. CRC Press, New York.

Frisina RD, Walton JP (2006) Age-related structural and functional changes in the cochlear nucleus. *Hear Res* 217: 216–33.

Frisina RD, Newman SR, Zhu X (2007) Auditory efferent activation in CBA mice exceeds that of C57s for varying levels of noise. *J Acoust Soc Am* 121: EL29–34.

Frisina ST, Mapes F, Kim S-H, Frisina DR, Frisina RD (2006) Characterization of hearing loss in aged type ii diabetics. *Hear Res* 211: 103–13.

Gordon-Salant S, Yeni-Komshian GH, Fitzgibbons PJ, Barrett J (2006) Age-related differences in identification and discrimination of temporal cues in speech segments. *J Acoust Soc Am* 119: 2455–66.

Grose JH, Hall JW 3rd, Buss E (2006) Temporal processing deficits in the pre-senescent auditory system. *J Acoust Soc Am* 119: 2305–15.

Guimaraes P, Zhu X, Cannon T, Kim S-H, Frisina RD (2004) Sex differences in distortion product otoacoustic emissions as a function of age in CBA mice. *Hear Res* 192: 83–9.

Guimaraes P, Frisina ST, Mapes F, Tadros SF, Frisina DR, Frisina RD (2006) Progestin negatively affects hearing in aged women. *Proc Nat Acad Sciences USA* 103: 14246–9.

He NJ, Horwitz AR, Dubno JR, Mills JH (1999) Psychometric functions for gap detection in noise measured from young and aged subjects. *J Acoust Soc Am* 106: 966–78.

Heinrich A, Schneider B (2006) Age-related changes in within- and between-channel gap detection using sinusoidal stimuli. *J Acoust Soc Am* 119: 2316–26.

Helfert RH, Sommer TJ, Meeks J, Hofstetter P, Hughes LF (1999) Age-related synaptic changes in the central nucleus of the inferior colliculus of the Fischer-344 rat. *J Comp Neurol* 406: 285–98.

Helfert RD, Krenning J, Wilson TS, Hughes LF (2003) Age-related synaptic changes in the anteroventral cochlear nucleus of Fischer-344 rats. *Hear Res* 183: 18–28.

Herman GE, Warren LR, Wagener JW (1977) Auditory lateralization: age differences in sensitivity to dichotic time and amplitude cues. *J Gerontol* 32: 187–91.

Hurley LM (2006) Different serotonin receptor agonists have distinct effects on sound-evoked responses in inferior colliculus. *J Neurophysiol* 96: 2177–88.

Hurley LM, Pollak GD (2001) Serotonin effects on frequency tuning of inferior colliculus neurons. *J Neurophysiol* 85: 828–42.

Hurley LM, Pollak GD (2005) Serotonin shifts first-spike latencies of inferior colliculus neurons. *J Neurosci* 25: 7876–86.

Idrizbegovic E, Canlon B, Bross LS, Willott JF, Bogdanovic N (2001a) The total number of neurons and calcium binding protein positive neurons during aging in the cochlear nucleus of CBA/CaJ mice: a quantitative study. *Hear Res* 158: 102–15.

Idrizbegovic E, Viberg A, Bogdanovic N, Canlon B (2001b) Peripheral cell loss related to calcium binding protein immunocytochemistry in the dorsal cochlear nucleus in CBA/CaJ mice during aging. *Audio Neuro-Otol* 6: 132–9.

Idrizbegovic E, Bogdanovic N, Viberg A, Canlon B (2003) Auditory peripheral influences on calcium binding protein immunoreactivity in the cochlear nucleus during aging in the C57BL/6J mouse. *Hear Res* 179: 33–42.

Idrizbegovic E, Bogdanovic N, Willott JF, Canlon B (2004) Age-related increases in calcium-binding protein immunoreactivity in the cochlear nucleus of hearing impaired C57BL/6J mice. *Neurobiol Aging* 25: 1085–93.

Idrizbegovic E, Salman H, Niu X, Canlon B (2006) Presbyacusis and calcium-binding protein immunoreactivity in the cochlear nucleus of BALB/c mice. *Hear Res* 216–217: 198–206.

Ison JR, Agrawal P, Pak J, Vaughn WJ (1998) Changes in temporal acuity with age and with hearing impairment in the mouse: a study of the acoustic startle reflex and its inhibition by brief decrements in noise level. *J Acoust Soc Am* 104: 1696–704.

Ison JR, Allen PD, O'Neill WE (2007) Age-related hearing loss in C57BL/6J mice has both frequency-specific and non-frequency-specific components that produce a hyperacusis-like exaggeration of the acoustic startle reflex. *J Assoc Res Otolaryngol* 8(4): 539–50.

Jacobson M, Kim S-H, Romney J, Zhu X, Frisina RD (2003) Contralateral suppression of distortion-product otoacoustic emissions declines with age: a comparison of findings in CBA mice with human listeners. *Laryngoscope* 113: 1707–13.

Kazee AM, West NR (1999) Preservation of synapses on principal cells of the central nucleus of the inferior colliculus with aging in the CBA mouse. *Hear Res* 133: 98–106.

Kazee AM, Han LY, Spongr VP, Walton JP, Salvi RJ, Flood DG (1995) Synaptic loss in the central nucleus of the inferior colliculus correlates with sensorineural hearing loss in the C57BL/6 mouse model of presbycusis. *Hear Res* 89: 109–20.

Kim SH, Frisina DR, Frisina RD (2002) Effects of age on contralateral suppression of distortion-product otoacoustic emissions in human listeners with normal hearing. *Audiol Neuro-Otol* 7: 348–57.

Krenning J, Hughes LF, Caspary DM, Helfert RH (1998) Age-related glycine receptor subunit changes in the cochlear nucleus of Fischer-344 rats. *Laryngoscope* 108: 26–31.

Le Beau FE, Rees A, Malmierca MS (1996) Contribution of GABA- and glycine-mediated inhibition to the monaural temporal response properties of neurons in the inferior colliculus. *J Neurophysiol* 75: 902–19.

Lister J, Besing J, Koehnke J (2002) Effects of age and frequency disparity on gap discrimination. *J Acoust Soc Am* 111: 2793–800.

Mazelova J, Popelar J, Syka J (2003) Auditory function in presbycusis: peripheral vs. central changes. *Exp Gerontol* 38: 87–94.

Mendelson JR, Ricketts C (2001) Age-related temporal processing speed deterioration in auditory cortex. *Hear Res* 158: 84–94.

Milbrandt JC, Caspary DM (1995) Age-related reduction of $[^3H]$strychnine binding sites in the cochlear nucleus of Fischer 344 rat. *Neuroscience* 67: 713–19.

Milbrandt JC, Albin RL, Caspary DM (1994) Age-related decrease in GABA$_B$ receptor binding in the Fischer 344 rat inferior colliculus. *Neurobiol Aging* 15: 699–703.

Milbrandt JC, Hunter C, Caspary DM (1997) Alterations of GABA$_A$ receptor subunit mRNA levels in the aging Fischer 344 rat inferior colliculus. *J Comp Neurol* 379: 455–65.

O'Neill WE, Zettel ML, Whittemore KR, Frisina RD (1997) Calbindin D-28k immunoreactivity in the medial nucleus of the trapezoid body declines with age in C57B1/6J, but not CBA/CaJ mice. *Hear Res* 112: 158–66.

Palombi P, Backoff PM, Caspary DM (2001) Responses of young and aged rat inferior colliculus neurons to sinusoidally amplitude modulated stimuli. *Hear Res* 153: 174–80.

Park TJ, Pollak GD (1993) GABA shapes sensitivity to interaural intensity disparities in the mustache bat's inferior colliculus: implications for encoding sound location. *J Neurosci* 13: 2050–67.

Park TJ, Pollak GD (1994) Azimuthal receptive fields are shaped by GABAergic inhibition in the inferior colliculus of the mustache bat. *J Neurophysiol* 72: 1080–102.

Pichora-Fuller MK, Schneider BA, Benson NJ, Hamstra SJ, Storzer E (2006) Effect of age on detection of gaps in speech and non-speech markers varying in duration and spectral symmetry. *J Acoust Soc Am* 119: 1143–55.

Pollak GD, Park TJ (1993) The effects of GABAergic inhibition on monaural response properties of neurons in the mustache bat's inferior colliculus. *Hear Res* 65: 99–117.

Poth EA, Boettcher FA, Mills JH, Dubno JR (2001) Auditory brainstem responses in younger and older adults for broadband noises separated by a silent gap. *Hear Res* 161: 81–6.

Schneider BA, Hamstra SJ (1999) Gap detection thresholds as a function of tonal duration for younger and older listeners. *J Acoust Soc Am* 106: 371–80.

Simon H, Frisina RD, Walton JP (2004) Age reduces response latency of mouse inferior colliculus neurons to AM sounds. *J Acoust Soc Am* 101: 469–77.

Snell KB (1997) Age-related changes in temporal gap detection. *J Acoust Soc Am* 101: 2214–20.

Snell KB, Frisina DR (2000) Relationships among age-related differences in gap detection and word recognition. *J Acoust Soc Am* 107: 1615–26.

Strouse A, Ashmead DH, Ohde RN, Grantham DW (1998) Temporal processing in the aging auditory system. *J Acoust Soc Am* 104: 2385–99.

Syka J (2002) Plastic changes in the central auditory system after hearing loss, restoration of function, and during learning. *Physiol Rev* 82: 601–36.

Tadros SF, Frisina ST, Mapes F, Frisina DR, Frisina RD (2005) High serum aldosterone levels correlate with lower hearing thresholds in aged humans: a possible protective hormone against presbycusis. *Hear Res* 209: 10–18.

Tadros SF, D'Souza M, Zettel ML, Zhu X, Lynch-Erhardt M, Frisina RD (2007a) Serotonin 2B receptor: upregulated with age and hearing loss in mouse auditory system. *Neurobiol Aging* 28: 1112–23.

Tadros SF, D'Souza M, Zettel ML, Zhu X, Waxmonsky NC, Frisina RD (2007b) Glutamate-related gene expression in CBA mouse inferior colliculus changes with age and hearing loss. *Brain Res* 1127: 1–9.

Thompson SK, Zhu X, Frisina RD (2006) Estrogen blockade reduces auditory feedback in CBA mice. *Otolaryngol Head Neck Surg* 135: 100–5.

Turner JG, Willott JF (1998) Exposure to an augmented acoustic environment alters auditory function in hearing-impaired DBA/2J mice. *Hear Res* 118: 101–13.

Walton JP, Frisina RD, Meierhans LR (1995) Sensorineural hearing loss effects recovery from short term adaptation in the CBA and C57 mouse models of presbycusis. *Hear Res* 88: 19–26.

Walton JP, Frisina RD, Ison JE, O'Neill WE (1997) Neural correlates of behavioral gap detection in the inferior colliculus of the young CBA mouse. *J Comp Physiol A* 181: 161–76.

Walton JP, Frisina, RD, O'Neill WE (1998) Age-related alteration in neural processing of silent gaps in the central nucleus of the inferior colliculus in the CBA mouse model of presbycusis. *J Neurosci* 18: 2764–76.

Walton J, Orlando M, Burkard R (1999) Auditory brainstem response forward-masking recovery functions in older humans with normal hearing. *Hear Res* 127: 86–94.

Walton JP, Simon H, Frisina RD (2002) Age-related alterations in the neural coding of envelope periodicities. *J Neurophysiol* 88: 565–78.

Willott J (1991) *Aging in the Auditory System: Anatomy, Physiology, and Psychophysics.* Singular, San Diego.

Willott JF, Bross LS (1990) Morphology of the octopus cell area of the cochlear nucleus in young and aging C57BL/6J and CBA/J mice. *J Comp Neurol* 300: 61–81.

Willott JF, Bross LS (1996) Morphological changes in the anteroventral cochlear nucleus that accompany sensorineural hearing loss in DBA/2J and C57BL/6J mice. *Dev Brain Res* **91**: 218–26.

Willott JF, Turner JG (1999) Prolonged exposure to an augmented acoustic environment ameliorates age-related auditory changes in C57BL/6J and DBA/2J mice. *Hear Res* **135**: 78–88.

Willott JF, Turner JG (2000) Neural plasticity in the mouse inferior colliculus: relationship to hearing loss, augmented acoustic stimulation, and prepulse inhibition. *Hear Res* **147**: 275–81.

Willott JF, Jackson LM, Hunter KP (1987) Morphometric study of the anteroventral cochlear nucleus of two mouse models of presbycusis. *J Comp Neurol* **260**: 472–80.

Willott JF, Parham K, Hunter KP (1988a) Response properties of inferior colliculus neurons in middle-aged C57BL/6J mice with presbycusis. *Hear Res* **37**: 15–28.

Willott JF, Parham K, Hunter KP (1988b) Response properties of inferior colliculus neurons in young and very old CBA/J mice. *Hear Res* **37**: 1–14.

Willott JF, Parham K, Hunter KP (1991) Comparison of the auditory sensitivity of neurons in the cochlear nucleus and inferior colliculus of young and aging C57BL/6J and CBA/J mice. *Hear Res* **53**: 78–94.

Willott JF, Bross LS, McFadden SL (1992) Morphology of the dorsal cochlear nucleus in C57BL/6J and CBA/J mice across the life span. *J Comp Neurol* **321**: 666–78.

Willott JF, Carlson S, Chen H (1994) Prepulse inhibition of the startle response in mice: relationship to hearing loss and auditory system plasticity. *Behav Neurosci* **108**: 703–13.

Willott JF, Milbrandt JC, Bross LS, Caspary DM (1997) Glycine immunoreactivity and receptor binding in the cochlear nucleus of C57BL/6J and CBA/CaJ mice: effects of cochlear impairment and aging. *J Comp Neurol* **385**: 405–14.

Willott JF, Turner JG, Carlson S, Ding D, Seegers Bross L, Falls WA. (1998) The BALB/c mouse as an animal model for progressive sensorineural hearing loss. *Hear Res* **115**: 162–74.

Willott JF, Turner JG, Sundin VS (2000) Effects of exposure to an augmented acoustic environment on auditory function in mice: roles of hearing loss and age during treatment. *Hear Res* **142**: 79–88.

Willott JF, Chisolm TH, Lister JJ (2001) Modulation of presbycusis: current status and future directions. *Audiol Neurootol* **6**: 231–49.

Willott JF, Bosch JV, Shimizu T, Ding DL (2006) Effects of exposing DBA/2J mice to a high-frequency augmented acoustic environment on the cochlea and anteroventral cochlear nucleus. *Hear Res* **216**: 138–45.

Zettel ML, Frisina RD, Haider S, O'Neill WE (1997) Age-related changes in the immunoreactivity of calbindin D28K and calretinin in the inferior colliculus of the CBA/J and C57/6J mouse. *J Comp Neurol* **386**: 92–110.

Zettel ML, O'Neill WE, Trang TT, Frisina RD (2001) Early bilateral deafening prevents calretinin up-regulation in the dorsal cortex of the inferior colliculus of aged CBA/CaJ mice. *Hear Res* **158**: 131–8.

Zettel ML, Trang TT, O'Neill WE, Frisina RD (2003) Activity-dependent age-related regulation of calcium-binding proteins in the mouse dorsal cochlear nucleus. *Hear Res* **183**: 57–66.

Zettel ML, Zhu X, O'Neill WE, Frisina RD (2007) Age-related declines in Kv 3.1b expression in the mouse auditory brainstem correlate with functional deficits in the medial olivocochlear efferent system. *J Assoc Res Otolaryngol* **8**: 280–93.

Zhu X, Vasilyeva ON, Kim, *et al.* (2007) Auditory efferent system declines precede age-related hearing loss: Contralateral suppression of otoacoustic emissions in mice. *J Comp Neurol* **503**: 593–604.

Section 5

Cognition and emotion in the auditory brain

Chapter 18

The cognitive auditory cortex

Norman M. Weinberger

18.1 Introduction

The auditory system subserves hearing, including the detection, analysis, and comprehension of sound. The traditional assumption has been that the primary auditory cortex (A1) is concerned with the *analysis of acoustic stimuli* but *not with the comprehension or behavioral relevance of sound*. Moreover, physiological plasticity in A1 (hereafter 'plasticity') was believed to be possible only during development, not in the adult. The conception of A1 as an auditory analyzer is deeply embedded in neuroscience. This entrenched view is the logical product of the long-established assumption that sensory processes and higher cognitive processes are separable within the cerebral cortex. Indeed, they are assumed to be 'in series'. In other words, the products of sensory analysis are presupposed to be 'passed on' to 'higher' cortical areas, where cognition takes place. Primary sensory cortices were termed, e.g., 'auditory sensory' while 'higher' sensory regions were termed, e.g., 'auditory psychic' (Campbell, 1905). 'Sensory' cortex was presumed to analyze stimuli while 'psychic' regions were presumed to provide the interpretation or assign psychological meaning to stimuli. In short, learning, memory, and other cognitive functions were thought to be engaged only after A1 had completed a hierarchically based analysis of the electrophysiological sequelae of patterns of traveling waves within the cochlea.

However, since the mid-twentieth century, extensive findings from behavioral neurophysiological and related experiments have been directly incompatible with this view of the auditory cortex. In the period 1955–1985, the 'pure analyzer' theory was rendered untenable by compelling documentation that the sound-elicited responses of A1 were governed by learning and memory, as well as by the physical parameters of sound. Nonetheless, auditory neuroscience did not recognize the cognitive functions of the auditory cortex until the mid-1990s, after the discovery that associative learning produced shifts of frequency receptive fields ('tuning curves') to favor the frequency of a sound that gained behavioral importance (Weinberger, 2004c). Subsequently, such learning-induced specific plasticity was rapidly embraced, so much so that the mature generation of auditory scientists generally takes it for granted while graduate students and younger workers have difficulty imagining a time when plasticity in the adult auditory cortex was not part of normal discourse.

At present, the study of systematic physiological plasticity in A1 (and to a lesser extent other auditory cortical fields) is burgeoning. Although studies of associative learning continue to hold a dominant position, inquiry has expanded to a variety of cognitive domains, including working and reference memory, attention, imagery, concept formation, preparatory set, motivation, learning strategy, cross-modality effects, and pre-motor processes. Despite the growing number of demonstrations of 'cognitive plasticity', the implications of this sea-change in conceptualization of A1 seldom have been addressed. They pose a challenge not only to the 'sensory analyzer' theory of the auditory cortex but also to the accepted conception of the functional organization of the entire cerebral cortex (see section 18.13).

This chapter reflects the amount of research on various aspects of cognitive processes in A1. While much of the background, technical, and conceptual issues are therefore necessarily discussed within the framework of associative learning, most of this material is equally relevant for other cognitive processes. Coverage of empirical findings focuses on studies of experimental animals because they afford precise control of stimuli, provide for strict localization of recording sites, and yield a variety of neurophysiological data, including unitary discharges. These three factors also enable comparison of the results of cognitive studies with the foundational animal literature on basic auditory neurophysiology.

This account summarizes major findings that are the basis for concluding that A1 has cognitive functions, includes a brief consideration of the mechanisms of A1 plasticity, and concludes with a discussion of the implications, challenges, and opportunities that make for an exciting and potentially illuminating research future. Tutorial material is interwoven where thought helpful for readers with little or no background in learning, memory, and other cognitive processes. Other related issues, such as the nature and importance of objective behavioral validation of cognitive functions and the advantages and limitations of various experimental designs, have been reviewed elsewhere (Weinberger, 2004c, 2008a, b)[1].

18.2 Learning and memory

Classical (Pavlovian) and instrumental (Thorndikian) conditioning are major types of associative learning. Classical conditioning concerns learning an association between two stimuli, specifically that an initially neutral stimulus (the conditioned stimulus, CS) predicts another stimulus (the unconditioned stimulus, US); the latter usually is of biological significance, i.e., a reward or aversive stimulus (Pavlov, 1927; see also Rescorla, 1988a). Instrumental conditioning involves learning an association between a behavioral response and a reinforcement, either a reward or the avoidance of a nociceptive stimulus.

Detailed explication of the fundamentals of learning is beyond the scope of this chapter. However, for purposes of this review, two factors must be kept in mind. First, learning cannot be observed directly; it must always be inferred from behavior. Therefore, placing a subject in a learning situation, such as repeated presentation of a CS paired with a US, is not sufficient for the conclusion that learning has taken place. Rather, learning is inferred from changes in behavior. In the case of classical conditioning, the major change occurs in the response to the CS as it becomes associated with the US rather than to the physical parameters of the sound itself. The subject comes to treat the CS as a signal or predictor of the US. This fundamental fact means that *neurophysiological plasticity cannot be used to validate that learning has occurred*. (As used here, 'plasticity' refers to any change in the activity of neurons, regardless of the method of recording, e.g., EEG, evoked potentials, unit discharges, metabolic activity. As generally understood, the minimum duration of change that is considered 'plasticity' is in the order of minutes, to distinguish it from purely sensory responses that may last seconds.)

This chapter concentrates on behaviorally validated cases of learning and memory rather than demonstrations of plasticity that are alleged to constitute 'learning' or 'memory'. Any specific instance of plasticity can, and should, be tested to determine if it could constitute an actual memory trace, that is, a substrate of information storage. This issue will be discussed later, when the *specificity* of plasticity is considered. For now, one should bear in mind that conflating neural plasticity with memory is empirically confusing and conceptually fallacious. While learning and

---

[1] This chapter relies to some extent on these previous reviews, particularly in summarizing particular experiments, there being a very limited number of ways to express the same findings.

memory, which are behavioral-level constructs, undoubtedly are caused by neural plasticity, equating the two constitutes a 'category error', i.e., attributing a property of the whole to one of its parts (Ryle, 1963).

Second, since learning is inferred, all causes of a change in behavior other than the formation of an association, must be ruled out. These include general changes in a subject's state of arousal or excitability (e.g., sensitization due to the presence of food or shock) and the possibility that the subject is 'timing' the next occurrence of the US and therefore not attending to the CS. Despite this 'bedrock' foundation of conditioning, fixed inter-trial intervals are still found in contemporary research (e.g., Suga and Ma, 2003). In classical conditioning a standard control for non-associative factors is to employ a second group that receives the CS and US unpaired or randomly, but with the same overall probability of occurrence as that used for the paired (conditioning) group. Another control for non-associative factors is afforded by discrimination training, which in classical conditioning consists of presenting a CS+ that is paired with a US and a CS– that is not followed by a US or any stimulus. Successful discrimination training demonstrates that an association has been formed between the CS+ and the US but not the CS– and the US. Such associative specificity cannot be explained by general factors such as sensitization.

Associative processes have a surprising richness. They include far more complex processes than simple conditioning, and they exhibit a remarkable ability to account for many 'higher cognitive processes' such as categorization and concept formation. There are many excellent and highly accessible accounts of associative learning (e.g., Mackintosh, 1974, 1983; Lieberman, 1990; Bouton, 2007).

18.2.1 Perceptual learning

One might expect that if any type of learning is characteristic of primary sensory cortices, it must be perceptual learning. Perceptual learning, as generally understood, is the increased ability to discriminate stimuli within a trained dimension, usually due to increasingly difficult discrimination training (Kellman, 2002). Perceptual learning usually requires extensive training, over days; for example, more than 4000 trials for frequency discrimination learning (Irvine *et al.*, 2000). The existence of perceptual learning is often erroneously thought to subsume the category of associative learning, so that all learning-induced plasticity in sensory systems is often incorrectly regarded as 'perceptual learning'. However, not all learning effects in A1 are 'perceptual' and associative learning is probably fundamental to perceptual learning.

The distinction becomes manifest by asking 'After an episode of *perceptual learning*, what is changed in the auditory cortex?' One answer is that the 'machinery' of A1 has been altered to enable greater acuity. However, in contrast to associative learning, perceptual learning does not seem to include '*perceptual memory*' in the same way that 'associative learning' is understood to produce '*associative memory*'. In perceptual learning, subjects apparently do not actually remember the specific details of their experiences during extensive discrimination training, that is, the particular stimuli or stimulus values given during certain of their multitude of trials. Thus, while perceptual learning *alters the gateway* to associative memory, *increased acuity* by itself is not necessary for memory, i.e., as the '*contents*' *of experience*. Of course, the level of acuity at any time can determine the *precision* with which auditory information is analyzed, and may then be encoded and stored.

A strong argument can be made that perceptual learning is actually a sub-class of associative learning because subjects first must learn an association between a sound stimulus and whatever comes next, which may be a different stimulus (classical conditioning) or a reward following a designated response (instrumental conditioning). Next, the discriminations simply become increasingly difficult. Because basic associative learning and its correlated cortical plasticity develop rapidly (e.g., in five trials; Edeline *et al.*, 1993), they may help elucidate mechanisms of subsequent perceptual learning. In summary, auditory learning and memory can develop rapidly, and can do so without an increase in perceptual acuity. Thus, the advantages that learning-induced plasticity in A1 confer may be mnemonic even if there is no accompanying perceptual learning.

18.2.2 Learning and plasticity in A1: 1956–1984

During the years 1956–1984, learning-induced plasticity in A1 was discovered, validated, and partially characterized. Virtually all assessments of the effects of learning were obtained from recordings taken during training trials. The importance of the distinction between recording *during* training trials vs recording *before* and *after* training trials will become evident later, when we consider contemporary research. Two learning phenomena were studied extensively: habituation and conditioning. We begin with the former.

Habituation

The literature on habituation during the first era of investigation yielded a singularly uniform finding. Repeated presentation of the same sound resulted in a reduction in the magnitude of evoked responses in A1, both for evoked potentials (hereafter 'local field potentials', LFPs) and neuronal discharges. Spontaneous recovery was observed after some minutes of silence. After decremental responses to a given sound had been established, presentation of a novel sound evoked normal responses. Continued presentation of the novel sound also resulted in response decrements (e.g., Marsh *et al.*, 1961).

These studies established the development of response plasticity in auditory cortex under the simplest possible circumstances, i.e., presentation of a single, isolated sound. This could indicate that the auditory cortex actively suppresses responses to sounds whose behavioral relevance or salience proves to be minimal. At the same time, it should be noted that the habituatory decrement is *selective* because responses are normal to novel sounds. Therefore, the auditory system appears to be continually evaluating current sounds with reference to prior experience, i.e., comparing the sound-of-the-moment with the *memory* of past sounds and the time period at which they occurred. Thus, although habituation appears to be a very basic and simple process, it does indicate the ongoing operation of cognition, i.e., the ongoing monitoring, comparison to memory, and decision whether to respond. In other words, habituation is based on *cognitive processes*.

Conditioning

Galambos and colleagues published the first Western study on learning and plasticity in A1. Cats received an auditory (click) conditioned stimulus paired with an immediately following puff of air to the face (unconditioned stimulus) (Galambos *et al.*, 1956). As a result of this classical conditioning procedure, CS-elicited LFPs in the auditory cortex increased in magnitude. A CS–US association was validated by development of behavioral conditioned responses. To eliminate inadvertent changes in CS level, the study was also conducted with subjects under neuromuscular blockade, thus preventing head and pinna movements and possible contractions of the middle ear muscles. Interestingly, the authors failed to include a non-associative control, such as a group that received the CS and US unpaired. However, subsequent investigations did include proper controls, confirming the associative nature of increased response magnitude of LFPs in A1 (e.g., Marsh *et al.*, 1961). LFP research was extended to different conditioning tasks and Pavlovian processes, with essentially the same findings of enhanced responses to sounds that became behaviorally important. Similar results were obtained for instrumental avoidance learning (reviewed in Weinberger and Diamond, 1987).

Subsequent studies of clusters of cells ('multiple-unit' activity) yielded similar results, i.e., increased discharges to an acoustic CS as animals formed conditioned responses (e.g., Buchwald *et al.*, 1966). In addition, both discrimination and discrimination reversal were obtained when the CS+ and CS– acoustic stimuli were interchanged after initial learning. Moreover, acoustic CS+ stimuli acquired the ability to elicit responses in the primary somatosensory cortex, which is the modality of the shock unconditioned stimulus (Oleson *et al.*, 1975).

Such 'cluster' recordings have the advantage over single unit recordings of yielding good data over many hours or days. They have the disadvantage of being unable to determine if single cells develop different directions of plasticity, i.e., either increased or decreased responses. That is, if associative processes produce both increased and decreased responses to the CS, but increased responses dominate, then the decreased responses would not be detected.

Study of single units in auditory cortex during learning also found plasticity. However, as suspected, despite the detection of many cells that developed increased responses to the CS, a substantial number of cells developed decreased responses, and yet others exhibited no change (e.g., Woody *et al.*, 1976). Similar heterogeneity of unit discharge plasticity was also found in auditory field A2 (Diamond and Weinberger, 1984). Such divergent results were not attributable to inadvertent changes in effective acoustic stimulus level in the auditory periphery, undetected movements or muscle contractions, or feedback from muscle spindles, because the same results were obtained when animals were trained while under neuromuscular blockade (Weinberger *et al.*, 1984b).

Although single unit plasticity was shown to be associative, the findings of opposite sign made little functional sense. Thus, while recordings in A1 during training trials had provided foundational information, this approach appeared to be yielding diminishing returns after almost 30 years of research.

18.2.3 Contemporary approaches: a synthesis of two disciplines

The contemporary era was initiated in the 1980s when a new question was posed. Instead of asking whether or not learning and memory *involved* the development of associative plasticity in A1, attention shifted to the issue of the *specificity* of such plasticity. 'Does learning cause a "re-tuning" of A1?'

This question not only altered the research agenda; it also necessitated the development of new experimental paradigms. While this 'paradigmatic shift' could take various forms, one factor was essential. It was now required that the new approach *combine the fields of auditory neurophysiology and learning/memory.*

Sounds (as all sensory stimuli) have 'two faces'. First, stimuli are described by their *physical parameters*. This is recognized universally. For example, a pure tone can be specified by its frequency, level, duration, etc. The physical parameters of sound can by-and-large be measured by off-the-shelf instruments, or their equivalent computer scripts. The complementary aspects of stimuli are their *psychological parameters*. This refers to the behavioral or psychological *meaning* of stimuli. The psychological parameters cannot be measured by standard engineering devices, but must be assessed through the careful analysis of behavior. Psychological parameters are not yet universally appreciated.

Auditory physiology (and other sensory physiologies) systematically varies the physical parameters of designated stimuli and records evoked neurophysiological responses. At the same time, it endeavors to hold constant the psychological parameters. This is often achieved by maintaining the subjects under general anesthesia. Of course, the latter maneuver was not devised for the purpose of preventing learning from occurring during the search for sensory codes, but this it nonetheless accomplished. In a complementary manner, experiments in learning concern the relationships between the acquired behavioral significance of stimuli and subsequent behavior. To accomplish this goal, it is necessary that the physical parameters of the stimuli be kept constant.

For both disciplines, simultaneous variation of both physical and psychological parameters would greatly complicate interpretation of the results. In this regard, the behavioral scientist has an easier time of it, because it is easy to *not change* the stimuli employed. For the sensory physiologist, there are potential problems when studying the unanesthetized subject. Waking animals and people have the opportunity to learn, including remembering the sounds that they are receiving and anticipating future sounds. In fact, learning cannot be prevented in awake animals or people, although some investigators may fail to appreciate this fact.

Limitations of relying on auditory cortical plasticity obtained during training trials

As noted previously, foundational studies on learning and the auditory cortex involved recording responses to the CS in simple conditioning experiments, or to the CS+ and CS– in acoustic discrimination studies. Naturally, this entailed obtaining cortical data during training trials. However, obtaining recordings during training trials has at least two major limitations: (1) they can be influenced by state factors; (2) they do not permit assessment of the degree of specificity of plasticity.

State factors Learning theorists have long recognized that there are two types of factors in any learning situation: (1) those involved in learning processes themselves and (2) non-learning factors that affect the process of learning, the behavioral expression of learning, or both. The latter are often referred to as 'performance' factors.

Non-learning factors are invariably present during training. They include, but are not limited to, changes in arousal level, selective attention, and motivational state. It is known that arousal level can alter sound-elicited responses in the auditory cortex (Teas and Kiang, 1964). Moreover, their effect can change during the course of training. Arousal may be high early in training, when subjects have not yet solved the problem (i.e., learned how to successfully perform the task at hand), but lower after they have done so and their performance improves.

It must be emphasized that cortical plasticity obtained during training trials is associative, given controls for sensitization, etc. That non-learning factors are operative in no way weakens the case for associativity. However, performance factors can modify the *expression* of associative plasticity, such that it may be difficult to obtain 'pure' associative effects. Rescorla has emphasized the dangers of relying on behavioral data obtained *during training trials* to infer the strength of learning and those aspects of an experience that enter into memory. These attributes are best determined by appropriate *post-training* assessments of behavior (Rescorla, 1988a). This counsel is equally applicable to neurophysiological plasticity that develops during training. One cannot assume that the neurophysiological plasticity observed in response to signal acoustic stimuli *during* training actually represents *exclusively* the product of learning.

Specificity of plasticity A second problem with relying on neurophysiological data obtained during training trials is that it cannot yield adequate information about the *specificity* of plasticity. Unlike the problem of state factors, which can be controlled by online monitoring of arousal level and other procedures, the limitation on specificity is endemic to the nature of the learning situation because the number of different stimulus values used in training is too small to permit determination of the specificity of plasticity. For example, in a two-tone discrimination study, increased responses to the CS+ and decreased responses to the CS– yield neurophysiological discriminative plasticity. However, this is insufficient to determine if frequency tuning has actually shifted, e.g., toward the frequency of the CS. To determine the overall degree of specificity of plasticity, it is necessary to present *many* stimuli, so that the frequency receptive field can be determined.

It might be thought that the problem could be solved by presenting several tones during training, only one of which is the CS+. However, all of the other tones would constitute CS– stimuli, so that the actual training would be that of a very complex discrimination. There would be no assessment of plasticity independent of discrimination learning. Moreover, one could not determine if single tone learning (or other acoustic stimulus parameters) modified the functional organization of the cortex.

Another tactic might be to present an extensive set of acoustic stimuli during training. In standard auditory neurophysiology studies, a matrix of different frequencies and stimulus levels is presented (with individual combinations given in random order) to obtain a 'frequency response area' (FRA). Such data yield not only tuning information (both for characteristic frequency (CF) at threshold and best frequency (BF) for each supra-threshold level), but also the absolute threshold itself (sound pressure level in decibels (dB SPL)), bandwidth (Q10 or octaves at 10–40 dB above threshold), and rate-level functions (monotonic or non-monotonic). Such comprehensive information would greatly increase the understanding of auditory cortical plasticity. However, these FRA stimuli would have to be presented in addition to the training stimuli themselves (e.g., CS in one-tone training, CS+ and CS– in two-tone discrimination training). To be *neutral*, FRA stimuli could not be followed by reinforcement, because they would *predict* reward or punishment and thus would constitute another CS+ that would require its own independent assessment, *ad infinitum*. On the other hand, the lack of reinforcement of FRA stimuli would render them CS– discriminative stimuli, i.e., sounds that signal the *absence* of reinforcement; that would constitute another type of learning which would have to be independently assessed, also *ad infinitum*. Therefore, interweaving FRA stimuli *during* training trials could not provide sufficiently independent assays of the specificity of developing plasticity. Complex sounds (e.g., ripple combinations) can be used to probe changes in response to pure tones *during attention performance following previous extensive learning* (e.g., Fritz *et al.*, 2003). However, they serve the animal *merely as a cue for a forthcoming detection trial*. Thus their use to study attention in the absence of learning does not violate the strictures explained in this section.

However, FRA assays or simply iso-level frequency receptive fields could be obtained *before* and *after* training trials. This brings us to the new experimental designs, which inaugurated the contemporary era.

18.2.4 Contemporary approaches: new paradigms and new controls

Two laboratories independently sought specificity simultaneously, although with complementary rather than similar experimental designs. They both first published their results in the same year, 1984. Henning Scheich's laboratory attacked the problem by the use of a metabolic technique, 2-deoxyglucose (2-DG) (Gonzalez-Lima and Scheich, 1984, 1986). Another laboratory studied the plasticity of frequency receptive fields (Diamond and Weinberger, 1986; Weinberger *et al.*, 1984a).

The metabolic approach relies on knowledge of the locus of representation of particular frequencies in the tonotopic map of A1. Typically, animals undergo fear conditioning, in which a CS sound is paired with an aversive US. *After* the completion of training, they are then exposed for several minutes to the CS before being sacrificed and processed for the detection of increased metabolic response in the auditory cortex. Increased metabolic activity in the cortical zone representing the CS frequency demonstrates associative CS-specific representational plasticity in A1.

The receptive field approach involves obtaining tuning curves of neurons in A1 *before* and *after* a learning experience. The training may be the same as used in metabolic studies, e.g., fear conditioning to a tone. However, the assessment approach is different. In receptive field (RF) studies, the RF obtained before training is subtracted from the receptive field obtained after training; the *difference* reflects the effects of conditioning, or some control treatment. Tuning shifts directed toward or to the CS frequency are indicative of associative CS-specific representational plasticity.

Both approaches are equally valid and interestingly use complementary experimental designs. The metabolic approach requires a 'between groups' design because the 2-DG technique can be performed only once on a subject. Thus, a paired group needs to be compared with an unpaired group to validate associative plasticity. The receptive field approach can use a 'within subjects' design because RFs can be obtained multiple times, before, immediately after learning, and at various later tests for retention. This permits within-subject tracking of the 'evolution' ('consolidation') of plasticity (see below). If a two-tone discrimination protocol is used, then differential effects for the CS+ and CS– obviate the need for a non-associative control group.

Finally, both approaches ameliorate or solve the 'state' problem. The metabolic line-of-attack reduces arousal, attention, motivational factors, and the like by presenting the CS frequency *outside* of the training situation, specifically *after* training has been completed. Thus, the absence of a motivational US, such as shock, should reduce general changes in arousal level, while attention to the CS should be consistent as training has been concluded. The receptive field methodology also obtains tuning data outside of the training situation. However, the situation is a bit more complicated because of the desire to avoid behavioral responses to the CS frequency when it is given as part of the stimulus set used to obtain RFs. Additionally, it is important to preclude *experimental extinction* during post-training of determination of receptive fields. This can occur if the subject regards presentations of the CS frequency (one of many tones in the RF stimulus set) as the original CS, and therefore learns that it no longer predicts the US. (The metabolic approach of prolonged post-training presentation of the CS does run the risk of some experimental extinction.)

The solution to these problems for RF (and similar) studies concerns *context*. This issue is both of considerable importance and often poorly understood. Given these considerations, and the need to understand the context before reviewing the literature, we need to consider it in some detail.

The importance of context: reduction or elimination of state factors and experimental extinction

How can state factors and experimental extinction be reduced or eliminated by obtaining receptive fields before and after training? The solution is to markedly *change the context of the training period from the context of the pre- and post-training assessments of receptive fields.* (The term 'receptive field' is a proxy for other measures of auditory neuronal response that may exhibit plasticity after learning, e.g., threshold, level, bandwidth.) If the contexts are sufficiently different, then subjects *do not* treat the same tonal frequency as the CS when it is presented *outside* of the training period.

Several changes in context are possible. While any one will be effective, together they provide exceptional control of state factors and prevent experimental extinction. The first difference in context is the *absence of a reinforcer* (food or shock), which also reduces and can even eliminate changes in state (see below). The second is a marked difference in the *acoustic environment*. Thus, training involves a CS tone presented in a discrete conditioning trial with standard parameters, e.g., a duration of 1–5 s, a long intertrial interval of 1–3 min, and a stimulus level that is well above threshold (60–80 dB SPL). In contrast, determination of receptive fields involves completely different parameters using many tones to cover the frequency spectrum, e.g., 24 tones at quarter-octave intervals, 100-ms duration, intertone intervals of 400 ms at stimulus levels of 0–80 dB SPL to cover the audible range. Also, these test tones can be repeated in a random sequence to obtain statistically reliable receptive fields. In short, the *acoustic context* of RF determination can be, and indeed must be, extremely different from that during conditioning trials. Third, one can conduct training and RF testing in completely different laboratory rooms under different conditions of general illumination (e.g., train in the light, obtain RFs in the dark).

State factors are reduced, if not eliminated, by minimizing similarities between the training context and the testing circumstances. The purpose of this maneuver is to oppose generalization from the training environment to the testing environment. For example, if an animal receives food or shock during training, it will also associate the location of the training with these reinforcers. If tested in the same place, its arousal level and expectations could be the same as those during training. Then, given the absence of the reinforcer, experimental extinction (i.e., loss of response to the CS frequency) would develop. However, testing in a different place prevents generalization based on location ('place'). Moreover, extinction is circumvented if the subjects do not respond to the CS frequency during RF determination, when it is presented as one of a large number of brief tone bursts.

These *differences in context* have proven to be sufficient to eliminate any behavioral or arousal response to the CS frequency when it is embedded as a brief tone in a series of test tones. Objective behavioral measures (e.g., pupillary size) indicate that subjects *do not regard* the CS frequency as a conditioned stimulus during determination of receptive fields. Moreover, because this frequency is not considered to be the CS, there is no experimental extinction (Diamond and Weinberger, 1989).

While the contexts between the periods of training and assessment of RFs must be *different*, so that the CS frequency is not regarded as a signal for reinforcement during the latter, the contexts during *pre-training* and *post-training* RF recordings must be the *same*. The rationale for this requirement is that subtraction of the pre-training from post-training RF data can reveal the effects of the intervening training only if there are no other differences between these two periods. The same states can be achieved by adapting subjects to the RF determination environment and also by recording the EEG, heart rate, or other physiological indices of state. It is also feasible to eliminate any possibility of arousal confounds by training subjects while they are awake (of course), but obtaining receptive fields while they are under general anesthesia. CS-specific plasticity is expressed with subjects under general anesthesia (Lennartz and Weinberger, 1992b; Weinberger *et al.*, 1993).

18.2.5 Contemporary approaches: specificity of associative plasticity

Habituation

Habituation is generally not considered an associative phenomenon, but at least one theory predicted it to be context-dependent, i.e., the repeated stimulus is associated with the environment within which it occurs (Wagner, 1981). Some authors dispute the context-dependence of habituation (e.g., Marlin and Miller, 1981), yet there is clear positive evidence. Apparently, some response systems exhibit context-dependent habituation while others fail to do so (e.g., Jordan *et al.*, 2000). Regardless of whether or not some or all cases of habituation have an associative component, the specificity of habituatory decrements of auditory cortical responses has received little attention.

Metabolic studies of acoustic habituation have used noise stimuli. Thus, they cannot provide evidence for putative frequency-specific reductions in auditory cortical 2-DG uptake at known loci within the tonotopic map (Gonzalez-Lima *et al.*, 1989a,b). Habituation to acoustic stimuli can develop when a sound is given repeatedly in a random or pseudorandom relationship to an unconditioned stimulus, e.g., shock. Under such circumstances, response decrements to noise have been observed in primary (TE1) and other auditory cortical fields (TE2, TE3) during decrements in behavioral responses to the noise. Interestingly, Poremba *et al.*'s study (1998) did find decrements in 2-DG uptake in the brainstem reticular arousal system, which is consistent with a state confound, i.e., a decrement in arousal during acoustic habituation.

The specificity of habituation with a 'built-in' control to preclude state confounds was first achieved during the early period of studies (Westenberg and Weinberger, 1976; Westenberg *et al.*, 1976). Although LFPs rather than unit discharges were used, this study was the first to use the basic design of determining auditory responses before and after a learning treatment. These findings were the first to demonstrate that repeated acoustic stimulation produces frequency-specific habituation in the auditory system.

There has been one study of auditory cortical habituation using receptive field analysis (Condon and Weinberger, 1991). After determining the tuning of unit clusters, and ensuring their stability, animals received single tone pips at the rate of 1.25 Hz for 5–7 min. The repetition of tones produced a decreased response that was *specific* to the frequency that had been repeatedly presented; frequencies 0.125 octaves from the habituated frequency exhibited no response decrement, showing a very high degree of specificity (Fig. 18.1). Consolidation, in the form of continued development of increasingly specific decrements, was often observed, for periods as long as an hour. The extreme degree of specificity is noteworthy and reveals that A1 tracks prior sounds with a great deal of precision, even in the absence of any biologically significant events.

Conditioning: initial studies and controls for reactive state confounds

As noted above, initial studies involved metabolic correlates of classical and instrumental conditioning (e.g., Gonzalez-Lima and Scheich, 1984, 1986). Analysis of patterns of 2-DG uptake in A1 revealed a CS-specific increase in metabolic activity for the cortical area that represented the CS frequency. The absence of similar effects in several control groups showed that the CS-specific plasticity was associative.

Receptive field analysis was first applied to behaviorally validated classical fear conditioning (tone–shock pairing) in the cat. Single unit discharges were recorded in two non-primary auditory fields, 'secondary' (A2), and ventral ectosylvian (VE) cortices (Diamond and Weinberger, 1986, 1989). CS-specific plasticity was found in a paired group, but not when tone and shock were unpaired. Extinction (additional CS presentation without the shock US) produced loss of the RF

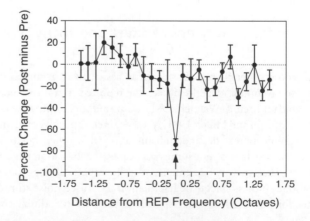

Fig. 18.1 The effects of habituation on frequency receptive fields in the primary auditory cortex of the guinea pig. Data are normalized to octave distance from the repeated frequency. Habituation produces frequency-specific decreased response. (From Condon and Weinberger, 1991.)

plasticity. The findings received little notice, probably because these 'non-primary' auditory fields were not well understood compared to A1.

Similar studies were then undertaken in A1 of the guinea pig with behavioral validation of associative learning, e.g., conditioned bradycardia. Following determination of frequency receptive fields ('frequency tuning'), a frequency other than the 'best frequency' (BF) was chosen as the CS to determine whether conditioning caused shifts of tuning toward the CS frequency. Animals then received 30–45 trials of tone paired with shock. A comparison of post-training with pre-training RFs revealed a dominance of CS-specific increased responses. Moreover, responses to the pre-training best frequency and other frequencies tended to decrease. These opposing changes were often sufficiently large to shift tuning toward, and even to, the frequency of the CS, which could become the new best frequency (Bakin and Weinberger, 1990; Fig. 18.2). RF plasticity is *associative*, as it requires stimulus pairing; sensitization training (no pairing) produces only a general increase in response to all frequencies across the RF (Bakin and Weinberger, 1990; Bakin *et al.*, 1992).

The independent and simultaneous discovery of CS-specific associative plasticity in A1 in metabolic and receptive field studies suggested that A1 might acquire and store specific information, that is, be a site of auditory memories. Mnemonic functions are in reality not easy to assign to neural tissue. Neural correlates of learning and memory might arise from many other sources. For example, animals might move closer to an acoustic source that provides sounds that are becoming behaviorally more important. Also, subjects are likely to pay greater attention to sounds that have become more interesting. Subjects may get more excited or aroused when meaningful sounds are likely to occur.

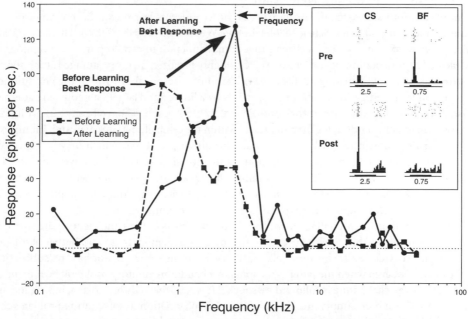

Fig. 18.2 Classical conditioning produces CS-specific facilitation and CS-directed tuning shifts. Shown is an example of a complete shift of frequency tuning of a single cell in A1 of the guinea pig, from a pre-training best frequency (BF) of 0.75 kHz to the CS frequency of 2.5 kHz after 30 trials of conditioning. *Inset* shows pre- and post-training post-stimulus time histograms (PSTHs) for the pre-training BF and the CS frequencies. (From Weinberger, 1997.)

We have already considered how the change in context between the training and testing parts of an experiment can prevent behavioral responses to a CS frequency when it is presented during RF determination. However, one can argue that contextual control must be verified rather than assumed. Furthermore, it is the case that except for the very first RF study (Diamond and Weinberger, 1986, 1989), such direct behavioral assessments have not been used. Yet, there is another line of defense against non-mnemonic confounds.

First, it is a simple matter to maintain acoustic control by keeping constant the relationship between the speaker and the external auditory meatus, e.g., by head-fixation, appropriate construction of the sound field, or earphones. More subtle are the controls for arousal and attention, because they are actually endemic to obtaining frequency receptive fields. This is because many different frequencies are given rapidly (e.g., 2/s) and repeatedly (often in a pseudo-random order) to generate enough responses across the frequency spectrum to enable the construction of frequency tuning curves. Arousal levels cannot increase and decrease sufficiently rapidly to 'track' the presentation of different tones. Attention might be paid to the CS frequency during RF determination, but attention would be invoked only after the tone had been processed and identified, far too late for attention to affect discharges that occur in the order of 10–50 ms after CS onset.

18.2.6 Does the primary auditory cortex 'hold' memory traces?

A specific memory trace (SMT) is an enduring neural record of a particular aspect of experience. How might one determine whether the development of specific RF plasticity does index actual memory traces? One might expect that destruction of A1 should remove its memory traces, which would in turn be revealed by behavioral tests showing a specific loss of auditory memories. This apparently simple and decisive test is neither.

Many authors assume that unless destruction of A1 prevents learning, it cannot hold specific memory traces (e.g., Ohl and Scheich, 2004; but see Weinberger, 2004b, 2007b). This assumption reflects a view of memory as a localized process, in distinction to contemporary conceptions of distributed representation of stored experience. Highly localized memory storage is typical only of stimulus–response learning of discrete skeletal motor responses in which the conditioned response under investigation can be produced only by a limited and largely stereotyped pattern of muscle actions. While studies of the conditioned eyeblink response have been extraordinarily successful in locating underlying memory traces within the cerebellum (Christian and Thompson, 2005), learning more often involves stimulus–stimulus associations, which may be expressed either at the time of learning or at a propitious future occasion, or both. Moreover, the same bit of knowledge may be communicated in innumerable ways. It matters not whether the typing of this sentence was produced by the action of one or many fingers, the skillful use of my nose, or by dictation via the stenographic talents of an extremely gifted monkey.

Further, distributed representation does not imply that parts of the same memory are stored in different locations, so that A1 is restricted to storing only a memory fragment. Rather, it is likely that the auditory cortex forms more elaborate SMTs of the same memory as the subcortical auditory system, even when the latter can completely handle an auditory problem, be it memory of a tone or even that a tone is followed by shock. However, the auditory cortex, having formed 'parallel' SMTs for even simple situations, can use this information to solve future problems that cannot be handled subcortically. It can do so because the auditory cortex has access to a *much greater range of information* than the subcortical auditory system. For example, while simple auditory conditioning does not require an intact A1 (e.g., DiCara *et al.*, 1970), as soon as two-tone discrimination is demanded, A1 is required (Teich *et al.*, 1988). An intact A1 is also obligatory to achieve experimental extinction (Teich *et al.*, 1989).

Therefore, the failure of a lesion of A1 to destroy some behavioral indication of learning cannot refute the manifold evidence that A1 forms and holds memory traces. The standard 'lesion logic' has legitimacy only for cases in which the entire substrate of a memory is localized to the destroyed brain matter. Such localization has not been demonstrated for any auditory memory.

Finally, as A1 is involved in both perceptual and learning processes, any lesion-induced behavioral impairments cannot be attributed simply to the destruction of memory. They could also reflect a perceptual deficit that is linked to acquired auditory information. The difficulty of interpreting lesions of the auditory cortex as disrupting either perceptual or mnemonic processes is underscored by the fact that the responses of a given individual neuron in A1 reflect both the physical acoustic stimulus and its acquired behavioral importance. Individual discharges of such cells cannot be attributed exclusively to either cause.

If not lesions, then what might be done? One approach is to attempt to defeat the proposal that memory traces form in A1. As A1 does form associative plasticity (see above), what line of attack might be taken? It could be argued that in addition to such plasticity, SMTs should possess the major characteristics of behavioral associative memory itself. This would impose a second level of criteria that have not previously been demanded of any neurophysiological studies of learning and memory. Nonetheless, this is not an unreasonable demand.

What are these characteristics? In addition to being associative, SMTs should also exhibit *specificity, fairly rapid formation, long-term retention,* and even *consolidation,* i.e., continued strengthening over time after training in the absence of additional reinforcement. Another feature of memory is that it can be formed in a wide variety of learning tasks, rather than being confined to, for example, classical conditioning. A further key feature of memory is that it transcends a particular type of motivation, but develops in both appetitive and aversive situations. Additionally, one would expect SMTs to be manifest for whatever the type of CS or signal stimuli used in training, as is the case for genuine associative memory. That is, SMTs should not be limited to plasticity of frequency representation, but should develop for any acoustic parameter that can serve as a signal for reward or punishment. Finally, as in the case of memory, SMTs should be biologically conserved, that is, they should develop across diverse taxa.

The findings from several laboratories support the conclusion that SMTs develop in A1. Moreover, as this is an active area of inquiry, new acoustic parameters are continually being studied. Although this chapter can never be up-to-date, at least one prediction can be made: 'If an acoustic parameter can serve as a signal or gain behavioral relevance through learning, then its processing in A1 (and perhaps other auditory cortical fields) will develop specific representational plasticity'.

Specificity of frequency plasticity

Let us first consider frequency tuning and representation, because it is has been studied most extensively. We have already noted that RF shifts are directed toward and to the CS frequency and that these are associative. Additionally, RF plasticity is *highly specific*; the maximum increase in response is at the CS frequency, while neighboring frequencies show no change or decreased response. Specificity is also evident in two-tone discrimination learning, in which a reinforced CS+ develops increased responses whereas a non-reinforced CS− has diminished responses (Fig. 18.3). Second, RF plasticity *develops very rapidly*, in as few as five training trials, as rapidly as the first behavioral (e.g., cardiac) signs of association (Edeline *et al.*, 1993; Fig. 18.4). Third, RF plasticity shows *long term retention*, enduring for the longest periods tested, up to 8 weeks after a single 30-trial conditioning session (Weinberger *et al.*, 1993). Fourth, RF plasticity *consolidates*, i.e., continues to develop increased responses to the frequency of the CS vs decreased responses to other frequencies in the absence of further training over hours (Edeline and Weinberger, 1993;

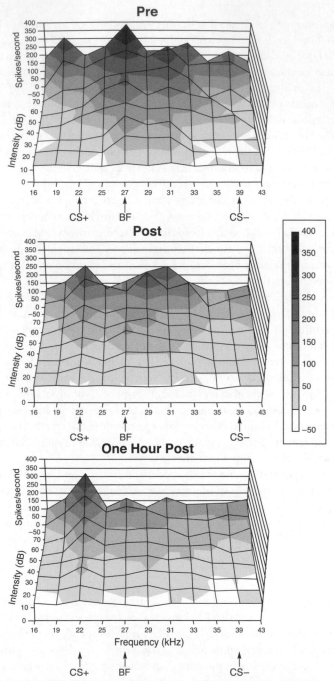

Fig. 18.3 Two-tone discrimination. Representation of neuronal responses in A1 before, immediately after, and 1 hour after two-tone discrimination training (30 each of CS+ (22.0 kHz) and CS– (39 kHz) intermixed trials). Displayed are rates of discharge (*Y-axis*) as a function of tonal frequency (*X-axis*) and level of testing stimuli (10–70 dB). Note that conditioning changed the 'topography' of neuronal response. The pre-training best frequency of 27.0 kHz suffered a reduction in response, as did the CS– frequency. In contrast, responses to the CS+ frequency increased. Note consolidation, in the form of a continued development of these changes; after 1 hour of silence, the only excitatory response is at the CS+ frequency. (From Edeline and Weinberger, 1993.)

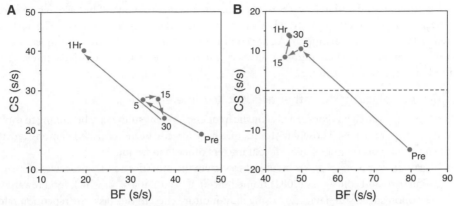

Fig. 18.4 Rapid induction of RF plasticity, shown as vector diagrams of changes in response to the pre-training best frequency (BF) and the CS frequency for two cases. **A** After five trials, responses to the BF had decreased while those to the CS increased. Changes were maintained after 15 and 30 trials, but further change developed after 1 hour (consolidation), at which time the CS frequency became the new BF. **B** Sign change in which the CS frequency was inhibitory pre-training but became excitatory after only five training trials; the initial response to the CS was too weak for it to become the new BF or exhibit consolidation in 1 hour. *X-axes*, rate of discharge for responses to pre-training BF; *Y-axes*, rate of discharge to the CS frequency. (From Edeline *et al.*, 1993.)

Weinberger *et al.*, 1993; Galván and Weinberger, 2002) and days (Weinberger *et al.*, 1993; Galván and Weinberger, 2002). 'Spontaneous' tuning shifts cannot account for the results because they are directed *toward* the CS frequency, whereas spontaneous changes would not favor the CS. Moreover, long-term tracking of tuning for 14–21 days showed that tuning does not drift over weeks; neither do thresholds nor bandwidths (Galván *et al.*, 2001; Galván and Weinberger, 2002).

RF plasticity also has other key features of memory. It develops in all tasks tested to date: in simple instrumental avoidance conditioning (Bakin *et al.*, 1996) as well as in simple classical conditioning (see above) and also in two-tone instrumental avoidance conditioning (Bakin *et al.*, 1996), as well as two-tone classical discrimination training (Edeline *et al.*, 1990a, b; Edeline and Weinberger, 1993), and in single tone appetitive classical conditioning in which the US was rewarding electrical stimulation of the ventral tegmental area (Kisley and Gerstein, 2001).

CS-specific associative tuning shifts develop in A1 of all species studied to date. First reported in the guinea pig (*Cavia porcellus*) (Bakin and Weinberger, 1990), it is also found in the echolocating big brown bat (*Eptesicus fuscus*) (Gao and Suga, 1998), the cat (*Felis catus*) (Diamond and Weinberger, 1986), and the rat (*Rattus rattus*) (Kisley and Gerstein, 2001). Additionally CS-specific expanded representations in the tonotopic map of A1, which are predicted from CS-directed RF shifts, have been found during perceptual learning in the owl monkey (*Aotus trivirgatus boliviensis*) (Recanzone *et al.*, 1993) and during instrumental bar-pressing for water reward in the rat (Rutkowski and Weinberger, 2005).

Learning-induced tuning plasticity is not limited to animals. The same paradigm of classical conditioning (tone paired with a mildly noxious stimulus) produces concordant CS-specific associative changes in A1 of humans (*Homo sapiens*) (Molchan *et al.*, 1994; Schreurs *et al.*, 1997; Morris *et al.*, 1998).

In summary, learning-induced CS-specific shifts of frequency tuning in A1 are not an artifact of spontaneous changes in tuning. Neither are they an artifact of state. We have reviewed above both empirical findings and design features of the experiments that rule out all but associative effects. This specific RF plasticity also meets all other criteria to constitute memory traces. The next issue is whether the effects of learning on A1 are confined to the domain of acoustic frequency or are general to whatever acoustic parameter serves as a signal for positive or negative reinforcement, i.e., food or a nociceptive stimulus.

Specificity of plasticity for other acoustic parameters

Although most research has concerned acoustic frequency, recent studies are beginning to explore other acoustic parameters. Those few studies that have already been published demonstrate that learning alters the processing of acoustic parameters other than frequency.

The *repetition rate of noise pulses* is subject to systematic modification by processes of associative learning. Bao and colleagues (2004) trained rats in a 'sound maze' in which food reward was contingent upon successful navigation using only auditory cues. In this task, the repetition rate of noise pulses increased as the distance between the rat and target location decreased. After subjects had learned this 'maze', the responses of neurons in A1 were investigated in a terminal session. A1 cells exhibited enhanced responses to high-rate noise pulses and stronger phase-locking of responses to the stimuli. The effects were due to learning because controls that had received identical sound stimulation, but were given free access to food, failed to exhibit such plasticity of temporal processing, and in fact were not different from naïve subjects. Thus, learning produced a shift in tuning to high repetition rates, i.e., the stimulus features that were most closely associated with procurement of food.

Similarly, owl monkeys trained to detect an increase in the *envelope frequency* of a sinusoidally modulated 1-kHz tone developed increased sensitivity to small changes in envelope frequency (Beitel *et al.*, 2003). The processing of *sound level* is also modified by learning (Polley *et al.*, 2004).

18.2.7 Summary: specific memory traces in A1

While the *fact* of associative CS-specific plasticity in A1 is now firmly established, some workers would consider this finding alone to be insufficient to conclude that A1 holds *specific memory traces*. Rather, they may require that plasticity should also satisfy several other criteria. It should (1) exhibit the major *attributes of memory* and show *generality* across (2) *tasks*, (3) *motivational valence*, (4) *acoustic stimulus parameters*, and (5) *species*.

The associative plasticity of frequency receptive fields *satisfies all of these criteria*. It does have the main attributes of associative memory: in addition to *associativity*, it is *highly specific, discriminative, rapidly acquired, develops consolidation* over hours and days, and exhibits *long-term retention* (over weeks). Moreover, this plasticity develops in *all tasks studied*, including habituation, both simple and discriminative classical and instrumental conditioning, and perceptual learning. Furthermore, RF tuning shifts exhibit *generality across both positive and negative motivational* circumstances. Also, specific plasticity develops for the several *acoustic stimulus parameters* tested to date. Finally, it shows *species generality* including *Homo sapiens*. In summary, the conclusion that *specific memory traces* form and are retained in A1 is extremely well justified.

Having 'survived' this 'gauntlet of criteria', one may ask what other structures in the brain have 'passed' the same level of scrutiny. Remarkably, it seems that *none except A1 has been evaluated to this extent*. The irony seems palpable. Neuroscience, having traditionally *excluded* primary sensory cortices from both conceptual and empirical legitimacy as loci of memory storage, now finds that A1 is apparently that part of the cerebral cortex for which the *storage of specific information is most extensively documented*.

18.2.8 **Working and reference memory**

Although research has concentrated on acquisition processes, various forms of memory also have been studied. Sakurai's laboratory has documented neural correlates of *working memory*, and also *reference memory* in A1 (Sakurai, 1990, 1992).

Working memory (WM) was studied when subjects had to remember whether the current tone was the same or different from the immediately preceding tone (i.e., immediate memory). Reference memory (RM) was studied when the subjects had to remember that a low tone required one type of behavioral response while the high tone required another type of response (i.e., long-term memory stores). Continual switching between the two tasks (demanding the two different types of memory) was not cued externally; subjects detected the switch in tasks by making errors after they had mastered each. About 20% of single units in A1 (and the medial geniculate) developed sustained differential activity during the delay period after exposure to the sample tone, leading the authors to conclude that the thalamocortical auditory system retains auditory information in working memory. Unit recordings also were obtained from the hippocampus (CA1, CA3, dentate gyrus). Cells in the hippocampal formation exhibited changes in firing related to *either* WM or RM but *not both*. In contrast, neurons in A1 could exhibit increased activity for *both* the WM and RM tasks, indicating the flexible involvement in memory of A1 (Sakurai, 1994). Further research, using cross correlations between pairs of neurons to detect 'cell assemblies', revealed that most correlated pairs in the hippocampal formation occurred during WM whereas correlated cells in A1 could participate equally in WM and RM (Sakurai, 1998). Thus, despite the accepted view that the hippocampus has mnemonic functions whereas A1 does not, in fact neurons in A1 exhibit more comprehensive involvement in auditory memory than do cells in the hippocampus.

18.3 **Auditory imagery**

If A1 networks are involved in memory storage and retrieval, then they should reveal themselves in the absence of relevant acoustic stimulation. That is, neural activation should occur when prior experiences of sound are recalled. Although probably less widely accepted than some other approaches, studies of imagery in humans support such involvement. Bearing in mind caveats concerning precise localization and the need to validate the presumptive imagery behaviorally, there is evidence for the involvement of A1 in musical imagery. For example, imagery for musical timbre activates A1 with some right side asymmetry, which is also the case for timbre perception (Halpern *et al.*, 2004).

18.4 **Auditory attention**

Attention has long been known to modulate the auditory cortex in humans (e.g., Alho, 1992). However, until recently, studies of attention had not been able to demonstrate the specificity of attentional modulation of A1. Fritz and colleagues (2003) devised a very clever and sensitive method of obtaining spectro-temporal receptive fields (STRFs) (see Chapter 5) 'on-line' while ferrets waited to detect a previously learned tone in order to avoid shock. They found that attention modulates A1 by facilitating responses to the target frequency while suppressing responses to other frequencies (Fig. 18.5). When trained in both simple frequency detection and frequency discrimination tasks, responses to the reinforced and target frequencies were enhanced, as might be expected. However, because the target during tone detection could be the non-reinforced (CS−) frequency during discrimination, the authors were able to show that responses to the

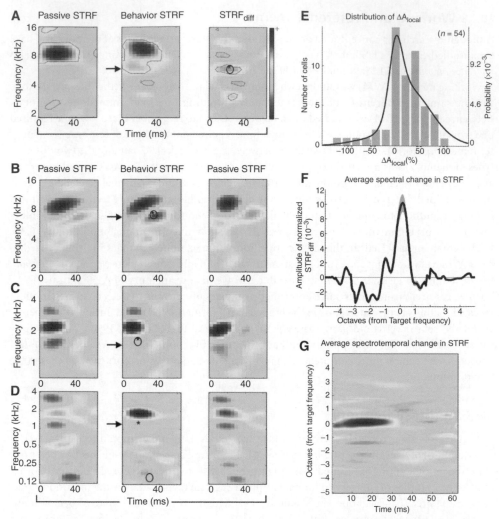

Fig. 18.5 Selective attention for a target tone involves specific modifications of spectro-temporal receptive fields (STRFs). Data from four single units in A1 show typical changes observed during performance of the detection task. **a** Comparison of a pre-behavior passive STRF (*left*) and a behavioral STRF (*middle*). *Color scale* represents increased (*red*) to suppressed (*blue*) firing about the mean firing rate (*green*). *Black arrow*, frequency of the target tone during the detection task. *Right*, the difference between the normalized passive and behavior STRF. An *asterisk* marks the location of maximal local change and a *circle* marks the global change. The local and global maximal changes were both at the target frequency in this case, as in about half of all cells. **b** Localized enhancement of an excitatory region in the STRF during behavior (*left* and *middle*). The post-behavior passive STRF (*right*) reverted immediately to its original shape. **c** Local decrease or elimination of inhibitory sidebands in the behavior STRF. **d** A global weakening of inhibitory fields during behavior. Immediately following behavior, the STRF recovered its pre-behavior shape. **e** Summary histogram and smoothed distribution of local STRF changes from all STRFs. The histogram (*left ordinate*) and distribution (*right ordinate*) are significantly skewed toward positive changes. **f** Average spectral change in the STRF at all frequencies relative to the target frequency. There was facilitation for about one octave around the target and asymmetric suppressive sidebands outside of this range. **g** Average spectrotemporal changes in the STRF derived from all units. The facilitative and suppressive changes near the target frequency, as well as the relatively rapid onset of these STRF changes, can be seen here. (From Fritz *et al.*, 2003.)

same physical stimulus could be facilitated or suppressed depending on the task (Fritz *et al.*, 2005b). In a third study, ferrets learned both tone detection and gap detection tasks. As expected, tone detection had the same target-specific enhancement. Additionally, during gap detection the STRF was changed along the temporal dimension; specifically, the temporal dynamics of discharge were sharpened (Fritz *et al.*, 2005a). In all of the studies, the effects could last for hours in some cases, suggesting an involvement in memory as well as in selective attention. Overall, the findings demonstrate that attention has a strong influence on A1. At least some of these influences are undoubtedly due to 'top-down' processes because switching tasks, and therefore the significance of a particular frequency, differentially affect responses to the same physical stimulus (see also Polley *et al.*, 2006).

18.5 Expectancy

Experiments on expectancy also demonstrate the involvement of A1 in cognitive processes. Subjects previously trained on a task form 'expectancies' that are based on the probability that a certain stimulus or event is likely to occur. In one such case, rats were trained in a visual reaction time task with a very brief (10-ms) warning tone, 1.4 s preceding the light stimulus. A subset of single neurons in A1 developed a significant sustained increase in discharge rate during the warning period which did not occur when the same warning stimulus was given by itself. The authors suggest that this activity constitutes a substrate of preparatory set (Shinba *et al.*, 1995). A phasic increase in arousal might have been responsible for increased cellular activity as preparatory set and expectancy often involve increased arousal. Direct measures of arousal level and recordings taken in arousing situations outside of the task would help resolve this issue.

A more elaborate study by Villa and co-workers provides compelling evidence for an expectancy function in A1 (Villa *et al.*, 1998). They obtained simultaneous single unit spike trains while rats performed a complex cognitive task, specifically a two-choice task (go/no go) with a two-component (pitch and location) auditory stimulus lasting 500 ms. They observed that functional interactions (cross correlations) are dynamically modified in the waiting period preceding the onset of auditory stimulation. Further, they found spatio-temporal firing patterns both within and across spike trains, several seconds before the actual stimulus delivery. These patterns had a very precise repetition of spike discharges separated by long intervals (up to several hundreds of milliseconds) in the absence of a change in mean rate. The authors suggest that network activity in A1 reflects '. . . participation of recurrent neuronal networks in processes anticipating the expected sensory input'.

18.6 Category learning and concept formation

Perceptual category formation often involves grouping sensory stimuli by abstract relationships based on some aspect of similar physical attributes. Ohl *et al.* (2001) trained rats to form the categories of 'rising' and 'falling' frequency modulation of tones, i.e., independent of their absolute frequencies. They detected category learning by a sudden change in learning strategy. Recordings from A1 revealed that the transition to category formation was correlated with the emergence of patterns of stimulus representation in the electroencephalogram (EEG) in which frequency-modulated tones are distinguished into the categories of 'rising' and 'falling' modulation (Fig. 18.6).

A recent related experiment extends this approach to humans. Subjects were required to classify sound on the basis of either the direction of change (rising or falling frequency modulation) or the duration of stimulation (short or long). Functional magnetic resonance imaging revealed

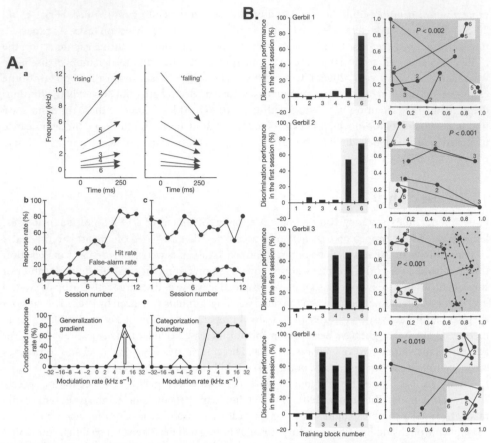

Fig. 18.6 A Stimuli and behavioral measures of category learning. **a** Rising (*red*) and falling (*blue*) frequency-modulated tones used in the six sequential training blocks (*numbers*). **b** Sample learning curve of gerbil 3 before transition to categorization. **c** Sample learning curve of same animal after transition to categorization. **d** Psychometric function for modulation rate obtained after training block shown in **b**. Peak modulation rate of 8 kHz s^{-1} (*arrow*) corresponds to modulation from 2–4 kHz in 250 ms used in this block. **e** Sigmoid psychometric function obtained after training block shown in **c**. **B** Behavioral transition to categorization (*left column*) parallels development of cortical spatial activity patterns (*right column*). *Left column*, discrimination performance in the first session of each of the six training blocks. *Yellow areas* indicate categorization phase (Wilcoxon's test, $P < 0.05$). *Right column*, similarity relations between spatial activity patterns during the marked states. Transition to category learning in the behavioral data correlates with clustering (*P*-values of resampling test given) of the marked states 'within category' (*yellow areas*). Only the activity pattern during the marked state that gave rise to the maximum peak value of the dissimilarity function for each category is plotted for each training block (*numbers*). For gerbil 3, marked states of later sessions in blocks 1 and 2 have been included (+) to demonstrate that these point clouds do not fall into the clusters found after the transition to categorization. Absolute coordinates of points have no particular meaning other than scaling relative distances between any pair of points. (From Ohl *et al.*, 2001.)

activation in the right auditory cortex for categorization by direction of change, while categorization by duration of stimulation activated the left auditory cortex (Brechmann and Scheich, 2005). The hemispheric specializations for the two types of stimulus parameters are consistent with prior studies of the human auditory cortex, but the linkage of the findings to categorization, rather than to the physical parameters of the stimuli *per se*, demonstrates that the human auditory cortex is involved in higher cognitive processes.

18.7 **Cross-modality effects**

Cognitive processes are also evident in 'cross-modal' effects, in which stimuli of a different sensory modality, or even behavioral responses, can elicit responses in A1. For example, monkeys were trained to perform a complex auditory discrimination. Following presentation of a cue light, they could initiate a sequence of tones by pressing a bar. Many neurons in A1 developed responses elicited by the bar press, of course prior to the presentation of the sounds. Moreover, presentation of the cue light itself became capable of eliciting responses in A1 (Brosch *et al.*, 2004).

Several studies have linked A1 of humans to speech in the absence of sound. Thus, the presentation of visual stimuli associated with language sounds, whether the sight of a letter or of silent speech, elicits neural activity in A1 (e.g., Pekkola *et al.*, 2005). This cross-modal effect might derive from earlier associative learning because the sight of the lips during speech is highly correlated with hearing the emitted speech. Related effects are not limited to putative associations. Visual stimuli can be transformed into a phonological code. Apparently, the left A1 is activated during such recoding (Suchan *et al.*, 2006). A recent anatomical study in the gerbil may provide an anatomical basis for some cross-modality effects. The authors found a surprisingly large number of inputs to A1 from non-auditory regions of both the cortex and the thalamus, arguing against the view that primary sensory cortices are unimodal (Budinger *et al.*, 2006).

18.8 **Motivation**

Several studies have found plasticity in A1 based on motivational level or the acquired behavioral importance of sensory stimuli. In a complex appetitive instrumental task, rats were trained in three phases and the amount of c-Fos expression was determined in different sub-groups at the end of each phase: (1) tone–food association, (2) two–tone discrimination, (3) two–tone discrimination contingent upon location of the sound source. Auditory stimuli were bursts of complex sounds lasting 500 ms. Compared to various control groups, successful animals exhibited no difference in the first phase but had significantly greater c-Fos activity in A1 during the next two phases. No subcortical auditory structures (cochlea through medial geniculate) differed from controls (Carretta *et al.*, 1999). The authors concluded that auditory cortex is involved in the coding of stimulus significance. Notably, they did not find plasticity after simple tone–food association, suggesting that not all associative learning involves A1 plasticity (see section 18.9).

While the previous study neither manipulated the level of motivation nor determined specificity of plasticity, a recent experiment addressed these issues directly. Rats were trained to bar press for water contingent upon the presence of a tone (6.0 kHz), at different levels of water deprivation and hence different levels of motivation and tone importance. Terminal mapping of A1 revealed a specific increase in the area of representation of the CS-frequency in the tonotopic map. More importantly, the amount of area was directly proportional to the level of correct performance, itself controlled by the level of motivation for water (Fig. 18.7; Rutkowski and Weinberger, 2005). These findings were predicted by the 'memory code hypothesis', viz. that the level of behavioral significance of a stimulus is encoded by the increase in the number of cells that become tuned to that stimulus (Weinberger, 2001).

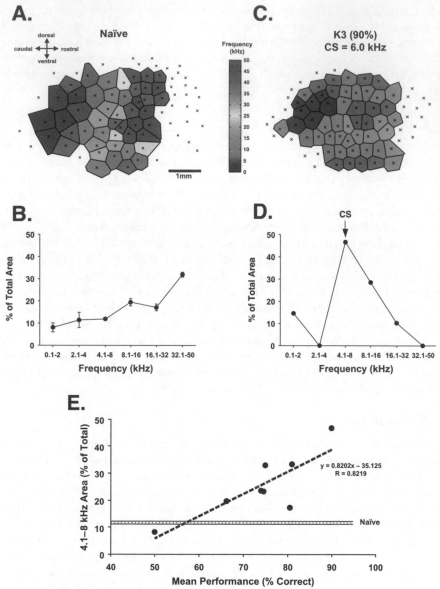

Fig. 18.7 The degree of acquired importance of a tone is correlated directly with the amount of area of frequency representation in the tonotopic map of A1. Trained rats received water reward for bar-presses in the presence of a 6.0 kHz tone. **A–D** Tonotopic maps and quantifications of percent of total area (octave frequency bands) for a naïve rat (*left*) and a rat that attained over 90% correct performance (*right*). Note that training greatly increased the area of representation for the frequency band containing the 6.0-kHz tone signal. **E** Evidence of a 'memory code' for the acquired behavioral importance of sound. The level of tone importance was controlled by the motivation for water (amount of water deprivation). Asymptotic performance was significantly correlated with motivation level. The area of representation of the frequency band containing the 6.0-kHz tone signal increases as a direct function of the level of behavioral importance of the tone, as operationally indexed by the level of correct performance. (From Weinberger, 2007a.)

18.9 **Learning strategy affects plasticity**

While learning modifies A1 to emphasize the processing and representation of behaviorally relevant sounds, the *factors that determine cortical plasticity* are poorly understood. One such factor that had escaped notice is the *learning strategy* used to solve a given problem. A recent study discovered that rats that solve the same problem, exhibit the same level of asymptotic perform-ance, and display the same specificity of learning about frequency *per se* either do or do not develop specific A1 plasticity, *depending upon the learning strategy* used to solve the task (Berlau and Weinberger, 2008). Rats were trained using the standard protocol to bar-press during a 5.0-kHz tone to receive a water reward and not bar-press during silent inter-trial intervals (ITI), when responses were signaled by a flashing light and a brief time-out penalty. This apparently simple auditory-cued problem *does not have a unique solution*. A strategy based on responding during the duration of the tone would solve the problem (*tone-duration strategy*, 'T-Dur'). However, animals could start responding at tone onset and continue to respond until they received the flashing light error signal without respect to the tone's ongoing presence (*tone-onset-to-error strategy*, 'TOTE'). Yet these alternatives cannot be distinguished because subjects receive the error signal for responses made immediately after tone offset. To distinguish between these strategies, one group received the standard training protocol (STD) while a second group (GRC) had the same protocol except for a 'post-tone grace period' (PTG) which was the 2 s immediately following tone offset, during which bar-presses were not punished (or rewarded). Thus, the *TOTE* strategy would be revealed as a pattern of behavior consisting of responding from tone-onset until receiving the error signal, i.e., bar-presses would continue after tone offset during the 2-s grace period.

The GRC group did continue to bar-press during the grace period after tone offset, showing that they used the *TOTE* strategy. Despite the fact that both groups solved the task to the same level, only the GRC group developed specific plasticity, which consisted in decreases in threshold and bandwidth in the CS-frequency band (Fig. 18.8). The results indicate that learning strategy can determine specific plasticity in A1, and be of greater impact than either the level of correct performance (magnitude of learning) or the learning about absolute frequency (specificity of learning). The *TOTE* strategy may indicate that GRC subjects used the cue of *tone onset* to solve the problem, whereas the STD subjects attended to the duration of the tone. Natural sounds are often brief, suggesting that the auditory system is adapted to extract information from transients (Masterton, 1993). Acoustic onsets appear to have a privileged status with respect to both percep-tion and auditory cortical discharge (Phillips *et al.*, 2002). Therefore, the formation of specific learning-induced cortical plasticity may depend on the use of learning strategies that best exploit cortical proclivities.

The effect of learning strategy may explain an apparent failure to replicate a study of perceptual learning. Owl monkeys trained to discriminate between two frequencies exhibited an increased area of representation for the training frequency band in the tonotopic map of A1 (Recanzone *et al.*, 1993). However, a similar study in the cat failed to find increased representation (Brown *et al.*, 2004). It is possible that the owl monkeys and cats employed different learning strategies. For example, given the rich vocal repertoire of these primates, and the fact that acoustic transients are particularly important for such vocalizations, the owl monkeys may have solved the tone dis-crimination problem by paying particular attention to tonal onset transients. In the absence of independent evidence of the strategy used, it may be difficult to understand why some auditory learning experiences induce cortical plasticity while others fail.

18.10 **Pre-motor processes**

While an intimate linkage between A1 and the motor functions apparent in behavior might seem most unlikely, there is evidence to support such a relationship. Within A1, patterns of neuronal

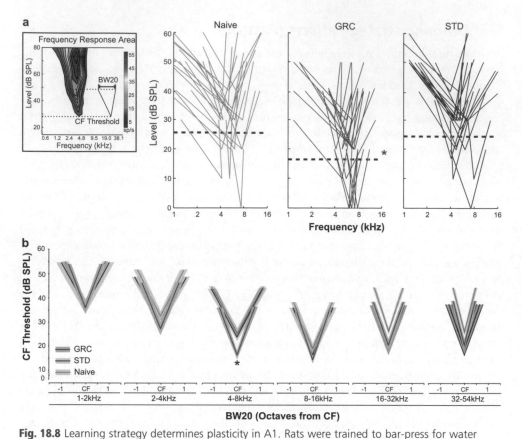

Fig. 18.8 Learning strategy determines plasticity in A1. Rats were trained to bar-press for water during presentation of a 6.0-kHz tone. Different groups used different strategies. One group (STD) used a 'tone-duration' strategy, ceasing bar-pressing at tone offset. Another group (GRC) started responding at tone onset and continued until receiving an error signal after tone offset ('tone-onset-to-error'). Only the GRC group developed specific plasticity, i.e., reduction of absolute threshold and bandwidth in the octave band (4.0–8.0 kHz) centered on the signal frequency. **a** Examples of frequency-response area (FRA) 'tuning tips' in each group: GRC, STD, and naive. Each 'V' shape delineates the CF threshold and BW20 of a recorded FRA (inset) that had a CF within the signal-tone frequency band (4–8 kHz) in each respective group. For sake of clarity, subsets of the total population of FRAs are depicted starting from the lowest threshold. Dashed lines represent the mean CF threshold for the entire population of each group. The asterisk shows that the GRC group had significantly lower CF thresholds than either naïve or STD groups, which did not differ from each other. **b** Plasticity in threshold and bandwidth in the GRC group is specific to the frequency band of the signal tone (asterisk). Both threshold and BW20 decreased only in the signal-tone frequency band. CF threshold and BW20 values are not significantly different from naïves in any frequency band in the STD group. Solid lines surrounded by shaded areas represent group means ± SE, respectively. (From Berlau and Weinberger, 2008.)

activity correlate with the animal's subsequent motor behavior. Rats were trained to distinguish between combinations of frequencies and two speaker locations. They had to make different motor responses to various combinations, e.g., a low tone from the left speaker might require one behavior while a high tone from the same speaker might require a different behavior. Patterns of unit discharges while waiting for the acoustic stimuli 'predicted' which response would be made.

The patterns in A1 might be parts of motor programs that are engaged in auditory tasks (Villa *et al.*, 1999). Of particular interest, mean discharge rates did not vary, emphasizing the importance of temporal parameters of cellular discharge that have too often been ignored (Edeline, 1996).

18.11 Mechanisms of associative plasticity

Consideration of the mechanisms of learning-induced specific plasticity in the auditory cortex may be profitably approached by beginning with proposed models. There are two. Both concern CS-directed shifts of tuning in auditory-cued fear conditioning. The first model proposed the *minimal* circuitry that would be *sufficient* to account for tuning shifts; it also predicted an increase in the representation of CS frequencies within the tonotopic map of A1 and otherwise has been tested by subsequent experiments (Weinberger *et al.*, 1990). The second model incorporated some key features of the first model, rejected others, and added descending projections from the auditory cortex to the inferior colliculus (Suga and Ma, 2003). For the sake of brevity, these are called the 'W' and 'S' models, respectively. An extended version of the 'S model' has been published recently (Suga, 2008), but it retains all of the essential features of the original model.

Because the 'W model' is a product of the author's laboratory, readers should be advised that the following discussion can be assumed to be biased in its favor despite attempts to be even-handed. Therefore, readers should consult the original relevant publications as well as the literature to draw their own conclusions about the relative validity and usefulness of the two models. In addition, exchanges of brief (Suga *et al.*, 2004; Weinberger, 2004a) and detailed (Suga, 2008; Weinberger, 2008c) letters provide a capsule of the major issues and mutual critiques. The following account is brief, given the ready availability of prior publications (in addition to those listed above, see Gao and Suga, 1998, 2000; Weinberger and Bakin, 1998; Suga *et al.*, 2002; Weinberger, 2004d, 2007a).

18.11.1 The 'W model'

This model was formulated to generate testable hypotheses regarding the minimal circuitry that could account for both behavioral signs of conditioned fear in Pavlovian associative learning (due to tone–shock pairing) and CS-specific tuning shifts in A1 (Fig. 18.9).

According to this model, the CS tone information is conveyed via the lemniscal system from the ventral medial geniculate nucleus (MGv) to the middle layers of A1, and also via the non-lemniscal auditory thalamus from the magnocellular medial geniculate (MGm) (and its affiliated posterior intralaminar nucleus, PIN) to the upper layers of A1. Initial associative plasticity develops in the MGm which also receives nociceptive afferentation via the spino-thalamic system, i.e., the CS and US converge in the MGm/PIN. The MGm develops CS-specific tuning shifts. However, because its cells are broadly and idiosyncratically tuned, the MGm cannot fully account for plasticity in A1, whose narrowly and systematically tuned cells develop RF shifts. Neither can the MGv, which, while having narrowly tuned cells, is hypothesized to not develop RF plasticity (but see below). However, the MGm does promote short-term tuning shifts in A1 by increasing its discharges to the CS frequency and therefore increasing the responses of A1 to the CS frequency. The MGm also projects to the amygdala, thus initiating behavioral signs of fear-conditioning (changes in heart rate, freezing, etc.). The amygdala also projects to the cholinergic nucleus basalis, which releases increased amounts of acetylcholine (ACh) into A1, thus inducing long-term plasticity, i.e., enduring CS-specific tuning shifts.

This model successfully predicted increased representation of CS frequencies in the tonotopic map of A1 (Recanzone *et al.*, 1993; Rutkowski and Weinberger, 2005), CS-specific associative tuning shifts in the MGm (Edeline and Weinberger, 1992), responses in the amygdala to MGm

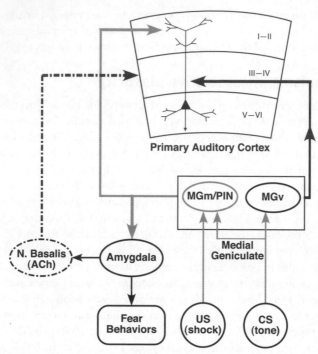

Fig. 18.9 The 'W model' of specific associative representational plasticity in A1, and autonomic conditioned responses in fear conditioning, based on convergence of the CS and US in the magnocellular medial geniculate. This model hypothesizes the minimal circuitry that would be *sufficient* to account for short- and long-term associative representational plasticity and rapidly acquired conditioned autonomic responses. See text for details. (From Weinberger, 1998.)

cells exhibiting auditory–somatosensory convergence (Bordi and LeDoux, 1994; Chapter 19), the development of CS-specific plasticity in the nucleus basalis prior to its appearance in A1 (Maho *et al.*, 1995), the induction of CS-specific plasticity in A1 by pairing a tone with stimulation of the nucleus basalis (Bakin and Weinberger, 1996; Kilgard and Merzenich, 1998) that is dependent upon the engagement of muscarinic receptors in A1 (Miasnikov *et al.*, 2001), and the induction of CS-specific behavioral memory by pairing a tone with stimulation of the nucleus basalis (McLin *et al.*, 2002; Miasnikov *et al.*, 2006, 2008; Weinberger *et al.*, 2006). However, the 'W model' incorrectly predicted the lack of CS-specific tuning shifts in the lemniscal MGv, which do in fact develop in this nucleus. However, in contrast to the MGm and A1, the tuning shifts in the MGv are very short-lived, having disappeared an hour after training (Edeline and Weinberger, 1991). Therefore, the long-term specific plasticity in A1 cannot simply be a passive reflection of tuning shifts in the MGv. The role of this transient MGv plasticity remains to be studied.

A test of the 'W model' using PET imaging in humans during discriminative (two-tone) fear conditioning found only five brain loci that exhibited associative plasticity: auditory cortex, medial geniculate, amygdala, nucleus basalis, and orbitofrontal cortex. Conditioning-related, frequency-specific modulation of tonotopic neural responses in the auditory cortex positively co-varied with activity in the amygdala, basal forebrain, and orbitofrontal cortex, and showed context-specific functional interactions with the medial geniculate nucleus. The authors conclude that 'These results accord with animal single-unit data and support neurobiological models of auditory conditioning and value-dependent neural selection' (Morris *et al.*, 1998). The 'W model' does not include the orbitofrontal cortex and PET imaging did not permit localization of plasticity within the medial geniculate nucleus, so whether the MGM/PIN was involved could not be determined.

18.11.2 The 'S model'

This model places convergence of information about the tonal CS and the shock US in the cerebral cortex rather than in the non-lemniscal medial geniculate complex (MGm/PIN). CS information goes to A1 via the lemniscal MGv and US information goes to S1 via the ventrobasal complex, presumably relayed by the ventral posterolateral (VPL) nucleus. Convergence then takes place in association cortex which then sends this information to the amygdala, or CS and US information may be sent independently to the amygdala where they converge. The amygdala then projects to the nucleus basalis, which releases ACh into the auditory cortex to promote long-term memory. This part of the 'S model' is identical to that of the 'W model'. Additionally, A1 projects to the inferior colliculus (IC), facilitating its responses to the CS frequency, and in turn the IC facilitates the responses of A1 to the CS frequency (presumably via the MGv). This positive feedback loop is halted by the thalamic reticular nucleus (TRN) which can inhibit thalamic sensory outflow to the cortex (Fig. 18.10).

The 'S model' is based on studies of tone–shock pairing in the big brown bat. Two features of frequency-specific plasticity in A1 of this animal differ from prior studies of other mammals. First, repetition of the *CS alone produces a tuning shift toward the repeated stimulus*. In contrast, virtually all other reports of the effects of repeated acoustic stimulation have found a decrement in response to repeated, non-reinforced sounds, which when properly investigated has proven to be habituation, i.e., learning not to respond to a stimulus of no behavioral significance. Second, conditioning augments the shift caused by presentation of the CS alone. This contrasts with the effect found in conditioning studies with other animals, in which an increased response due to pairing a CS and a US reverses the decrement of CS alone presentations. These differences might reflect the fact that the CS in these studies consists of a series of brief, high-frequency tone bursts that resemble the echolocating signal of the big brown bat. Therefore, they probably have behavioral salience prior to training. The tuning shifts during the CS-alone presentation may be a species-specific strategy to identify the source (i.e., another bat) of the CS sounds. Pairing this echo-locating signal with shock might then augment this process. In any event, the 'S model' and the experimental findings with the big brown bat might be best suited to understand its particular adaptations rather than serve as a general model of mammalian auditory learning.

A striking difference between the 'S' and 'W' models is that the former does not accept CS–US convergence in the MGm/PIN (Weinberger, 1982). The 'S model' holds that the MGm/PIN serves as a global alerting or activating influence on the auditory cortex (Suga, 2008), rather than having an associative role. This is not in accordance with the literature. At least 25 studies from many laboratories have found such convergence and associative plasticity, including CS-specific tuning shifts (e.g., Disterhoft and Stuart, 1976).

18.11.3 Neuromodulators in frequency-specific plasticity

Both the 'W' and 'S' models agree on the importance of nucleus basalis release of ACh for frequency-specific plasticity in the primary auditory cortex. Of all of the potential mechanisms involved in such A1 plasticity, the NB/ACh hypothesis has the greatest support among laboratories (e.g., Metherate and Ashe, 1993).

Recall that the 'W model' specifies a hypothesized minimal circuitry that could be *sufficient* for CS-specific tuning shifts. This does not imply that the NB/ACh system is *necessary* for plasticity, although there is evidence to support necessity. For example, fear conditioning in humans produces CS-specific plasticity in the auditory cortex that is blocked by scopolamine, a cholinergic

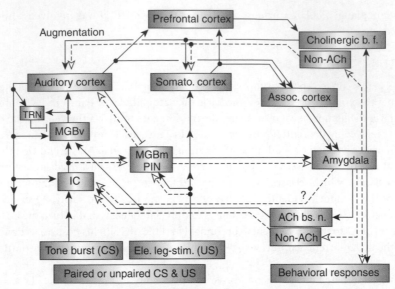

Fig. 18.10 The 'S model' of fear conditioning. Simplified neural circuits for tone-specific plasticity (BF shifts) elicited by paired CS–US and for non-specific plasticity (non-specific augmentation) elicited by unpaired CS–US (working hypothesis). *Solid arrows* indicate the neural circuit for BF shifts elicited by paired CS–US (conditioning). *Dashed arrows* indicate the neural circuit for non-specific augmentation, including the broadening of tuning, elicited by unpaired CS–US (pseudoconditioning). ACh Acetylcholine; b.f. basal forebrain (nucleus basalis); bs. n. brainstem nucleus; CS conditioned stimulus (tone bursts); IC inferior colliculus; MGBm medial division of the medial geniculate body; MGBv ventral division of the medial geniculate body; PIN posterior intralaminar nucleus in the thalamus; TRN thalamic reticular nucleus; US unconditioned stimulus (electric leg-shock). *Arrows* indicate excitatory projections; *projection with a short bar at the end* indicates inhibitory projection. An identical CS tone evokes tone-specific or non-specific changes in the central auditory system depending on whether it is paired or unpaired with a US. When the cortical BF shift is evoked by the cortical neural net, corticofugal feedback, and cholinergic basal forebrain, the auditory cortex probably reduces the signals from the MGBm and PIN which evoke the non-specific augmentation (*solid line with a bar at the end*). The cholinergic system augments the BF shift, whereas a non-cholinergic neuromodulatory system augments the non-specific augmentation evoked by the signals from the MGBm and PIN. For simplicity, the neural circuit for eliciting the non-specific augmentation of subcortical auditory neurons is not included in this model. (From Suga, 2008.)

antagonist (Thiel *et al.*, 2002). In any event, although much less studied, other neuromodulatory systems are also capable of promoting at least some features of specific plasticity in the auditory cortex: nor-adrenergic (Edeline, 1995), dopaminergic (Bao *et al.*, 2001), and serotonergic (Stark and Scheich, 1997). Therefore, while additional study of the cholinergic system is certainly warranted, increased research on other neuromodulatory systems is sorely needed to better establish their functions and determine how various modulators interact (Atzori *et al.*, 2005).

18.12 Conclusions

18.12.1 The primary auditory cortex is 'cognitive'

A1 exhibits many *cognitive processes*. While this is a simple enough conclusion, the observant reader will have noticed that nowhere has the term 'cognitive processes' been defined. This was intentional. The issue was avoided because it cannot be definitively resolved because of the lack of universal agreement regarding the meaning of the term. Thus, to enter into an adequate consideration of 'What is cognition?' at the outset would have clouded the review of findings that support the 'cognitive' conclusion. Instead, by omission, readers were encouraged to apply their own sense of 'cognition' to the material reviewed.

Why does the term 'cognition' pose such a problem? Isn't it merely a matter of semantics? Doesn't 'cognition' simply have the core meaning of 'knowing' or 'knowledge'? Doesn't it refer in some sense to 'higher mental processes'? Well, yes, but 'knowing' and 'higher mental processes' have different meanings to different groups of workers. For example, cognitive scientists take no issue with considering language to be a cognitive process, but most might look unkindly upon including 'classical (Pavlovian) conditioning'. After all, the conclusion that the auditory cortex is cognitive rests largely on studies of conditioning, as reviewed above.

Classical conditioning is generally considered to refer to 'reflexive', stimulus–response (S–R) 'habits', that are considered within the domain of 'procedural memory' (Squire, 1987). The term conjures an image of 'Pavlov's drooling dog'; 'ring the bell, see it drool'. However, if this picture ever applied to Pavlovian conditioning, it would have to be limited to the minority of cases in which the learning consists of a stimulus–response association. It had long been suspected that conditioning involves at least two stages – stimulus–stimulus (S–S) followed by S–R learning – and this is now an accepted characteristic (Lennartz and Weinberger, 1992a). Briefly stated, S–S learning rapidly permits an organism to predict the US given the CS. S–R learning allows that same organism to make a behavioral response either toward or away from the US, depending upon whether it is rewarding or potentially punishing. Most importantly, the pairing of a CS and a US is *not sufficient* for a Pavlovian association to form; there is nothing automatic or inevitable about forming an association. *Contingency*, rather than *temporal contiguity*, is necessary. In short, the CS must be a valid predictor of the US and may even have to provide information about the US that is not provided by other stimuli. Thus, conditioning, far from being automatic or 'reflexive', is a means for assessing a situation and permitting a subject to free itself from simply *reacting* to events in the environment. Rather, conditioning enables proactive behavior, based on an organism's ability to learn the 'causal fabric' of its environment (Rescorla, 1988a, b).

In toto, studies of Pavlovian conditioning, in which A1 develops CS-specific plasticity of frequency tuning and other acoustic parameters, are not demonstrations of 'low level', 'reflexive', or 'automatic' processes, but rather of *cognitive processes*. When combined with the growing research on the involvement of A1 with attention and concept formation, the conclusion is inescapable that accepted views of A1 as non-cognitive are no longer tenable.

18.12.2 The primary auditory cortex is not merely an 'adaptive' sound analyzer

This chapter has summarized findings that implicate A1 not only in attention and concept formation, but also in auditory imagery, expectancy, cross-modality effects, motivation, learning strategy, working and reference memory, and pre-motor processes. Why have these processes been separated from attention and concept formation at this juncture? Because the argument might still be made that all of these processes are actually *components of learning and memory*. Thus, to the extent that learning and memory can be reconciled with A1 as a sound analyzer, the argument for 'cognitive auditory cortex' fails. On the contrary, it has been argued that while learning and memory constitute the major evidence that A1 is cognitive, even this conclusion must be consigned to contemporary limbo because specific memories have not been destroyed by cortical lesions (Irvine, 2007). (Irvine did not review the many other topics and processes included in this chapter.) The basis for challenging this 'lesion position' has been presented above, so all that need be said now is that some researchers remain skeptical about even mnemonic functions of A1.

To return to the argument against the 'cognitive auditory cortex', how might one argue that, notwithstanding the evidence summarized above, A1 remains an acoustic analyzer, albeit operating on slightly different principles? The argument goes as follows: 'A1 is an *adaptive acoustic analyzer*', i.e., its function is still the analysis of sounds, but it does so in an adaptive manner, adjusting its analyses on the basis of experience. All of the learning and memory phenomena simply are components of the 'adaptive tuning' aspect of A1'.

For the sake of argument, let us grant the premise that learning and memory are not cognitive processes. (But what is more 'knowing' than storing the details of daily experience?) In rebuttal, we might point out that 'adaptive analysis' has to include the acceptance of memory, including long-term specific memory traces in A1.

However, the acceptance of long-term memory traces transforms the concept of acoustic analysis beyond all recognition, as it saves 'analysis' by keeping its label but discarding its core meaning of unambiguously identifying a sound. How could a system perform pure acoustic analysis, even if its parameter-evaluating 'weightings' are 'tweaked' or 'retuned' to optimize the analysis of behaviorally important sounds? How could the system determine whether the acoustic stimulus received is a loud unimportant sound or a quiet important sound, since 'importance' stored in the cortex could produce the same discharge to a quiet important sound and a loud unimportant sound? One answer might be by not relying on a discharge-rate code, but on something else. But then, one still must face a considerable problem: an acoustic (or other sensory) analysis system that also stores non-acoustic information (which alters representations) engenders conflations between the two domains and hence sacrifices analytic precision. So to show that A1 is an 'adaptive analyzer', unencumbered with 'cognitive' processes, proponents of this view will have to both formulate an adequate novel algorithm that prevents conflation of, e.g., sound level and behavioral importance and devise appropriate experimental tests.

Finally, there is no actual justification for granting the premise that learning and memory are not cognitive processes, that is processes that concern the interpretation and understanding of sound, once it has been analyzed and identified. Nor is there actual justification for treating, e.g., 'learning strategy' as a sub-class of the actual processes of learning and memory. After all, learning strategy is more closely related to selective attention, i.e., what aspects of sound should be attended, than to learning *per se*. Similarly, motivation and cross-modality effects are factors that can affect learning-induced plasticity in A1, but they are hardly part and parcel of the learning process itself. Thus, the conclusion that A1 is not simply an acoustic analyzer, whether operating adaptively or not, is strongly supported by the available evidence.

18.13 Implications

If A1 is cognitive, but is not simply an adaptive acoustic analyzer, what might it be? To arrive at a reconceptualization of A1, it will be helpful to consider three major implications.

First, the traditional view of the functional organization of the cerebral cortex is that it operates as a sequence of functions: (1) sensory analysis, (2) sensory interpretation, and (3) motor performance, carried out by anatomically distinct areas. However, as A1 is certainly involved in both analysis and interpretation, this schema is no longer tenable. Moreover, and to reiterate one final time, 'primary auditory cortex', as purely sensory–analytic, *does not exist*. By extension, neither does primary somatosensory nor visual cortex, because, although less extensively studied, they both exhibit learning and memory-related processes (reviewed in Weinberger, 2008a).

Second, while A1 is certainly concerned with the processing of sounds, the fact that it also involves auditory concepts and category formation (Wetzel *et al.*, 1998) demonstrates that it has '*supra-stimulus*' functions. This term refers to the fact that categories, such as 'ascending frequency', denote a higher level construct than any particular physical parameters.

Third, and a related point, as the degree of plasticity reflects the level of acquired behavioral importance (Rutkowski and Weinberger, 2005), motivational information that is presumably not assessed in A1 is nonetheless represented therein. (A similar process has been found in primary visual cortex (Shuler and Bear, 2006).) Therefore, A1 appears to serve '*extra-stimulus*' functions.

In summary, while the functions of A1 most certainly do involve the analysis of sound, they also involve *supra-stimulus* and *extra-stimulus* functions. If we keep these three functions in mind, a certain reconceptualization of A1 begins to take form.

18.14 **Reconceptualizing the primary auditory cortex**

To start, the modality specialization of A1 has to be foremost. Regardless of cross-modality influences, A1 is specialized for audition. However, given its supra-stimulus and extra-stimulus functions, its domain of concern with sound is considerably broader than heretofore believed. I suggest that the overall function of A1 is to *attempt to solve higher auditory problems and challenges that face an organism*.

By 'higher auditory problems' I mean 'non-reflexive' situations. For example, A1 would not be important for the acoustic startle reflex, but would be involved in 'constructing' acoustic space in the service of locating the source of the loud sound that elicited startle. Also, if a specific motor act is required with respect to acoustic stimulation, then the auditory cortex would integrate (unknown aspects of) motor function with the analysis, acquisition, and storage of information about the relevant sounds. The result would not be confined to auditory information but rather auditory information combined with relevant motor and spatial information for the situation in question. This may explain why selective lesions of frequency bands within the tonotopic map of A1 in the cat produce selective impairment of locomotion to the source of the corresponding sound frequency in the cat (Jenkins and Merzenich, 1984).

In no case would A1 *execute* the requisite behavioral act. Nor would it assess or determine the motivational state or determine the nature of the goal object, such as food, water, or opportunity for sex. Nonetheless, A1 would be a major site in which the relevant information is integrated. Of course, A1 would be working in concert with other auditory cortical fields, but so little is known about their functions in behavior that no more can be said at this time. In fact, the manner in which A1 interacts with 'belt' and 'higher' fields, with both feed forward and feed back interactions, remains a central problem in auditory neuroscience.

Clearly, this liberalized view of A1 is preliminary and really little more than an 'outline of an idea'. However, even in its nascent state, it offers an alternative to the traditional auditory analytic role of the primary auditory cortex. If this reconceptualization does nothing more than provoke thought and experiment, it will have served a beneficial purpose.

18.15 **A future research emphasis for the auditory cortex**

That A1 has cognitive functions which cannot be reduced to adaptive acoustic analysis forces us to confront our limited state of understanding. If our deeply implicit assumptions about the differential localization of stimulus analysis and stimulus meaning are no longer tenable, then our comprehension of what the auditory system does and how it does it is sadly wanting. However, we are also confronted with virtually unlimited opportunities. Auditory neuroscience should embrace this prospect of new frontiers of research. The creative exploitation of our wealth of foundational knowledge of the auditory system together with asking new types of questions about its functions and mechanisms will reveal how we come to know and to comprehend sounds. We will need to expand our domains of thought and experiment while achieving a symbiosis of auditory and behavioral neuroscience.

Acknowledgements

Sincere thanks to Gabriel K. Hui and Jacquie Weinberger for assistance in the preparation of this chapter. This work was supported by research grants from the National Institutes of Health/National Institute on Deafness and Other Communication Disorders (NIDCD), DC-02938 and DC-05592 to N.M.W.

References

Alho K (1992) Selective attention in auditory processing as reflected by event-related brain potentials. *Psychophysiology* 29(3): 247–63.

Atzori M, Kanold PO, Pineda JC, Flores-Hernandez J, Paz RD (2005) Dopamine prevents muscarinic-induced decrease of glutamate release in the auditory cortex. *Neuroscience* 134(4): 1153–65.

Bakin JS, Weinberger NM (1990) Classical conditioning induces CS-specific receptive field plasticity in the auditory cortex of the guinea pig. *Brain Res* 536(1–2): 271–86.

Bakin JS, Weinberger NM (1996) Induction of a physiological memory in the cerebral cortex by stimulation of the nucleus basalis. *Proc Natl Acad Sci USA* 93(20): 11219–24.

Bakin JS, Lepan B, Weinberger NM (1992) Sensitization induced receptive field plasticity in the auditory cortex is independent of CS-modality. *Brain Res* 577(2): 226–35.

Bakin JS, South DA, Weinberger NM (1996) Induction of receptive field plasticity in the auditory cortex of the guinea pig during instrumental avoidance conditioning. *Behav Neurosci* 110(5): 905–13.

Bao S, Chan VT, Merzenich MM (2001) Cortical remodelling induced by activity of ventral tegmental dopamine neurons. *Nature* 412(6842): 79–83.

Bao S, Chang EF, Woods J, Merzenich MM (2004) Temporal plasticity in the primary auditory cortex induced by operant perceptual learning. *Nat Neurosci* 7(9): 974–81.

Beitel RE, Schreiner CE, Cheung SW, Wang X, Merzenich MM (2003) Reward-dependent plasticity in the primary auditory cortex of adult monkeys trained to discriminate temporally modulated signals. *Proc Natl Acad Sci USA* 100(19): 11070–5.

Berlau KM, Weinberger NM (2008) Learning strategy determines auditory cortical plasticity. *Neurobiol Learn Mem* 89(2): 153–66.

Bordi F, LeDoux JE (1994) Response properties of single units in areas of rat auditory thalamus that project to the amygdala. II. Cells receiving convergent auditory and somatosensory inputs and cells antidromically activated by amygdala stimulation. *Exp Brain Res* 98(2): 275–86.

Bouton ME (2007) *Learning and Behavior: A Contemporary Synthesis.* Sinauer Associates, Sunderland, Massachusetts.

Brechmann A, Scheich H (2005) Hemispheric shifts of sound representation in auditory cortex with conceptual listening. *Cereb Cortex* 15(5): 578–87.

Brosch M, Selezneva E, Bucks C, Scheich H (2004) Macaque monkeys discriminate pitch relationships. *Cognition* 91(3): 259–72.

Brown M, Irvine DR, Park VN (2004) Perceptual learning on an auditory frequency discrimination task by cats: association with changes in primary auditory cortex. *Cereb Cortex* 14(9): 952–65.

Buchwald JS, Halas ES, Schramm S (1966) Changes in cortical and subcortical unit activity during behavioral conditioning. *Physiol Behav* 1(1): 11–22.

Budinger E, Heil P, Hess A, Scheich H (2006) Multisensory processing via early cortical stages: connections of the primary auditory cortical field with other sensory systems. *Neuroscience* 143(4): 1065–83.

Campbell AW (1905) *Histological Studies on the Localization of Cerebral Function*. Cambridge University Press, Cambridge.

Carretta D, Herve-Minvielle A, Bajo VM, Villa AE, Rouiller EM (1999) c-Fos expression in the auditory pathways related to the significance of acoustic signals in rats performing a sensory-motor task. *Brain Res* 841(1–2): 170–83.

Christian KM, Thompson RF (2005) Long-term storage of an associative memory trace in the cerebellum. *Behav Neurosci* 119(2): 526–37.

Condon CD, Weinberger NM (1991) Habituation produces frequency-specific plasticity of receptive fields in the auditory cortex. *Behav Neurosci* 105(3): 416–30.

Diamond DM, Weinberger NM (1984) Physiological plasticity of single neurons in auditory cortex of the cat during acquisition of the pupillary conditioned response: II. Secondary field (AII). *Behav Neurosci* 98(2): 189–210.

Diamond DM, Weinberger NM (1986) Classical conditioning rapidly induces specific changes in frequency receptive fields of single neurons in secondary and ventral ectosylvian auditory cortical fields. *Brain Res* 372(2): 357–60.

Diamond DM, Weinberger NM (1989) Role of context in the expression of learning-induced plasticity of single neurons in auditory cortex. *Behav Neurosci* 103(3): 471–94.

DiCara LV, Braun JJ, Pappas BA (1970) Classical conditioning and instrumental learning of cardiac and gastrointestinal responses following removal of neocortex in the rat. *J Comp Physiol Psychol* 73(2): 208–16.

Disterhoft JF, Stuart DK (1976) Trial sequence of changed unit activity in auditory system of alert rat during conditioned response acquisition and extinction. *J Neurophysiol* 39(2): 266–81.

Edeline J-M (1995) The alpha 2-adrenergic antagonist idazoxan enhances the frequency selectivity and increases the threshold of auditory cortex neurons. *Exp Brain Res* 107(2): 221–40.

Edeline J-M (1996) Does Hebbian synaptic plasticity explain learning-induced sensory plasticity in adult mammals? *Journal of Physiology Paris* 90(3–4): 271–6.

Edeline J-M, Weinberger NM (1991) Thalamic short-term plasticity in the auditory system: associative retuning of receptive fields in the ventral medial geniculate body. *Behav Neurosci* 105(5): 618–39.

Edeline J-M, Weinberger NM (1992) Associative retuning in the thalamic source of input to the amygdala and auditory cortex: receptive field plasticity in the medial division of the medial geniculate body. *Behav Neurosci* 106(1): 81–105.

Edeline J-M, Weinberger NM (1993) Receptive field plasticity in the auditory cortex during frequency discrimination training: selective retuning independent of task difficulty. *Behav Neurosci* 107(1): 82–103.

Edeline J-M, Neuenschwander-El Massioui N, Dutrieux G (1990a) Discriminative long-term retention of rapidly induced multiunit changes in the hippocampus, medial geniculate and auditory cortex. *Behav Brain Res* 39(2): 145–55.

Edeline J-M, Neuenschwander-El Massioui N, Dutrieux G (1990b) Frequency-specific cellular changes in the auditory system during acquisition and reversal of discriminative conditioning. *Psychobiology* 18(4): 382–93.

Edeline J-M, Pham P, Weinberger NM (1993) Rapid development of learning-induced receptive field plasticity in the auditory cortex. *Behav Neurosci* 107(4): 539–51.

Fritz J, Shamma S, Elhilali M, Klein D (2003) Rapid task-related plasticity of spectrotemporal receptive fields in primary auditory cortex. *Nat Neurosci* 6(11): 1216–23.

Fritz J, Elhilali M, Shamma S (2005a) Active listening: task-dependent plasticity of spectrotemporal receptive fields in primary auditory cortex. *Hear Res* 206(1–2): 159–76.

Fritz JB, Elhilali M, Shamma SA (2005b) Differential dynamic plasticity of A1 receptive fields during multiple spectral tasks. *J Neurosci* **25**(33): 7623–35.

Galambos R, Sheatz G, Vernier V (1956) Electrophysiological correlates of a conditioned response in cats. *Science* **123**(3192): 376–7.

Galván VV, Weinberger NM (2002) Long-term consolidation and retention of learning-induced tuning plasticity in the auditory cortex of the guinea pig. *Neurobiol Learn Mem* **77**(1): 78–108.

Galván VV, Chen J, Weinberger NM (2001) Long-term frequency tuning of local field potentials in the auditory cortex of the waking guinea pig. *J Assoc Res Otolaryngol* **2**(3): 199–215.

Gao E, Suga N (1998) Experience-dependent corticofugal adjustment of midbrain frequency map in bat auditory system. *Proc Natl Acad Sci USA* **95**(21): 12663–70.

Gao E, Suga N (2000) Experience-dependent plasticity in the auditory cortex and the inferior colliculus of bats: Role of the corticofugal system. *Proc Natl Acad Sci USA* **97**(14): 8081–6.

Gonzalez-Lima F, Scheich H (1984) Neural substrates for tone-conditioned bradycardia demonstrated with 2-deoxyglucose: I. Activation of auditory nuclei. *Behav Brain Res* **14**(3): 213–33.

Gonzalez-Lima F, Scheich H (1986) Neural substrates for tone-conditioned bradycardia demonstration with 2-deoxyglucose: II. Auditory cortex plasticity. *Behav Brain Res* **20**(3): 281–93.

Gonzalez-Lima F, Finkenstadt T, Ewert JP (1989a) Learning-related activation in the auditory system of the rat produced by long-term habituation: a 2-deoxyglucose study. *Brain Res* **489**(1): 67–79.

Gonzalez-Lima F, Finkenstadt T, Ewert JP (1989b) Neural substrates for long-term habituation of the acoustic startle reflex in rats: a 2-deoxyglucose study. *Neurosci Lett* **96**(2): 151–6.

Halpern AR, Zatorre RJ, Bouffard M, Johnson JA (2004) Behavioral and neural correlates of perceived and imagined musical timbre. *Neuropsychologia* **42**(9): 1281–92.

Irvine DR (2007) Auditory cortical plasticity: does it provide evidence for cognitive processing in the auditory cortex? *Hear Res* **229**(1–2): 158–70.

Irvine DR, Martin RL, Klimkeit E, Smith R (2000) Specificity of perceptual learning in a frequency discrimination task. *J Acoust Soc Am* **108**(6): 2964–8.

Jenkins WM, Merzenich MM (1984) Role of cat primary auditory cortex for sound-localization behavior. *J Neurophysiol* **52**(5): 819–47.

Jordan WP, Strasser HC, McHale L (2000) Contextual control of long-term habituation in rats. *J Exp Psychol Anim Behav Process* **26**(3): 323–39.

Kellman PJ (2002) Perceptual learning. In: *Learning, Motivation and Emotion*, 3rd edn (eds Pashler H, Gallistel R), pp. 259–99. John Wiley, Hoboken.

Kilgard MP, Merzenich MM (1998) Cortical map reorganization enabled by nucleus basalis activity. *Science* **279**(5357): 1714–8.

Kisley MA, Gerstein GL (2001) Daily variation and appetitive conditioning-induced plasticity of auditory cortex receptive fields. *Eur J Neurosci* **13**(10): 1993–2003.

Lennartz RC, Weinberger NM (1992a) Analysis of response systems in Pavlovian conditioning reveals rapidly versus slowly acquired conditioned responses: support for two factors, implications for behavior and neurobiology. *Psychobiology* **20**(2): 93–119.

Lennartz RC, Weinberger NM (1992b) Frequency-specific receptive field plasticity in the medial geniculate body induced by Pavlovian fear conditioning is expressed in the anesthetized brain. *Behav Neurosci* **106**(3): 484–97.

Lieberman DA (1990) *Learning: Behavior and Cognition*. Wadsworth Publishing, Belmont, California.

Mackintosh NJ (1974) *The Psychology of Animal Learning*. Academic Press, New York.

Mackintosh NJ (1983) *Conditioning and Associative Learning*. Oxford University Press, New York.

Maho C, Hars B, Edeline J-M, Hennevin E (1995) Conditioned changes in the basal forebrain: relations with learning-induced cortical plasticity. *Psychobiology* **23**(1): 10–25.

Marlin NA, Miller RR (1981) Associations to contextual stimuli as a determinant of long-term habituation. *J Exp Psychol Anim Behav Process* **7**(4): 313–33.

Marsh JT, McCarthy DA, Sheatz G, Galambos R (1961) Amplitude changes in evoked auditory potentials during habituation and conditioning. *Electroencephalog Clin Neurophysiol* 13: 224–34.

Masterton RB (1993) Central auditory system. *J Oto-rhino-laryngol Related Spec* 55(3): 159–63.

McLin DE 3rd, Miasnikov AA, Weinberger NM (2002) Induction of behavioral associative memory by stimulation of the nucleus basalis. *Proc Natl Acad Sci USA* 99(6): 4002–7.

Metherate R, Ashe JH (1993) Nucleus basalis stimulation facilitates thalamocortical synaptic transmission in the rat auditory cortex. *Synapse* 14(2): 132–43.

Miasnikov AA, McLin D 3rd, Weinberger NM (2001) Muscarinic dependence of nucleus basalis induced conditioned receptive field plasticity. *NeuroReport* 12(7): 1537–42.

Miasnikov AA, Chen JC, Weinberger NM (2006) Rapid induction of specific associative behavioral memory by stimulation of the nucleus basalis in the rat. *Neurobiol Learn Mem* 86(1): 47–65.

Miasnikov AA, Chen JC, Gross N, Poytress BS, Weinberger NM (2008) Motivationally neutral stimulation of the nucleus basalis induces specific behavioral memory. *Neurobiol Learn Mem* 90(1): 125–37.

Molchan SE, Sunderland T, McIntosh AR, Herscovitch P, Schreurs BG (1994) A functional anatomical study of associative learning in humans. *Proc Nat Acad Sci USA* 91(17): 8122–6.

Morris JS, Friston KJ, Dolan RJ (1998) Experience-dependent modulation of tonotopic neural responses in human auditory cortex. *Proc R Soc Lond Ser B Biol Sci* 265(1397): 649–57.

Ohl FW, Scheich H (2004) Fallacies in behavioural interpretation of auditory cortex plasticity. *Nat Rev Neurosci* 5(4). Published online 20 November 2004, http://www.nature.com/nrn/journal/v5/n4/full/nrn1366-c1.html.

Ohl FW, Scheich H, Freeman WJ (2001) Change in pattern of ongoing cortical activity with auditory category learning. *Nature* 412(6848): 733–6.

Oleson TD, Ashe JH, Weinberger NM (1975) Modification of auditory and somatosensory system activity during pupillary conditioning in the paralyzed cat. *J Neurophysiol* 38(5): 1114–39.

Pavlov IP (1927) *Conditioned Reflexes*. Dover, New York.

Pekkola J, Ojanen V, Autti T, *et al.* (2005) Primary auditory cortex activation by visual speech: an fMRI study at 3T. *NeuroReport* 16(2): 125–8.

Phillips DP, Hall SE, Boehnke SE (2002) Central auditory onset responses, and temporal asymmetries in auditory perception. *Hear Res* 167(1–2): 192–205.

Polley DB, Heiser MA, Blake DT, Schreiner CE, Merzenich MM (2004) Associative learning shapes the neural code for stimulus magnitude in primary auditory cortex. *Proc Natl Acad Sci USA* 101(46): 16351–6.

Polley DB, Steinberg EE, Merzenich MM (2006) Perceptual learning directs auditory cortical map reorganization through top-down influences. *J Neurosci* 26(18): 4970–82.

Poremba A, Jones D, Gonzalez-Lima F (1998) Classical conditioning modifies cytochrome oxidase activity in the auditory system. *Eur J Neurosci* 10(10): 3035–43.

Recanzone GH, Schreiner CE, Merzenich MM (1993) Plasticity in the frequency representation of primary auditory cortex following discrimination training in adult owl monkeys. *J Neurosci* 13(1): 87–103.

Rescorla RA (1988a) Behavioral studies of Pavlovian conditioning. *Annu Rev Neurosci* 11: 329–52.

Rescorla RA (1988b) Pavlovian conditioning: it's not what you think it is. *Am Psychol* 43(3): 151–60.

Rutkowski RG, Weinberger NM (2005) Encoding of learned importance of sound by magnitude of representational area in primary auditory cortex. *Proc Natl Acad Sci USA* 102(38): 13664–9.

Ryle G (1963) *The Concept of Mind*. Hutchinson, London.

Sakurai Y (1990) Cells in the rat auditory system have sensory-delay correlates during the performance of an auditory working memory task. *Behav Neurosci* 104(6): 856–68.

Sakurai Y (1992) Auditory working and reference memory can be tested in a single situation of stimuli for the rat. *Behav Brain Res* 50(1–2): 193–5.

Sakurai Y (1994) Involvement of auditory cortical and hippocampal neurons in auditory working memory and reference memory in the rat. *J Neurosci* 14(5 Part 1): 2606–23.

Sakurai Y (1998) The search for cell assemblies in the working brain. *Behav Brain Res* **91**(1–2): 1–13.

Schreurs BG, McIntosh AR, Bahro M, Herscovitch P, Sunderland T, Molchan SE (1997) Lateralization and behavioral correlation of changes in regional cerebral blood flow with classical conditioning of the human eyeblink response. *J Neurophysiol* **77**(4): 2153–63.

Shinba T, Sumi M, Iwanami A, Ozawa N, Yamamoto K (1995) Increased neuronal firing in the rat auditory cortex associated with preparatory set. *Brain Res Bull* **37**(2): 199–204.

Shuler MG, Bear MF (2006) Reward timing in the primary visual cortex. *Science* **311**(5767): 1606–9.

Squire LR (1987) *Memory and Brain*. Oxford University Press, New York.

Stark H, Scheich H (1997) Dopaminergic and serotonergic neurotransmission systems are differentially involved in auditory cortex learning: a long-term microdialysis study of metabolites. *J Neurochem* **68**(2): 691–7.

Suchan B, Linnewerth B, Koster O, Daum I, Schmid G (2006) Cross-modal processing in auditory and visual working memory. *Neuroimage* **29**(3): 853–8.

Suga N (2008) The neural circuit for tone-specific plasticity in the auditory system elicited by conditioning. *Learn Mem* **15**(4): 198–201.

Suga N, Ma X (2003) Multiparametric corticofugal modulation and plasticity in the auditory system. *Nat Rev Neurosci* **4**(10): 783–94.

Suga N, Xiao Z, Ma X, Ji W (2002) Plasticity and corticofugal modulation for hearing in adult animals. *Neuron* **36**(1): 9–18.

Suga N, Ji W, Ma X (2004) Criticisms of 'Specific long-term memory traces in primary auditory cortex'. *Nat Rev Neurosci* **5**(4). Published online 20 November 2004, http://www.nature.com/nrn/journal/v5/n4/full/nrn1366-c3.html.

Teas DC, Kiang NY (1964) Evoked responses from the auditory cortex. *Exp Neurol* **10**(2): 91–119.

Teich AH, McCabe PM, Gentile CG, *et al.* (1988) Role of auditory cortex in the acquisition of differential heart rate conditioning. *Physiol Behav* **44**(3): 405–12.

Teich AH, McCabe PM, Gentile CC, *et al.* (1989) Auditory cortex lesions prevent the extinction of Pavlovian differential heart rate conditioning to tonal stimuli in rabbits. *Brain Res* **480**(1–2): 210–8.

Thiel CM, Friston KJ, Dolan RJ (2002) Cholinergic modulation of experience-dependent plasticity in human auditory cortex. *Neuron* **35**(3): 567–74.

Villa AE, Hyland B, Tetko IV, Najem A (1998) Dynamical cell assemblies in the rat auditory cortex in a reaction-time task. *Biosystems* **48**(1–3): 269–77.

Villa AE, Tetko IV, Hyland B, Najem A (1999) Spatiotemporal activity patterns of rat cortical neurons predict responses in a conditioned task. *Proc Natl Acad Sci USA* **96**(3): 1106–11.

Wagner A (1981) SOP: a model of automatic memory processing in animal behavior. In: *Information Processing in Animals* (eds Spear NE, Miller RR), pp. 5–47. Erlbaum, Hillsdale, New Jersey.

Weinberger NM (1982) Sensory plasticity and learning: the magnocellular medial geniculate nucleus of the auditory system. In: *Conditioning: Representation of Involved Neural Functions (Advances in Behavioral Biology*, Vol. 26) (ed. Woody CD), pp. 697–710. Plenum Press, New York.

Weinberger NM (1997) Learning-induced receptive field plasticity in the primary auditory cortex. *Sem Neurosci* **9**(1–2): 59–67.

Weinberger NM (1998) Physiological memory in primary auditory cortex: characteristics and mechanisms. *Neurobiol Learn Mem* **70**(1–2): 226–51.

Weinberger NM (2001) Memory codes: new concept for old problem. In: *Memory Consolidation: Essays in Honor of James L. McGaugh* (eds Gold PE, Greenough WT), pp. 321–42. American Psychological Association, Washington, DC.

Weinberger NM (2004a) Consequences of failures to meet standards in learning and memory. *Nat Rev Neurosci* **5**(4). Published online 20 November 2004, http://www.nature.com/nrn/journal/v5/n4/full/nrn1366-c4.html.

Weinberger NM (2004b) Correcting misconceptions of tuning shifts in auditory cortex. *Nat Rev Neurosci* 5(4). Published online 20 November 2004, http://www.nature.com/nrn/journal/v5/n4/full/nrn1366-c2.html.

Weinberger NM (2004c) Experience-dependent response plasticity in the auditory cortex: issues, characteristics, mechanisms, and functions. In: *Plasticity of the Auditory System (Springer Handbook of Auditory Research*, Vol. 23) (eds Parks TN, Rubel EW, Fay RR, Popper AN), pp. 173–227. Springer, New York.

Weinberger NM (2004d) Specific long-term memory traces in primary auditory cortex. *Nat Rev Neurosci* 5(4): 279–90.

Weinberger NM (2007a) Associative representational plasticity in the auditory cortex: a synthesis of two disciplines. *Learn Mem* 14(1–2): 1–16.

Weinberger NM (2007b) Auditory associative memory and representational plasticity in the primary auditory cortex. *Hear Res* 229(1–2): 54–68.

Weinberger NM (2008a) Cortical plasticity in associative learning and memory. In: *Learning and Memory: A Comprehensive Reference*, Vol. 3 (ed. Byrne JH), pp. 187–218. Academic Press, New York.

Weinberger NM (2008b) Reconceptualizing the auditory cortex: learning, memory and specific plasticity. In: *The Auditory Cortex* (eds Winer JA, Schreiner CE). Springer, New York.

Weinberger NM (2008c) Retuning the brain by learning, literature, and logic: reply to Suga. *Learn Mem* 15(4): 202–7.

Weinberger NM, Bakin JS (1998) Learning-induced physiological memory in adult primary auditory cortex: receptive fields plasticity, model, and mechanisms. *Audiol Neuro-otol* 3(2–3): 145–67.

Weinberger NM, Diamond DM (1987) Physiological plasticity in auditory cortex: rapid induction by learning. *Progr Neurobiol* 29(1): 1–55.

Weinberger NM, Diamond DM, McKenna TM (1984a) Initial events in conditioning: plasticity in the pupillomotor and auditory systems. In: *Neurobiology of Learning and Memory* (eds Lynch G, McGaugh JL, Weinberger NM), pp. 197–227. Guilford Press, New York.

Weinberger NM, Hopkins W, Diamond DM (1984b) Physiological plasticity of single neurons in auditory cortex of the cat during acquisition of the pupillary conditioned response: I. Primary field (AI). *Behav Neurosci* 98(2): 171–88.

Weinberger NM, Ashe JH, Metherate R, McKenna TM, Diamond DM, Bakin JS (1990) Retuning auditory cortex by learning: a preliminary model of receptive field plasticity. *Concept Neurosci* 1(1): 91–131.

Weinberger NM, Javid R, Lepan B (1993) Long-term retention of learning-induced receptive-field plasticity in the auditory cortex. *Proc Natl Acad Sci USA* 90(6): 2394–8.

Weinberger NM, Miasnikov AA, Chen JC (2006) The level of cholinergic nucleus basalis activation controls the specificity of auditory associative memory. *Neurobiol Learn Mem* 86(3): 270–85.

Westenberg IS, Weinberger NM (1976) Evoked potential decrements in auditory cortex. II: Critical test for habituation. *Electroencephalog Clin Neurophysiol* 40(4): 356–69.

Westenberg IS, Paige G, Golub B, Weinberger NM (1976) Evoked potential decrements in auditory cortex: I. Discrete-trial and continual stimulation. *Electroencephalog Clin Neurophysiol* 40(4): 337–55.

Wetzel W, Wagner T, Ohl FW, Scheich H (1998) Categorical discrimination of direction in frequency-modulated tones by Mongolian gerbils. *Behav Brain Res* 91(1–2): 29–39.

Woody CD, Knispel JD, Crow TJ, Black-Clewerth PA (1976) Activity and excitability to electrical current of cortical auditory receptive neurons of awake cats as affected by stimulus association. *J Neurophysiol* 39: 1045–61.

Chapter 19

Emotional responses to auditory stimuli

Jorge L. Armony and Joseph E. LeDoux

19.1 Introduction

The ability to quickly detect and accurately decode emotional stimuli arising in the environment is critical for an organism's survival. Some of these stimuli are species-specific and their affective value innate, genetically determined throughout evolution. In contrast, other signals have no intrinsic meaning and only acquire a particular emotional value through experience; their meaning may thus vary from individual to individual, and depends on the specific spatial and temporal context in which they appear. Although all sensory modalities can carry emotional information, acoustic stimuli are particularly well suited for efficiently conveying biologically relevant information, such as information about predators. For instance, the sound made by an approaching predator can be detected well before the animal enters the potential prey's field of view. This is due to the ability of auditory stimuli to signal distant events and their rapid transmission through the nervous system. However, acoustic signals are also useful in communicating between members of a species. In both human and non-human species, vocalizations are relied upon extensively in intra-species communication. In spite of the necessity of the sensory systems in processing biologically significant stimuli, emotional meaning requires that processing extend beyond the traditional sensory systems to structures such as the amygdala.

In this chapter, we describe what is currently known about the neural structures and mechanisms associated with the processing of emotional auditory information for stimuli with intrinsic or learned affective value. We focus on the amygdala, as this structure has been consistently shown to be a crucial component of the emotional brain, across several sensory modalities, in particular, within the auditory domain.

19.2 Fear conditioning

Most of what is known about the neural bases and mechanisms of auditory emotional processing has been learned through the use of aversive classical or Pavlovian conditioning. In this paradigm, also referred to as fear conditioning, an emotionally neutral stimulus (the conditioned stimulus; CS), such as a simple tone, is paired with an intrinsically noxious stimulus (the unconditioned stimulus; US), such as a mild electric shock, which elicits unconditioned defensive responses. Before conditioning, the CS does not elicit any overt behavioral reaction (except an initial orienting response). However, after a few pairings, sometimes as little as one, an association between the conditioned and unconditioned stimuli is formed, such that when the CS is presented alone, the individual will now exhibit a host of species-specific conditioned fear responses. That is, through conditioning, new stimuli that become warning signals for impending threat can gain access to evolutionary shaped defensive responses, allowing the individual to rapidly respond to, or even avoid, the dangerous situation.

In rats, conditioned fear responses include 'freezing' (i.e., absence of any movement except those associated with breathing), vocalizations, increase of heart rate, blood pressure, defecation, and the potentiation of reflexes such as the acoustic startle response (Blanchard and Blanchard, 1969; Kapp et al., 1979; LeDoux et al., 1988; Davis, 1992; Borszcz, 1995). In humans, some of the conditioned responses that are typically measured are muscle tension, pupil dilation, changes in heart rate, blood pressure, respiration and, most often, electrodermal or skin conductance responses, which are mediated by the sympathetic nervous system.

Fear conditioning not only is a powerful paradigm to study the neurobiology of emotional processing and learning in the healthy brain, but also has been proposed as a model to account, at least in part, for some of the key features associated with the development of certain psychiatric disorders involving a dysregulation of the fear system, such as phobias and post-traumatic stress disorder (Davis, 1992; Armony and LeDoux, 1997; Rasmusson and Charney, 1997; Brewin, 2001).

19.2.1 Neural circuits

There is a large body of literature pointing towards the amygdala as a critical structure for auditory fear conditioning. Disruption of this structure by permanent lesions or temporary inactivation disrupts the learning of the CS–US association and hence the development of conditioned fear. Interestingly, while bilateral lesions completely abolish conditioning, unilateral lesions result in a substantial, though partial, reduction of fear responses to the CS, with no significant differences between lesions in the right or left hemispheres (LaBar and LeDoux, 1996; Baker and Kim, 2004).

The amygdala is a relatively heterogeneous conglomerate of cells located in the depth of the anteromedial temporal lobe. Although there is still no consensus on its exact borders or the nomenclature of its nuclei, most researchers now agree that the amygdala is composed of about a dozen nuclei, each of them in turn subdivided into several subregions with unique architectonic, histochemical, and physiological characteristics (Pitkanen, 2000; De Olmos, 2004). The main features of the amygdala appear to have been highly conserved throughout evolution. Indeed, its basic structure and function is strikingly similar across mammals, including rodents, monkeys, and humans (Fig. 19.1). In fact, it has been suggested that other species, such as birds (Lowndes and Davies, 1994) and fish (Portavella et al., 2004), also have amygdala-like structures which mediate some aspect of their emotional behavior, in particular the acquisition and expression of conditioned fear responses.

An acoustic CS is transmitted from cochlear receptors through the brainstem to the auditory thalamus, the medial geniculate body (MGB). Information is then conveyed to the amygdala by way of two parallel routes (LeDoux, 1996). A direct projection originates primarily in the medial division of the MGB (MGm) and the associated posterior intralaminar nucleus (PIN). A second, indirect pathway involves projections from all areas of the MGB to the auditory cortex, from where, via several cortico-cortical links, information about the CS reaches the amygdala (see Fig. 19.2).

Both pathways terminate primarily in the lateral nucleus of the amygdala (LA), its main sensory input (LeDoux, 1990; Amaral et al., 1992; Bordi and LeDoux, 1992a; Romanski and LeDoux, 1993; Doron and LeDoux, 1999). Anatomical tracing and electrophysiological studies in rats have shown that projections from the MGm/PIN and auditory cortex often converge onto the same cells in LA (Li et al., 1996). These cells also receive somatosensory information about the US (Romanski et al., 1993), thus being well suited to integrate information about the CS (from both pathways) and the US during fear conditioning. Indeed, as we will see below, cells in LA exhibit conditioning-induced plasticity which is likely to be critical for learning the CS–US association. Interestingly, a substantial proportion of cells in PIN contribute to both pathways, that is, they project both to LA and to auditory cortex (Doron and LeDoux, 2000). Therefore, some of the information transmitted from the thalamus to the amygdala via the direct and indirect pathway

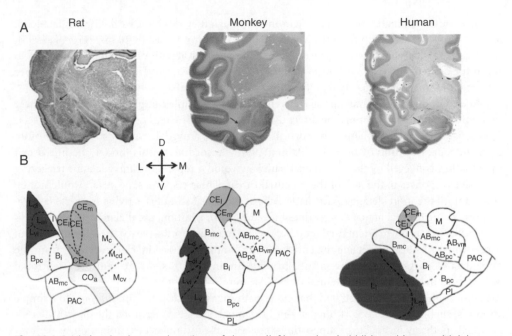

Fig. 19.1 A Nissl-stained coronal sections of the rat (*left*), monkey (*middle*), and human (*right*) brains, showing the location of the amygdala (*arrows* indicate the position of the lateral nucleus). **B** Schematic representation of the location of some of the main divisions of the amygdala in the three species. (Adapted with permission from Pitkanen and Kemppainen, 2002.) L Lateral nucleus; L_{dl} dorsolateral; L_{vl} ventrolateral; L_m medial; L_d dorsal; L_d dorsal intermediate; L_v ventral; L_{vi} ventral intermediate; L_l lateral; L_m medial; B basal nucleus; B_i intermediate; B_{pc} parvicellular; B_{mc} magnocellular; AB accessory basal nucleus; AB_{mc} magnocellular; AB_{pc} parvicellular; AB_{vm} ventromedial; M medial nucleus; M_c caudal; M_{cd} central, dorsal part; M_{cv} central, ventral part; CE central nucleus; CE_l lateral; CE_m medial; CE_i intermediate; CE_c capsular; PAC periamygdaloid cortex; CO_a anterior cortical nucleus; I intercalated nuclei; PL paralaminar nucleus.

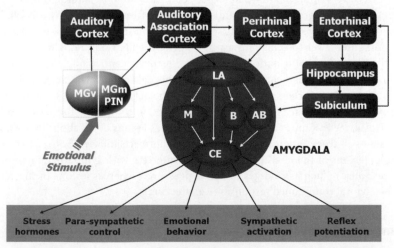

Fig. 19.2 Simplified diagram of the neural circuit involved in the processing of emotional auditory stimuli. LA Lateral nucleus of the amygdala; CE central nucleus of the amygdala.

originates and terminates in the same neurons, although they reach LA with different latencies. Monosynaptic transmission from the MGm/PIN to LA neurons is fast (< 10 ms) (Li *et al.*, 1995), whereas acoustic signals traveling through the indirect cortical pathway require longer time to reach the amygdala (>20 ms) (Quirk *et al.*, 1997). In contrast, this latter pathway has higher information processing capacity than the direct subcortical one.

These anatomical and physiological differences suggest possible complementary roles for these two routes in fear conditioning: the direct thalamic pathway provides rapid, but not very precise emotional information, whereas the cortical inputs to the amygdala convey a slower but more detailed representation of the CS (LeDoux, 1996). According to this model, the initial fast information conveyed by the subcortical pathway would 'prepare' the amygdala for triggering defensive responses in the face of the potential threat. These responses, however, would not be elicited until the more detailed information about the threat stimulus arriving from the cortical pathway confirms that actual danger does indeed exist. In addition, the thalamic pathway is less susceptible to top-down attentional modulation and may therefore serve to detect the presence of threat when this occurs outside the current focus of attention. Feedback projections from the amygdala to cortical areas may in turn provide an 'interrupt' signal to redirect attentional resources to the origin of the potential threat (Armony and LeDoux, 2000).

Lesion studies have demonstrated that either pathway is sufficient for conditioning to a simple stimulus, such as a pure tone (Romanski and LeDoux, 1992). Furthermore, the direct thalamo-amygdala pathway is capable of supporting some aspects of stimulus discrimination, as demonstrated by intact conditioning-induced frequency generalization behavioral gradients in animals with complete removal of auditory cortex (Armony *et al.*, 1997b). However, cortical inputs are likely to become crucial for higher levels of processing involving complex sounds, such as rising and falling FM tones (Whitfield, 1980; Rybalko *et al.*, 2006; Allen *et al.*, 2007). Further work is necessary to determine the full capacity and precise contribution of each pathway to fear conditioning.

For instance, in a recent study, Boatman and Kim (2006) showed that post-training lesions of the auditory cortex completely abolished freezing responses to a previously learned CS, whereas lesions of the MGm resulted in a significant, but not complete, reduction of fear responses. The authors concluded that, in the intact brain, it is the cortical pathway that mediates fear conditioning. It is important to point out, however, that these results were obtained after the animals had undergone extensive training: 30 CS–US pairings, compared to most studies which only use 1–10 conditioning trials. Furthermore, significant differences in freezing between cortical and thalamic animals were only observed during the first minute of an 8-min CS. Thus, the effects of post-training lesions after fewer CS–US pairings, and shorter CS durations, remain to be explored.

Within the amygdala, information flows from LA to the central nucleus (CE in Fig. 19.2) through direct projections as well as indirect intra-amygdala circuits (Pitkanen *et al.*, 1997; Pare *et al.*, 2004). The central nucleus can be thought of as the output module of the fear conditioning system, providing the interface with the systems involved in controlling the various conditioned responses (Davis, 1992; Kapp *et al.*, 1992). Thus, whereas lesions of CE abolish the expression of fear responses of all types, lesions of areas to which CE projects interfere with specific responses. For example, lesions of the lateral hypothalamus interfere with sympathetic nervous system mediated responses (such as changes in blood pressure), whereas lesions of the central gray eliminate behavioral conditioned responses (e.g., freezing).

19.3 Amygdala physiology

In rats, cells in LA, particularly those in the dorsal division, respond to simple auditory stimuli with short latencies (12–20 ms), which most likely correspond to direct inputs from the thalamus.

These early bursts are often followed by longer-latency responses (>20, often 60–100 ms) (Bordi and LeDoux, 1992b). Cells in LA tend to have very low spontaneous activity (<1 Hz) and relatively high thresholds (about 30–50 dB above the primary auditory system). Most LA neurons in the rat display broad frequency receptive fields, with a preference to high frequencies (>10 kHz). Interestingly, this range corresponds to that of the warning calls emitted by these animals when they are threatened (Blanchard et al., 1991). These observations suggest that amygdala cells may be tuned preferentially to respond to species-specific stimuli, particularly those with emotional content.

Consistent with their hypothesized role in emotional processing, amygdala cells usually habituate quickly to repeated presentations of the same neutral stimulus, but they respond strongly if the stimulus is changed, becomes less predictable (Herry et al., 2007), or if it acquires affective value (e.g., through conditioning). That is, these cells act as emotional novelty detectors: they respond quickly and strongly to new stimuli in the environment, but learn to ignore them if these have no biologically relevant consequences. Their low baseline rate and high threshold may serve as a safety mechanism to minimize the chances of false alarms. Indeed, it has been suggested that a hypersensitive amygdala may underlie some of the psychiatric disorders associated with a dysfunction of the fear system in humans (e.g., post-traumatic stress disorder, panic attacks, and phobias).

This proposed selectivity of amygdala cells for species-specific stimuli with affective value is also present in other species. For instance, conspecifics' meows are the most effective auditory stimuli to drive amygdala cells in a cat (Sawa and Delgado, 1963). Similarly, monkey vocalizations, especially those associated with distress (isolation peep and snake calls), elicit stronger neural responses in the monkey amygdala than other auditory stimuli, even after lesions of the inferior temporal cortex (Kling et al., 1987). Furthermore, as in rats, most auditory neurons in the lateral and basal nuclei of the monkey amygdala have a preference for unfamiliar stimuli, to which they habituate quickly (2 or 3 repetitions) if these sounds have no meaningful consequences (Nishijo et al., 1988). Although most neurons in the monkey amygdala respond preferentially to visual stimuli, a large proportion of them, especially those located within the central nucleus, are modulated by auditory information. For example, their responses to monkey dynamic facial expressions can be enhanced by the simultaneous presentation of the corresponding auditory vocalization (Kuraoka and Nakamura, 2007), an effect that is most pronounced in the case of fear-related stimuli (i.e., scream). These findings support the notion that the amygdala can integrate information from different sensory modalities to produce a supramodal representation of the stimuli in the environment and, in particular, their affective value.

19.4 Conditioning-induced plasticity

Complementing the findings from lesion studies, electrophysiological experiments have shown that neurons in the amygdala change their responses to the CS after fear conditioning. In particular, cells in the dorsal aspect of LA (LAd), the main target of MGm/PIN projections (Doron and LeDoux, 1999) and a site of CS–US convergence (Romanski et al., 1993), develop short-latency increases in response to a tone CS after it has been paired with a footshock US (Fig. 19.3A). The shortest latency of this plasticity is within 10–20 ms after tone onset (Quirk et al., 1995), most likely corresponding to inputs from the direct thalamo-amygdala pathway. These enhanced responses to the CS can already be observed after a few CS–US pairings (Quirk et al., 1997) and they persist even after extensive over-training (75 pairings) (Maren, 2001).

The majority of neurons exhibiting short-latency plasticity are located in the dorsal tip of LAd. These cells typically show a maximal response to the CS after a few conditioning trials and then

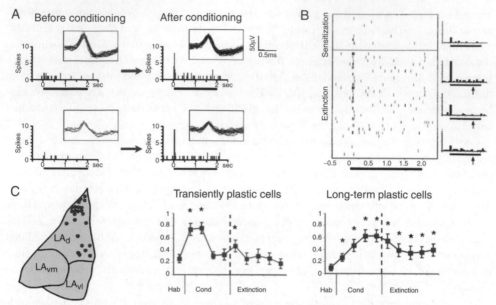

Fig. 19.3 A Peri-stimulus time histograms (PSTHs) and representative waveforms from two neurons recorded simultaneously in the lateral amygdala of a freely behaving rat before and after fear conditioning. Each histogram represents the sum of the cell's responses to 10 CSs (a 2-s pure tone, represented by the *black bar*). (Data from Quirk *et al.*, 1997.). **B** Raster plot showing the time course of the responses of an LA neuron to the CS across the conditioning experiment (pre-conditioning: 10 sensitization trials; post-conditioning: 30 extinction trials; conditioning phase not shown). Unit firing is summarized for 10-trial blocks in the PSTHs shown to the right of the raster plot (bin width, 100 ms). The *arrow* indicates the time of US presentation during conditioning. (Reproduced with permission from Quirk *et al.*, 1997.) **C** *Left* Anatomical recording locations for transiently plastic cells (*blue circles*) and long-term plastic cells (*red circles*) in the lateral nucleus of the amygdala. *Right* Mean CS-response for transiently and long-term plastic cells (*n* = 12 cells per group) throughout the three phases of the conditioning experiment. Each data point represents the average of four consecutive trials (except for the first point, which is the average of the final six trials of the pre-conditioning, habituation, session). *Error bars* represent the standard error of the mean. *Asterisks* indicate trial blocks during which the response was significantly greater than habituation levels (p < 0.05). (Adapted with permission from Repa *et al.*, 2001.)

again at the beginning of extinction (i.e., when the CS is presented alone, in the absence of the US (Fig. 19.3B; Quirk *et al.*, 1995). That is, neurons in the dorsal LAd respond strongly when the CS–US contingency is changing (at the beginning of conditioning and extinction), but return to their baseline levels when this relation remains constant (at the end of the conditioning and extinction phases). Thus, these 'transiently plastic cells' appear to signal the degree of CS–US association in relation to its recent history, acting as a differentiator or error detector between the predicted and experienced outcomes associated with the CS presentation (Quirk *et al.*, 1997). Interestingly, a group of cells further downstream in LAd exhibit a complementary behavior to that of the transiently plastic cells (Repa *et al.*, 2001). These 'long-term plastic cells', located mostly in the ventral portion of LAd, have longer latency responses to the CS (30–40 ms), suggesting they receive intra-amygdala and/or cortico-amygdala inputs, rather than direct monosynaptic thalamic information, and take a larger number of trials to reach their maximal firing rates.

In contrast, these cells maintain enhanced responses to the CS throughout conditioning and even during extinction (Fig. 19.3C).

Critically, plasticity in both cell types tends to precede changes in behavioral fear responses, demonstrating that physiological changes in LAd are not simply a reflection of the behavioral fear responses. This important issue was more directly investigated in a series of elegant experiments by Goosens *et al.* (2003). In the first one, rats initially underwent differential fear conditioning to two tones. In this paradigm, one stimulus is paired with the US and therefore becomes a conditioned stimulus (CS+), whereas another stimulus is also presented, but never paired with the US (the CS–). One group of animals (the control group) was later presented with the two CSs in a neutral (new) environment, whereas a second group (the experimental group) was tested in the chamber in which the original conditioning training took place. Because this context had itself acquired aversive value through contextual conditioning, rats in this latter group were in a state of fear and arousal during the presentation of both CSs. However, changes in LA firing were observed only for the CS+, while responses to CS– remained at the preconditioning levels, despite the high levels of behavioral fear. In fact, the degree of neural discrimination between CS+ and CS– in both groups was almost identical. In a second experiment, Goosens and colleagues showed that temporary inactivation of the central nucleus of the amygdala abolishes conditioned freezing, but does not interfere with the learning-related enhanced responses to the CS in LA. Taken together, these experiments demonstrate that behavioral fear is neither necessary nor sufficient for the expression of conditioning-induced changes in CS-elicited activity in LA neurons.

Importantly, the increase in responsivity of LA neurons to the CS is not due to a non-specific sensitization effect, but, rather, it depends on its direct association with the US. Neural responses to the CS are greater when this stimulus is explicitly paired with the US than when the CS and US are presented in an unpaired (random) fashion. That is, plasticity in LA neurons depends on the associative contingency between the CS and US. Furthermore, this conditioning-induced enhancement of auditory responses is specific to the CS (and similar stimuli). To directly asses this stimulus specificity, Pare and colleagues (Collins and Pare, 2000) conducted a differential conditioning experiment in awake cats while recording single unit activity and local field potentials in LA. They found that, in agreement with previous studies, the CS+ elicited greater neural firing and larger field potentials after conditioning. In contrast, conditioning caused a decrease in spike firing and field potentials in response to the CS–. This increase in firing rates to the CS+ accompanied by a decrease in response to other non-paired stimuli is consistent with the conditioning-induced shift in frequency receptive field previously reported in the LA (Bordi and LeDoux, 1993), MGm (Edeline and Weinberger, 1992), inferior colliculus (Xiao and Suga, 2005), and auditory cortex (Xiao and Suga, 2005; Weinberger, 2007; Chapter 18).

19.5 **Cellular mechanisms**

As described in the previous section, LA responses to a CS before conditioning are relatively weak, especially after a few repetitions of the same stimulus. In contrast, the same cell may exhibit robust and reliable activity when an aversive US is presented (Blair *et al.*, 2003). After a few CS–US pairings, however, CS inputs become stronger and therefore more efficient in driving LA neurons. These cells, in turn, can activate other circuits and structures downstream that will generate the appropriate fear responses to the CS in the absence of the US.

This associative change in the ability of the CS to drive LA neurons is very reminiscent of the notion of Hebbian plasticity. This rule, as originally postulated by D.O. Hebb, states that 'when an axon of cell A is near enough to excite a cell B and repeatedly or persistently takes part in firing it, some growth process or metabolic change takes place in one or both cells such that A's efficiency, as one of the cells firing *B*, is increased' (Hebb, 1949). In other words, *cells that fire together, wire together*. Hebbian plasticity has been proposed as a cellular mechanism for learning and memory, especially in classical conditioning. In particular, since its discovery about 30 years ago, long-term potentiation (LTP) has gained acceptance as an experimental model of Hebb's rule underlying memory formation (for a review see Sigurdsson *et al.*, 2007).

Indeed, some forms of LTP satisfy the key requirements of Hebb's theory: (1) it is associative, requiring simultaneous pre- and postsynaptic activity; (2) it is input-specific, in that synaptic strengthening occurs only at those synapses of the input cell that are coactive with the postsynaptic neuron; and (3) it can be long lasting, thus being a possible substrate of long-term memory storage. Although most of our understanding of LTP comes from studies in the hippocampus and neocortex, the main features of LTP have also been observed in the amygdala.

LTP has been shown to develop in LA following high-frequency stimulation of the auditory thalamic inputs in anesthetized animals (reviewed in Rodrigues *et al.*, 2004), and of both the thalamic and cortical pathways in awake freely behaving rats (Doyere *et al.*, 2003). Interestingly, LTP at the two pathways appears to have different properties. Soon after induction, LTP at cortical inputs is larger than at thalamic sites, but this difference disappears after 24 hours. Furthermore, it has been observed that while LTP decayed to baseline levels at the cortical input within 3 days, the thalamic pathway remained significantly potentiated for about a week (Fig. 19.4A,B). Whether these findings reflect intrinsic differences in the plasticity of the two pathways or, rather, they represent a differential sensitivity to experimental parameters remains to be determined. For instance, some stimulation protocols selectively induce LTP at the cortical but not thalamic inputs to LA (Humeau *et al.*, 2003), whereas the opposite pattern is obtained with others (Humeau *et al.*, 2005).

LTP has also been induced *in vitro* by stimulating the internal and external capsules, the putative sources of thalamic and cortical auditory inputs to LA, respectively. LTP has also been demonstrated by pairing a weak stimulation at either pathway with a strong depolarization of LA neurons. This form of LTP is of particular relevance for fear conditioning, as it could be thought to mimic the association between the auditory CS (the weak presynaptic stimulation) and the US (the strong postsynaptic depolarization). Further support for LTP as a plausible mechanism underlying auditory fear conditioning comes from studies showing that LTP produces an enhancement of auditory-evoked field potentials in LA, indicating that natural stimuli can make use of artificially induced plasticity (Fig. 19.4C). Most important, though, natural learning (e.g., fear conditioning) also enhances the processing of auditory stimuli in the same way. In summary, although further work remains to be conducted, there is currently strong evidence to support the hypothesis that LTP or LTP-like processes may underlie the synaptic plasticity observed in LA neurons during auditory fear conditioning.

19.6 **Other structures**

In addition to the amygdala, fear conditioning induces plasticity in other regions within the auditory system, such as the MGB and auditory cortex. Given that auditory information is conveyed by these structures to the amygdala, in particular the LA, it is possible that the observed plasticity in this region could be passively transmitted from either the auditory thalamus or cortex (for a more detailed review, see Maren and Quirk, 2004). In terms of cortical plasticity, Quirk and colleagues (1997) showed that the shortest-latency conditioning-induced changes in temporal area Te3, the first auditory cortical area in rat that projects to LA, happen at around 30–50 ms after CS onset, which is later than the earliest changes observed in LA (10–20 ms) (Fig. 19.5A). Furthermore, whereas LAd neurons develop significant changes within the first three CS–US

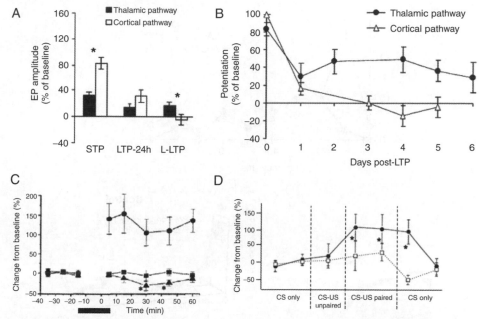

Fig. 19.4 A Mean potentiation of the thalamic (*black bars*) and cortical (*white bars*) afferents to LA in freely moving rats, 10 min (short-term potentiation, STP), 24 hours (long-term potentiation, LTP-24h), and 4–5 days (L-LTP) after stimulation. Potentiation was significantly larger in the cortical pathway after 10 min, but this effect was reversed after 4–5 days (* $p < 0.05$); no significant difference between pathways was present at 24 hours post-tetanus **B** Time course of LTP as a function of the number of days following high-frequency stimulation for the thalamic (*filled circles*) and cortical (*open triangles*) pathways. Each point represents the mean amplitude of the evoked potential, expressed as a percentage of the maximum potentiation for each pathway. (Adapted with permission from Doyere *et al.*, 2003.) **C** Group data showing percentage change from baseline of the slope of the auditory-evoked potentials in the lateral amygdala following electrical high-frequency simulation (*black bar*) of the MGm/PIN (*circles*). Control conditions consisted of recordings in the caudate/putamen (*triangles*), as well as in the lateral amygdala after low-frequency stimulation (*squares*). Only the high-frequency amygdala group showed a significant increase of evoked potential, relative to the pretreatment baseline measurement ($p < 0.05$), whereas a small transient decrease was observed in the caudate/putamen group (* $p < 0.05$). (Adapted with permission from Rogan and LeDoux, 1995.) **D** Slope of the negative-going CS-evoked potentials, normalized as a percentage of the mean pre-conditioning values. CS–US pairing resulted in a significant increase in slope in the experimental group ($n = 6$, *filled circles*) relative to pre-training levels, as well as compared to the control group ($n = 6$, *open squares*), in which the CS and US were never paired (* $p < 0.05$). *Error bars* represent the standard error of the mean. (Adapted with permission from Rogan *et al.*, 1997.)

pairings, cortical cells require between six and nine trials. These results rule out the possibility that LAd plasticity is simply a reflection of that of auditory cortex, as cells in the latter structure respond more slowly and need more pairings to exhibit similar plastic changes during conditioning than those in LA.

Moreover, in a follow-up experiment (Armony *et al.*, 1998), it was shown that some aspects of cortical plasticity are amygdala-dependent, as they are abolished in amygdalectomized animals. Namely, although short-latency (<50 ms) plasticity was still observed in auditory cortex (Te1, Te1v,

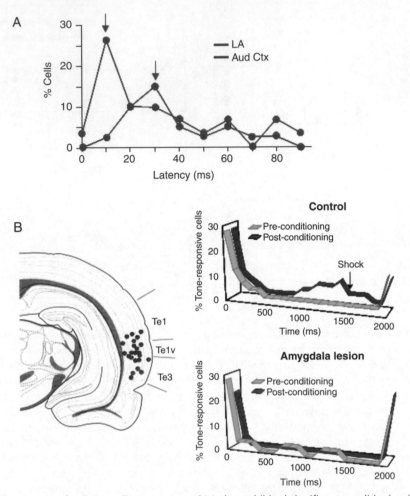

Fig. 19.5 A Percent of cells in auditory cortex and LA that exhibited significant conditioning-induced increased responses to the CS, plotted as a function of latency from tone onset. *Arrows* indicate peak conditioning latency for each region. (Adapted with permission from Quirk *et al.*, 1997.).
B *Left* Electrode placements within auditory cortex in control (*blue circles*) and amygdalectomized (*red circles*) animals undergoing fear conditioning. *Right* Plots showing the percentage of tone-responsive neurons in auditory cortex in control (*top*) and lesion (*bottom*) groups before and after fear conditioning, as a function of latency from CS onset (100 ms bin size). An increase in the proportion of cells showing an anticipatory response to the expected presentation of the US developed in control animals, even though no US was presented during the testing phase. In contrast, no conditioning-induced late responses were observed in rats with bilateral lesion of the amygdala. (Reproduced from Armony *et al.*, 1998.)

and Te3), long-latency responses (>500 ms) anticipating the delivery of the US were absent, together with any behavioral expression of fear (Fig. 19.5B). Although the behavioral significance of short- and long-latency plasticity in auditory cortex remains to be determined, it is possible that the former, amygdala-independent changes may correspond to a more 'cognitive' representation of the CS–US association (Weinberger, 2004), whereas the latter could reflect an amygdala-mediated interruption of ongoing processing in order to redirect processing and/or attentional resources to the imminent threat (Armony and LeDoux, 1997, 2000; Armony *et al.*, 1997a).

Thalamic plasticity also appears to be dependent on a functioning amygdala, as temporary inactivation of its basolateral complex during fear conditioning interferes with the development of plasticity in the MGm/PIN (Poremba and Gabriel, 1997, 2001; Maren *et al.*, 2001). Finally, it is important to point out that conditioning-induced plasticity is also observed in other amygdala subnuclei, such as the basal and central nuclei (Pascoe and Kapp, 1985; Muramoto *et al.*, 1993). Plasticity in these areas, however, occurs at later times than in LA (e.g., 30–50 ms after CS onset in the central nucleus (Pascoe and Kapp, 1985)).

19.7 **Computational model of fear conditioning**

Several of the key anatomical and physiological features of the fear conditioning circuit were incorporated into a computational model (Armony *et al.*, 1995), in order to derive a formal mathematical framework in which to explore, in a quantitative fashion, the relation between neurophysiology and behavior, as well as to make testable predictions. Computational units consisted of non-linear summation elements whose output was meant to represent the time-averaged firing rate of a neuron or small neural assembly. The units were organized in separate interconnected modules corresponding to the main neural structures of the auditory fear conditioning circuit, namely the lemniscal (MGv) and non-lemniscal (MGm/PIN) regions of the auditory thalamus, the auditory cortex, and the amygdala (Fig. 19.6A). Connections between units within a module were bidirectional and inhibitory (negative), whereas connections between modules were feedforward and excitatory (positive). The strength of the lateral inhibition was externally set for each module, and was used to capture the differences in the receptive fields (RFs) of the neurons of the different structures, namely broadly tuned units in the MGm/PIN and amygdala, and narrowly tuned ones in the MGv and auditory cortex.

The magnitude of the excitatory connections between pairs of units across layers were modified using a Hebbian learning rule with multiplicative normalization, so that connection strengths were increased between correlated units and decreased in the case of uncorrelated units. This rule, together with the nonmodifiable inhibitory connections between units within a module, results in a 'soft' competition between units so that the most active strengthen their weights at the expense of the weaker ones (Rumelhart and Zipser, 1986).

Auditory stimuli consisted of a set of pure tones of contiguous frequencies and equal intensities, along an arbitrary scale. They were represented by overlapping patterns of activations in the input layer. A noxious input, representing an aversive unconditioned stimulus (US) was modeled as an external ON/OFF unit projecting to the MGm/PIN and amygdala modules, providing an excitatory input of equal (fixed) intensity to all units in these modules. Behavioral response was modeled as the sum of the activations of the units in the amygdala module. Although admittedly simplistic, this output was intended to capture the fact that amygdala activation plays a key role in the behavioral expression of conditioned fear responses.

At the beginning of simulations, all modifiable weights were set to random values between zero and one, so that units responded, on average, equally but weakly to all input patterns. Training proceeded in three phases. During *development*, all auditory inputs were randomly presented, and the modifiable weights adjusted according to the rule described above until units developed stable receptive fields, mirroring those observed in actual cells in the different structures modeled. The US was not presented during this phase. During *conditioning* all auditory stimuli were presented again, but this time one of the tones was arbitrarily chosen as the CS, and thus paired with the presentation of the US. Finally, a *testing* phase took place where all the inputs were presented

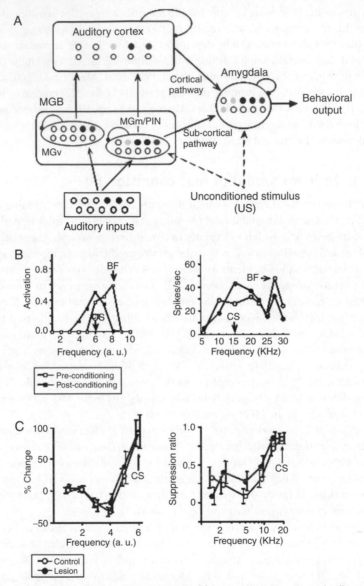

Fig. 19.6 A Architecture of a computational model of fear conditioning. *Gray shading* represents the magnitude of the activation of a unit (*black*: maximum activation; *white*: zero activation). *Dashed arrows* indicate excitatory, nonmodifiable connections. *Circular arrowheads* indicate mutual nonmodifiable inhibitory connections between units in each layer. (Adapted from Armony *et al.*, 1995, with permission of the American Psychological Association.) **B** Examples of conditioning-induced changes in receptive fields (RFs) of amygdala units in the computational model (*left*) and in rats (*right*). (Based on data from Bordi and LeDoux, 1993.) **C** Effects of auditory cortex lesions on the stimulus generalization gradient in the model (*left*) and in rats (*right*). (Adapted with permission from Armony *et al.*, 1997b.) MGv Ventral division of the medial geniculate body (MGB); MGm/PIN medial division of the MGB and posterior intralaminar nucleus; a.u. arbitrary units.

once, and receptive fields and behavioral responses measured in the absence of the US presentation. Weights were not modified during this session.

Comparison of receptive fields between development and testing phases revealed that, as a result of conditioning, several units developed frequency-specific changes in their RFs. Specifically, units in the MGm/PIN, auditory cortex, and amygdala modules whose RFs prior to conditioning included the CS showed a substantial increase in their response to the CS during testing, while their response to other stimuli either remained unchanged or decreased. In many cases, these changes resulted in a retuning of the RF, so that the BF shifted towards the CS (Fig. 19.6B). In contrast, those units whose original BFs were relatively distant from the CS, and thus did not respond to the CS before conditioning, did not show a significant change in their receptive fields. Because units in the MGv module did not receive US input either directly (i.e., MGM/PIN and amygdala) or indirectly (i.e., auditory cortex), they showed no significant changes following conditioning. In terms of behavior, the conditioning induced a significant increase in the model's response to the CS and neighboring frequencies, in the form of a stimulus generalization gradient (Fig. 19.6C). Notably, these results closely reproduced the physiological and behavioral findings observed in animal experiments (Fig. 19.6B).

In a follow-up experiment, designed to explore the relative contributions of the cortical and subcortical pathways to conditioning-induced amygdala plasticity and behavior, a lesion of the auditory cortex was simulated by setting the connections between the auditory cortex and amygdala units to zero throughout the conditioning phase. Interestingly, removal of the cortico-amygdala pathway did not significantly affect the width of the behavioral-stimulus generalization gradient (Fig. 19.3C). This result was somewhat surprising as once the auditory cortex was removed the only input to the amygdala came from the broadly tuned units in the MGm/PIN module and therefore should have resulted in the conditioned responses to generalize more broadly to auditory stimuli other than the CS. This counter-intuitive finding could be explained in terms of population coding; even though individual units in the MGm/PIN were poor frequency discriminators, the structure as a whole could provide a sufficient degree of stimulus discrimination and thus compensate for the loss of detailed stimulus information provided by the cortex. Notably, this prediction of the model was later verified experimentally (Armony et al., 1997b). Other anatomically based computational models have recently been developed to further explore the contribution of the subcortical and cortical inputs to the amygdala during emotional processing (den Dulk et al., 2003).

19.8 Human studies

Although most of our knowledge on the neurobiology of auditory emotional processing, in particular fear conditioning, comes from studies conducted in experimental animals, especially rodents, recent studies have confirmed that analogous brain regions and mechanisms are responsible for the processing of emotional information in humans.

19.8.1 Fear conditioning

Studies in patients with temporal lobe resection due to intractable epilepsy have provided direct support for the involvement of medial temporal lobe structures, including the amygdala in fear conditioning (LaBar et al., 1995). In a series of important studies, Damasio and colleagues further investigated the specific role of the amygdala in emotion in a patient suffering from lipoid proteinosis (Urbach-Wiethe disease), a very rare congenital syndrome characterized by the deposition of hyaline material in the skin and mouth areas, and which often causes bilateral calcifications in the medial temporal lobes. This particular patient, known as S.M., exhibited a complete and selective damage to both amygdalae, with a small lesion in the anterior entorhinal cortex (Tranel and Hyman, 1990). Importantly, neuropsychological evaluations revealed normal general intellect, language, and verbal memory function. In two differential fear conditioning experiments, using auditory and visual CSs (Bechara *et al.*, 1995), respectively, they showed that this patient was impaired in the acquisition of conditioned autonomic responses to the CS+, as measured by electrodermal activity, although she exhibited intact declarative memory for the conditioning procedure (e.g., which stimulus was paired with the US). Interestingly, the opposite pattern was found in a patient with hippocampal damage but intact amygdala, who developed normal conditioned physiological responses to the CS but showed no episodic memory of the CS–US pairing.

The critical role of the amygdala in human fear conditioning has also been demonstrated in the healthy brain through the use of hemodynamic-dependent functional neuroimaging techniques, especially positron emission tomography (PET) and functional magnetic resonance imaging (fMRI). These studies have consistently shown amygdala activation during fear conditioning across different modalities, including audition (for a review see Phelps and LeDoux, 2005). In contrast to electrophysiological techniques, however, fMRI and PET cannot be used to investigate the latencies of these conditioned responses, due to their limited temporal resolution. Nonetheless, the use of so-called event-related paradigms in fMRI has enabled researchers to investigate the time course of amygdala responses across conditioning trials. Interestingly some of these studies (Büchel *et al.*, 1998; LaBar *et al.*, 1998) reported an enhanced amygdala response to the CS only at the beginning of the conditioning session, as the activity returned to baseline levels in the later stages of the procedure. This temporal pattern of amygdala activation appears to be consistent with the behavior of the transiently plastic cells in LAd described in single-unit recordings in rats. Unfortunately, the source of these activations cannot be localized to particular amygdala subnuclei given the spatial resolution that is currently available with these neuroimaging methods (in the order of a few millimeters).

Fear conditioning also induces changes in human auditory cortex (Morris *et al.*, 1998; Armony and Dolan, 2001; Thiel *et al.*, 2002). Although the exact origin of this plasticity remains to be determined, connectivity analyses suggest that it may be amygdala-dependent (Morris *et al.*, 1998). A more direct test of this hypothesis would require measuring conditioning-induced plasticity in auditory cortex in patients with amygdala damage. Although this experiment has not been conducted yet, an fMRI experiment using visual threat-related stimuli (fearful faces) showed that the normally enhanced responses observed in the fusiform gyrus, a visual association area thought to be important for face processing, was abolished in individuals with amygdala sclerosis due to temporal lobe epilepsy (Vuilleumier *et al.*, 2004).

19.9 **Emotional vocalizations**

Most animals, including humans, use vocalizations to inform their conspecifics about important events and signals that arise in their environment (e.g., presence of food or a predator). In addition, vocalizations, together with facial expressions, represent a significant source of information about the emotional state, and intention, of the speaker. As such, the ability to accurately decode the emotional information carried by a vocalization is an essential aspect of social interactions and can even become crucial for survival. Nonlinguistic vocalizations constitute one type of vocalization that is particularly effective for this. Emotional nonlinguistic vocalizations – such as laughs, groans, or screams – are part of innate behaviors to communicate emotional states (Kreiman, 1997; Barr *et al.*, 2000) and can thus be thought of as the auditory equivalent of facial expressions (Belin *et al.*, 2004). Despite their importance, and in contrast to the large literature on facial expressions, nonlinguistic vocalizations have not been extensively studied in humans.

In particular, until recently, the question of whether the amygdala is involved in the evaluation of these stimuli, as it has been found to be the case in other animals, remained unanswered, as inconsistent findings had been reported both in lesion and neuroimaging studies.

For example, one study found that a patient with bilateral amygdala lesions (extending into the basal ganglia) due to epilepsy was impaired in the recognition of vocalizations of fear and anger (Scott et al., 1997), whereas another patient with bilateral gliosis in the region of amygdala (more pronounced in the right hemisphere) and a left thalamic lesion was only impaired on fear recognition. In fact, this patient was significantly better than controls in the recognition of vocalizations of anger (Sprengelmeyer et al., 1999). Finally, another patient was reported as showing intact recognition of vocalization of fear even though she was severely impaired in the evaluation of fearful facial expressions (Anderson and Phelps, 1998). Because of the varied nature and extent of the lesions in these three patients, it is difficult to draw definitive conclusions from these studies as to the role of the amygdala in the processing of negative emotional nonspeech vocalizations (see also Fowler et al., 2006).

The few functional neuroimaging studies of nonlinguistic emotional vocalizations conducted to date have also yielded conflicting results in terms of amygdala involvement. In an fMRI study, Phillips et al. (1998) found that the amygdala was activated bilaterally in response to both visual and auditory fearful expressions when compared to stimuli depicting mildly happy states, providing support for a supramodal role of this structure in the detection of threat-related stimuli. In contrast, a PET experiment by Morris et al. (1999) revealed decreased responses in the right amygdala to fear vocalizations, compared to the combination of happy, sad, and neutral sounds. The authors hypothesized that this decrease could reflect inhibitory signals to the amygdala from other structures, possibly prefrontal cortex. Given their previous findings of enhanced amygdala responses to fearful faces (Morris et al., 1996), they suggested, in contrast to the conclusions by Phillips et al., that differential, modality-specific neuronal dynamics are associated with the amygdala responses to fearful stimuli.

The role of the amygdala in the processing of other emotional vocalizations, especially laughter and crying, has also been subject to investigation, and controversy, using functional neuroimaging. In a series of experiments using slightly different paradigms and tasks, Sander and Scheich observed right (Sander et al., 2003b), left (Sander and Scheich, 2005), and bilateral (Sander and Scheich, 2001) amygdala activation to vocalizations of happiness and sadness. In contrast, Morris et al. (1999) found no significant activation in this structure in response to sad or happy sounds, as compared to neutral ones. Similarly, using event-related fMRI, Meyer et al. (2005) reported no significant changes in amygdala activity when contrasting laughs to either neutral speech or nonvocal sounds.

A number of technical issues are important to consider when interpreting the results from these studies. Most of them (Phillips et al., 1998; Morris et al., 1999; Sander and Scheich, 2001) used a block design in which vocalizations for each emotion were presented repeatedly for 30–60 s and in all studies only two speakers produced the stimuli. As mentioned earlier, neuroimaging studies have reported that the amygdala is sensitive to habituation when the same emotional category is continuously presented (Breiter et al., 1996; Büchel et al., 1998, 1999; Fischer et al., 2000), and neural habituation has been observed when the same speaker produces the stimuli (Belin and Zatorre, 2003). Moreover, most neuroimaging techniques rely on a subtractive approach, where the experimental condition is compared to a control. It has been shown that brain activation, including that of the amygdala, depends strongly on the specific control stimulus used (Sergerie et al., 2008). The studies described here used different control conditions, such as mildly happy vocalizations (Phillips et al., 1998), voiced nasal sounds (Morris et al., 1999), silence (Sander and Scheich, 2001), and speech or nonvocal sounds (Meyer et al., 2005).

In addition, individual differences may influence amygdala responses to nonlinguistic emotional vocalizations, and thus partly account for the apparent inconsistencies in the literature. For instance, whereas in women natural infant crying and laughing elicits stronger amygdala activation than un-natural (control) stimuli, the opposite pattern is observed for men (Sander *et al.*, 2007). In addition, parental status (and thus experience) may play a role: infant crying activates the right amygdala more than laughing in parents, while the reverse is true for nonparents (Seifritz *et al.*, 2003). The importance of control stimuli in neuroimaging to isolate the specific contribution of emotion to a stimulus-induced activation was highlighted by Lorberbaum *et al.* (2002) in a study of breast-feeding first-time mothers who showed significant amygdala activation to infant cries compared to silence. However, a similar activation was observed when contrasting the control stimuli (white noise) to silence, so that no significant effect was obtained when comparing crying to control sounds.

In a recent study, Fecteau *et al.* (2007) conducted an event-related fMRI experiment that attempted to overcome some of the limitations of previous studies. They used a large set of brief vocalizations which had been previously validated (Fecteau *et al.*, 2005) and that represented positive (happiness and sexual pleasure) or negative (fear and sadness) emotions, as well as emotionally neutral vocalizations (e.g., yawning, coughing). Critically, and unlike previous studies, each vocalization was produced by a different speaker, thus minimizing the chances of speaker-specific habituation effects, and presented in a pseudo-random order to reduce potential emotional priming, habituation, or expectation effects. In addition, they used neutral vocalizations as control stimuli to specifically identify the emotional contributions to any observed activations. Several acoustic parameters were also measured, including duration, mean energy, percent of unvoiced segments, fundamental frequency, harmonics-to-noise-ratio, etc. As expected, in some cases the neutral sounds differed from one or two of the emotional subcategories in terms of an acoustic parameter, a necessary compromise in order to keep the emotional stimuli ecologically valid. Importantly, however, the neutral stimuli were not significantly different from all the emotional categories for any single physical parameter, nor were they different from any emotional subcategory across all parameters. In contrast, neutral vocalizations were significantly different from all emotional sounds in terms of valence and emotional intensity.

Significant bilateral amygdala activation was associated with the presentation of emotional vocalizations (Fig. 19.7), when compared to neutral ones, which, as explained above, could not be due solely to acoustic differences. Post-hoc analyses revealed that the amygdala activation was equally driven by negative and positive vocalizations. The observed amygdala activation for vocalizations of fear and sadness was thus in agreement with some of the previous studies (Phillips *et al.*, 1998; Sander and Scheich, 2001, 2005; Sander *et al.*, 2003b), but inconsistent with another (Morris *et al.*, 1999). However, as mentioned earlier, this latter study compared vocalizations of fear with the combination of sad, happy, and neutral vocalizations. Given that the amygdala responds significantly to auditory expressions of happiness and sadness, as well as fear, the observed deactivation could instead reflect an activation associated with the opposite contrast (Gusnard *et al.*, 2001).

In summary, the observed amygdala activation to vocalizations of fear and sadness in several studies, together with electrophysiological recordings in experimental animals, provides further support for an involvement of this structure in the processing of negative emotional information, regardless of modality. This, however, does not imply the absence of any differences between sensory modalities in the neural responses to emotional stimuli. Indeed, as mentioned earlier, there is some evidence suggesting that in primates the amygdala responds preferentially to visual stimuli.

In contrast, the strong amygdala activation to positive vocalizations, including pleasure and laughter, appears to be at odds with the standard view of the amygdala as involved only in threat

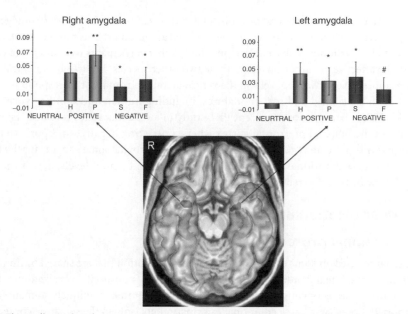

Fig. 19.7 Three-dimensional reconstruction of the significant bilateral amygdala activation associated with the presentation of nonlinguistic emotional vocalizations (*bottom*). Parameter estimates for the five sound categories. *Symbols* indicate the level of significance associated with the paired t-test between each emotional category and the neutral vocalizations: # $p < 0.1$; * $p < 0.05$; ** $p < 0.005$. H Happy; P pleasure; S sad; F fear. (Adapted with permission from Fecteau *et al.*, 2007.)

detection. However, the role of the amygdala in positive emotions, even within the visual domain, is still under debate (Baxter and Murray, 2002; Burgdorf and Panksepp, 2006). Indeed, an important literature has begun to emerge supporting an involvement of the amygdala in the processing of positive information across different modalities, such as static and dynamic facial expressions, linguistic nonauditory material, olfactory stimuli, taste, erotic film excerpts, and food stimuli (Murphy *et al.*, 2003; Phan *et al.*, 2004). Taken together, these findings appear to support a model in which the amygdala acts as a supramodal 'relevance detector' for biologically salient or meaningful events, independent of their valence (Sander *et al.*, 2003a).

An enhanced response to emotional vocalizations is also seen in cortical regions along the temporal lobes, including auditory cortex, superior temporal sulcus (STS), and superior temporal gyrus (STG). The activations in the STS are particularly interesting, as the anterior and middle aspects of this region have been shown to selectively respond to the human voice, with or without linguistic content (Belin *et al.*, 2000; Fecteau *et al.*, 2004). In particular, the right anterior STS has been shown to be involved in the analysis of nonverbal features of speech, such as the speaker's identity (Belin and Zatorre, 2003; Von Kriegstein *et al.*, 2003; Kriegstein and Giraud, 2004). Some of these findings have been integrated into a model (Schirmer and Kotz, 2006) proposing that emotional acoustic information is integrated in regions within the STS and STG, especially in the right hemisphere, to form an emotional 'gestalt,' which is then made accessible for higher-order cognitive processes, possibly taking place in the prefrontal cortex. As is the case of fear conditioning, further investigation is required to understand the exact causal relation between the responses to emotional vocalizations in temporal cortical regions and the amygdala.

Interestingly, some brain regions appear to support the processing of emotional vocalizations produced by different species. In a recent fMRI study, Belin and colleagues (2008) found an area within the human right ventrolateral orbitofrontal cortex that responded more strongly to negative than positive vocalizations of other humans, as well as cats and rhesus monkeys. Intriguingly, this differential activation was observed despite the fact that participants were unable to correctly categorize the affective vocalizations from these two other species. Electrophysiological recordings in macaques have shown that cells in the ventrolateral prefrontal cortex respond to complex stimuli in both visual and auditory modalities, including human and monkey vocalizations (Romanski, 2007). Furthermore, a recent PET study in awake macaques revealed a significant activation in ventromedial prefrontal cortex when contrasting negative and positive monkey vocalizations (Gil-da-Costa *et al.*, 2004). Thus, these results provide some support for the hypothesized continuity of emotional expression, at behavioral and neural levels, across the animal kingdom (Darwin, 1872, Owren and Rendall, 2001).

19.10 Other emotional stimuli

19.10.1 Emotional prosody

We have so far focused on some of the aspects of auditory emotion that are shared by humans and other animals, namely fear conditioning and the perception of conspecific vocalizations. There is, however, another means of conveying emotional information that is uniquely human: language (see Chapter 9). Speech can carry emotional information not only in the semantic content of the utterances (i.e., *what* is being said) but also in the modulation of intonation (i.e., *how* it is being said). Affective prosody refers to our ability to detect emotion in speech based on variations in pitch, loudness, and rhythm, regardless of the actual words being spoken. An influential model proposed by Ross (1981) posits that while language is lateralized to the left hemisphere (in the majority of people), prosody is processed in homologous regions within the right hemisphere. Although this model has received considerable experimental support, especially from lesion studies, several recent neuroimaging studies have suggested that decoding emotional prosody engages both hemispheres (Schirmer and Kotz, 2006). Studies in patients with focal brain lesions (Adolphs *et al.*, 2002) show that recognition of emotional information through prosody engages a distributed network of areas, mostly within the (right) frontal and parietal lobes (Fig. 19.8A). These conclusions are supported by the neuroimaging literature, which has reported activations in frontal areas, either in the right hemisphere or bilaterally, during evaluation of affective prosody (Kotz *et al.*, 2006).

There is relatively little support for a specific involvement of the amygdala in decoding emotional prosody. Although Scott *et al.* (1997) reported one patient who had impaired perception of positive (happiness) and negative (sadness, anger, fear) prosody, other patients with bilateral amygdala damage showed normal recognition of positive (Adolphs and Tranel, 1999; Adolphs *et al.*, 2001) and negative (Anderson and Phelps, 1998; Adolphs and Tranel, 1999; Adolphs *et al.*, 2001) prosody. In particular, patient S.M., who was severely impaired in auditory fear conditioning (see above), did not show any deficits in the evaluation of emotional prosody (Fig. 19.8C). Similarly, the majority of neuroimaging studies have failed to observe significant amygdala activity associated with emotional prosody recognition (Imaizumi *et al.*, 1997; Royet *et al.*, 2000, Pourtois *et al.*, 2005), although a small right amygdala activation in response to anger prosody has recently been reported (Sander *et al.*, 2005).

Deficits in recognition of emotional prosody have been observed in psychiatric populations. Individuals suffering from schizophrenia are impaired in the perception and expression of affective prosody. Whether this impairment is specific to emotional processing or a reflection of a more generalized deficit in auditory sensory processing is still under debate. Furthermore, there is some evidence, albeit conflicting, for a deficit in these patients in the recognition of emotional

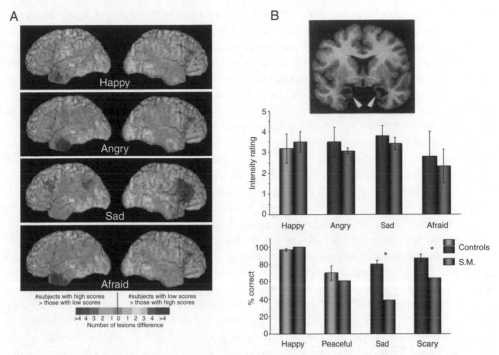

Fig. 19.8 A Lesion density maps comparing individuals with performances in the top half and bottom half of the distribution of the intensity ratings of the intended emotion conveyed by prosodic stimuli (e.g., how 'happy' a happy voice sounded). The *color* of each voxel represents the difference in the overlaps of lesions from the two groups. Cold colors (*green* to *blue*) indicate areas with a larger lesion overlap in individuals with performances in the top half of the rating distribution, whereas warm colors (*green* to *red*) represent larger overlap of lesions in participants in the bottom half. Data are derived from 55 individuals with unilateral brain lesions. (Adapted from Adolphs *et al.*, 2002, with permission of the American Psychological Association.) **B** MRI coronal section of patient S.M. showing her circumscribed and complete bilateral amygdala lesion. (Reproduced with permission from Adolphs *et al.*, 1994.) **C** Performance of S.M. and control subjects in the recognition of emotional prosody (*top*) and music (*bottom*). In the case of prosody, patient data represent the mean and standard deviation of three separate experiments. *Error bars* in the bottom graph represent the standard error of the mean. * $p < 0.001$. (Based on Adolphs and Tranel, 1999, and Gosselin *et al.*, 2007, respectively.)

facial expressions. Structural neuroimaging studies suggest that the impairments in emotional prosody in schizophrenia may be associated with abnormalities in the white matter tracts connecting the medial geniculate body and auditory cortex, as well as in the fibers communicating auditory cortical regions with temporal and frontal areas, along the so-called ventral and dorsal auditory streams (Leitman *et al.*, 2007).

19.10.2 Music

Another class of emotional acoustic stimuli that is arguably unique to humans is music. The past few years have seen a growing interest in the neural correlates of music perception and, in particular, the use of musical stimuli to induce emotions. Blood *et al.* (1999) conducted a PET experiment to investigate the brain correlates of emotional perception of novel musical melodies along the pleasantness/unpleasantness dimension (determined by the degree of dissonance of the stimuli) in individuals without professional musical training. Activations in right parahippocampal gyrus and precuneus were associated with increased unpleasantness (dissonance), whereas activity in frontal regions, including bilateral orbitofrontal cortex, was correlated with the degree of pleasantness (consonance) of the musical melodies.

In a more recent experiment (Koelsch *et al.*, 2006), employing a similar paradigm (although the original stimuli were natural music excerpts), unpleasant music was associated with activations in the medial temporal lobes, including the hippocampus and parahippocampal gyrus, the temporal poles, and, interestingly, the amygdala (Fig. 19.9). Pleasant music elicited enhanced responses in the insula and the ventral striatum, as well as several frontal cortical regions. The ventral striatum activation, also observed in other studies using pleasant music (Blood *et al.*, 1999; Brown *et al.*, 2004; Mitterschiffthaler *et al.*, 2007) and normal vs scrambled music (Menon and Levitin, 2005), is consistent with the established role of this structure (specifically the nucleus accumbens) in the processing of reward-related stimuli (Knutson and Cooper, 2005).

In contrast to the study of Koelsch *et al.* (2006), Blood and colleagues did not observe amygdala activation in response to unpleasant music. However, in another study by the same group (Blood and Zatorre, 2001), amygdala *deactivation* was found to be associated with the experience of 'chills' (shivers down the spine) evoked by highly pleasant music (Fig. 19.9). These findings thus suggest that the role of the amygdala in (negative) emotional processing of auditory stimuli may also apply to music. Further support for this notion comes from studies of individuals with temporal lobe lesions (Gosselin *et al.*, 2005) and a patient with bilateral amygdala damage (Gosselin *et al.*, 2007) showing impaired recognition of 'scary' music (Fig. 19.8C). In the latter case, a deficit in recognition of sad music was also observed, consistent with a recent fMRI study reporting amygdala activation to sad musical stimuli (Mitterschiffthaler *et al.*, 2007; Fig. 19.9). Thus, although there is some evidence for an involvement of the amygdala in the perception of emotional, particularly negative, music, the results are so far inconclusive. Further research is therefore necessary to resolve this outstanding question. In particular, it would be very interesting to assess the similarities and differences in the neural processing of the emotional information conveyed by prosody and music.

19.11 **Conclusions**

One of the most important roles of sensory processing is the conveyance of biologically significant information to the brain. Danger, sex, food, and safety are all signaled by sensory events. However, the emotional significance of such events requires processing beyond the traditional sensory system in areas such as the amygdala. Indeed, the amygdala responds preferentially to innate, species-specific affective vocalizations, as well as to stimuli that have acquired biological relevance through learning (e.g., fear conditioning). In humans, emotional information can also be carried by other means within the auditory domain, such as prosody and music, although the role of the amygdala in the processing of these stimuli remains unclear. Interestingly, much of emotional information processing by the amygdala appears to be similar between different sensory modalities, particularly audition and vision (although some differences do exist), and between species. This suggests that the amygdala may be part of a supramodal emotional brain network that has remained fairly conserved throughout evolution. Future studies should help further identify the similarities and differences in the neural processing of emotional information across modalities and species.

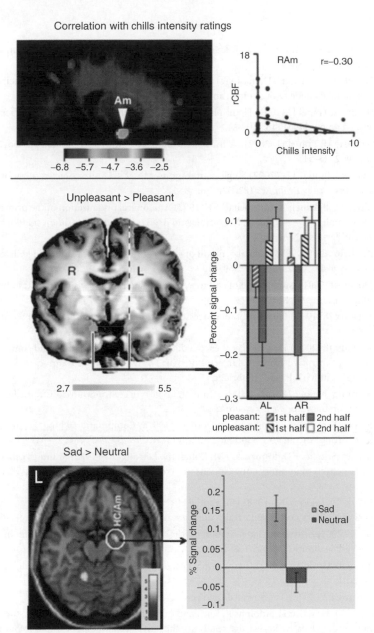

Fig. 19.9 Statistical parametric maps showing amygdala activation associated with emotional music. **A** Negative correlation between regional cerebral blood flow (rCBF) in the right amygdala and subjects' ratings of 'chills' (see text) intensity for musical pieces. (Reproduced with permission from Blood and Zatorre, 2001, copyright 2001 National Academy of Sciences, USA.) **B** Bilateral amygdala activation associated with the contrast unpleasant vs pleasant music. (Reproduced with permission from Koelsch *et al.*, 2006.) **C** Right amygdala activation for the comparison of sad vs neutral music. (Reproduced with permission from Mitterschiffthaler *et al.*, 2007.)

References

Adolphs R, Tranel D (1999) Intact recognition of emotional prosody following amygdala damage. *Neuropsychologia* **37**: 1285–92.

Adolphs R, Tranel D, Damasio H, Damasio A (1994) Impaired recognition of emotion in facial expressions following bilateral damage to the human amygdala. *Nature* **372**: 669–72.

Adolphs R, Jansari A, Tranel D (2001) Hemispheric perception of emotional valence from facial expressions. *Neuropsychology* **15**: 516–24.

Adolphs R, Damasio H, Tranel D (2002) Neural systems for recognition of emotional prosody: a 3-D lesion study. *Emotion* **2**: 23–51.

Allen TA, Furtak SC, Brown TH (2007) Single-unit responses to 22 kHz ultrasonic vocalizations in rat perirhinal cortex. *Behav Brain Res* **182**: 327–36.

Amaral DG, Price JL, Pitkanen A, Carmichael ST (1992) Anatomical organization of the primate amygdaloid complex. *The Amygdala: Neurobiological Aspects of Emotion, Memory, and Mental Dysfunction*. Wiley-Liss, New York.

Anderson AK, Phelps EA (1998) Intact recognition of vocal expressions of fear following bilateral lesions of the human amygdala. *NeuroReport* **9**: 3607–13.

Armony JL, Dolan RJ (2001) Modulation of auditory neural responses by a visual context in human fear conditioning. *Neuroreport* **12**: 3407–11.

Armony JL, LeDoux JE (1997) How the brain processes emotional information. *Ann N Y Acad Sci* **821**: 259–70.

Armony JL, LeDoux JE (2000) How danger is encoded: towards a systems, cellular, and computational understanding of cognitive-emotional interactions. In: *The New Cognitive Neurosciences*, 2nd edn (ed. Gazzaniga MS). The MIT Press, Cambridge.

Armony JL, Servan-Schreiber D, Cohen JD, LeDoux JE (1995) An anatomically constrained neural network model of fear conditioning. *Behav Neurosci* **109**: 246–57.

Armony JL, Servan-Schreiber D, Cohen JD, Le Doux JE (1997a) Computational modeling of emotion: explorations through the anatomy and physiology of fear. *Trends Cogn Sci* **1**: 28–34.

Armony JL, Servan-Schreiber D, Romanski LM, Cohen JD, LeDoux JE (1997b) Stimulus generalization of fear responses: effects of auditory cortex lesions in a computational model and in rats. *Cereb Cortex* **7**: 157–65.

Armony JL, Quirk GJ, LeDoux JE (1998) Differential effects of amygdala lesions on early and late plastic components of auditory cortex spike trains during fear conditioning. *J Neurosci* **18**: 2592–601.

Baker KB, Kim JJ (2004) Amygdalar lateralization in fear conditioning: evidence for greater involvement of the right amygdala. *Behav Neurosci* **118**: 15–23.

Barr RG, Hopkins B, Green JA (2000) *Crying as a Sign, a Symptom, and a Signal*. Cambridge University Press, New York.

Baxter MG, Murray EA (2002) The amygdala and reward. *Nat Rev Neurosci* **3**: 563–73.

Bechara A, Tranel D, Damasio H, Adolphs R, Rockland C, Damasio AR (1995) Double dissociation of conditioning and declarative knowledge relative to the amygdala and hippocampus in humans. *Science* **269**: 1115–8.

Belin P, Zatorre RJ (2003) Adaptation to speaker's voice in right anterior temporal lobe. *Neuroreport* **14**: 2105–9.

Belin P, Zatorre RJ, Lafallie P, Ahad P, Pike B (2000) Voice-selective areas in human auditory cortex. *Nature* **403**: 309–12.

Belin P, Fecteau S, Bedard C (2004) Thinking the voice: neural correlates of voice perception. *Trends Cogn Sci* **8**: 129–35.

Belin P, Fecteau S, Charest I, Nicastro N, Hauser MD, Armony JL (2008) Human cerebral response to animal affective vocalizations. *Proc R Soc B* **275**: 473–81.

Blair HT, Tinkelman A, Moita MA, LeDoux JE (2003) Associative plasticity in neurons of the lateral amygdala during auditory fear conditioning. *Ann N Y Acad Sci* **985**: 485–7.

Blanchard RJ, Blanchard DC (1969) Crouching as an index of fear. *J Comp Physiol Psychol* **67**: 370–5.

Blanchard RJ, Weiss S, Agullana R, Flores T, Blanchard DC (1991) Antipredator ultrasounds: sex differences and drug effects. *Neurosci Abstr* **17**: 878.

Blood AJ, Zatorre RJ (2001) Intensely pleasurable responses to music correlate with activity in brain regions implicated in reward and emotion. *Proc Natl Acad Sci USA* **98**: 11818–23.

Blood AJ, Zatorre RJ, Bermudez P, Evans AC (1999) Emotional responses to pleasant and unpleasant music correlate with activity in paralimbic brain regions. *Nat Neurosci* **2**: 382–7.

Boatman JA, Kim JJ (2006) A thalamo-cortico-amygdala pathway mediates auditory fear conditioning in the intact brain. *Eur J Neurosci* **24**: 894–900.

Bordi F, LeDoux J (1992a) Sensory tuning beyond the sensory system: an initial analysis of auditory properties of neurons in the lateral amygdaloid nucleus and overlying areas of the striatum. *J Neurosci* **12**: 2493–503.

Bordi F, LeDoux J (1992b) Sensory tuning beyond the sensory system: an initial analysis of auditory response properties of neurons in the lateral amygdaloid nucleus and overlying areas of the striatum. *J Neurosci* **12**: 2493–503.

Bordi F, LeDoux JE (1993) Sensory-specific conditioned plasticity in lateral amygdala neurons. *Soc Neurosci Abstr* **19**: 1227.

Borszcz GS (1995) Pavlovian conditional vocalizations of the rat: a model system for analyzing the fear of pain. *Behav Neurosci* **109**: 648–62.

Breiter HC, Etcoff NL, Whalen PJ, *et al.* (1996) Response and habituation of the human amygdala during visual processing of facial expression. *Neuron* **17**: 875–87.

Brewin CR (2001) A cognitive neuroscience account of posttraumatic stress disorder and its treatment. *Behav Res Ther* **39**: 373–93.

Brown S, Martinez MJ, Parsons LM (2004) Passive music listening spontaneously engages limbic and paralimbic systems. *NeuroReport* **15**: 2033–7.

Büchel C, Morris J, Dolan RJ, Friston KJ (1998b) Brain systems mediating aversive conditioning: an event-related fMRI study. *Neuron* **20**: 947–57.

Büchel C, Dolan RJ, Armony JL, Friston KJ (1999) Amygdala-hippocampal involvement in human aversive trace conditioning revealed through event-related functional magnetic resonance imaging. *J Neurosci* **19**: 10869–76.

Burgdorf J, Panksepp J (2006) The neurobiology of positive emotions. *Neurosci Biobehav Rev* **30**: 173–87.

Collins DR, Pare D (2000) Differential fear conditioning induces reciprocal changes in the sensory responses of lateral amygdala neurons to the CS(+) and CS(−). *Learn Mem* **7**: 97–103.

Darwin C (1872) *The Expression of the Emotions in Man and Animals*. John Murray, London.

Davis M (1992) The role of the amygdala in fear-potentiated startle: implications for animal models of anxiety. *Trend Pharmacol Sci* **13**: 35–41.

De Olmos JS (2004) Amygdala. In: *The Human Nervous System*, 2nd edn (eds Paxinos G, Mai J). Elsevier Academic Press, San Diego.

Den Dulk P, Heerebout BT, Phaf RH (2003) A computational study into the evolution of dual-route dynamics for affective processing. *J Cogn Neurosci* **15**: 194–208.

Doron NN, LeDoux JE (1999) Organization of projections to the lateral amygdala from auditory and visual areas of the thalamus in the rat. *J Comp Neurol* **412**: 383–409.

Doron NN, LeDoux JE (2000) Cells in the posterior thalamus project to both amygdala and temporal cortex: a quantitative retrograde double-labeling study in the rat. *J Comp Neurol* **425**: 257–74.

Doyere V, Schafe GE, Sigurdsson T, LeDoux JE (2003) Long-term potentiation in freely moving rats reveals asymmetries in thalamic and cortical inputs to Edeline J-M, Weinberger NM (1992) Associative retuning in the thalamic source of input to the amygdala and auditory cortex: receptive field plasticity in the medial division of the medial geniculate body. *Behav Neurosci* **106**: 81–105.

Fecteau S, Armony JL, Joanette Y, Belin P (2004) Is voice processing species-specific in human auditory cortex? An fMRI study. *NeuroImage* **23**: 840–8.

Fecteau S, Armony JL, Joanette Y, Belin P (2005) Judgment of emotional nonlinguistic vocalizations: age-related differences. *Appl Neuropsychol* **12**: 40–8.

Fecteau S, Belin P, Joanette Y, Armony JL (2007) Amygdala responses to nonlinguistic emotional vocalizations. *Neuroimage* **36**: 480–7.

Fischer H, Furmark T, Wik G, Fredrikson M (2000) Brain representation of habituation to repeated complex visual stimulation studied with PET. *NeuroReport* **11**: 123–6.

Fowler HL, Baker GA, Tipples J, *et al.* (2006) Recognition of emotion with temporal lobe epilepsy and asymmetrical amygdala damage. *Epilep Behav* **9**: 164–72.

Gil-da-Costa R, Braun A, Lopes M, *et al.* (2004) Toward an evolutionary perspective on conceptual representation: species-specific calls activate visual and affective processing systems in the macaque. *Proc Natl Acad Sci USA* **101**: 17516–21.

Goosens KA, Hobin JA, Maren S (2003) Auditory-evoked spike firing in the lateral amygdala and Pavlovian fear conditioning: mnemonic code or fear bias? *Neuron* **40**: 1013–22.

Gosselin N, Peretz I, Noulhiane, *et al.* (2005) Impaired recognition of scary music following unilateral temporal lobe excision. *Brain* **128**: 628–40.

Gosselin N, Peretz I, Johnsen E, Adolphs R (2007) Amygdala damage impairs emotion recognition from music. *Neuropsychologia* **45**: 236–44.

Gusnard DA, Raichle ME, Raichle ME (2001) Searching for a baseline: functional imaging and the resting human brain. *Nat Rev Neurosci* **2**: 685–94.

Hebb DO (1949) *The Organization of Behavior*. John Wiley, New York.

Herry C, Bach DR, Esposito F, *et al.* (2007) Processing of temporal unpredictability in human and animal amygdala. *J Neurosci* **27**: 5958–66.

Humeau Y, Shaban H, Bissiere S, Luthi A (2003) Presynaptic induction of heterosynaptic associative plasticity in the mammalian brain. *Nature* **426**: 841–5.

Humeau Y, Herry C, Kemp N, *et al.* (2005) Dendritic spine heterogeneity determines afferent-specific Hebbian plasticity in the amygdala. *Neuron* **45**: 119–31.

Imaizumi S, Mori K, Kiritani S, Yumoto M (1997) Observation of neural processes of auditory scene analysis by magnetoencephalography. *Acta Oto-Laryngol Suppl* 106–8.

Kapp BS, Frysinger RC, Gallagher M, Haselton JR (1979) Amygdala central nucleus lesions: effect on heart rate conditioning in the rabbit. *Physiol Behav* **23**: 1109–17.

Kapp BS, Whalen PJ, Supple WF, Pascoe JP (1992) Amygdaloid contributions to conditioned arousal and sensory information processing. In: *The Amygdala: Neurobiological Aspects of Emotion, Memory, and Mental Dysfunction* (ed. Aggleton JP). Wiley-Liss, New York.

Kling AS, Lloyd RL, Perryman KM (1987) Slow wave changes in amygdala to visual, auditory, and social stimuli following lesions of the inferior temporal cortex in squirrel monkey (*Saimiri sciureus*). *Behav Neural Biol* **47**: 54–72.

Knutson B, Cooper JC (2005) Functional magnetic resonance imaging of reward prediction. *Curr Opin Neurol* **18**: 411–7.

Koelsch S, Fritz T, Dy VC, Muller K, Friederici AD (2006) Investigating emotion with music: an fMRI study. *Hum Brain Mapp* **27**: 239–50.

Kotz SA, Meyer M, Paulmann S (2006) Lateralization of emotional prosody in the brain: an overview and synopsis on the impact of study design. *Prog Brain Res* **156**: 285–94.

Kreiman J (1997) Listening to voices: theory and practice in voice perception research. In: *Talker Variability in Speech Research* (eds Johnson K, Mullenix J). Academic Press, New York.

Kriegstein KV, Giraud AL (2004) Distinct functional substrates along the right superior temporal sulcus for the processing of voices. *Neuroimage* **22**: 948–55.

Kuraoka K, Nakamura K (2007) Responses of single neurons in monkey amygdala to facial and vocal emotions. *J Neurophysiol* **97**: 1379–87.

LaBar KS, LeDoux JE (1996) Partial disruption of fear conditioning in rats with unilateral amygdala damage: correspondence with unilateral temporal lobectomy in humans. *Behav Neurosci* **110**: 991–7.

LaBar KS, LeDoux JE, Spencer DD, Phelps EA (1995) Impaired fear conditioning following unilateral temporal lobectomy in humans. *J Neurosci* **15**: 6846–55.

LaBar KS, Gatenby JC, Gore JC, LeDoux JE, Phelps EA (1998) Human amygdala activation during conditioned fear acquisition and extinction: a mixed-trial fMRI study. *Neuron* **20**: 937–45.

LeDoux JE (1990) Information flow from sensation to emotion: plasticity in the neural computation of stimulus value. In: *Learning and Computational Neuroscience: Foundations of Adaptive Networks* (eds Gabriel M, Moore J). MIT Press, Cambridge.

LeDoux JE (1996) *The Emotional Brain*. Simon and Schuster, New York.

LeDoux JE, Iwata J, Cicchetti P, Reis DJ (1988) Different projections of the central amygdaloid nucleus mediate autonomic and behavioral correlates of conditioned fear. *J Neurosci* **8**: 2517–29.

Leitman DI, Hoptman MJ, Foxe JJ, *et al.* (2007) The neural substrates of impaired prosodic detection in schizophrenia and its sensorial antecedents. *Am J Psychiatry* **164**: 474–82.

Li XF, Phillips R, LeDoux JE (1995) NMDA and non-NMDA receptors contribute to synaptic transmission between the medial geniculate body and the lateral nucleus of the amygdala. *Exp Brain Res* **105**: 87–100.

Li XF, Stutzmann GE, LeDoux JE (1996) Convergent but temporally separated inputs to lateral amygdala neurons from the auditory thalamus and auditory cortex use different postsynaptic receptors: *in vivo* intracellular and extracellular recordings in fear conditioning pathways. *Learn Mem* **3**: 229–42.

Lorberbaum JP, Newman JD, Horwitz AR, *et al.* (2002) A potential role for thalamocingulate circuitry in human maternal behavior. *Biol Psychiatry* **51**: 431–45.

Lowndes M, Davies DC (1994) The effects of archistriatal lesions on one-trial passive avoidance learning in the chick. *Eur J Neurosci* **6**: 525–30.

Maren S (2001) Is there savings for Pavlovian fear conditioning after neurotoxic basolateral amygdala lesions in rats? *Neurobiol Learn Mem* **76**: 268–83.

Maren S, Quirk GJ (2004) Neuronal signalling of fear memory. *Nat Rev Neurosci* **5**: 844–52.

Maren S, Yap SA, Goosens KA (2001) The amygdala is essential for the development of neuronal plasticity in the medial geniculate nucleus during auditory fear conditioning in rats. *J Neurosci* **21**: RC135.

Menon V, Levitin DJ (2005) The rewards of music listening: response and physiological connectivity of the mesolimbic system. *Neuroimage* **28**: 175–84.

Meyer M, Zysset S, von Cramon DY, Alter K (2005) Distinct fMRI responses to laughter, speech, and sounds along the human peri-sylvian cortex. *Cogn Brain Res* **24**: 291–306.

Mitterschiffthaler MT, Fu CH, Dalton JA, Andrew CM, Williams SC (2007) A functional MRI study of happy and sad affective states induced by classical music. *Hum Brain Mapp* **28**: 1150–62.

Morris JS, Frith CD, Perrett DI, *et al.* (1996) A differential neural response in the human amygdala to fearful and happy facial expressions. *Nature* **383**: 812–5.

Morris JS, Friston KJ, Dolan RJ (1998) Experience-dependent modulation of tonotopic neural responses in human auditory cortex. *Proc Biol Sci* **265**: 649–57.

Morris JS, Scott SK, Dolan RJ (1999) Saying it with feeling: neural responses to emotional vocalizations. *Neuropsychologia* **37**: 1155–63.

Muramoto K, Ono T, Nishijo H, Fukuda M (1993) Rat amygdaloid neuron responses during auditory discrimination. *Neuroscience* **52**: 621–36.

Murphy FC, Nimmo-Smith I, Lawrence AD (2003) Functional neuroanatomy of emotions: a meta-analysis. *Cogn Affect Behav Neurosci* **3**: 207–33.

Nishijo H, Ono T, Nishino H (1988) Single neuron responses in amygdala of alert monkey during complex sensory stimulation with affective significance. *J Neurosci* **8**: 3570–83.

Owren MJ, Rendall D (2001) Sound on the rebound: bringing form and function back to the forefront in understanding nonhuman primate vocal signaling. *Evol Anthrop* **10**: 58–71.

Pare D, Quirk GJ, LeDoux JE (2004) New vistas on amygdala networks in conditioned fear. *J Neurophysiol* **92**: 1–9.

Pascoe JP, Kapp BS (1985) Electrophysiological characteristics of amygdaloid central nucleus neurons during Pavlovian fear conditioning in the rabbit. *Behav Brain Res* **16**: 117–33.

Phan KL, Wager TD, Taylor SF, Liberzon I (2004) Functional neuroimaging studies of human emotions. *CNS Spectr* **9**: 258–66.

Phelps EA, LeDoux JE (2005) Contributions of the amygdala to emotion processing: from animal models to human behavior. *Neuron* **48**: 175–87.

Phillips ML, Young AW, Scott SK, *et al.* (1998) Neural responses to facial and vocal expressions of fear and disgust. *Proc R Soc Biol Sci Ser B* **265**: 1809–17.

Pitkanen A (2000) Connectivity of the rat amygdaloid complex. In: *The Amygdala. A Functional Analysis* (ed. Aggleton JP). Oxford University Press, New York.

Pitkanen A, Kemppainen S (2002) Comparison of the distribution of calcium-binding proteins and intrinsic connectivity in the lateral nucleus of the rat, monkey, and human amygdala. *Pharmacol Biochem Behav* **71**: 369–77.

Pitkanen A, Savander V, LeDoux JE (1997) Organization of intra-amygdaloid circuitries in the rat: an emerging framework for understanding functions of the amygdala. *Trends Neurosci* **20**: 517–23.

Poremba A, Gabriel M (1997) Amygdalar lesions block discriminative avoidance learning and cingulothalamic training-induced neuronal plasticity in rabbits. *J Neurosci* **17**: 5237–44.

Poremba A, Gabriel M (2001) Amygdalar efferents initiate auditory thalamic discriminative training-induced neuronal activity. *J Neurosci* **21**: 270–8.

Portavella M, Torres B, Salas C (2004) Avoidance response in goldfish: emotional and temporal involvement of medial and lateral telencephalic pallium. *J Neurosci* **24**: 2335–42.

Pourtois G, De Gelder B, Bol A, Crommelinck M (2005) Perception of facial expressions and voices and of their combination in the human brain. *Cortex* **41**: 49–59.

Quirk GJ, Repa C, LeDoux JE (1995) Fear conditioning enhances short-latency auditory responses of lateral amygdala neurons: parallel recordings in the freely behaving rat. *Neuron* **15**: 1029–39.

Quirk GJ, Armony JL, LeDoux JE (1997) Fear conditioning enhances different temporal components of tone-evoked spike trains in auditory cortex and lateral amygdala. *Neuron* **19**: 613–24.

Rasmusson AM, Charney DS (1997) Animal models of relevance to PTSD. *Ann N Y Acad Sci* **821**: 332–51.

Repa JC, Muller J, Apergis J, Desrochers TM, Zhou Y, LeDoux JE (2001) Two different lateral amygdala cell populations contribute to the initiation and storage of memory. *Nat Neurosci* **4**: 724–31.

Rodrigues SM, Schafe GE, LeDoux JE (2004) Molecular mechanisms underlying emotional learning and memory in the lateral amygdala. *Neuron* **44**: 75–91.

Rogan MT, LeDoux JE (1995) LTP is accompanied by commensurate enhancement of auditory-evoked responses in a fear conditioning circuit. *Neuron* **15**: 127–36.

Rogan MT, Staubli UV, LeDoux JE (1997) Fear conditioning induces associative long-term potentiation in the amygdala. *Nature* **390**: 604–7.

Romanski LM (2007) Representation and integration of auditory and visual stimuli in the primate ventral lateral prefrontal cortex. *Cereb Cortex* **17**(1): i61–69.

Romanski LM, LeDoux JE (1992) Equipotentiality of thalamo-amygdala and thalamo-cortico-amygdala circuits in auditory fear conditioning. *J Neurosci* **12**: 4501–9.

Romanski LM, LeDoux JE (1993) Information cascade from primary auditory cortex to the amygdala: corticocortical and corticoamygdaloid projections of temporal cortex in the rat. *Cereb Cortex* **3**: 515–32.

Romanski LM, LeDoux JE, Clugnet MC, Bordi F (1993) Somatosensory and auditory convergence in the lateral nucleus of the amygdala. *Behav Neurosci* **107**: 444–50.

Ross ED (1981) The aprosodias. Functional-anatomic organization of the affective components of language in the right hemisphere. *Arch Neurol* **38**: 561–9.

Royet JP, Zald D, Versace R, *et al.* (2000) Emotional responses to pleasant and unpleasant olfactory, visual, and auditory stimuli: a positron emission tomography study. *J Neurosci* **20**: 7752–9.

Rumelhart DE, Zipser D (1986) Feature discovery by competitive learning. In: *Parallel Distributed Processing. Volume 1: Foundations* (eds Rumelhart DE, Mcclelland JL). The MIT Press, Boston.

Rybalko N, Suta D, Nwabueze-Ogbo F, Syka J (2006) Effect of auditory cortex lesions on the discrimination of frequency-modulated tones in rats. *Eur J Neurosci* **23**: 1614–22.

Sander K, Scheich H (2001) Auditory perception of laughing and crying activates human amygdala regardless of attentional state. *Brain Res Cogn Brain Res* **12**: 181–98.

Sander K, Scheich H (2005) Left auditory cortex and amygdala, but right insula dominance for human laughing and crying. *J Cogn Neurosci* **17**: 1519–31.

Sander D, Grafman J, Zalla T (2003a) The human amygdala: an evolved system for relevance detection. *Rev Neurosci* **14**: 303–16.

Sander D, Grandjean D, Pourtois G, *et al.* (2005) Emotion and attention interactions in social cognition: brain regions involved in processing anger prosody. *NeuroImage* **28**: 848–58.

Sander K, Brechmann A, Scheich H (2003b) Audition of laughing and crying leads to right amygdala activation in a low-noise fMRI setting. *Brain Res Brain Res Protoc* **11**: 81–91.

Sander K, Frome Y, Scheich H (2007) FMRI activations of amygdala, cingulate cortex, and auditory cortex by infant laughing and crying. *Hum Brain Mapp* **28**(10): 1007–22.

Sawa M, Delgado JM (1963) Amygdala unitary activity in the unrestrained cat. *Electroencephalogr Clin Neurophysiol* **15**: 637–50.

Schirmer A, Kotz SA (2006) Beyond the right hemisphere: brain mechanisms mediating vocal emotional processing. *Trend Cogn Sci* **10**: 24–30.

Scott SK, Young AW, Calder AJ, Hellawell DJ, Aggleton JP, Johnson M (1997) Impaired auditory recognition of fear and anger fellowing bilateral amygdala lesions. *Nature* **385**: 254–7.

Seifritz E, Esposito F, Neuhoff JG, *et al.* (2003) Differential sex-independent amygdala response to infant crying and laughing in parents versus nonparents. *Biol Psychiatry* **54**: 1367–75.

Sergerie K, Chochol C, Armony JL (2008) The role of the amygdala in emotional processing: a quantitative meta-analysis of functional neuroimaging studies. *Neurosci Biobehav Rev* **32**: 811–30.

Sigurdsson T, Doyere V, Cain CK, LeDoux JE (2007) Long-term potentiation in the amygdala: a cellular mechanism of fear learning and memory. *Neuropharmacology* **52**: 215–27.

Sprengelmeyer R, Young AW, Schroeder U, *et al.* (1999) Knowing no fear. *Proc Biol Sci* **266**: 2451–6.

Thiel CM, Friston KJ, Dolan RJ (2002) Cholinergic modulation of experience-dependent plasticity in human auditory cortex. *Neuron* **35**: 567–74.

Tranel D, Hyman BT (1990) Neuropsychological correlates of bilateral amygdala damage. *Arch Neurol* **47**: 349–55.

Von Kriegstein K, Eger E, Kleinschmidt A, Giraud AL (2003) Modulation of neural responses to speech by directing attention to voices or verbal content. *Cogn Brain Res* **17**: 48–55.

Vuilleumier P, Richardson MP, Armony JL, Driver J, Dolan RJ (2004) Distant influences of amygdala lesion on visual cortical activation during emotional face processing. *Nat Neurosci* **7**: 1271–8.

Weinberger NM (2004) Specific long-term memory traces in primary auditory cortex. *Nat Rev Neurosci* **5**: 279–90.

Weinberger NM (2007) Associative representational plasticity in the auditory cortex: a synthesis of two disciplines. *Learn Mem* **14**: 1–16.

Whitfield IC (1980) Auditory cortex and the pitch of complex tones. *J Acoust Soc Am* **67**: 644–7.

Xiao Z, Suga N (2005) Asymmetry in corticofugal modulation of frequency-tuning in mustached bat auditory system. *Proc Natl Acad Sci USA* **102**: 19162–7.

Section 6

Pathology of the auditory brain and its treatment

Chapter 20

Disorders of the auditory brain

Timothy D. Griffiths, Doris-Eva Bamiou, and
Jason D. Warren

20.1 Introduction

For the purposes of this chapter we define the auditory brain or central auditory system as the auditory system beyond the cochlea. In clinical practice we do not have the precision of workers studying the normal anatomy, physiology, and regional organization of the auditory system using invasive techniques. Nevertheless, we argue that a systematic approach to disordered processing in the ascending pathway and cortex allows characterization of disorders in terms that are congruent with ideas developed in the rest of this book.

The current exercise might be represented as the study of abnormal *auditory cognition*. During normal auditory cognition the incoming sound information in temporal, spectral, and spatial domains must be organized into a form that allows perception, recognition, attention, working memory, learning, and anterograde memory. The normal bases for perception and recognition are much better understood than the other processes. Like most syntheses we focus primarily on disorders of perception and recognition, whilst acknowledging the likely existence of other types of disorder of the auditory brain that are not currently understood in such detail.

20.2 Clinical assessment of disorders of the auditory brain

20.2.1 History and neurological examination

As in any other neurological disorder the history and physical examination is critical and can of itself allow valuable information about diagnosis. Many of the diagnoses considered in this chapter can be made on the basis of a clear and detailed history from the patient and his/her relatives, where this is supported by further tests that are determined by the initial assessment. The tests are rarely sufficient in themselves to establish the diagnosis, and even when they are, the correct test has to be chosen based on the history. A good example of this is in the case of auditory agnosia following stroke. The history will often suggest problems with single word, music, or environmental sound comprehension in the absence of new deafness before any detailed behavioural testing, which will realistically need to be targeted on the relevant symptoms in a clinical setting.

It is important to obtain the history and neurological examination before the detailed psychophysical testing: the latter is time consuming and it is not realistic in real clinical settings to carry out screening psychoacoustic testing using all possible measures. A robust battery for the assessment of adult disorders (Griffiths *et al.*, 2001) has not been widely taken up, primarily because of the inflexibility of this approach. The approach currently under development in our joint clinic is based on modular assessment with audiological evaluation at its core to which additional acoustic tests are added based on the history. As such, the added tests represent tests of hypotheses about affected domains that arise from the clinical history. The approach is directly comparable with other aspects of cognitive neurology in which there are core neuropsychological tasks, like the Wechsler Adult Intelligence Scale (Wechsler, 1997) to which other measures of domains such as memory and executive dysfunction might be added depending on the clinical scenario. A maxim from cognitive neurology also applies, that the proper assessment of (auditory) cognition requires testing of (auditory) cognition, and that brain imaging is not an adequate investigation in itself. We describe a number of disorders of auditory cognition below that are not accompanied by abnormal structural imaging.

The assessment of disorders of the central auditory system in our clinic is a multidisciplinary exercise, involving a key collaboration between neurology and audiological medicine. We do not feel in any sense dogmatic, however, about the way in which these disorders 'should' be approached. The assessment of these disorders may require a number of different inputs, for example from audiology, otolaryngology, speech and language therapy, clinical neurophysiology, and psychiatry. These different specialties employ different models of patient assessment and that might be an argument for the development of standardized interviews for assessment. However, such interviews can be unwieldy and all we would stress here is the need to consider symptoms carefully before embarking on investigations.

Any assessment of a suspected disorder of the central auditory system should begin with an assessment of symptomatic deficits that suggest dysfunction of the cochlear or vestibular end organs (deafness, difficulty hearing talkers in noise, recruitment, tinnitus, or vertigo). Deficits within particular domains should also be sought, such as deficits in speech, music, and environmental sound comprehension, and also deficits in spatial analysis.

20.2.2 Audiological assessment

Patients with a suspected disorder of the central auditory system require audiological evaluation of middle ear and cochlear function to exclude disordered processing at this level as an explanation for the symptoms. This is not always as straightforward as it sounds. Audiological assessment also includes tests of auditory nerve function and the integrity of the auditory brainstem.

A pure tone audiogram (PTA) can identify hearing loss due to external or middle ear pathology (conductive), or to pathology of the cochlea and auditory nerve. However, an abnormal PTA will not distinguish between hearing loss due to cochlea and auditory nerve dysfunction, and normal results do not guarantee intact cochlear or auditory nerve function. Moreover, abnormal audiometry is not an exclusion criterion for central auditory pathology. First, an abnormal PTA may co-exist with, but be unrelated to, a central auditory disorder: acquired disorders of auditory perception following cortical stroke tend to occur in an elderly population with separate cochlear damage. Second, in rare cases, the abnormal PTA may be directly caused by the central auditory lesion, as in deafness due to brainstem, midbrain, or bilateral cortical lesions.

Speech audiometry assesses the ability of subjects to recognize words (consonant-vowel-consonant sounds) as a function of intensity by repetition or pointing to pictures. Normal subjects show a sigmoid function that can be shifted to the right in conductive or cochlear deafness. Speech audiometry can be helpful in acoustic nerve lesions such as auditory neuropathy, when there may be a normal PTA and an abnormal speech audiogram, but that can also occur in disorders affecting other points in that pathway up to and including cortex. In auditory neuropathy a 'rollover' in speech audiometry (speech recognition scores becoming worse at higher sound levels than the level of the optimal speech recognition score) can be a helpful additional diagnostic feature.

Assessment of cochlear function may include otoacoustic emissions (OAEs) and electrical tests of cochlear function. OAEs are emitted sounds recorded in the ear canal that reflect outer hair cell function (provided middle ear function is satisfactory) (Kemp, 2002). They can even be recorded if the auditory nerve has been sectioned (Martin *et al.*, 1999). Electrocochleography records the electrical responses of the cochlea and auditory nerve to sound. It has components related to basilar member motion and hair cell function (cochlear microphonic and summating potential) and the action potential in the proximal auditory nerve (compound action potential).

The audiological assessment of patients with a suspected disorder of the central auditory system will also often include brainstem reflexes. OAE suppression by noise tests the reduction in the OAE due to noise stimulation of the ipsi- or contralateral ear. This tests the integrity of the efferent olivocochlear system. Acoustic stimulation reduces the amplitude of OAEs, via afferent fibers from the cochlea to the superior olivary complex and efferent fibers from the superior olivary complex, mostly via the medial olivocochlear bundle to the ipsi- and contralateral cochlea (Ryan *et al.*, 1991). The acoustic or stapedial reflex involves sound-elicited stapedius contraction via a pathway comprising the auditory nerve, cochlear nucleus, superior olivary complex, and ipsi- and contra-lateral medial facial nerve motoneurons. Acoustic (or stapedial) reflexes are recorded using a tympanometer. The reflexes can be absent or require louder evoking stimuli than normal in acoustic nerve lesions (Cohen and Prasher, 1988).

Brainstem processing can also be tested using auditory evoked potentials to clicks. These are electrical recordings from the scalp reflecting sequential activity in the ascending auditory pathway in the 10–15 ms following click stimulation. The waveform consists of seven major peaks, with wave I corresponding to the compound action potential recorded using electrocochleography and wave II arising from the proximal part of the auditory nerve. The later waves may have multiple generators; however, wave III is thought to arise from the cochlear nucleus, wave IV mainly from the superior olivary complex, wave V from the lateral lemniscus, and waves VI and VII from the inferior colliculus (Moller and Jannetta, 1983). A delay between waves I and III would thus indicate possible pathology of the auditory nerve, while a delay between waves III and V would indicate a brainstem lesion.

The responses depend on synchronized firing in nerves and tracts and can therefore be degraded by loss of synchrony (for example, due to demyelination in auditory neuropathy, which if severe can lead to conduction block). An early evoked response to clicks can still occur in auditory neuropathy, when it reflects the cochlear microphonic response (Berlin and Hood, 2001). In addition to these responses to clicks, the potential usefulness of brainstem responses to speech stimuli in central disorders has been emphasized (Johnson *et al.*, 2007).

20.2.3 Psychoacoustics

There is no general psychoacoustic schedule that is appropriate for any patient with a suspected disorder of the central auditory system. In clinical practice, as opposed to research settings, a major limitation is the amount of time that can be realistically spent on assessment. Most psychoacoustic techniques are developed by using normal volunteers: it is a very different proposition to assess, say, children with suspected developmental disorder or patients after neurological insult, neither of whom are prepared to spend large amounts of time in a sound-proof booth. Part of the possible solution is the targeting of tests based on the features brought up in the history. The other part of the solution is the use of appropriate psychoacoustic measures for the deficit sought.

Criterion-free methods, in which there is always a reference sound to allow an objective measure of the perceived change in a sound, allow the robust assessment of the perception of auditory cues. Cues such as frequency change (Foxton *et al.*, 2004; Moore *et al.*, 2008) modulation detection (Witton *et al.*, 1998; Talcott *et al.*, 2000), gap detection (Musiek *et al.*, 2005), and forward and backward masking (Wright *et al.*, 1997; Amitay *et al.*, 2006; Johnson *et al.*, 2007) have been assessed in a number of disorders in which abnormal central auditory function is implicated.

These cues can be varied continuously and assessed using robust criterion-free methods based on multiple intervals, including one 'target' interval containing a change. Methods include two-interval-two-alternative forced choice (2I2AFC) (e.g. Griffiths *et al.*, 2001) and three-interval designs. Three-interval designs are well suited to naïve listeners and patients: subjects do not need to remember the acoustic features they are listening out for from trial to trial. One type of three-interval design called AXB is based on two alternatives and includes a central reference (X) and preceding (A) and following (B) intervals containing either a sound that matches the reference or a sound that differs from it (e.g. Hill *et al.*, 2005; Amitay *et al.*, 2006). Another type of three-interval design is a three-alternative 'odd one out' task (e.g. Amitay *et al.*, 2006; Moore *et al.*, 2008) where any of three intervals can contain the altered cue.

A number of psychoacoustic paradigms can be used to determine measures of perception and attention from two- and three-interval designs. The method of constant stimuli is based on varying the cue change in the target interval randomly. The method allows fitting of psychometric functions using maximum likelihood estimation (Wichmann and Hill, 2001) from which detection thresholds (75% in the case of two-alternative designs) can be calculated. If the method is being used to measure perceptual threshold, 20 trials per point may be sufficient (Treutwein and Stasburger, 1999). In addition to estimates of the perceptual threshold, the method can yield measures of attention in terms of the lapse rate for large stimulus change and measures of the variance of the threshold, but these require greater numbers of trials per point to be reliable than for threshold.

The method of constant stimuli can be time consuming and requires naïve listeners to apply themselves for extended periods. It also requires an initial estimate of the appropriate range of stimulus change and it is not robust to rapid changes in threshold that can occur during initial assessment (Hawkey *et al.*, 2004). More widely used in clinical work than the method of constant stimuli are adaptive tracking ('staircase') procedures. These can also be based on two- or three-interval designs and start with a large stimulus change. The task is made harder after a certain number of correct responses and easier after a number of incorrect ones, so that a typical track will move to increasingly smaller stimulus change and then fluctuate up and down around a given threshold. The main advantage of adaptive tracking paradigms is that they can give quicker estimates of threshold than full functions.

Most natural sounds contain a number of cues: the criterion-free measures described above can only be applied to single cues varied continuously. Criterion-free techniques are valuable for investigating the analysis of sound cues such as frequency, temporal structure, intensity, and lateralization that are relevant to the perception of the acoustic world. However, patients do not complain of problems with frequency, temporal structure, intensity, and lateralization: they complain of difficulties with the distinction, recognition, and localization of natural sounds such as speech and environmental sounds.

These types of deficit can be investigated in robust ways, but the investigation is a significant departure from usual criterion-free methods. Natural sounds differ from each other in a number of dimensions that can be characterized using the technique of multidimensional scaling (MDS) (Grey, 1977; Caclin *et al.*, 2005). Essentially, this involves pairwise judgements of the degree of difference between sounds that are then arranged in an *n* dimensional space where the degree of dissimilarity between sounds is represented by the degree of physical separation. The technique is not dependent on any assumptions about what aspects of sounds cause them to sound different. However, the dimensions determined by MDS can be examined to determine whether the dimension corresponds to any systematic variation of acoustic properties. For musical sounds with the same pitch, the dimensions of timbre space have been argued to correspond to the spectrum of the sound (characterized by the spectral centroid), the temporal envelope (attack and decay), and changes in spectral centroid over time. Caclin *et al.* (2005) also emphasized the relevance of the fine-spectral structure.

Multidimensional scaling has not been widely used to assess the perception of natural sounds in clinical populations, although one study (Samson *et al.*, 2002) has assessed the effect of temporal lobectomy on timbre analysis using the technique, and suggested a deficit in the analysis of both temporal envelope and spectrum due to right temporal lobe lesions in a well-defined research group. More generally in clinical studies, the perception of sound objects can be assessed by the use of 'random pair' designs where subjects make same/different discriminations between pairs of sounds without quantification of the difference as in multidimensional scaling. Such designs do not allow the calculation of thresholds, but do allow the use of ethological sounds and the rapid assessment of high-level deficits that might occur in cortical disorders.

The assessment of auditory agnosia (impaired recognition of sounds in the absence of deafness) requires the assessment of both discrimination and recognition. Problems with discrimination occur in apperceptive agnosia, a perceptual form of agnosia, when there will also be associated deficits in recognition. In associative agnosia, discrimination is intact, but there will be a dissociated deficit in recognition due to a deficit in the attribution of semantic labels to sounds in the absence of any deficit in perception.

In addition to the use of random-pair design, the perception of ethological sounds can be investigated using sounds that have similar complexity in frequency and time structure to natural sounds, but where such sounds are created synthetically in such a way that specific dimensions of timbre can be explored systematically. Using such an approach (which might be called the investigation of 'prototimbre') we have characterized a deficit in timbre perception (Griffiths *et al.*, 2007) in a patient following a right temporal lobe stroke. The approach can allow the determination of thresholds for the detection of dimensions of timbre processing in the same way as the detection of auditory cues such as frequency or temporal gaps.

Disorders of the central auditory system will often affect speech perception. A number of aphasia batteries are available for the analysis of speech that are beyond the scope of this chapter. Essentially, these systematize the clinical assessment of speech comprehension, repetition, and naming in a way that is appropriate for patients with acquired lesions and degenerative disorders. It is worth pointing out, however, that the assessment of these two types of speech disorder are not necessarily both characterized adequately by a single type of assessment, and that clinical schedules for aphasia have been primarily developed for use in aphasia following stroke (Hillis, 2007).

The assessment of musical analysis is problematic for a number of reasons. Unlike speech and language, where a certain baseline of common experience and aptitude can be assumed, this is not the case with music, where subjects have a wide variety of background training and exposure. It is therefore difficult to develop a musical equivalent of standard aphasia batteries. A battery that has been employed widely is the Montreal Battery for the Evaluation of Amusia (MBEA) (Peretz *et al.*, 2003). The tests are based on a same/different random-pairs design based on novel melodies to overcome issues related to previous musical exposure. The tests were developed based on considerations from musicology. Dowling and Harwood (1985) developed a theory of melodic perception in which the assessment of contour (the pattern of 'ups' and 'downs' in pitch, often referred to as global structure in much of the literature) and the absolute of pitch values (often referred to as local structure) are processed serially. The MBEA contains subtests that assess contour analysis (where the different pairs of melodies have different contour), absolute pitch value analysis (where the different pairs of melodies have the same contour), and key structure (where the different pairs of melodies show key violation).

20.2.4 Cortical evoked potentials and EEG

In addition to EEG responses to clicks that correspond to brainstem analysis, responses corresponding to cortical analysis can be helpful in localizing deficits in disorders of the central auditory system. The earliest middle latency response recorded using surface EEG, Na, arises from primary auditory cortex in the medial part of Heschl's gyrus: responses at a similar latency of about, 20 ms have been recorded directly from primary cortex in patients with depth electrodes for epilepsy investigation (Howard *et al.*, 2000). Middle latency responses may be absent in patients with central deafness, when the brainstem responses will be preserved. The later N1 response to clicks and tones arises from the planum temporale (Lutkenhoner and Steinstrater, 1998) and has a latency of approximately 100 ms. The N1 is a robust response and useful indicator of the presence of an intact pathway up to and including auditory association cortex.

'Oddball' paradigms, based on streams of acoustic stimuli comprising common 'standards' and rare 'deviants', elicit two types of difference response: the early mismatch negativity (MMN) at about 130 ms and the later P3 response with a latency of 300 ms. The MMN can be characterized as an online sensory memory trace (for a comprehensive review see Naatanen, 2003) and has a large component that is independent of attention, whilst the P300 is highly influenced by attention. Both measures have been used to assess a number of neurological and psychiatric conditions that involve the cortex, and the responses have been useful in clinical research settings to characterize disorders in terms of online auditory processing and auditory attention. The clinical application is limited to the level of individual patients, however, by the fact that normal subjects can sometimes have absent MMN responses, preventing robust single-subject inference based on the absence of these responses. Other measures of auditory cognition that have been used to assess cortical clinical disorders include steady-state responses to modulated sound (Stefanatos *et al.*, 1997).

Continuous EEG is sometimes needed to seek evidence of abnormal epileptic activity that might be associated with auditory processing disorders. Rarely, auditory phenomena may be the primary manifestation of focal seizure activity, as in musical hallucinations due to epilepsy (Erkwoh *et al.*, 1993). In children with acquired disorders of complex sound perception and language, EEG is important to exclude the rare condition of Landau-Kleffner syndrome or acquired epileptic aphasia. In that case a sleep study may be required (Smith and Hoeppner, 2003). Other examples of links between auditory phenomena and epilepsy are given in the section below on 'Epilepsy'. In all cases in which an association between transient central auditory phenomena and epilepsy is sought the association can only be confirmed or refuted absolutely if a recording is made at the same time as the phenomenon, which might require EEG telemetry. In general, however, there is no routine indication for EEG in the evaluation of central auditory disorders in adults.

20.2.5 Structural MRI

Structural imaging is essential in the assessment of subjects with suspected disorders of the central auditory system. The history, clinical evaluation, and acoustic tests will yield a characterization of auditory abnormalities and hypotheses about their cause that can be tested by the use of structural imaging. Vascular and inflammatory lesions are best demonstrated by specific MRI sequences (high resolution T2 and proton-density weighted), and the sensitivity may be further increased by the use of Gadolinium contrast. As noted above, however, disorders of the central auditory system are not necessarily accompanied by any abnormality of structural imaging (e.g. see section 20.3.5).

20.2.6 Functional imaging

A criticism of functional imaging techniques (functional MRI and magnetoencephalography, MEG) applied to auditory analysis is that these have not led to direct immediate clinical applications. That criticism is reasonable, although we would argue that functional imaging has lead to significant advances in our understanding of the brain analysis of complex sound that provides an anatomical and functional framework within which cortical disorders (in particular) can be understood. The argument is developed in detail in the case of musical disorders in Stewart *et al.* (2006). Such frameworks, in turn, allow the development of behavioural measures of auditory cortical disorders. In general, however, there is no current routine clinical application for auditory functional imaging.

20.3 **Specific auditory deficits**

We consider here a number of disorders that are defined on the basis of deficits in auditory cognition, before considering in section 20.4 disorders defined on the basis of positive auditory symptoms. Section 20.5 discusses abnormal auditory cognition in common clinical disorders in which the auditory features do not define the disorder. In the current section we have made an effort to define auditory deficits in terms of the level in the system at which they are caused. That is not always straightforward and we consider in section 20.3.5 the need for a diagnostic category to describe disorders of central auditory processing for which a clear neural substrate has not been identified.

20.3.1 **Auditory nerve**

Auditory neuropathy

Auditory neuropathy (AN) or auditory dys-synchrony refers to the disorder of listening caused by disordered conduction in the auditory nerve with relatively preserved outer hair cell function and cochlear amplification (Starr *et al.*, 1996; Berlin *et al.*, 2003). Diagnosis of AN is made on the basis of all three of the following criteria, as well as exclusion of other potential causes by appropriate investigations, such as a brain MRI (Sininger and Oba, 2001): (1) poor auditory nerve function demonstrated by abnormal auditory evoked potentials and elevated or absent stapedial reflexes; (2) normal outer hair cell function demonstrated by normal otoacoustic emissions or cochlear microphonics on electrocochleography; and (3) poor hearing demonstrated by either abnormal pure tone audiometry or normal pure tone audiometry, but poor speech perception, particularly in noise.

In the PTA, hearing thresholds may range from normal to profoundly impaired (Rance *et al.*, 1999). Speech perception may also be impaired, with severe degradation in background noise being a hallmark of this condition (Zeng and Liu, 2006). In addition, patients with AN may have characteristic psychoacoustic deficits, with preserved loudness discrimination, pitch discrimination at high frequencies, and sound localization using interaural level differences, but with severe deficits in all aspects of temporal processing (temporal integration, resolution, and masking), sound localization using interaural time differences, as well as pitch discrimination at low frequencies (Zeng and Liu, 2006).

Post-mortem biopsy studies indicate that AN is characterized by two processes, demyelination and axonal loss (Starr *et al.*, 2003). Demyelination of the auditory nerve leads to disruption of temporal synchronization within the auditory nerve and explains the particular deficit in psychoacoustic tasks requiring accurate temporal coding, and the marked deficit in speech perception that can sometimes be seen even in the presence of a normal pure tone audiogram. Axonal loss and reduced numbers of auditory fibres are also described. However, the clinical picture of AN may also be seen due to a disorder of the synapse between inner hair cell and the auditory nerve, as seen in cases with mutations in the otoferlin gene, which encodes a protein at the base of the inner hair cells thought to be involved in recycling synaptic vesicles (Varga *et al.*, 2003).

Finally, AN may be due to selective inner hair cell loss, as demonstrated by animal models of AN (Salvi *et al.*, 1999).

AN can be inherited (in isolation or as part of a syndrome) or acquired due to a number of causes, including infections, toxins, and neonatal illness. Non-syndromic genetic causes include mutations of the otoferlin gene (Varga *et al.*, 2003) and the gene that encodes the neuronal protein pejvakin (Delmaghani *et al.*, 2006). Syndromic presentations in combination with other peripheral neuropathies are caused by mutations in genes that encode gap junction channels such as Connexin 31 (Lopez-Bigas *et al.*, 2001) and Connexin 32 (Senderek *et al.*, 1999) and by mutations of the gene for peripheral myelin protein 22 (Kovach *et al.*, 2002) and the NDRG1 gene (Kalaydjieva *et al.*, 2000). AN is associated with optic atrophy in mutations of the OPA1 gene (Amati-Bonneau *et al.*, 2005). AN may also be associated with cerebellar abnormalities in forms of spinocerebellar degeneration, including Friedreich's ataxia.

Management of AN is extremely difficult, given that disorder affects transduction and synchronous firing in the auditory nerve: sophisticated hearing aids and cochlear implants have been tried with varying success. Auditory training strategies may help to overcome the functional deficit. Many patients will need detailed evaluation and family assessment by specialist genetic services.

20.3.2 Brainstem and midbrain

Deafness due to brainstem and midbrain lesions

Deafness due to processes affecting the brainstem and midbrain is rare. This reflects the need for an extensive bilateral lesion because of the partial decussation of the ascending pathway, and such lesions are rarely compatible with life. Deafness has been reported due to lesions of the pons in the brainstem (Egan *et al.*, 1996) and bilateral lesions affecting the inferior colliculus in the midbrain (Hoistad and Hain, 2003; Musiek *et al.*, 2004).

Abnormal auditory perception due to brainstem and midbrain lesions

Abnormal auditory perception without deafness can occur in a number of disorders affecting the brainstem and midbrain, and is commoner than brainstem or midbrain deafness.

Multiple sclerosis (MS) can lead to deficits in speech perception in noisy environments (Lewis *et al.*, 2006) and a number of deficits in temporal analysis (Quine *et al.*, 1984; Hendler *et al.*, 1990; Rappaport *et al.*, 1994). As a white matter disorder commonly affecting the brainstem it is reasonable to ascribe such deficits in MS to the brainstem or midbrain, although disease affecting the auditory radiation might also be relevant. Recent work on MS also highlights a disorder of the efferent system, even in the absence of brainstem lesions demonstrated by MRI (Coelho *et al.*, 2007): this may be relevant to symptomatic problems with selective listening in MS.

A tumour infiltrating the midbrain can cause abnormal perception of music, environmental sounds, and speech with a normal PTA (Pan *et al.*, 2004).

Deficits in binaural analysis due to brainstem lesions are predicted by the fact that this is the first point of convergence of the binaural pathway. Such deficits have been demonstrated in a number of studies based on psychoacoustics and lateralization-related potentials arising in the brainstem (e.g. Van der Poel *et al.*, 1988; Furst *et al.*, 1995; Litovsky *et al.*, 2002).

20.3.3 Cortex

Cortical deafness

Table 20.1 describes cases of adult cortical deafness selected on the basis of a clear description of the lesion and deficit. Figure 20.1 shows the responsible vascular lesion in one of our patients.

Table 20.1 Reports of acquired cortical deafness

Report (number of cases)	Hearing loss	AEP	Evolution	Lesion
Bahls, 1988 (1) *Neurology* **38**: 1490–3	No consistent response to tones up to 100 dB	Normal wave I–V response Normal mid-latency responses (10–50 ms) Absent longer-latency potentials (to 300 ms)	Total deafness persisted for 20 months	R superior temporal lobe infarction involving HG.and adjacent frontal and inferior parietal cortex L superior temporal lobe infarction involving HG and adjacent parietal cortex
Leicester, 1980 (1) *Brain Lang* **10**: 224–42	Bilateral and increasing with frequency from 25 dB at 20 Hz to 100 dB at 8 kHz	Not done	Sudden onset without recovery	R hemisphere infarct involving superior temporal gyrus and insula L hemisphere infarct involving lateral HG Discrete right occipital and left motor strip infarcts
Mendez, 1988 (2) *J Neurol Neurosurg Psychiatry* **51**: 1–9	Apparent loss of > 70 dB initially Thresholds of 30–40 (R) and 20–25 (L) after 2 weeks	Normal brainstem responses Absent mid-latency responses	Much apparent recovery of deafness within 2 weeks Developed into generalized auditory agnosia	R/L superior temporal gyrus infarcts
	No initial response to sounds to audiometry limit At 3 weeks bilateral loss of < 50 dB at most frequencies	Normal brainstem responses Absent mid-latency responses	Much improvement in deafness within 3 weeks Developed into agnosia for primarily speech and music, with further recovery to residual sound sequencing deficit	R hemisphere infarct involving frontoparietotemporal regions L temporoparietal infarct
Szirmai, 2003 (2) *Brain Lang* **85**: 159–65		Normal wave I–V	Deafness after successive haemorrhages on R then L after 4-year interval. Persistent loss	R hemisphere haemorrhage involving superior temporal gyrus and underlying white matter(first event) L hemisphere subinsular infarct (second event)
		Normal wave I–V	Deafness after successive haemorrhages on L then R with 4-year interval. Persistent loss	L hemisphere subinsular (first event) R hemisphere subinsular infarct (second event)

Table 20.1 (continued) Reports of acquired cortical deafness

Report (number of cases)	Hearing loss	AEP	Evolution	Lesion
Tanaka, 1991 (2) *Brain* **114**: 2385–401	Severe loss (~ 90 dB at all frequencies between 250 Hz and 8 kHz) with marked variability in threshold)	Normal brainstem reponses Main component mid-latency response not recorded Variable and inconsistent long latency responses	Persistent loss	R deep white matter infarcts of temporal lobe below insula, especially posterior part – HG partially involved L deep white matter infarcts of temporal lobe below insula, especially posterior part – HG spared
	Severe loss with marked variability in threshold	Normal brainstem reponses Main component mid-latency response not recorded Variable and inconsistent long latency responses	Persistent loss	R/L deep white matter lesions below insula. HG involved on both sides
Woods, 1984 (1) *EEG Clin Neurophysiol* **57**: 208–20	Initially no response to sound After 1 month increasing loss with frequency to 70/100 dB (L/R) at 6 kHz	Normal brainstem responses Normal later responses (latency ~ 100 ms), even to subthreshold stimuli	Some recovery in 1 month after initial total unresponsiveness	R/L superior temporal lobe infarcts (more extensive on right and extending to temporoparietal junction) involving HG on both sides

AEP Auditory evoked potentials; HG Heschl's gyrus; R/L right/left

These patients typically have deafness following bilateral vascular lesions involving primary and secondary cortices in Heschl's gyrus (HG) and association cortex in the planum temporale (PT), in the absence of any evidence of a lesion in the cochlea, auditory nerve, or brainstem auditory pathway based on normal auditory-evoked potentials to clicks. Patients often demonstrate both abnormal hearing level and variability in hearing level (Tanaka *et al.*, 1991): the disorder is likely to have an attentional component. However, when attention is taken into account there is a hearing loss that cannot be accounted for by attentional effects. This often takes the form of a profound initial loss followed by partial recovery. A similar pattern is seen in macaque models of cortical deafness due to bilateral lesions affecting the superior temporal plane (Heffner and Heffner, 1986). There is debate as to whether the critical lesion is in the cortex or auditory radiation, which is often also affected by the associated vascular lesions.

Cortical agnosias

Auditory agnosia is the loss of auditory recognition in the absence of deafness. It is often associated with cortical lesions. Table 20.2 describes adult cases associated with cortical lesions. Responsible lesions are usually strokes affecting the superior temporal cortex, which are commonly bilateral. It can also occur after temporal lobe damage due to herpes simplex encephalitis

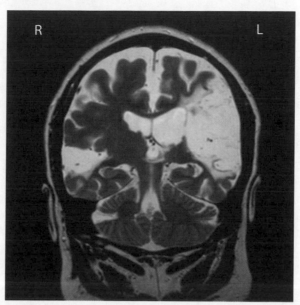

Fig. 20.1 Structural imaging of a patient with cortical deafness. This patient sustained bilateral cerebral infarcts due to emboli at the age of 36, 6 years before these magnetic resonance images were acquired. After the event she demonstrated no response to any sounds (even a fire alarm going off next to her) and she was unable to read despite normal visual acuity. Communication was achieved with a set of visual symbols to which she and carers pointed to in order to indicate her needs. She has normal spontaneous and induced otoacoustic emissions and normal auditory evoked potential to clicks (*waves I–V*). The imaging demonstrates an extensive left hemisphere lesion that has destroyed the whole of Heschl's gyrus (in addition to the perisylvian language areas on the left), and a lesion on the right that, although more restricted, has also destroyed the whole of Heschl's gyrus. Coronal T2 images. (Personal observation by T.D.G.)

in adults (Buchman *et al.*, 1986) and children (Kaga *et al.*, 2003). It should be emphasized that, although auditory agnosia is often considered to be a cortical disorder, the definition above does not require this, and abnormal auditory recognition in the absence of deafness can occur in auditory neuropathy (Kaga *et al.*, 2002; Pinard *et al.*, 2002), lesions affecting the midbrain (Pan *et al.*, 2004), and lesions affecting the auditory radiation (Tanaka *et al.*, 2002). Table 20.2 demonstrates that many cases of auditory agnosia reported after cortical lesions do not actually meet a strict definition of agnosia based on the presence of normal hearing. This may reflect the evolution from cortical deafness to auditory agnosia that is observed in a number of cases. In addition, many patients with auditory agnosia due to stroke are from an elderly population in which deafness due to cochlear dysfunction is common.

Table 20.2 also demonstrates overlap between the domains in which acquired agnosia is manifest. Deficits in the recognition of single words (word deafness), environmental sounds (environmental sound agnosia), and music (amusia) commonly coexist, especially in patients with agnosia due to bilateral superior temporal lobe lesions. This may reflect apperceptive agnosia in such patients where the profile of deficits depends on the particular aspect of spectrotemporal analysis that is affected by the cortical lesions. This argument is developed in detail in Griffiths *et al.* (1999). The degree of overlap between domains affected by agnosia is likely to be underestimated in view of the practical difficulty of carrying out a comprehensive and rigorous assessment

Table 20.2 Reports of acquired auditory agnosia

Report (number of cases)	Symptomatic deafness	Audiogram (AEP)	General language deficit	Single word comprehension deficit	Environmental sound deficit	Music deficit	Lesion
Auerbach 1982 (1) *Brain* **105**: 271–300	No	Mild bilateral loss up to 2 KHz and more severe loss above this (AEP normal)	No aphasia except rare paraphrasic errors	Yes	Yes – mild	Yes – profound	R infarct extending from middle superior temporal lobe to parietal lobe; L infarct involving posterior and deep superior temporal lobe sparing HG on left
Buchman 1986 (3) *J Neurol Neruosurg Psychiatry* **49**: 489–99	Yes	Moderate to severe bilateral loss	Mild fluent aphasia (WAB)	Yes	No	No	Multiple infarcts; R temporal lobe infarct; L temporoparietal lobe infarcts; Additional changes consistent with Alzheimer's disease on autopsy
	No	Mild to severe bilateral loss (AEP normal)	No aphasia (BDAE)	Yes	Not systematically tested	Not reported	R temporoparietal lobe infarct; L superior temporal lobe infarct
	Yes	Audiogram and brainstem responses not reported	No clear aphasia	Yes	Yes	Not reported	Normal CT; R/L epileptiform discharges in temporal lobes attributed to HSV encephalitis
Buchtel 1989 (1) *Brain Lang* **37**: 12–25		Moderate bilateral loss	Aggramatism and decreased verbal fluency	Yes	Yes	Not reported	R posterior temporal lobe infarct; L temporal lobe infarcts (2)
Caramazza 1983 (1) *Brain Lang* **18**: 128–74	No	Mild L high tone loss	Severe fluent aphasia	Yes	No	Not reported	L posterior superior temporal lobe infarct

Reference		Audiogram	Aphasia			Deficit	Lesion
Coslett 1984 (1) Neurology 34: 347–52	No	Normal audiogram	No discrete aphasia	Yes	No	No deficit in melody perception but impaired rhythm	R middle and superior temporal gyrus infarct; L superior temporal gyrus infarct (both involving HG)
Engelien 1995 (1) Brain 118: 1395–409	Yes	Mild R loss above 4 kHz (AEP normal)	Initial global aphasia Residual Broca's aphasia	Yes	Yes, with partial recovery between 2 and 8 years after second event	Not reported	R posterior superior temporal gyrus and insula infarct; L temporal lobe infarct involving HG and insula extending to parietal and frontal lobes
Eustache 1990 (2) Neuropsychologia 28: 257–70		Normal audiogram		Yes	No	Yes, identification	L temporoparietal lobe infarct
		High tone loss		No	Yes	Yes, discrimination	R anterior temporal lobe and frontal infarct
Fujii 1990 (1) Cortex 26: 263–8	No	Mild L loss above 2 kHz (AEP normal)	No aphasia	No	Yes, with complete recovery	Yes, profound	R posterior temporal lobe haemorrhage
Godefroy 1995 (1) Cortex 31: 149–59	Yes	Profound initial deafness at onset haemorrhage with recovery to average 20 dB (500 Hz to 2 kHz) loss in 2 weeks (AEP normal)	No discrete aphasia (BDAE)	Yes, with partial resolution in 8 weeks	Yes, with complete resolution in 8 weeks	Yes, with complete resolution in 2 weeks	R/L external capsule haemorrhage affecting auditory radiation
Griffiths 1997 (1) Brain 120: 785–94	No	Normal audiogram	No aphasia (WAB)	No	No	Yes, moderate	R posterior hemisphere infarct involving posterior superior temporal lobe, inferior parietal lobe. and anterolateral occipital lobe
Griffiths 2007 (1) Hear Res 229: 46–53	No	Normal audiogram	No aphasia	No	No	Yes, with marked timbral deficit	R posterior superior temporal lobe infarct

Table 20.2 (continued) Reports of acquired auditory agnosia

Report (number of cases)	Symptomatic deafness	Audiogram (AEP)	General language deficit	Single word comprehension deficit	Environmental sound deficit	Music deficit	Lesion
Habib 1995 (1) Neuropsychologia **33**: 327–39	Yes	Normal audiogram (AEP normal)	1 month mutism with no residual aphasia except decreased verbal fluency (BDAE)	No	Yes	Yes	R/L infarct affecting insula
Kohlmetz 2003 (1) Neurocase **9**: 86–93	No	Bilateral mild high frequency loss	No aphasia (AAB)	No	No	Specific musical timbre deficit	R anterior superior and medial temporal infarct
Lambert 1989 (1) Cortex **25**: 71–82	Yes	Profound initial bilateral loss worse on L improved to mild bilateral loss within 3 months (AEP normal)	No discrete aphasia (FAB)	Yes, with partial recovery within 3 months	Yes, persistent	Yes, persistent	Initial imaging after head trauma showed intraventricular haemorrhage without parenchymal lesion Follow-up imaging at 5 months showed ventricular enlargement only
Mendez and Geehan 1988 (2) J Neurol Neurosurg Psychiatry **51**: 1–9	Yes	Bilateral moderate loss with partial resolution	No clear discrete aphasia	Yes	Yes	Yes	R/L superior temporal infarcts
	Yes	Abnormal audiogram with partial resolution		Yes	Mild	Mild	R frontoparietotemporal infarct L parietotemporal infarct

Reference							
Metz-Lutz 1984 (1) Brain Lang 23: 13–25	Yes	Mild R loss (AEP normal)	Wernicke's aphasia (BDAE)	Yes	No	Yes – rhythm perception affected more than melody	Left temporal lobe infarction attributed to arteritis
Miceli 1982 (1) Neuropsychologia 20: 5–20		Initial severe loss with partial recovery	Fluent aphasia	Yes	Yes	Yes	R/L infarctions involving superior temporal lobes
Motomura 1986 (1) Brain 109: 379–91	No	Moderate to severe loss at high and low frequency and mild loss (~40 dB) between 250 and 4 KHz (AEP normal)	No	Yes, with rapid partial resolution	Yes, with partial resolution in 6 weeks	Yes, with partial resolution in 2 weeks	R/L posterior thalamic vascular events (mixed infarct/bleed) extending to left auditory thalamus and right internal capsule
Oppenheimer 1978 (1) Arch Neurol 35: 712–19	Yes	Not tested	Mild fluent dysphasia	Yes	Yes	Yes	R/L superior temporal lobe infarct sparing part of right HG
Peretz 1994 (2) Brain 117: 1283–301	No	Normal audiogram	No discrete aphasia (BDAE)	No	No	Yes, profound	R/L superior temporal vascular insults related to aneurysms with sparing HG
	No	Normal audiogram	Wernicke's aphasia (BDAE)	Yes, with recovery	No	Yes, profound	R/L middle cerebral infarcts related to known bilateral aneurysms HG involved on R and spared on L
Peretz 1999 (1) Neurocase 5: 21–30	No	Normal audiogram	No discrete aphasia	No	No	Yes, profound	R/L bilateral middle cerebral artery vascular events related to known aneurysms, involving most of superior temporal gyrus on R and anterior two-thirds on L

Table 20.2 (continued) Reports of acquired auditory agnosia

Report (number of cases)	Symptomatic deafness	Audiogram (AEP)	General language deficit	Single word comprehension deficit	Environmental sound deficit	Music deficit	Lesion
Praamstra 1991 (1) *Brain* **114**: 1197–225	No	Mild high-frequency loss (AEP normal)	Wernicke's aphasia (AAB)	Yes	Slight impairment	Yes (not systematically tested)	R/L middle cerebral infarcts involving superior temporal lobes including HG
Satoh 2007 (1) *Eur Neurol* **58**: 70–7	No	Mild high-frequency loss (AEP normal)	Receptive aphasia with resolution	Yes (speech audiogram)	Yes	Yes – abnormal melody perception and singing	R middle temporal gyrus infarct L extensive temporal infarct
Takahashi 1992 (1) *Cortex* **28**: 295–303	No	Normal up to 2 kHz (AEP normal)	No discrete aphasia (WAB)	Yes	No	Mild deficit in melody and rhythm	L infarct extending from left posterior thalamus and adjacent internal capsule to left temperoparietal white matter – HG spared
Tanaka 1987 (1) *Brain* **110**: 381–403	No	Mild loss (<20 dB) between 250 Hz and 4 kHz (AEP normal)	No	Yes	Mild	Yes – mild melody deficit and more severe tone-sequencing deficit and *supramodal* rhythm perception deficit	R/L superior temporoparietal lesions with partial sparing of HG on left
Taniwaki 2000 (1) *Clin Neurol Neurosurg* **102**: 156–62	Yes initially	Severe bilateral loss with partial resolution (AEP normal)	Mild	Yes	Yes	Not systematically tested	R/L deep haemorrhages in putaminal region affecting auditory radiation especially on left

Study					
von Stockert 1982 (1) *Brain Lang* **16**: 133–46	Not reported	No clear aphasia	Yes	Yes	Unclear (but no output amusia)	R/L temporal lobe damage from self-inflicted gunshot wound (CT)
Wang 2000 (1) *Brain Lang* **73**: 442–55	Mild L loss Mild to moderate R loss	Yes	Yes	Not reported	Not reported	L superior temporal lobe infarct involving parietal and frontal lobe
Yaqub 1988 (1) *Brain* **111**: 457–66	Mild bilateral loss up to 2 kHz and moderate high-frequency loss (AEP normal)	No discrete aphasia	Yes	No	No	R/L subcortical superior temporal gyrus infarcts (CT)

AEP Auditory evoked potentials; AAB Aachen Aphasia Battery (Huber, 1984: *Adv Neurol* **42**: 291–303); BDAE Boston Diagnostic Aphasia battery (Goodgrass, 1972: Lea and Febiger, Philadelphia); FAB French Aphasia battery (Ducarne, 1976: Centre de Psychologie Appliquée, Paris); HG Heschl's gyrus; R/L right/left; WAB Western Aphasia battery

General language deficit refers to any evidence of aphasia over and above any deficit in auditory verbal comprehension of all of these, and because it is unusual for patients to undergo a systematic assessment of complex sound analysis.

A number of the studies in Table 20.2 have assessed aspects of complex sound analysis based on measures that are crude compared to approaches developed in the rest of this book. There have been a number of studies of temporal analysis, especially in cases of word deafness, using approaches that include click counting, click-fusion threshold, tone-sequence, and rhythm discrimination (for discussion see Griffiths *et al.* 1999). Many of the reported patients with word deafness in which such temporal deficits have been described also suffered deficits in other domains, as would be predicted on the basis of an apperceptive agnosia due to a deficit in temporal analysis. Deficits in spectral analysis have not been systematically explored in agnosia, but might be relevant to deficits in musical perception in particular, which is less robust than speech to degraded spectral structure (Shannon, 2001). There is an ongoing need for an efficient and robust means of characterizing the analysis of spectrotemporal structure and sound sequences in cortical disorders.

The substrate for acquired apperceptive auditory agnosia is similar to that for auditory deafness, from which it commonly evolves: lesions are usually bilateral and affect primary and secondary cortices in HG and association cortex in PT. Human imaging studies that suggest a systematic increase in preferred temporal 'windows' of analysis as you move further from primary cortex (Giraud *et* al., 2000; Boemio *et al.*, 2005), or a difference in temporal analysis between the right and left auditory cortices (Zatorre and Belin, 2001), suggest mechanisms by which lesions differentially affecting the two sides or primary and secondary cortex might produce different temporal deficits that might be more manifest in particular domains. In the spectral domain, differences in bandwidth preference between auditory cortices in primates (Petkov *et al.*, 2006) are another means by which lesions affecting different cortical areas might produce differences in the domains affected. The existence of attentional deficits in agnosia due to bilateral superior temporal lesions has not been systematically assessed; given the frequent evolution from cortical deafness in which attentional deficits are common, an auditory attentional deficit would be expected in a number of cases.

The distinction between acquired apperceptive and associative agnosia has been emphasized most in the word-deafness literature. Associative forms of word deafness, where word discrimination is intact but word recognition impaired, can occur with unilateral left temporal lesions (although unilateral lesions can also produce apperceptive deficits Wang *et al.*, 2000). A similar distinction has been made in the case of phonagnosia: agnosia for voices. Reports of symptomatic deficits in voice recognition are rare in the case literature. Van Lancker and colleagues (1989) described a series of patients assessed with left and right hemisphere lesions: apperceptive phonagnosia was associated with right or left temporal lobe damage and right parietal damage was associated with associative phonagnosia. A temporal lobe basis for apperceptive deficits fits with the ideas developed above, in particular the association of environmental-sound agnosia with unilateral or bilateral superior temporal lobe lesions. However, the parietal lesions are difficult to reconcile with normal imaging data that suggest a pathway for voice identification running anteriorly in the right temporal lobe (Belin *et al.*, 2000).

Acquired amusia has been studied in a number of patients following unilateral or bilateral temporal lobe stroke. In Stewart *et al.* (2006) the argument is developed that musical deficits, due to acquired cortical lesions, can be considered in terms of the components of music in the pitch or rhythm domain. In the pitch domain, for example, deficits can occur in the perception of the pitch of individual notes, simple pitch patterns such as pitch-interval direction between pairs of notes, contour (the patterns of 'ups' and 'downs' in a melody), and tonal structure. Neuropsychological models suggest that these are successive levels in a hierarchy of pitch and pitch-pattern analysis, and normal functional imaging suggests that the substrate for such analysis becomes increasingly distributed (involves areas increasingly distant from primary and secondary cortex in HG) further up the perceptual hierarchy. The disorder commonly coexists with a deficit in the perception of prosody in speech at a similar level of temporal structure to the critical level in music (changes in pitch, stress, and rhythm within a temporal 'window' of hundreds of milliseconds). The disorder is best characterized as an apperceptive agnosia before the level of deficits in tonal analysis, when learned associations with pitch patterns are made and a form of associative deficit might be argued.

Figure 20.2 shows areas that are commonly associated with deficits at different levels in the pitch hierarchy. The schematic shows that, for the pitch domain, there is a tendency for deficits at higher levels in the pitch hierarchy to be caused by lesions that are more remote from primary and secondary cortex in HG, consistent with a number of functional imaging studies. The illustrative use of Fig. 20.2 has to be borne in mind: right hemisphere lesions causing deficits are more commonly reported and are therefore emphasized in the figure, but left hemisphere lesions *can* produce deficits in mechanisms for the analysis of pitch and pitch pattern. In part this might reflect a bias in subjects selected for study: subjects with acquired amusia due to left-hemisphere damage may also have aphasia, making behavioural assessment more difficult (and reports rarer).

There has been recent interest in lifelong disorders of musical perception (also reviewed in Stewart *et al.* 2006). Lifelong disorders of singing have been recognized for over a century, and work using the Montreal Battery for the Assessment of Amusia (MBEA) (Peretz *et al.*, 2003) demonstrates that the deficit is commonly associated with a deficit in musical perception that can be demonstrated by impaired discrimination of novel melodies (Ayotte *et al.*, 2002). The disorder can therefore be characterized as a congenital form of apperceptive agnosia. The disorder is particularly associated with deficits in the pitch domain. Rhythm deficits can also occur in the context of a melody (Foxton *et al.*, 2006). Behavioural studies have demonstrated deficits in pitch discrimination and pitch-direction analysis, suggesting a fundamental deficit in the analysis of pitch pattern.

Based on the acquired lesion data shown in Fig. 20.2, and consideration of the normal cortical mechanisms for pitch-pattern analysis demonstrated by functional imaging (reviewed in Stewart *et al.*, 2006), a cortical basis for the disorder would be predicted. Although abnormalities of brain structure are not seen at the individual level, group studies of cortical thickness provide evidence for a cortical disorder (Hyde *et al.*, 2007; Fig. 20.3). Figure 20.3 implicates right superior temporal and right inferior frontal cortices that may be important in working memory for pitch, although left-hemisphere bases have been suggested by other work (Mandell *et al.*, 2007).

20.3.4 Lesions affecting emotional sound analysis

Emotional sound analysis is considered in Chapter 19 and, like pitch and melody analysis, cannot be considered as a unitary entity. The emotional effects of a loud bang or nails scraping down a blackboard, for example, are difficult to consider in the same way as the effect on some people of certain passages in a Mahler symphony (the 'shiver down the spine' or chill) or the effect of hearing the music played at the funeral of a loved one. The argument is developed in Chapter 19 that there are direct projections to amygdala from auditory thalamus (a second auditory pathway), in addition to an indirect route to the amygdala via the auditory cortices. There are therefore two routes to the amygdala and limbic circuits that might be more concerned with automatic emotional reactions, or with more cognitive aspects of emotional experience.

The hypersensitivity to sounds in certain disorders, including autism, could have a low-level basis. At a cognitive level of emotion, a patient has been described with normal musical recognition,

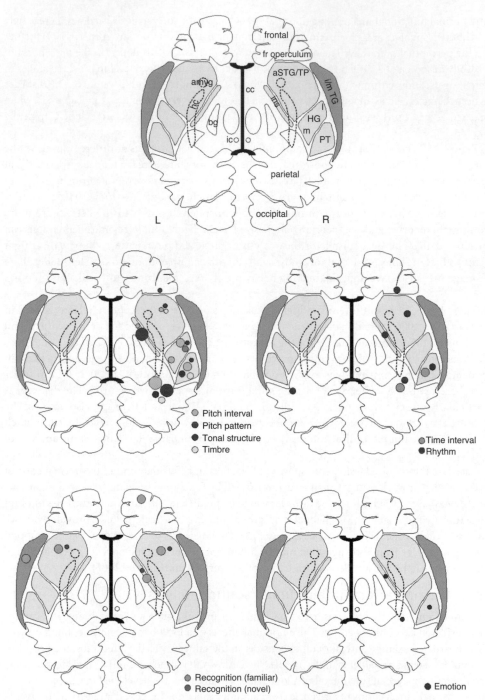

Fig. 20.2 Brain lesions in acquired musical agnosia. Five cartoons are shown, each depicting the brain in a schematic axial projection that includes all key anatomical areas involved in music listening (identified on the *upper cartoon*). Musical functions have been grouped as follows: pitch processing (pitch interval, pitch pattern, tonal structure, timbre); temporal processing (time interval, rhythm); musical memory (familiar and novel material); and emotional response to music.

Fig. 20.2 (*continued*) Each group of functions is assigned to a separate cartoon; individual functions are identified to the right of the corresponding cartoon. The data summarize the case literature using a form of thresholding procedure in which the presence of a *coloured circle* corresponding to a particular function in a region indicates that at least 50% of reported studies of the function implicate that region. The size of each *circle* is scaled according to the proportion of studies of the function implicating that region. Note that the absence of any *circle* does not exclude the area from that function: it means the area has been implicated in less than 50% of the case reports of that function. In the case of pitch the figure shows a tendency for lesions at different levels in the pitch hierarchy (pitch interval, pitch pattern, and tonal structure) to affect areas more remote from Heschl's gyrus. Note that left hemisphere causes of deficits in pitch and pitch-pattern analysis are described, but in less than 50% of published cases. amyg Amygdala; aSTG anterior superior temporal gyrus; bg basal ganglia; cc corpus callosum; fr frontal; HG Heschl's gyrus; ic inferior colliculi; inf inferior; ins insula; mid middle; thal thalamus; PT planum temporale; TG temporal gyrus. (From Stewart *et al.*, 2006.)

but a loss of the learned emotional effect of certain music (Griffiths *et al.*, 2004). The deficit cannot be called an agnosia because there is no perceptual loss, and the substrate is likely in the limbic system rather than in the cortex. Such cases are unusual, but the abnormal analysis of sound emotion at this cognitive level might be relevant to a number of common psychiatric disorders.

20.3.5 Auditory processing disorder without a clear associated structural lesion

In the previous sections we have considered a number of disorders of the central auditory system that are associated with a clear neurological event and anatomical lesion. The question arises whether it is useful to have a diagnostic category for disorders of auditory cognition where this is not the case. The area is controversial because of difficulties in defining any core syndrome or syndromes based on the pattern of deficits in auditory cognition, and because of the absence of clear-cut defining pathophysiology in these cases. However, a number of observations have suggested a developmental form of auditory processing disorder that is not explained by a cochlear deficit and is not due to a generalized cognitive deficit.

Myklebust (1954) originally proposed that central auditory function ought to be assessed in children with communication disorders, and it has long been recognized that some children have particular problems with speech in noisy conditions despite normal hearing levels. This can also be a feature of auditory neuropathy, but that disorder is too rare to provide a general explanation. A number of studies since Myklebust have described subjects (usually in childhood) with normal peripheral hearing but who display uncertainty about what is heard, difficulty listening in the presence of competing sounds, difficulty following oral instructions, and difficulty understanding rapid or degraded speech (ASHA, 1996; Jerger and Musiek, 2000). The term auditory processing disorder (APD) has been applied to such subjects: the term is most commonly used to refer to a developmental disorder in the absence of a clearly defined event or lesion. The disorder may be common with a prevalence of 5% (Chermak and Musiek, 1997), which is similar to that of developmental dyslexia.

A number of groups have suggested definitions of APD. In the UK, the Auditory Processing Disorder Interest Group proposed that APD 'results from impaired neural function and is characterized by poor recognition, discrimination, separation, grouping, localization, or ordering of *non-speech* sounds. It does not solely result from a deficit in general attention, language or

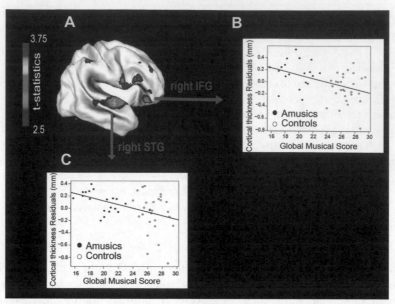

Fig. 20.3 Structural brain changes in developmental musical agnosia. The figure shows changes in cortical thickness in a cohort of subjects with developmental musical agnosia from Canada and the UK. The right hemisphere surface representation shows areas in which cortical thickness varies with the severity of the musical deficit (as shown in accompanying plots with linear regression: decreasing 'global musical score' corresponds to worsening musical perception). Areas are demonstrated in the right superior temporal gyrus and right inferior frontal gyrus in which cortical thickness increases as a function of the severity of the musical deficit. (From Hyde *et al.*, 2007, with permission.)

other cognitive processes'. In the USA, the American Speech-Language-Hearing Association (ASHA) Working Group on Auditory Processing Disorders (ASHA, 2005) proposed that the term 'central' should precede the term APD, since 'most definitions of the disorder focus on the central auditory nervous system'. Thus, (C)APD was defined as 'a deficit in neural processing of auditory stimuli that is not due to higher order language, cognitive, or related factors'. According to the ASHA definition (ASHA, 1996) patients with APD may show deficits in a number of psychoacoustic tasks and their electrophysiological correlates: (1) sound localization and lateralization; (2) auditory pattern recognition; (3) auditory discrimination; (4) temporal aspects of hearing (masking, ordering, integration, resolution); (5) processing degraded auditory signals; and (6) processing the auditory signal when embedded in competing acoustic signals.

Although APD is being increasingly diagnosed in the UK and North America there are a number of issues related to the definition (Jerger and Musiek, 2000; Hind, 2006). First, although many would argue that the deficit is central (beyond the cochlea), the use of the term central has not been applied by the UK group because of possible peripheral factors that might cause a subsequent central deficit: in particular, the condition of recurrent otitis media in childhood. Second, although a number of tests that have been applied to APD have incorporated speech and phonemes (e.g. Musiek, 1983; Keith, 2000), others have argued that the disorder should be defined using measures that are independent of speech (Rosen, 2005; Moore, 2006), and this is incorporated into the current UK definition. Third, a major issue is that the list of possible deficits in the ASHA definition might be due to a large number of disorders affecting sensory representation, perceptual analysis, and attention at a number of points in the ascending pathway to the auditory cortex, and beyond. Indeed, the definitions suggested by groups in both the UK and USA would define deficits described in association with known lesions at several levels as APD. This calls into question the utility of a single diagnosis, and some groups (Bellis and Ferre, 1999) would actually argue that there are a number of subtypes of APD that can be anatomically localized based on comparison with the effect of known lesions. Finally, whilst definitions from the UK and USA have both stressed differentiation from 'higher-order' factors, the argument has been made that such a differentiation cannot be achieved with tests that are commonly used (Cacace and McFarland, 2005) and that tests based on other modalities should also be used to exclude a general deficit. Whether the definition of APD should require the exclusion of problems in other modalities is a moot point: it is straightforward to come up with disorders that might affect both auditory processing and general cortical analysis (e.g. disorders of the normal myelination process (Moore *et al.*, 1995)). All of these issues highlight a need to define more precisely behavioural syndrome(s) that might constitute APD and clarify the underlying neural bases.

Both the ASHA (2005) and the Auditory Processing Disorder Interest Group in the UK have proposed that the diagnosis of APD requires a test battery approach that assesses different auditory processes, in addition to language, attention and memory. The ASHA (2005) proposes that otoacoustic emissions, acoustic reflexes, and event-related potentials are also measured.

An issue with test batteries mentioned in section 20.2 is the difficulty in designing a comprehensive battery that might define any given component of auditory processing with rigor. The difficulty is compounded by the suggestion based on recent work that there may be subtypes of APD defined on the basis of perceptual (Bellis and Ferre, 1999) or attentional measures (Moore *et al.*, 2008). A unifying diagnosis based on one test battery may therefore turn out to be unrealistic.

A primary motivation for defining APD rigorously is to help subjects with deficits in auditory perception. If the diagnosis can be clearly established at the syndromic and pathological level this will have significant resource implications at the population level, considering the suggested high prevalence, and at the individual level, as a 'label' that might attract targeted resources. Possible intervention strategies for APD might include environmental modifications (such as minimizing background noise), signal enhancement strategies (such as personal FM systems), teacher/speaker based adaptations, auditory training, and non-auditory communication strategies.

20.4 Specific positive auditory experiences

20.4.1 Tinnitus

Tinnitus is defined as the perception of phantom sounds in the absence of an auditory stimulus. The disorder is dealt with in Chapter 21 and can be characterized as a disorder due to abnormal activity within the structures of the ascending auditory pathway or cortex, usually concerned with the normal perception of the tones and noises that are experienced by these patients.

20.4.2 Musical hallucinations

Musical hallucinations can occur in psychosis, as a form of focal epilepsy, and in association with brain lesions. The most common situation in which this occurs, however, is in psychiatrically normal subjects with acquired deafness in middle to later life, where the degree of deafness is usually moderate to severe (Griffiths, 2000). It has been argued, based on the hallucinations that are described by these patients, that the disorder can be characterized as an amplification of normal mechanisms for the perception and imagery of music. As such, the disorder might be thought of as having a similar basis to forms of tinnitus in which abnormal activity occurs in processing mechanisms for noise and tones in the region of primary cortex, but where the

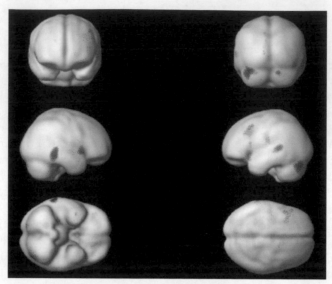

Fig. 20.4 Substrate for musical hallucinations associated with deafness. The figure shows areas where brain activity in a group of sufferers (measured by regional cerebral blood flow, shown in *red*) increases as a function of the intensity of the musical experience. Those areas are rendered onto a surface map of the brain, which has been smoothed in the same way as the blood flow data to allow group averaging. (From Griffiths, 2000, with permission.)

substrate for musical hallucinations requires 'higher' cortex representing more complex structure that evolves over a timescale of seconds. Consistent with the hypothesis, functional imaging of patients with musical hallucinations (Fig. 20.4) demonstrates a network of areas that have been implicated in the normal perception and imagery of melodies.

20.5 Abnormal auditory processing in general brain disorder

We now consider a range of brain disorders that are not defined by an abnormality of auditory cognition, but in which abnormal auditory cognition is a feature of the disorder.

20.5.1 Acute brain disorders

Coma

Behavioural testing of auditory processing in coma is impossible, but there has been considerable interest in whether other measures of auditory analysis at different levels of the system can allow comment on the prognosis for coma. Evoked potentials to clicks arising from the brainstem can allow a measure of brainstem integrity. Persistent absence of these can be caused by irreversible brainstem damage and is associated with poor outcome: death or a permanent vegetative state (Young *et al.*, 2004). Note, however, that a cochlear cause for the absent responses needs to be excluded. Evoked potentials reflecting higher levels of auditory processing are useful in predicting return to wakefulness: the MMN and P3 responses can both be reliable predictors of awakening in comatose patients (Daltrozzo *et al.*, 2007). Additionally, these measures may predict the return to useful function, a measure of more interest to physicians and carers. Note, however, that the absence of MMN or P3 has to be interpreted with caution. MMN, in particular, can be absent in normal patients.

20.5.2 Chronic brain disorders

Dementia

The dementias are a group of disorders characterized by progressive cognitive decline with a number of different cognitive profiles and associated patterns of brain abnormality. We consider here the effects of dementia on auditory cognition as an aspect of those profiles. Most dementias do not affect the cochlea (one important exception to this generalization is mitochondrial disease, which can produce cochlear hearing loss in association with a variety of neurological and cognitive deficits: (Chinnery *et al.*, 2000)). In the ascending pathway, pathological changes in the inferior colliculus and medial geniculate nucleus have been described in Alzheimer's disease (AD) (Sinha *et al.*, 1993). A corresponding *functional* deficit of ascending pathway pathology has not been established in AD or any other common degenerative dementia. Histopathological involvement of primary auditory cortex has been demonstrated in a number of dementias including AD (Baloyannis *et al.*, 1992), the frontotemporal lobar degenerations (FTLD) (Baloyannis *et al.*, 2001), vascular dementia (Baloyannis, 2005), and Creutzfeldt-Jakob disease (CJD) (Baloyannis *et al.*, 1995). However, pathological changes in these diseases are generally more pronounced in non-primary and association cortex.

The auditory deficits that develop in AD and the other prototypical dementias reflect the patterns of pathological involvement above. Whereas cortical deafness is rare in dementia (Kaga *et al.*, 2004), forms of agnosia may be relatively common, and can be interpreted using a framework similar to that developed in the section on 'Cortical agnosias'. Auditory agnosia is rarely the leading feature of a dementia, as in cases of progressive word deafness due to FTLD (Kuramoto *et al.*, 2002). In AD, forms of word deafness (Kurylo *et al.*, 1993; Eustache *et al.*, 1995), environmental sound agnosia (Rapcsak *et al.*, 1989; Eustache *et al.*, 1995), and defective recognition of affective prosody (Testa *et al.*, 2001) have all been described. Deficits in auditory duration analysis have been described in both AD (Hellstrom and Almkvist, 1997) and FTLD (Wiener and Coslett, 2008). Defective recognition of environmental sounds (Bozeat *et al.*, 2000; Uttner *et al.*, 2006) and familiar voices (Gainotti *et al.*, 2003) can also occur in FTLD and may reflect abnormal semantic analysis in anterior temporal-lobe mechanisms. Conversely, there is a suggestion that certain aspects of complex sound processing (such as recognition of familiar music) might be selectively spared in the dementias.

Auditory dysfunction is an important practical issue in the common dementias. These deficits can impair communication and reduce available sensory information, thereby compounding the effects of other cognitive deficits. Examples would include disproportionate difficulty with conversations involving more than one speaker, or over a telephone line, commonly experienced by patients with AD. Deficits in a related 'competing message' test (requiring selective processing of one of two simultaneous speech information streams) predicted the subsequent development of AD in a cohort of older individuals (Gates *et al.*, 2002). Attentional impairments are likely to contribute to such deficits in the dementias, reflecting both direct involvement of cortical attentional networks by the disease process and disruption of ascending and cortico-cortical modulation of attention. There is an extensive literature on auditory evoked potentials with an attentional component in dementia (Polich and Corey-Bloom, 2005).

Whereas most auditory processing disorders in the dementias reflect loss of function, 'positive' auditory symptoms may also occur in certain contexts. Patients with cortical Lewy body disease, in which cognitive decline is accompanied by parkinsonism, visual hallucinations, and visual perceptual distortions, may also experience poorly defined auditory hallucinations and misperceptions, often described as indistinct or 'muffled' sounds and voices (rather than the frank verbal hallucinations of psychosis). The pathophysiological basis for these experiences has not been defined; however, (analogous with visual hallucinations) deficiency of cortical acetylcholine with abnormal release of spontaneous cortical activity is likely to play a key role (Collerton *et al.*, 2005).

Developmental disorders

Dyslexia and specific language impairment are developmental disorders of reading and language respectively. There is enormous interest in central auditory processing in these disorders. In the case of dyslexia, a prominent theory places deficits in phonological analysis (spoken word representation) at the core of the syndrome (Snowling, 2000). From first principles, a number of deficits of auditory analysis might be relevant to phonological impairment. Relevant abnormalities might occur at the level of perception, attention, working memory for sound features, and supramodal cognition. For a recent review that summarizes work seeking deficits in temporal aspects of auditory perception and suggests a particular problem at the level of encoding of sensory information, see Ahissar (2007). Auditory deficits that might be relevant have been sought using psychoacoustic techniques or evoked potentials (especially MMN (Bishop, 2007)).

A problem with many studies of auditory analysis in dyslexia is that abnormalities have generally only been demonstrated *at a group level of inference*, in certain studies, whilst the diagnosis can be made *in individual subjects* based on reading and phonological ability that is below the level expected based on non-verbal intelligence measures. In the rest of this chapter we have developed an approach in which profiles of auditory deficits in individual subjects based on systematic testing can be characteristic of specific disorders. No reliable auditory profile has emerged for the diagnosis of dyslexia at the individual level. That is not to dismiss the possible relevance of auditory abilities during early language acquisition (and the possible benefits from auditory intervention at that stage), but it does limit the possible diagnostic usefulness of auditory testing in defining the disorder.

One issue with auditory assessment in dyslexia is the age of testing, with a number of studies focusing on older schoolchildren and adults. A recent study has demonstrated that pre-school measures of frequency-modulation perception do predict first-grade phonological skills, based on group-level inference (Boets *et al.*, 2008). Another issue is that the measures of temporal analysis that have been used in studies to date focus on simple temporal cues such as gap detection or sinusoidal frequency modulation of a narrow band carrier. Phonological analysis involves the analysis of multiple cues with a more complex structure. Thus, another question related to auditory assessment in dyslexia is whether the assessment of more complex sounds, closer to those present in speech, might show stronger association with phonological skill at the individual subject level.

Autism is a developmental disorder characterized by deficits in social interaction, communication, and imagination, and is accompanied by restricted, repetitive interests and behavioural patterns. Subjects can have mildly increased hearing levels (despite normal cochlear function and frequent reports of sound hypersensitivity in this group (Tharpe *et al.*, 2006)). A number of reports have investigated the cognitive style in autism, in particular the analysis of fine detail (local structure) and global structure, and the interactions between these. The ideas were originally developed in the visual domain. The idea that there are changes in the analysis of the local and global structure of pitch sequences in autism is discussed in Foxton *et al.* (2003).

Psychosis

Abnormal auditory perception can be a defining feature of psychosis in the form of auditory hallucinations. Auditory verbal hallucinations ('voices') are common in schizophrenia and bipolar affective disorder. Functional imaging studies (reviewed in Allen *et al.*, 2008) suggest involvement of auditory cortex (more commonly non-primary) in addition to a number of other areas including mesiofrontal cortex. These findings are congruent with the idea that auditory verbal hallucinations are associated with abnormal activity in areas that are usually active during auditory perception.

A similar argument was suggested in section 20.4.2 as an explanation of tinnitus and auditory musical hallucinations, which might be due to the amplification of mechanisms for normal sound perception and imagery. In auditory verbal hallucinations the additional activity beyond auditory cortex (especially mesiofrontal cortex) might be relevant to the context associated with the perceived voices. In particular, the voices experienced in psychosis can be considered to be a form of abnormal imagery or abnormal metarepresentation (Frith, 1992) where the imagined voice and speech are misattributed to external speakers. Hunter and colleagues (2006) demonstrated spontaneous activity in auditory cortex (in silence) that is modulated by the anterior cingulate in health, arguing that auditory hallucinations derive from a combination of 'top-down' and 'bottom-up' processes. In their model, endogenous activity within auditory cortex provides the substrate upon which attentional processes operate to generate the perceived product of what the person expects to hear.

Epilepsy

Epilepsy is a syndrome not a diagnosis, defined as recurrent abnormal electrical (usually cortical) discharges associated with paroxysmal brain dysfunction that can be produced by a variety of disease processes. The interface between epilepsy and the auditory brain takes four general forms: the effects of epilepsy and its treatment on auditory function; abnormal auditory experiences that occur in the context of seizures; disease processes that produce both seizures and inter-ictal auditory dysfunction; and seizures triggered by auditory phenomena.

Altered auditory perception taking the form of a systematic distortion of pitch perception (usually heard as a lower pitch) has been described chiefly by patients taking the anticonvulsant medication carbamazepine (Konno *et al.*, 2003). This usually arises as a clinical issue in musicians, and particularly those with absolute pitch. The mechanism is uncertain.

Seizures with auditory features are most frequently due to pathological processes involving the temporal lobes. However, it is unusual for auditory features to dominate seizure semiology. Palinacousis, the episodic, illusory perceptual perseveration of an auditory stimulus, is a rare auditory phenomenon that may occur as an ictal or post-ictal phenomenon with seizures arising from the temporal lobes (Di Dio *et al.*, 2007). The perseverated stimulus is most often vocal but may be another environmental sound; it is usually fragmentary, may be distorted (patients may describe hearing an 'echo'), and often localized in space contralateral to the brain lesion. Auditory hallucinations due to seizures can be complex and sustained and are often mixed-modality with a prominent affective context. Auditory hallucinations typically accompany temporal lobe seizures involving the mesial temporal lobes and limbic structures (Gloor *et al.*, 1982). The recently described entity of 'partial epilepsy with auditory features' is characterized by prominent auditory symptoms (with or without accompanying sensory or psychic manifestations or aphasia) that herald the onset of seizures arising from the temporal lobe (Bisulli *et al.*, 2004). Patients may describe simple auditory hallucinations of hissing or buzzing, complex sounds such as music or voices, or loss of hearing. It has been suggested that Joan of Arc had this condition (d'Orsi and Tinuper, 2006). The disorder may be sporadic or familial, due to mutations in the LGI1 'epitempin' gene which has been proposed to play a role in neuronal migration.

The paradigmatic illustration of brain disease causing both seizures and persistent auditory dysfunction is Landau-Kleffner syndrome, a rare acquired encephalopathy of childhood. In this condition regression of language abilities (both comprehension and output) is accompanied by seizures of variable semiology, often with posterior superior temporal origin, and progressive inter-ictal non-verbal auditory agnosia and behavioural disturbance (Smith and Hoeppner, 2003). Structural images are abnormal in a minority of cases, though there is evidence of focal cortical dysplasia radiologically or histopathologically in some. However, the pathogenetic relation between seizures and cognitive decline remains contentious: in principle, seizures could produce a 'functional ablation' of cortex with secondary structural damage, or alternatively a common process might underpin both seizures and cortical damage. Lasting cognitive dysfunction is usual even following remission of seizures, though the outlook may be improved by early treatment with anticonvulsants, corticosteroids, and surgical resection of abnormal cortex in selected cases.

Seizures precipitated by auditory stimuli are rare in humans, and fall into the more general category of seizures evoked by a specific sensory input or activity: the 'reflex epilepsies'. Although various environmental sounds may act as triggers (Bisulli *et al.*, 2004), the most fully described are seizures provoked by music: 'musicogenic epilepsy' (Kaplan, 2003). A variety of musical stimuli (ranging from single instrumental timbres, bells, and sirens to complex orchestral and operatic pieces) have been implicated, but generally the patient describes some degree of emotional engagement with the stimulus. Seizures may arise from either temporal lobe; however, limited functional imaging evidence suggests that a right temporo-limbic network including the anterior temporal lobe, limbic structures, and insula may be critical (Cho *et al.*, 2007). This is consistent with emerging evidence in healthy individuals indicating that this brain network mediates the affective response to music.

20.6 **Conclusions**

Similar principles can be applied to the assessment of developmental, acquired, and degenerative disorders of the central auditory system, whether or not the auditory abnormality is the defining feature of the condition.

1 A systematic approach to these disorders based on the history and appropriately targeted behavioural tests can allow diagnosis as a first step in management. In view of the large range of possible auditory symptoms there is no panacea and no behavioural assessment schedule will be appropriate for all situations.

2 Any assessment of a suspected disorder of central auditory function must include tests of cochlear function to disambiguate peripheral disorders from central disorders: such disambiguation is often not straightforward even when the appropriate cochlear tests are used.

3 Beyond the cochlea, assessment of the anatomical level at which a disorder affects auditory cognition can also be difficult based on behavioural assessment alone. For example, auditory neuropathy and cortical agnosia have a number of common behavioural features.

4 In addition to behavioural assessment, structural imaging and auditory event-related potentials can be helpful in the evaluation of these disorders. However, at the single-subject level, developmental disorders of auditory cognition can occur in the absence of any clear structural lesion defined by imaging, and routine event-related responses to click will not capture all types of disorder.

5 There is a clear need for behavioural and other measures of auditory cognition that bridge the gap between those using simple stimuli that easily allow robust inference, and more complex measures based on ethological assessments that might better characterize the symptoms with which patients present.

References

Ahissar M (2007) Dyslexia and the anchoring-deficit hypothesis. *Trends Cog Sci* 11: 458–65.

Allen P, Laroi F, McGuire PK, Aleman A (2008) The hallucinating brain: a review of structural and functional neuroimaging studies of hallucinations. *Neurosci Biobehav Rev* 32: 175–91.

Amati-Bonneau P, Guichet A, Olichon A, *et al.* (2005) OPA1 R445H mutation in optic atrophy associated with sensorineural deafness. *Ann Neurol* 58: 958–63.

Amitay S, Irwin A, Hawkey DJ, Cowan JA, Moore DR (2006) A comparison of adaptive procedures for rapid and reliable threshold assessment and training in naive listeners. *J Acoust Soc Am* 119: 1616–25.

ASHA (1996) *Central Auditory Processing*. http://www.asha.org/members/deskref-journals/deskref/default.

ASHA (2005) *(Central) Auditory Processing Disorders*. American Speech–Language–Hearing Association, Rockville.

ASHA (2006) Central auditory processing: current status of research and implications for clinical practice. *Am J Audiol* 5: 41–54.

Ayotte J, Peretz I, Hyde K (2002) Congenital amusia. A group study of adults afflicted with a music-specific disorder. *Brain* 125: 238–51.

Baloyannis SJ (2005) The acoustic cortex in vascular dementia: a Golgi and electron microscope study. *J Neurol Sci* 229–230: 51–5.

Baloyannis SJ, Manolidis SL, Manolidis LS (1992) The acoustic cortex in Alzheimer's disease. *Acta Otolaryngol Suppl* 494: 1–13.

Baloyannis SJ, Manolidis SL, Manolidis LS (1995) Synaptic alterations in acoustic cortex in Creutzfeldt-Jacob disease. *Acta Otolaryngol* 115: 202–5.

Baloyannis SJ, Manolidis SL, Manolidis LS (2001) The acoustic cortex in frontal dementia. *Acta Otolaryngol* 121: 289–92.

Belin P, Zatorre RJ, Lafaille P, Ahad P, Pike B (2000) Voice-selective areas in human auditory cortex. *Nature* 403: 309–12.

Bellis TJ, Ferre JM (1999) Multidimensional approach to the differential diagnosis of central auditory processing disorders in children. *J Am Acad Audiol* 10: 319–28.

Berlin CI, Hood L (2001) Auditory neuropathy (auditory desynchrony) disables efferent suppression of otoacoustic emissions. In: *Auditory Neuropathy* (eds Sininger Y, Starr A). Singular, San Diego.

Berlin CI, Hood L, Morlet T, Rose K, Brashears S (2003) Auditory neuropathy/dys-synchrony: diagnosis and management. *Ment Retard Dev Disabil Res Rev* 9: 225–31.

Bishop DV (2007) Using mismatch negativity to study central auditory processing in developmental language and literacy impairments: where are we, and where should we be going?. *Psychol Bull* 133: 651–72.

Bisulli F, Tinuper P, Avoni P (2004) Idiopathic partial epilepsy with auditory features (IPEAF): a clinical and genetic study of 53 sporadic cases. *Brain* 127: 1343–52.

Boemio A, Fromm S, Braun A, Poeppel D (2005) Hierarchical and asymmetric temporal sensitivity in human auditory cortices. *Nat Neurosci* 8: 389–95.

Boets B, Wouters J, van Wieringen A, De Smedt B, Ghesquière P (2008) Modelling relations between sensory processing, speech perception, orthographic and phonological ability, and literacy achievement. *Brain Lang* 106: 29–40.

Bozeat S, Lambon-Ralph MA, Patterson K, Garrard P, Hodges J (2000) Non-verbal semantic impairment in semantic dementia. *Neuropsychologia* 38: 1207–15.

Buchman AS, Garron DC, Trost-Cardamone JE, Wichter MD, Schwartz M (1986) Word deafness: a hundred years later. *J Neurol Neruosurg Psychiatry* 49: 489–99.

Cacace AT, McFarland DJ (2005) The importance of modality specificity in diagnosing central auditory processing disorder. *Am J Audiol* 14: 112–23.

Caclin A, McAdams S, Smith BK, Winsberg S (2005) Acoustic correlates of timbre space dimensions: a confirmatory study using synthetic tones. *J Acoust Soc Am* 118: 471–82.

Chermak GD, Musiek FE (1997) Central auditory processing disorders. In: *New Perspectives*. Singular, San Diego.

Chinnery PF, Elliott C, Green GR (2000) The spectrum of hearing loss due to mitochondrial DNA defects. *Brain* 123 (Part 1): 82–92.

Cho JW, Seo DW, Joo EY, Tae WS, Lee J, Hong SB (2007) Neural correlates of musicogenic epilepsy: SISCOM and FDG-PET. *Epilepsy Res* 77: 169–73.

Coelho A, Ceranic B, Prasher D, Miller DH, Luxon LM (2007) Auditory efferent function is affected in multiple sclerosis. *Ear Hear* 28: 593–604.

Cohen M, Prasher D (1988) The value of combining auditory brainstem responses and acoustic reflex threshold measurements in neuro-otological diagnosis. *Scand Audiol* 17: 153–62.

Collerton D, Perry E, McKeith I (2005) Why people see things that are not there: a novel perception and attention deficit model for recurrent complex visual hallucinations. *Behav Brain Sci* 28: 737–57.

Daltrozzo J, Wioland N, Kotchoubey B (2007) Sex differences in two event-related potentials components related to semantic priming. *Arch Sex Behav* 36: 555–68.

Delmaghani S, del Castillo FJ, Michel V (2006) Mutations in the gene encoding pejvakin, a newly identified protein of the afferent auditory pathway, cause DFNB59 auditory neuropathy. *Nat Genet* 38: 770–8.

Di Dio AS, Fields MC, Rowan AJ (2007) Palinacousis – auditory perseveration: two cases and a review of the literature. *Epilepsia* 48: 1801–6.

Dowling WJ, Harwood DL (1985) *Music and Cognition*. Academic Press, London.

Egan CA, Davies L, Halmagyi GM (1996) Bilateral total deafness due to pontine haematoma. *J Neurol Neurosurg Psychiatry* 61: 628–31.

Erkwoh R, Ebel H, Kachel F (1993) 18FDG-PET and electroencephalographic findings in a patient suffering from musical hallucinations. *Nuclear Medizin* 32: 159–63.

Eustache F, Lambert J, Cassier C (1995) Disorders of auditory identification in dementia of the Alzheimer type. *Cortex* 31: 119–27.

Foxton JM, Stewart ME, Barnard L (2003) Absence of auditory 'global interference' in autism. *Brain* 126: 2703–9.

Foxton JM, Dean JL, Gee R, Peretz I, Griffiths TD (2004) Characterization of deficits in pitch perception underlying 'tone deafness'. *Brain* 127: 801–10.

Foxton JM, Nandy RK, Griffiths TD (2006) Rhythm deficits in 'tone deafness'. *Brain Cogn* 62: 24–9.

Frith CD (1992) *The Cognitive Neuropsychology of Schizophrenia*. Lawrence Erlbaum, Hove.

Furst M, Levine RA, Korczyn AD, Fullerton BC, Tadmore R, Algom D (1995) Brainstem lesions and click lateralisation in patients with mutiple sclerosis. *Hear Res* 82: 109–24.

Gainotti G, Barbier A, Marra C (2003) Slowly progressive defect in recognition of familiar people in a patient with right anterior temporal atrophy. *Brain* 126: 792–803.

Gates GA, Beiser A, Rees TS, D'Agostino RB, Wolf PA (2002) Central auditory dysfunction may precede the onset of clinical dementia in people with probable Alzheimer's disease. *J Am Geriatr Soc* 50: 482–8.

Giraud A-L, Lorenzi C, Ashburner J (2000) Representation of the temporal envelope of sounds in the human brain. *J Neurophysiol* 84: 1588–98.

Gloor P, Olivier A, Quesney LF, Andermann F, Horowitz S (1982) The role of the limbic system in experiential phenomena of temporal lobe epilepsy. *Ann Neurol* 12: 129–44.

Grey JM (1977) Multidimensional perceptual scaling of musical timbres. *J Acoust Soc Am* 61: 1270–7.

Griffiths TD (2000) Musical hallucinosis in acquired deafness. Phenomenology and brain substrate. *Brain* 123: 2065–76.

Griffiths TD, Rees A, Green GGR (1999) Disorders of human complex sound processing. *Neurocase* 5: 365–78.

Griffiths TD, Dean JL, Woods W, Rees A, Green GGR (2001) The Newcastle Auditory Battery (NAB). A temporal and spatial test battery for use on adult naive subjects. *Hear Res* 154: 165–9.

Griffiths TD, Warren JD, Dean JL, Howard D (2004) "When the feeling's gone": a selective loss of musical emotion. *J Neurol Neurosurg Psychiatry* **75**: 344–5.

Griffiths TD, Kumar S, Warren JD, Stewart L, Stephan KE, Friston KJ (2007) Approaches to the cortical analysis of auditory objects. *Hear Res* **229**: 46–53.

Hawkey DJ, Amitay S, Moore DR (2004) Early and rapid perceptual learning. *Nat Neurosci* **7**: 1055–6.

Heffner HE, Heffner RS (1986) Hearing loss in Japanese macaques following bilateral auditory cortex lesions. *J Neurophysiol* **55**: 256–71.

Hellstrom A, Almkvist O (1997) Tone duration discrimination in demented, memory-impaired, and healthy elderly. *Dement Geriatr Cogn Disord* **8**: 49–54.

Hendler T, Squires WK, Emmerich DS (1990) Psychophysical measures of central auditory dysfunction in multiple sclerosis: neurophysiological and neuroanatomical correlates. *Ear Hear* **11**: 403–16.

Hill PR, Hogben JH, Bishop DM (2005) Auditory frequency discrimination in children with specific language impairment: a longitudinal study. *J Speech Lang Hear Res* **48**: 1136–46.

Hillis AE (2007) Aphasia: progress in the last quarter of a century. *Neurology* **69**: 200–13.

Hind SE (2006) Survey of care pathway for auditory processing disorder. *Audiol Med* **7**: 12–24.

Hoistad DL, Hain TC (2003) Central hearing loss with a bilateral inferior colliculus lesion. *Audiol Neurootol* **8**: 111–13.

Howard MA, Volkov IO, Mirsky R (2000) Auditory cortex on the human posterior superior temporal gyrus. *J Comp Neurol* **416**: 79–92.

Hunter MD, Eickhoff SB, Miller TW, Farrow TF, Wilkinson ID, Woodruff PW (2006) Neural activity in speech-sensitive auditory cortex during silence. *Proc Natl Acad Sci USA* **103**: 189–94.

Hyde KL, Lerch JP, Zatorre RJ, Griffiths TD, Evans AC, Peretz I (2007) Cortical thickness in congenital amusia: when less is better than more. *J Neurosci* **27**: 13028–32.

Jerger J, Musiek F (2000) Report of the Consensus Conference on the Diagnosis of Auditory Processing Disorders in School-Aged Children. *J Am Acad Audiol* **11**: 467–74.

Johnson KL, Nicol TG, Zecker SG, Kraus N (2007) Auditory brainstem correlates of perceptual timing deficits. *J Cogn Neurosci* **19**: 376–85.

Kaga K, Kaga M, Tamai F, Shindo M (2003) Auditory agnosia in children after herpes encephalitis. *Acta Otolaryngol* **123**: 232–5.

Kaga K, Nakamura M, Takayama Y, Momose H (2004) A case of cortical deafness and anarthria. *Acta Otolaryngol* **124**: 202–5.

Kaga M, Kon K, Uno A, Horiguchi T, Yoneyama H, Inagaki M (2002) Auditory perception in auditory neuropathy: clinical similarity with auditory verbal agnosia. *Brain Dev* **24**: 197–202.

Kalaydjieva L, Gresham D, Gooding R (2000) N-myc downstream-regulated gene 1 is mutated in hereditary motor and sensory neuropathy-Lom. *Am J Hum Genet* **67**: 47–58.

Kaplan PW (2003) Musicogenic epilepsy and epileptic music: a seizure's song. *Epilepsy Behav* **4**: 464–73.

Keith RW (2000) Development and standardization of SCAN-C test for auditory processing disorders in children. *J Am Acad Audiol* **11**: 438–45.

Kemp DT (2002) Otoacoustic emissions, their origin in cochlear function, and use. *Br Med Bull* **63**: 223–41.

Konno S, Yamazaki E, Kudoh M, Abe T, Tohgi H (2003) Half pitch lower sound perception caused by carbamazepine. *Intern Med* **42**: 880–3.

Kovach MJ, Campbell KC, Herman K (2002) Anticipation in a unique family with Charcot-Marie-Tooth syndrome and deafness: delineation of the clinical features and review of the literature. *Am J Med Genet* **108**: 295–303.

Kuramoto S, Hirano T, Uyama E, *et al.* (2002) A case of slowly progressive aphasia accompanied with auditory agnosia]. *Rinsho Shinkeigaku* **42**: 299–303.

Kurylo DD, Corkin S, Allard T, Zatorre RJ, Growden JH (1993) Auditory function in Alzheimer's disease. *Neurology* **43**: 1893–9.

Lewis MS, Lilly DJ, Hutter M, Bourdette DN, Saunders J, Fausti SA (2006) Some effects of multiple sclerosis on speech perception in noise: preliminary findings. *J Rehabil Res Dev* **43**: 91–8.

Litovsky RY, Fligor BJ, Tramo MJ (2002) Functional role of the human inferior colliculus in binaural hearing. *Hear Res* **165**: 177–88.

Lopez-Bigas N, Olive M, Rabionet R (2001) Connexin 31 (GJB3) is expressed in the peripheral and auditory nerves and causes neuropathy and hearing impairment. *Hum Mol Genet* **10**: 947–52.

Lutkenhoner B, Steinstrater O (1998) High-precision neuromagnetic study of the functional organisation of the human auditory cortex. *Audiol Neurootol* **3**: 191–213.

Mandell J, Schulze K, Schlaug G (2007) Congenital amusia: an auditory-motor feedback disorder?. *Restor Neurol Neurosci* **25**: 323–34.

Martin GK, Stagner BB, Jassir D, Telischi FF, Lonsbury-Martin BL (1999) Suppression and enhancement of distortion-product otoacoustic emissions by interference tones above f(2). I. Basic findings in rabbits. *Hear Res* **136**: 105–23.

Moller AR, Jannetta PJ (1983) Interpretation of brainstem auditory evoked potentials: results from intracranial recordings in humans. *Scand Audiol* **12**: 125–33.

Moore DR (2006) Auditory processing disorder (APD): definition, diagnosis, neural basis, and intervention. *Audiolog Med* **4**: 4–11.

Moore DR, Ferguson MA, Halliday LF, Riley A (2008) Frequency discrimination in children: perception, learning and attention. *Hear Res* **238**: 147–54.

Moore JK, Perazzo LM, Braun A (1995) Time course of axonal myelination in the human brainstem auditory pathway. *Hear Res* **87**: 21–31.

Musiek FE (1983) Assessment of central auditory dysfunction: the dichotic digit test revisited. *Ear Hear* **4**: 79–83.

Musiek FE, Charette L, Morse D, Baran JA (2004) Central deafness associated with a midbrain lesion. *J Am Acad Audiol* **15**: 133–51; quiz 172–3.

Musiek FE, Shinn JB, Jirsa R, Bamiou DE, Baran JA, Zaida E (2005) GIN (Gaps-In-Noise) test performance in subjects with confirmed central auditory nervous system involvement. *Ear Hear* **26**: 608–18.

Myklebust H (1954) *Auditory Disorders in Children: A Manual for Differential Diagnosis*. Grune & Stratton, New York.

Naatanen R (2003) Mismatch negativity: clinical research and possible applications. *Int J Psychophysiol* **48**: 179–88.

d'Orsi G, Tinuper P (2006) "I heard voices…": from semiology, a historical review, and a new hypothesis on the presumed epilepsy of Joan of Arc. *Epilepsy Behav* **9**: 152–7.

Pan CL, Kuo MF, Hsieh ST (2004) Auditory agnosia caused by a tectal germinoma. *Neurology* **63**: 2387–9.

Peretz I, Champod AS, Hyde K (2003) Varieties of musical disorders. The Montreal Battery of Evaluation of Amusia. *Annal N Y Acad Sci* **999**: 58–75.

Petkov CI, Kayser C, Augath M, Logothetis NK (2006) Functional imaging reveals numerous fields in the monkey auditory cortex. *PLoS Biol* **4**: e215.

Pinard M, Chertkow H, Black S, Peretz I (2002) A case study of pure word deafness: modularity in auditory processing?. *Neurocase* **8**: 40–55.

Polich J, Corey-Bloom J (2005) Alzheimer's disease and P300: review and evaluation of task and modality. *Curr Alzheimer Res* **2**: 515–25.

Quine DB, Regan D, Beverly KI, Murray TJ (1984) Patients with multiple sclerosis experience hearing loss for shifts of tone frequency. *Arch Neurol* **41**: 506–7.

Rance G, Beer DE, Cone-Wesson B (1999) Clinical findings for a group of infants and young children with auditory neuropathy. *Ear Hear* **20**: 238–52.

Rapcsak SZ, Kentros M, Rubens AB (1989) Impaired recognition of meaningful sounds in Alzheimer's disease. *Arch Neurol* **46**: 1298–300.

Rappaport JM, Gulliver JM, Phillips DP, Van Dorpe RA, Maxner CE, Bhan V (1994) Auditory temporal resolution in multiple sclerosis. *J Otolaryngol* 23: 307–24.

Rosen S (2005) "A riddle wrapped in a mystery inside an enigma": defining central auditory processing disorder. *Am J Audiol* 14: 139–42.

Ryan S, Kemp DT, Hinchcliffe R (1991) The influence of contralateral acoustic stimulation on click-evoked otoacoustic emissions in humans. *Br J Audiol* 25: 391–7.

Salvi RJ, Wang J, Ding D, Stecker N, Arnold S (1999) Auditory deprivation of the central auditory system resulting from selective inner hair cell loss: animal model of auditory neuropathy. *Scand Audiol Suppl* 51: 1–12.

Samson S, Zatorre RJ, Ramsay JO (2002) Deficits of musical timbre perception after unilateral temporal-lobe lesion revealed with multidimensional scaling. *Brain* 125: 511–23.

Senderek J, Hermanns B, Bergmann C, *et al.* (1999) X-linked dominant Charcot-Marie-Tooth neuropathy: clinical, electrophysiological, and morphological phenotype in four families with different connexin 32 mutations. *J Neurol Sci* 167: 90–101.

Shannon RV (2001) The relative importance of temporal and spectral cues for recognition of speech and music. Proc 6th Biennial Symp, Center for Neural Science at New York Univ, 10–11 June.

Sinha UK, Hollen KM, Rodriguez R, Miller CA (1993) Auditory system degeneration in Alzheimer's disease. *Neurology* 43: 779–85.

Sininger Y, Oba S (2001) Patients with auditory neuropathy: who are they and what can they hear?. In: *Auditory Neuropathy* (eds Sininger Y, Starr A). Singular, San Diego.

Smith MC, Hoeppner TJ (2003) Epileptic encephalopathy of late childhood: Landau-Kleffner syndrome and the syndrome of continuous spikes and waves during slow-wave sleep. *J Clin Neurophysiol* 20: 462–72.

Snowling MJ (2000) *Dyslexia*. Blackwell, Oxford.

Starr A, Picton TW, Sininger Y, Hood LJ, Berlin CI (1996) Auditory neuropathy. *Brain* 119 (Part 3): 741–53.

Starr A, Michalewski HJ, Zeng FG (2003) Pathology and physiology of auditory neuropathy with a novel mutation in the MPZ gene (Tyr145->Ser). *Brain* 126: 1604–19.

Stefanatos GA, Foley C, Grover W, Doherty B (1997) Steady-state auditory evoked responses to pulsed frequency modulations in children. *EEG Clin Neurophys* 104: 31–42.

Stewart L, von Kriegstein K, Warren JD, Griffiths TD (2006) Music and the brain: disorders of musical listening. *Brain* 129: 2533–53.

Talcott JB, Witton C, McLean MF, *et al.* (2000) Dynamic sensory sensitivity and children's word decoding skills. *Proc Natl Acad Sci USA* 97: 2952–7.

Tanaka Y, Kamo T, Yoshida M, Yamadori A (1991) "So-called" cortical deafness. Clinical, neurophysiological and radiological observations. *Brain* 114: 2385–401.

Tanaka Y, Nakano I, Obayashi T (2002) Environmental sound recognition after unilateral subcortical lesions. *Cortex* 38: 69–76.

Testa JA, Beatty WW, Gleason AC, Orbelo DM, Ross ED (2001) Impaired affective prosody in AD: relationship to aphasic deficits and emotional behaviors. *Neurology* 57: 1474–81.

Tharpe AM, Bess FH, Sladen DP, Schissel H, Couch S, Schery T (2006) Auditory characteristics of children with autism. *Ear Hear* 27: 430–41.

Treutwein B, Stasburger H (1999) Fitting the psychometric function. *Percept Psychophys* 61: 87–106.

Uttner I, Mottaghy FM, Schreiber H, Riecker A, Ludolph AC, Kassubek J (2006) Primary progressive aphasia accompanied by environmental sound agnosia: a neuropsychological, MRI and PET study. *Psychiatry Res* 146: 191–7.

Van der Poel JC, Jones SJ, Miller DH (1988) Sound lateralisation, brainstem auditory evoked potentials and magnetic resonance imaging in multiple sclerosis. *Brain* 111: 1453–74.

Van Lancker DR, Kreiman J, Cummings J (1989) Voice perception deficits: neuroanatomical correlates of phonagnosia. *J Clin Exp Neuropsychol* 11: 665–74.

Varga R, Kelley PM, Keats BJ, *et al.* (2003) Non-syndromic recessive auditory neuropathy is the result of mutations in the otoferlin (OTOF) gene. *J Med Genet* **40**: 45–50.

Wang E, Peach RK, Xu Y, Schneck M, Manry C 2nd (2000) Perception of dynamic acoustic patterns by an individual with unilateral verbal auditory agnosia. *Brain Lang* **73**: 442–55.

Wechsler D (1997) *Wechsler Adult Intelligence Scale – Third Edition, Technical Manual.* The Psychological Corporation, San Antonio.

Wichmann FA, Hill NJ (2001) The psychometric function: I. Fitting, sampling, and goodness of fit. *Percept Psychophys* **63**: 1293–313.

Wiener M, Coslett HB (2008) Disruption of temporal processing in a subject with probable frontotemporal dementia. *Neuropsychologia* **46**(7): 1927–39.

Witton C, Talcott JB, Hansen PC (1998) Sensitivity to dynamic auditory and visual stimuli predicts nonword reading ability in both dyslexic and normal readers. *Curr Biol* **8**: 791–7.

Wright BA, Lombardino LJ, King WM, Puranik CS, Leonard CM, Merzenich MM (1997) Deficits in auditory temporal and spectral resolution in language-impaired children. *Nature* **387**: 176–8.

Young GB, Wang JT, Connolly JF (2004) Prognostic determination in anoxic-ischemic and traumatic encephalopathies. *J Clin Neurophysiol* **21**: 379–90.

Zatorre RJ, Belin P (2001) Spectral and temporal processing in human auditory cortex. *Cereb Cortex* **11**: 946–53.

Zeng FG, Liu S (2006) Speech perception in individuals with auditory neuropathy. *J Speech Lang Hear Res* **49**: 367–80.

Chapter 21

Tinnitus

Jos J. Eggermont

21.1 Introduction

Tinnitus is an auditory sensation (ringing of the ears) experienced when no external sound is present. Although a ringing sound is one of the forms tinnitus takes, other forms include sounds of hissing, buzzing, chirping, and even like roaring ocean waves. Tinnitus is commonly divided into objective and subjective tinnitus. Tinnitus that can be attributed to an internal sound source, such as a pulsating blood vessel adjacent to the auditory nerve, is called objective tinnitus and can generally be ameliorated by surgery. This chapter only considers subjective tinnitus, which is a phantom sound sensation (Jastreboff *et al.*, 1988) often accompanying hearing loss and head and neck injuries, or manifesting itself as a hypersensitivity to various drugs. Most, but not all, cases of tinnitus are associated with hearing loss induced by noise exposure or aging. Typically the sensation is associated with a reversible cause – for instance after listening to loud music, fever, use of aspirin or quinine, or transient perturbations of the middle ear – and subsides over a period of time ranging from a few seconds to a few days. However, in 5–15% of the general population, the tinnitus sensation is persistent (Heller, 2003). Chronic tinnitus is more prevalent among seniors (12% after age 60) than in young adults (5% in the 20–30 age group), but can occur at any age. In 1–3% of the general population, the tinnitus sensation is sufficiently annoying to affect the quality of life, involving sleep disturbance, work impairment, and psychiatric distress. The prevalence of tinnitus is likely to increase as the senior population grows and as young people are increasingly exposed to regulated industrial noise and unregulated recreational noise levels.

21.2 Peripheral or central tinnitus?

Is tinnitus in the ear or in the brain? Tinnitus sensations associated with hearing loss are nearly always localized towards the affected ear(s). Does this mean that tinnitus is generated in the ear? This somewhat contentious issue, which has implications for the types of treatment that should be developed, can only be resolved in animal models that are conditioned to signal the presence of tinnitus following application of either salicylate or excessive noise. Tinnitus resulting from head and neck injury localizes to the ipsilateral ear and in general there are no sensitivity changes in that ear (Levine *et al.*, 2003).

There is limited support for the assumption that tinnitus is the result of increased spontaneous firing rates (SFR) in auditory nerve fibers: evidence is only found in cases with loss restricted to outer hair cells, i.e., in the absence of any damage to inner hair cell stereocilia (Liberman and Dodds, 1987), and after acute high-dose application of salicylate in cats (Evans *et al.*, 1981). However, low doses in the same species do not increase the SFR (Stypulkowski, 1990), even though tinnitus can be demonstrated behaviorally with chronic application of low doses (Bauer *et al.*, 2000). Other drugs that cause tinnitus, such as quinine (Mulheran, 1999) and aminoglycosides (Kiang *et al.*, 1970), produced a consistent decrease in the SFR of auditory nerve fibers. A similar decrease was reported after noise-induced hearing loss (Liberman and Kiang, 1978). These results, showing reduced SFR in auditory nerve fibers following noise exposure or ototoxicity, point to a central cause of tinnitus, possibly related to changes in the balance of excitatory and inhibitory inputs conveyed to central auditory structures.

Two important qualifications are that behavioral signs of tinnitus can be prevented if NMDA receptor blockers are infused into the cochlea before salicylate application (Guitton *et al.*, 2003), and that prior administration of NMDA receptor blockers can limit hearing loss resulting from noise trauma (Duan *et al.*, 2000). It seems that by reducing the extent of the hearing loss, probably by preventing neurotoxic effects on AMPA or NMDA receptors in auditory nerve fiber synapses with inner hair cells, the tinnitus is also prevented. These findings are consistent with the insightful early view that the origin of tinnitus may be an imbalance of firing patterns across the tonotopic array of auditory nerve fibers (Kiang *et al.*, 1970), but not with the alternative view that tinnitus reflects increased spontaneous activity generated in auditory nerve fibers. Tinnitus sensations often persist even when input from the ear is removed by section of the auditory nerve in humans (House and Brackmann, 1981) or animals (Zacharek *et al.*, 2002).

21.3 **Tinnitus-inducing agents**

Tinnitus-inducing agents in humans have been listed on the basis of epidemiological and clinical studies. Noise trauma is the single most common cause of tinnitus (18%), followed by head and neck injury (8%), and ear infections and related illnesses (8%). In contrast, commonly used drugs such as aminoglycosides, cisplatin, salicylate, and quinine only account for 2% of known causes of persistent and bothersome tinnitus (Henry *et al.*, 2005).

This suggests that most often tinnitus is related to hearing loss and potentially exacerbated by aging. One has to realize that hearing loss only causes tinnitus in, at most, half of cases, so other aspects such as traumatic vs a gradually acquired loss may play a role. Head and neck injury may cause tinnitus by increasing or modulating spontaneous neural activity in the extra-lemniscal auditory pathways. The tinnitus-inducing agents that are most commonly used in animal studies are noise trauma (either acute or chronic) and salicylate. Salicylates have side effects when used in high acute dosages and typically produce changes in the cochlea as well as in the brain. These effects are quite different from those caused by noise trauma. This has to be kept in mind when results of animal studies for these two agents are compared or generalized.

21.3.1 **Tinnitus in humans**

Listening to tinnitus

Tinnitus is a percept that can be quantified for pitch and loudness by psychoacoustic means (Eggermont and Roberts, 2004). Changes in cortical tonotopic maps and in neural dynamics occurring after exposure to noise or the application of tinnitus-inducing drugs should relate to what the tinnitus subject perceives. However, which neural changes in the brain correlate with the perception of tinnitus? One possibility is that over-representation in the cortical tonotopic map (see below) of edge frequencies (i.e., those frequencies at the low-frequency and/or high-frequency borders of the hearing loss that have near-normal thresholds) is itself responsible for the tinnitus sensation (Rauschecker, 1999).

However, if this over-representation of edge frequencies is underlying tinnitus it implies that people with tinnitus should equate their tinnitus pitch with that of the edge frequency of hearing loss in the audiogram (typically 2–4 kHz in tinnitus associated with noise-induced hearing loss in humans). Psychoacoustic measurements do not support this hypothesis. For tonal tinnitus, Konig *et al.* (2006) did find a clear association between the tinnitus pitch and the edge of the audiogram, however, with the tinnitus pitch on average 1.5 octaves above the edge frequency. In addition, tinnitus subjects generally give variable pitch matches, between and within test sessions, when asked to match pure tones to the pitch of their tinnitus. This would be expected if the tinnitus were comprised of a range of frequencies even when perceived as tonal rather than hissing. The tonal or hissing character could then be largely determined by the bandwidth of the hearing loss. This is supported by results obtained when tinnitus subjects were asked to rate pure tones covering a wide range of frequencies for similarity to their tinnitus sensation. Tinnitus sufferers typically identified a range of frequencies spanning the region of their hearing loss as resembling their tinnitus sensation (Noreña et al., 2002). This implies that, even though expansion of the cortical representation for edge frequencies appears to be functional, the expanded representation is not itself the neural substrate of tinnitus. The activity of the affected neurons is heard in accordance with their original frequency tuning and location in the cortical place map and this defines tinnitus as a phantom sensation. Underpinning these observations with controlled animal experiments and modeling studies is one of the aspects that will be reviewed in this chapter.

Imaging tinnitus

Positron emission tomography (PET) studies in gaze-induced tinnitus (a condition often found after vestibular schwannoma surgery in which gaze direction modulates the strength of tinnitus) suggest various correlates of tinnitus indicated by the increase of regional cerebral blood flow in the temporal-parietal auditory association areas (Brodman areas 22, 40, and 42), but excluding primary auditory cortex (Brodman area 41) (Giraud et al., 1999; Lockwood et al., 2001). The absence of a regional cerebral blood flow increase in primary auditory cortex rules out significantly increased SFR, but not increased neural synchrony (in the absence of increased SFR) as a correlate of tinnitus (Fig. 21.1). In the case of enhanced neural synchrony the same number of neurons could have the same SFR as in asynchronous firing of the same neurons, but their firing times would be different. Neural synchrony increase does not increase the energy demands of the synapses involved, and hence will not be reflected in increased regional cerebral blood flow. It is known that increased synchrony between the firings of a pair of neurons increases the probability of activating the higher-order neurons to which the synchronized pair project, and therefore one may expect, and indeed find, increased regional cerebral blood flow in non-primary auditory cortical areas.

Using functional magnetic resonance imaging (fMRI) to determine the correlation of tinnitus and neural activity in the inferior colliculus, Melcher et al. (2000) found a specific effect of noise stimulation: in unilateral tinnitus binaural noise produced an abnormally low activation in the inferior colliculus contralateral to the tinnitus ear. Since the amount of activation was calculated by comparing the brain oxygen level dependent response in the noise condition to that without noise (but with tinnitus), one can interpret this by assuming that the tinnitus condition has an increased SFR in the inferior colliculus and that the noise stimulus can only produce little extra activation in firing rate. This finding suggests a highly spontaneously active inferior colliculus in tinnitus subjects. The authors note that increased neural synchrony without increased SFR could not produce this effect. Smits et al. (2007) found the same effect of sound stimulation in auditory midbrain, thalamus, and auditory cortex. So, indirectly, this points to increased SFR from the inferior colliculus to cortex, although it is not clear if this applies to all subdivisions of these auditory centers.

Electro- and magneto-encephalography

The spontaneous magneto-encephalogram in a group of individuals with tinnitus is characterized by a marked reduction in alpha (8–12 Hz) power together with an enhancement in delta (1.5–4 Hz)

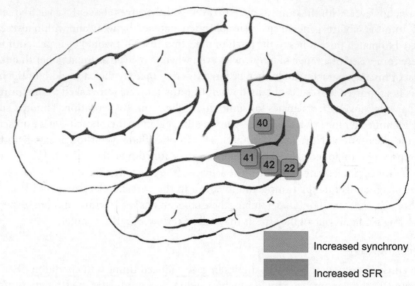

Fig. 21.1 Auditory cortical areas that show increased spontaneous firing rates according to positron emission tomography and functional magnetic resonance imaging (*pink color*) and those that show only increased neural synchrony (according to evoked potentials or magnetic fields; *blue color*). *Numbers* indicate Brodmann areas.

power compared to normal hearing controls. This pattern was especially pronounced over the temporal cortex, including the auditory areas. Moreover, this spectral pattern, particularly in right temporal and left frontal areas, correlated with tinnitus-related distress (Weisz *et al.*, 2005b).

Tinnitus as an auditory phantom sensation suggests similarities with the better-known phantom limb sensation. Phantom limb pain has been associated with changes in the body-surface map in sensorimotor cortex as deduced from magneto-encephalogram recordings. Suggested tonotopic map changes in auditory cortex of individuals experiencing tinnitus could also underlie tinnitus. However, unambiguous demonstration of auditory topographic map changes based on evoked potentials or magnetic fields has been difficult. Most of the techniques used are based on recording the N_{100} component of the magnetic field, and the tonotopic map is then constructed on the basis of equivalent dipole source locations for a series of tone frequencies. The equivalent dipole source location and strength is computed from the scalp distribution of activity in response to auditory stimulation. The auditory cortex in humans has several tonotopically organized areas in both the core and belt. Because the frequency gradient of these tonotopic maps reverses at the map borders (Formisano *et al.*, 2003), the common practice of reducing scalp activity to only one equivalent dipole to summarize tonotopic map changes in auditory cortical areas is fraught with pitfalls (Lütkenhöner *et al.*, 2003).

In tinnitus subjects the long-latency auditory evoked potential components (e.g., N_{100}) originate largely in secondary and association cortex (Brodman areas 40, 42, and 22; cf. Fig. 21.1) and were reduced in amplitude compared to those in a group of controls matched for hearing loss and age (Attias *et al.*, 1993). This could again point to increased spontaneous activity in secondary and association cortex so that stimulation can recruit fewer non-refractory neurons. Weisz *et al.* (2005a) compared tinnitus subjects with normal controls and used edge-frequency stimuli and stimuli with a frequency one octave below the edge. They found that the N_{100} amplitude for tinnitus subjects and controls was not different for edge-frequency tones, but that the N_{100} responses were significantly larger for tonal stimuli one octave below the edge frequency.

The enlarged N_{100} was found in the right hemisphere of the tinnitus subjects, regardless of the localization of the tinnitus. The source location for the edge-frequency dipole was abnormal, but in contrast to their earlier findings, the deviation from the control position was not related to tinnitus distress. This suggests that changes in the tonotopic map, if this is what causes the deviant position of the dipole, are unrelated to the strength of the tinnitus percept. The data from Weisz *et al.* (2005a) do suggest increased neural synchrony (larger N_{100}), but in the normal hearing frequency range, partially in contrast to the interpretation by Attias *et al.* (1993).

High-frequency (gamma) oscillations have been linked to conscious sensory perception and positive symptoms in a variety of neurological disorders. Weisz *et al.* (2007) examined gamma band activity during brief periods of marked enhancement of slow-wave (delta) activity, and found that both control and tinnitus groups showed significant increases in gamma band activity after the appearance of slow waves. However, gamma activity was more prominent in tinnitus subjects than in controls. The hemispheric lateralization of the gamma activity did correlate with the lateralization of the perceived tinnitus.

Otoacoustic emissions and tinnitus

Spontaneous otoacoustic emissions are low-level sounds of very precise and constant frequency emitted by the healthy normal ear, and are recordable with sensitive microphones inserted in the ear canal. In about 6–12% of tinnitus suffers with normal hearing, spontaneous otoacoustic emissions are considered to be at least partially responsible for the tinnitus. In most cases, however, spontaneous otoacoustic emissions and tinnitus are independent phenomena (Lonsbury-Martin and Martin, 2003). In this respect it is interesting to note that acute salicylate administration abolishes spontaneous otoacoustic emissions, and this could function as a simple test for the co-occurrence of emissions and tinnitus.

In audiometrically normal individuals with tinnitus, distortion-product otoacoustic emission amplitudes were reduced compared to normal hearing controls (Ozimek *et al.*, 2006). This suggests that standard audiometry is insensitive to minor changes in hearing sensitivity caused by outer hair cell loss that may be at the origin of tinnitus. In tinnitus resulting from head trauma, again in subjects with normal audiograms, transient otoacoustic emission amplitudes were increased, the incidence of spontaneous acoustic emissions was doubled, and contralateral tinnitus suppression was reduced, all pointing to a potential deficit in the medial olivocochlear bundle activity (Ceranic *et al.*, 1998). Thus, otoacoustic emissions are useful in the delineation of some mechanisms involved in cochlear functioning that might accompany tinnitus, but they do not generally relate to tinnitus itself.

Multimodal effects

Head and neck injuries are a frequent cause of tinnitus; moreover head and neck contractions can modulate existing tinnitus in 80% of patients. In 60% of individuals without tinnitus at the time of testing such contractions could induce tinnitus even in the profoundly deaf (Levine *et al.*, 2003). This suggests an important multimodal aspect in the perception of tinnitus and points to various sites along the extra-lemniscal pathway (indicated by orange in Fig. 21.2), including the olivo-cochlear bundle (see above), dorsal cochlear nucleus, and inferior colliculus, as important ignition sites in the generation of tinnitus (Zhou and Shore, 2006).

Neural correlates of tinnitus suggested by observations in humans

All in all, this overview of findings in humans with tinnitus suggests that elevated delta waves in the spontaneous electro- or magneto-encephalogram may be accompanying tinnitus. Increased evoked-potential or evoked-magnetic field amplitudes suggest that increased neural synchrony

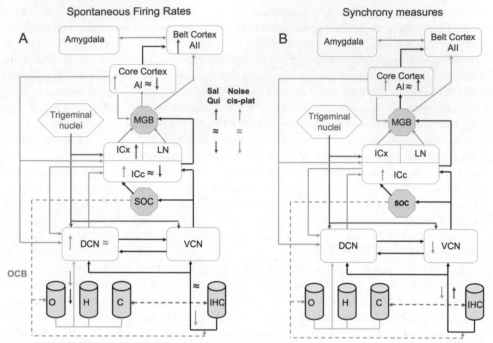

Fig. 21.2 Overview of changes in spontaneous firing rates (**A**) and neural synchrony (**B**) in animal studies after application of salicylate and quinine (*red symbols*) and noise trauma and cis-platin (*green symbols*). *Up and down arrows* indicate increase and decrease respectively; the ≈ *symbol* indicates no significant changes. The lemniscal pathway is indicated in *black;* the extra-lemniscal pathway is in *orange;* corticofugal and other feedback pathways are in *green*. Somatic influences are illustrated by the pathways (in *blue*) from the trigeminal nuclei to brainstem and midbrain nuclei.

may also be a factor. There may be tonotopic map changes in auditory cortex that accompany tinnitus. Increased spontaneous firing rates from the inferior colliculus to higher order cortex are also putative correlates of tinnitus in humans. Underlying all this are changes at the receptor and ion-channel level that disrupt the balance between excitation and inhibition in the brain (see below).

Neural correlates of tinnitus should be similar to neural correlates of audible sound if there is a unique coding of loudness. Thus, when a sound is made louder, the neurons in the auditory cortex typically increase their firing rates, suggesting that increased spontaneous firing rates could reflect the presence of tinnitus. However, the number of activated neurons also increases with increasing sound level. In addition raising the sound level from sub- to supra-threshold increases the neural synchrony in auditory cortex, so one could postulate that increased neural synchrony is also a correlate of tinnitus. It is, however, not *a priori* clear if the changes need to happen in primary cortical areas or if the neural correlate of tinnitus should be restricted to the extra-lemniscal pathway and thus to the secondary auditory cortex.

21.3.2 **Do animals have tinnitus?**

The findings in animal studies are reviewed below first of all with respect to changes in SFR, changes in neural synchrony, and changes in tonotopic maps. Subsequently, some underlying molecular changes in the auditory system are discussed. Finally, similarities of central nervous system mechanisms putatively involved in tinnitus with those underlying neuropathic pain and epilepsy are presented.

The neural substrate of tinnitus can only be adequately studied in animal models that show behavioral evidence of tinnitus under conditions similar to those that cause tinnitus in humans. Behavioral test models have been devised for rats, hamsters, guinea pigs, and mice (Turner, 2007). The findings have been taken as evidence that agents causing tinnitus in humans and these particular animal models also cause tinnitus in other common experimental animals, such as cats (Eggermont, 2005). In cats, rats, mice, and hamsters, changes in spontaneous neural activity in auditory nerve fibers, the dorsal cochlear nucleus, the inferior colliculus, and the auditory cortex have been recorded following the application of tinnitus-inducing agents – mostly noise trauma or application of salicylate. The issue of awake vs anesthetized animals is of some importance here as well (Yang *et al.*, 2007). Tinnitus-inducing agents may show potentially larger effects in awake animals, and different levels of corticofugal activity at subcortical structures cannot be excluded, albeit that anesthesia effects on corticofugal activity appear to be small (Yan and Ehret, 2002). The findings from recordings of single cells and neuronal population activity in animal models are shown in Fig. 21.2 and reviewed below.

21.3.3 Neural substrates of tinnitus in animals

Changes in spontaneous firing rate

A potential neural correlate of tinnitus is increased SFR (Fig. 21.2A). Typically, SFR does not change in aging animals, neither in dorsal cochlear nucleus (Caspary *et al.*, 2005) nor in auditory cortex (Turner *et al.*, 2005). Thus, aging in itself is unlikely to be a tinnitus-inducing factor, albeit it may enhance pre-existing tinnitus given the increased incidence of tinnitus with age.

Noise trauma After noise trauma, the SFR in cat auditory nerve fibers was significantly reduced (Liberman and Kiang, 1978), and the SFR was significantly enhanced *in vitro* in chinchilla dorsal cochlear nucleus (Brozoski *et al.*, 2002), but not in rat dorsal cochlear nucleus (Chang *et al.*, 2002). *In vivo* experiments in hamster dorsal cochlear nucleus indicate massive increases in SFR 5–180 days after noise exposure (Kaltenbach *et al.*, 2000). Complete or nearly complete section of ascending (Zacharek *et al.*, 2002) or descending inputs (Zhang *et al.*, 2006) did not significantly affect the magnitude of SFR in the dorsal cochlear nucleus, suggesting that increased SFR is either a self-contained neural network phenomenon or reflects intrinsic cell changes. The increase in SFR in hamster dorsal cochlear nucleus correlated with the strength of the behavioral index of tinnitus (Kaltenbach *et al.*, 2004). In mice inferior colliculus, noise trauma significantly increased SFR (Ma *et al.*, 2006). In cat primary auditory cortex, a significant increase in SFR occurred at least 2 hours after the trauma, but not immediately (< 15 min) following it (Noreña and Eggermont, 2003). At least 3 weeks after the trauma, the SFR was significantly higher than in controls at all characteristic frequencies (CFs) tested, so increased SFR is not restricted to the region of the hearing loss, although that region showed a more pronounced increase (Noreña and Eggermont, 2006).

Cisplatin About 1 month after daily cisplatin application that caused a high-frequency hearing loss, increased SFRs in the dorsal cochlear nucleus of hamsters were found when there was severe outer hair cell loss, and slightly less so when this was also accompanied by inner hair cell loss. No effect was found in the absence of or only minor outer hair cell loss (Kaltenbach *et al.*, 2002).

Salicylate Chronic salicylate application in doses that did not cause hearing loss, but can cause tinnitus (Bauer *et al.*, 2000), did increase the spontaneous activity of the auditory nerve measured as electric noise at the round window (Cazals *et al.*, 1998). This was interpreted as reflecting increased spontaneous firing synchrony in auditory nerve fibers. Interestingly, the amplitude of otoacoustic emissions increased, after an initial drop, with continued low-dose salicylate application (Huang *et al.*, 2005), suggesting a link between otoacoustic emissions and tinnitus, and thus a potential cochlear origin in this condition. However, it is surprising that the initial depressing effect of salicylate on the outer hair cell motor (and on otoacoustic emissions) reverses with time.

Guitton and Puel (2004) suggested that salicylate-induced tinnitus resulted from inhibition of cyclo-oxygenase activity, thereby causing an altered arachidonic acid metabolism and potentiating NMDA receptor currents in the cochlea. The increased opening probability of NMDA receptors can result in burst-firing activity in auditory nerve fibers, potentially leading to tinnitus. Such bursting activity has been found in some auditory nerve fibers after severe noise trauma (Liberman and Kiang, 1978). However, acute administration of moderate doses of salicylate failed to increase SFR in cat (Stypulkowski, 1990) and gerbil auditory nerve fibers (Müller *et al.*, 2003). In rats, salicylate in moderate to high dose resulted in decreased mean inter-spike intervals (suggestive for either increased SFR or burst firing) in the external nucleus of the inferior colliculus (Chen and Jastreboff, 1995). In mice, a moderate to high dose decreased SFR significantly in the central nucleus of the inferior colliculus (Ma *et al.*, 2006), suggesting a species difference or a difference in susceptibility of the central nucleus and the external nucleus of the inferior colliculus. In cat auditory cortex, salicylate did produce increased SFRs for high CFs in secondary auditory cortex, but did not have an effect in primary auditory cortex, and even caused decreased SFRs in the anterior auditory field for all CFs (Eggermont and Roberts, 2004). In awake rats, salicylate levels that induced behavioral signs of tinnitus decreased SFR in auditory cortex (Yang *et al.*, 2007).

Quinine In guinea pig auditory nerve fibers, quinine reduced the SFR significantly and increased the CF thresholds (Mulheran, 1999). Quinine administered to the cat significantly increased SFRs in secondary auditory cortex but not in primary auditory cortex or anterior auditory field (Eggermont, 2005).

This all suggests that there are species–dose interactions likely related to salicylate metabolism and tolerance. In addition, anesthesia levels may play a role. This makes salicylate studies in animals difficult to generalize to humans.

21.3.4 Changes in neural synchrony

The degree to which spike firing from two different neurons is time-locked or synchronized can be quantified by the cross-correlogram (Eggermont, 2000). The neural synchrony of spontaneous firing (Fig. 21.2B) studied in the same single-neuron pairs in primary auditory cortex of the cat before and after application of salicylate was not changed. In contrast to the effects produced by salicylate, and despite the same average hearing loss produced, the cross-correlation of single-unit pairs in primary auditory cortex increased after quinine administration (Eggermont and Roberts, 2004).

Effects of acute noise trauma on neural synchrony were studied by Noreña and Eggermont (2003) in primary auditory cortex. A significant increase in peak cross-correlation coefficients was apparent within 15 min of the trauma, and increased by a further 50% at 2 hours after the trauma. Several weeks to months after the trauma all neuron pairs in the reorganized region of auditory cortex showed significant neural correlations.

Despite a reduction in the compound action potential amplitude of the auditory nerve and in the local field potential of the cochlear nucleus following noise trauma in the rat (Fig. 21.2B), the local field potential amplitude in the inferior colliculus was typically enhanced at higher intensity levels (Wang *et al.*, 2002), and so was the local field potential in auditory cortex (Yang *et al.*, 2007).

21.3.5 **Changes in cortical tonotopic maps**

Tonotopic maps are representations of the distribution of characteristic frequency as a function of spatial coordinates in an auditory nucleus or cortex. Local mechanical damage to the cochlea, ototoxic-drug damage to the cochlea, and noise-induced hearing loss all cause tonotopic map changes in primary auditory cortex (Eggermont and Roberts, 2004). The map changes (Fig. 21.3) are not causally related to the hearing loss (Noreña and Eggermont, 2005), but are always accompanied by increased SFR and increased neural synchrony.

Map changes do not occur if immediately after noise trauma a compensatory complex sound that mimics the frequency range of the hearing loss in bandwidth and level is presented for several weeks (Noreña and Eggermont, 2005). It is assumed that during the presentation of this compensatory sound the downregulation of inhibition that usually follows noise-induced hearing loss (Milbrandt *et al.*, 2000) does not occur, and that the unmasking of new excitatory inputs (Noreña and Eggermont, 2003) does not happen or is reversed. When this 'unmasking" trigger for tonotopic map reorganization is absent, map changes do not occur, despite a remaining hearing loss.

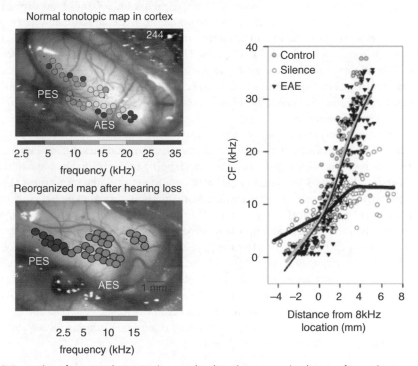

Fig. 21.3 Examples of a normal tonotopic map (*top*) and a reorganized map after noise trauma (*bottom, left hand column*).*Right* the CF of AI neurons is plotted according to location of the recording site along the anteroposterior axis relative to the CF 8 kHz location in each cat. Noise trauma cats reared in silence after the exposure show a clear deviation in the CF-distance map, largely the result of the absence of high CFs. In contrast, cats reared in an enriched acoustic environment (4–20 kHz) after the noise trauma show a CF-distance map that is indistinguishable from the control map. Silence reared cats, enriched acoustic environment (EAE) reared cats, and control cats are represented by *open circles, filled triangles*, and *filled gray circles*, respectively. *Lines* represent locally weighted regression lines (*solid gray line*, control; *thin black line*, EAE; *thick black lines*, silence). (After Noreña and Eggermont, 2005.)

21.4 **Tinnitus: a hypersynchrony disorder?**

Ever since we included changes in neural synchrony in our description of the effects produced by tinnitus-inducing agents, there have been questions as to why neural synchrony would play a role in the perception of tinnitus.

21.4.1 **Neural synchrony and perception**

There is a large body of literature, mainly originating from studies of the visual cortex, that suggests a role of neural synchrony in perceptual binding (Singer and Gray, 1995). Typically, neurons that simultaneously respond to a particular stimulus feature show synchrony in their firing. This synchrony in the visual system is often accompanied by oscillations in the local field potentials in the frequency range around 40 Hz, and spontaneous oscillations at that frequency in the human EEG accompany tinnitus (Weisz *et al.*, 2007).

Although neural cross-correlation studies in auditory cortex are not performed routinely, one can summarize the findings as showing a significant increase in synchrony between neural spiking in separate cortical areas during stimulation compared with spontaneous firing. The amount of cortical neural synchrony in the cat auditory cortex (Eggermont, 2000) did not depend on the stimulus level. Thus, the stepwise change in neural synchrony between sub- and supra-threshold conditions, together with the increase in firing rate, may help to signal both a change from silence to sound and the presence of an ongoing stimulus. The latter may be important in the perception of tinnitus. Recently, it was found that neural synchronization plays a critical role in the transmission of sensory information from the thalamus to the cortex. It is likely that increased synchronization of auditory cortical neurons will similarly enhance the transmission of information to subsequent stages in auditory processing.

Horizontal fiber activity in auditory cortex can also induce strong neural correlations. Cortico-cortical fibers largely connect cell groups with characteristic frequencies differing by more than one octave. Such neurons have generally non-overlapping receptive fields, but can still have sizeable correlated firings. Correlated neural activity and neural interconnections (Lee *et al.*, 2004) are presented as the substrates for cortical reorganization; increased neural synchrony and tonotopic map reorganization go hand in hand. This links cortical reorganization with hypersynchrony and can be considered as an important driving force underlying tinnitus. In our studies, increased neural synchrony was correlated with increased SFR. This can be interpreted in two ways: the first is that changes in neural synchrony are determined largely by changes in SFR. However, our previous studies into the immediate effects of an acoustic trauma indicate that the initial increases in neural synchrony occurred in the absence of SFR changes, whereas a few hours after the trauma neural synchrony and increased SFR became correlated (Noreña and Eggermont, 2003). I interpret this to indicate that neural synchrony changes are priming subsequent changes in firing rate, likely by the mechanisms suggested above.

21.4.2 **Tinnitus, epilepsy, and neuropathic pain**

Loss of peripheral input to central neurons can promote the development of synchronous spiking activity (Noreña and Eggermont, 2003) by prolonging postsynaptic depolarization and increasing the likelihood of temporally coincident inputs converging on synapses. In the normal central auditory system, the inhibition surrounding the excitatory part of the receptive field of a neuron produced by thalamo-cortical input would be expected to restrict synchronous activity to neurons tuned to properties of the acoustic stimulus, thereby leading to normal auditory perception. However, when intra-cortical inhibition is weakened, widely distributed synchronous spike-firing activity can develop and lead to the perception of sounds that are physically absent, i.e., tinnitus.

A highly persistent modification of brain functioning occurs after repeated application of electrical stimulation (kindling) and results in the development and spread of epileptiform activity (Valentine *et al.*, 2004). Hearing sensitivity measured by the auditory brainstem response, and as reflected in the thresholds at the CF of cortical neurons, was not affected by the kindling sessions. Recordings were obtained from primary auditory cortex contralateral to the kindled site the day after the last kindling session. Spontaneous neural synchrony, as measured by spike cross-correlation, was enhanced by 40% compared to sham controls. This was accompanied by a profound alteration of the tonotopic map in primary auditory cortex, with a large area becoming tuned to a narrow frequency range that was related to the location of the kindling electrodes.

Noise trauma acting at the periphery and kindling interfering at a central level both cause profound changes in the tonotopic map in primary auditory cortex and both induce a strong increase in spontaneous neural synchrony. These correspondences suggest a role of neural synchrony in tinnitus and epilepsy, indicating that tinnitus could result from an epileptiform-like pattern of activity in auditory cortex.

As reviewed in Valentine *et al.* (2004) the changes in GABA and glutamate receptors in kindling and noise-induced hearing loss are also comparable. Kindling has been associated with a loss in GABAergic inhibition. It has also been hypothesized that kindling stimulation in cortex produces an accumulation of glutamate that triggers altered NMDA channel functions and long-lasting changes in synaptic efficacy of long-range horizontal connections. In cat primary auditory cortex horizontal connections generally follow a course parallel to the iso-frequency contours (Read *et al.*, 2001), but 10–15% project in directions orthogonal to the iso-frequency contours and may even extend as far as the anterior and posterior auditory fields (Wallace *et al.*, 1991; Lee *et al.*, 2004). Strengthening of the horizontal connections after kindling may explain the larger percentage of double-tuned frequency tuning curves that we observed. If these horizontal connections become stronger than those of the specific thalamic inputs, they could elicit an outward migration of glutamate hyperactivity and subsequent synaptic changes. This process would likely stop when all the neurons in the stimulated cortical area (and its projection region) were combined into one large neural assembly.

Chronic tinnitus and chronic pain also display considerable similarities, including plastic changes in the central nervous system leading to hypersensitivity to sensory stimuli and a change in the way those stimuli are perceived (Møller, 1997). Tinnitus has been classified among the positive symptoms that arise after lesions of the nervous system, sharing with neurogenic pain the phenomenon of low-threshold calcium spike-burst firing in the medial thalamus (Weisz *et al.*, 2007). Another example of the similarities between tinnitus and pain is that the vanilloid receptor type I (VR1) is expressed in the spiral ganglion of rats (Balaban *et al.*, 2003). VR1 is commonly expressed in dorsal root and trigeminal ganglion cells and allows us to appreciate the painfully pleasant effect of hot peppers. In the case of an inflammatory response, arachidonic acid can be metabolized by lipo-oxygenase, and its metabolites act as agonists at the VR1-binding site. This could provide a mechanism for hyperacusis and tinnitus. Epilepsy, neuropathic pain, and tinnitus all may result from an imbalance of excitatory and inhibitory transmitter efficacy (Fig. 21.2B).

21.5 **Molecular aspects**

21.5.1 **Ion channels**

The inner hair cells in the cochlea are equipped with only one type of Ca^{2+} channel, namely the L-type. These Ca^{2+} channels regulate the release of glutamate from the inner hair cells, and blocking these L-type channels with nimodipine results in a decrease in spontaneous and stimulus-driven firing rates in auditory nerve fibers (Robertson and Paki, 2002). Systemic salicylate does not block these channels because only the low-intensity segment of the input–output function is affected. The low-intensity effect on the input–output function points to an action of salicylate on the outer hair cell-mediated cochlear amplifier.

Quinine is a K^+ channel blocker, and results in broadening of the action potential (Lin *et al.*, 1998), which could result in enhanced transmitter release and thus likely increased SFR. However, the concurrent increase in the refractory period in auditory nerve fibers appears to offset this (Mulheran, 1999). At higher dose, quinine also blocks the Na^+ current, which may cause the often-observed threshold increase. Quinine does not affect Ca^{2+} currents, but blocks Ca^{2+}-activated K^+ currents. The observed threshold increase could, just as following noise trauma, start central loss of inhibition and central unmasking of previously silent excitatory inputs.

Lidocain can relieve tinnitus temporarily by blocking the fast voltage-sensitive Na^+ channels, but probably only in the central nervous system, since tinnitus could be suppressed with lidocain in patients with sectioned auditory nerve after vestibular schwannoma removal (Baguley *et al.*, 2005).

21.5.2 Receptor systems

An overview of the changes in transmitter activity separated into neuromodulators and more traditional excitatory and inhibitory transmitters is presented in Fig. 21.4.

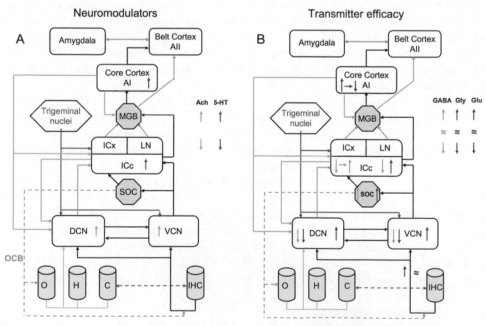

Fig. 21.4 Actions of neuromodulators (**A**) and common transmitters (**B**) after induction of tinnitus in animals. The neuromodulators that are affected are acetylcholine (ACh, *green symbols*) and serotonin (5-HT, *red symbols*). Transmitter efficacy can be transient as indicated by the ↓→↑ sequence (first reduced, then increased) for GABA (*green symbols* in ICc), and as indicated by the ↑→↓ sequence (first increased, then reduced) for glutamate (*red symbols* in core cortex). Generally, there are opposite effects for GABA or glycine (*blue symbols*) and glutamate.

AMPA and NMDA

AMPA is the dominant glutamate receptor type in auditory nerve fiber endings below the inner hair cells. AMPA receptors also mediate the excitotoxic effect of noise trauma that causes excessive amounts of glutamate in the synaptic cleft, thereby allowing excessive Ca^{2+} influx into the nerve fiber endings and resulting in neurite loss. This neurite loss may be reversible under certain conditions (Puel *et al.*, 1998).

Salicylate amplifies cochlear NMDA-mediated responses but has little or no effect on AMPA- and kainate-mediated responses (Peng *et al.*, 2003). NMDA antagonists protect from aminoglycoside ototoxicity (Basile *et al.*, 1996) and prevent excitotoxicity induced by acoustic trauma (Duan *et al.*, 2000). Behavioral effects of tinnitus induced by salicylate, but not the resulting hearing loss, were abolished by NMDA receptor antagonists, and tinnitus-like behavior could be induced by NMDA receptor agonists (Guitton *et al.*, 2003). This suggests an important role of NMDA receptors in the initial stages of tinnitus both in the cochlea and in cortex (Wang *et al.*, 2005).

GABA

Following noise trauma, significant decreases in glutamic acid decarboxylase (the rate-limiting enzyme in the formation of GABA) were found in the inferior colliculus in the first 42 hours after the trauma; however, complete recovery occurred after 30 days (Milbrandt *et al.*, 2000). Decreases were also found for glycine- and GABA-related activity in the cochlear nucleus (Milbrandt and Caspary, 1995) and inferior colliculus (Caspary *et al.*, 1999) as a result of aging. In contrast, following auditory deprivation, glycine- and GABA-related activity was upregulated in the superior olivary complex (Suneja *et al.*, 1998).

Acetylcholine

Acetylcholine receptors come in two flavors: muscarinic (mAChR) and nicotinic (nAChR). nAChR subunits are located on the cochlear hair cells and mediate the medial efferent olivocochlear bundle response. These nAChRs are ligand-mediated ion channels (Lustig, 2006). After noise trauma, choline-acetyl transferase increased by 74% in ipsilateral antero-ventral cochlear nucleus and by somewhat less in ipsilateral dorsal cochlear nucleus at 8 days post trauma. By 2 months post trauma, the level was still increased in the dorsal cochlear nucleus on the exposed side (Jin *et al.*, 2006). In rat dorsal cochlear nucleus, intense noise exposure resulted in an upregulation of cholinergic receptors (Kaltenbach and Zhang, 2007).

Serotonin

Serotonergic activity increases the perception of chronic pain and phantom limb pain and thus may play a role in the perception of tinnitus (Simpson and Davies, 2000). Indeed, serotonin receptor agonists exacerbate the behavioral index of salicylate-induced tinnitus (Guitton *et al.*, 2005). Salicylate in itself increases the serotonergic activity in the rat for up to 6 hours post injection in inferior colliculus and primary auditory cortex (Liu *et al.*, 2003).

21.5.3 Conclusion

Animal studies suggest that tinnitus may be accompanied by increased NMDA receptor-mediated responses and/or decreased efficacy of GABA in the central auditory system. Acetylcholine and serotonin may play a role as well.

21.6 Homeostatic mechanisms as a cause for tinnitus?

Homeostatic mechanisms stabilize the mean activity of a neuron around a certain target level over time scales in the order of days, and typically do so by scaling the efficacy of the neuron's synapses

(Turrigiano, 1999). Schaette and Kempter (2006) modeled the effects of homeostatic plasticity by a change in a gain factor proportional to the deviation of the mean activity from a certain target rate. In their model, homeostatic plasticity restores the mean firing rate of a neuron in the dorsal cochlear nucleus after hearing loss. This mean firing rate includes both driven and spontaneous parts, and both are scaled upwards to the target level. This applies to all neurons along the auditory pathway. Restoring the mean rate therefore likely increases the spontaneous rate throughout the auditory system. Interestingly, Schaette and Kempter's model also allows the evaluation of how the pathologic changes could be reversed through additional sensory stimulation. Noreña and Eggermont (2005) demonstrated that stimulation, which restores the spatial distribution of firing rates in auditory nerve fibers, is indeed effective at reversing the effects of noise trauma (see section 21.3.5).

21.7 Tinnitus in the brain: a summary

In the search for bottom-up mechanisms of tinnitus, increased SFR and increased neural synchrony have attracted most of the attention. It is doubtful whether increased SFRs in subcortical structures alone will lead to increased SFR in cortex, despite the action of homeostatic mechanisms. It is far more likely that increased neural synchrony in subcortical structures will propagate effectively along the auditory pathway and ultimately result in increased synchrony and/or increased SFRs in cortex. Increased neural synchrony combined with increased SFR would be very powerful indeed. Human studies using fMRI that find increased activation in certain brain regions suggest an increased spontaneous firing rate in those regions. Enlarged evoked potential or magnetic fields in addition imply increased neural synchrony as its cause. The fMRI data point to increased SFR in the midbrain, thalamus, and cortex, whereas evoked potential data point to increased synchrony in these same structures. It is likely that both conditions co-occur as both may result from downregulated inhibition levels. The laterality of the strongest activity in the gamma band corresponded clearly with the laterality of the tinnitus percept. Gamma activity being a consequence of enhanced neural synchrony was more prominent in tinnitus subjects than in controls. In that sense gamma activity may play a similar role as it has been posited to do in normal auditory perception. All these changes may be the result of an imbalance in the two major transmitter systems: the glutamatergic and GABAergic ones. These imbalances may cause tonotopic map changes, increased SFR, and increased neural synchrony, which all have been suggested to be a neural substrate of tinnitus. Speedy intervention, at least following noise trauma, by applying an enhanced acoustic environment that compensates for loss of neural activity in the hearing loss range appears to prevent the occurrence of these imbalances.

Acknowledgements

This study was supported by the Alberta Heritage Foundation for Medical Research, a grant from the Canadian Institutes of Health Research – New Emerging Teams, and the Campbell McLaurin Chair for Hearing Deficiencies.

References

Attias J, Urbach D, Gold S, Shemesh Z (1993) Auditory event related potentials in chronic tinnitus patients with noise induced hearing loss. *Hear Res* 71: 106–13.

Baguley DM, Jones S, Wilkins I, Axon PR, Moffat DA (2005) The inhibitory effect of intravenous lidocaine infusion on tinnitus after translabyrinthine removal of vestibular schwannoma: a double-blind, placebo-controlled, crossover study. *Otol Neurotol* 26: 169–76.

Balaban CD, Zhou J, Li HS (2003) Type 1 vanilloid receptor expression by mammalian inner ear ganglion cells. *Hear Res* 175: 165–70.

Basile AS, Huang JM, Xie C, Webster D, Berlin C, Skolnick P (1996) N-methyl-D-aspartate antagonists limit aminoglycoside antibiotic-induced hearing loss. *Nat Med* 2: 1338–43.

Bauer CA, Brozoski TJ, Holder TM, Caspary DM (2000) Effects of chronic salicylate on GABAergic activity in rat inferior colliculus. *Hear Res* 147: 175–82.

Brozoski TJ, Bauer CA, Caspary DM (2002) Elevated fusiform cell activity in the dorsal cochlear nucleus of chinchillas with psychophysical evidence of tinnitus. *J Neurosci* 22: 2383–90.

Caspary DM, Holder TM, Hughes LF, Milbrandt JC, McKernan RM, Naritoku DK (1999) Age-related changes in GABA(A) receptor subunit composition and function in rat auditory system. *Neuroscience* 93: 307–12.

Caspary DM, Schatteman TA, Hughes LF (2005) Age-related changes in the inhibitory response properties of dorsal cochlear nucleus output neurons: role of inhibitory inputs. *J Neurosci* 25: 10952–9.

Cazals Y, Horner KC, Huang ZW (1998) Alterations in average spectrum of cochleoneural activity by long-term salicylate treatment in the guinea pig: a plausible index of tinnitus. *J Neurophysiol* 80: 2113–20.

Ceranic BJ, Prasher DK, Raglan E, Luxon LM (1998) Tinnitus after head injury: evidence from otoacoustic emissions. *J Neurol Neurosurg Psychiatry* 65: 523–9.

Chang H, Chen K, Kaltenbach JA, Zhang J, Godfrey DA (2002) Effects of acoustic trauma on dorsal cochlear nucleus neuron activity in slices. *Hear Res* 164: 59–68.

Chen GD, Jastreboff PJ (1995) Salicylate-induced abnormal activity in the inferior colliculus of rats. *Hear Res* 82: 158–78.

Duan M, Agerman K, Ernfors P, Canlon B (2000) Complementary roles of neurotrophin 3 and a N-methyl-D-aspartate antagonist in the protection of noise and aminoglycoside-induced ototoxicity. *Proc Natl Acad Sci USA* 97: 7597–602.

Eggermont JJ (2000) Sound induced correlation of neural activity between and within three auditory cortical areas. *J Neurophysiology* 83: 2708–22.

Eggermont JJ (2005) Tinnitus: neurobiological substrates. *Drug Discov Today* 10: 1283–90.

Eggermont JJ, Roberts LE (2004) The neuroscience of tinnitus. *Trends Neurosci* 27: 676–82.

Evans EF, Wilson JP, Borerwe TA (1981) Animal models of tinnitus. *Ciba Found Symp* 85: 108–38.

Formisano E, Kim DS, Di Salle F, van de Moortele PF, Ugurbil K, Goebel R (2003) Mirror-symmetric tonotopic maps in human primary auditory cortex. *Neuron* 40: 859–69.

Giraud AL, Chery-Croze S, Fischer G, *et al.* (1999) A selective imaging of tinnitus. *Neuroreport* 10: 1–5.

Guitton MJ, Puel JL (2004) Cochlear NMDA receptors and tinnitus. *Audiolog Med* 2: 3–7.

Guitton MJ, Caston J, Ruel J, Johnson RM, Pujol R, Puel JL (2003) Salicylate induces tinnitus through activation of cochlear NMDA receptors. *J Neurosci* 23: 3944–52.

Guitton MJ, Pujol R, Puel JL (2005) m-Chlorophenylpiperazine exacerbates perception of salicylate-induced tinnitus in rats. *Eur J Neurosci* 22: 2675–8.

Heller AJ (2003) Classification and epidemiology of tinnitus. *Otolaryngol Clin N Am* 36: 239–48.

Henry JA, Dennis KC, Schechter MA (2005) General review of tinnitus: prevalence, mechanisms, effects, and management. *J Speech Lang Hear Res* 48: 1204–35.

House JW, Brackmann DE (1981) Tinnitus: surgical treatment. *Ciba Found Symp* 85: 204–16.

Huang ZW, Luo Y, Wu Z, Tao Z, Jones RO, Zhao HB (2005) Paradoxical enhancement of active cochlear mechanics in long-term administration of salicylate. *J Neurophysiol* 93: 2053–61.

Jastreboff PJ, Brennan JF, Coleman JK, Sasaki CT (1988) Phantom auditory sensation in rats: an animal model for tinnitus. *Behav Neurosci* 102: 811–22.

Jin YM, Godfrey DA, Wang J, Kaltenbach JA (2006) Effects of intense tone exposure on choline acetyltransferase activity in the hamster cochlear nucleus. *Hear Res* 216–217: 168–75.

Kaltenbach JA, Zhang J (2007) Intense sound-induced plasticity in the dorsal cochlear nucleus of rats: evidence for cholinergic receptor upregulation. *Hear Res* **226**: 232–43.

Kaltenbach JA, Zhang J, Afman CE (2000) Plasticity of spontaneous neural activity in the dorsal cochlear nucleus after intense sound exposure. *Hear Res* **147**: 282–92.

Kaltenbach JA, Rachel JD, Mathog TA, Zhang J, Falzarano PR, Lewandowski M (2002) Cisplatin-induced hyperactivity in the dorsal cochlear nucleus and its relation to outer hair cell loss: relevance to tinnitus. *J Neurophysiol* **88**: 699–714.

Kaltenbach JA, Zacharek MA, Zhang J, Frederick S (2004) Activity in the dorsal cochlear nucleus of hamsters previously tested for tinnitus following intense tone exposure. *Neurosci Lett* **355**: 121–5.

Kiang NY, Moxon EC, Levine RA (1970) Auditory-nerve activity in cats with normal and abnormal cochleas. *Ciba Foundation Symposium – Sensorineural Hearing Loss*. John Wiley, Hoboken, pp 241–73.

Konig O, Schaette R, Kempter R, Gross M (2006) Course of hearing loss and occurrence of tinnitus. *Hear Res* **221**: 59–64.

Lee CC, Schreiner CE, Imaizumi K, Winer JA (2004) Tonotopic and heterotopic projection systems in physiologically defined auditory cortex. *Neuroscience* **128**: 871–87.

Levine RA, Abel M, Cheng H (2003) CNS somatosensory–auditory interactions elicit or modulate tinnitus. *Exp Brain Res* **153**: 643–8.

Liberman MC, Dodds LW (1987) Acute ultrastructural changes in acoustic trauma: serial-section reconstruction of stereocilia and cuticular plates. *Hear Res* **26**: 45–64.

Liberman MC, Kiang NY (1978) Acoustic trauma in cats. Cochlear pathology and auditory-nerve activity. *Acta Otolaryngol Suppl* **358**: 1–63.

Lin X, Chen S, Tee D (1998) Effects of quinine on the excitability and voltage-dependent currents of isolated spiral ganglion neurons in culture. *J Neurophysiol* **79**: 2503–12.

Liu J, Li X, Wang L, Dong Y, Han H, Liu G (2003) Effects of salicylate on serotoninergic activities in rat inferior colliculus and auditory cortex. *Hear Res* **175**: 45–53.

Lockwood AH, Wack DS, Burkard RF, *et al.* (2001) The functional anatomy of gaze-evoked tinnitus and sustained lateral gaze. *Neurology* **56**: 472–80.

Lonsbury-Martin BL, Martin GK (2003) Otoacoustic emissions. *Curr Opin Otolaryngol Head Neck Surg* **5**: 361–6.

Lustig LR (2006) Nicotinic acetylcholine receptor structure and function in the efferent auditory system. *Anat Rec A Discov Mol Cell Evol Biol* **288**: 424–34.

Lütkenhöner B, Krumbholz K, Seither-Preisler A (2003) Studies of tonotopy based on wave N100 of the auditory evoked field are problematic. *Neuroimage* **19**: 935–49.

Ma WL, Hidaka H, May BJ (2006) Spontaneous activity in the inferior colliculus of CBA/J mice after manipulations that induce tinnitus. *Hear Res* **212**: 9–21.

Melcher JR, Sigalovsky IS, Guinan JJ Jr, Levine RA (2000) Lateralized tinnitus studied with functional magnetic resonance imaging: abnormal inferior colliculus activation. *J Neurophysiol* **83**: 1058–72.

Milbrandt JC, Caspary DM (1995) Age-related reduction of [^{3}H]strychnine binding sites in the cochlear nucleus of the Fischer 344 rat. *Neuroscience* **67**: 713–19.

Milbrandt JC, Holder TM, Wilson MC, Salvi RJ, Caspary DM (2000) GAD levels and muscimol binding in rat inferior colliculus following acoustic trauma. *Hear Res* **147**: 251–60.

Møller AR (1997) Similarities between chronic pain and tinnitus. *Am J Otol* **18**: 577–85.

Mulheran M (1999) The effects of quinine on cochlear nerve fibre activity in the guinea pig. *Hear Res* **134**: 145–52.

Müller M, Klinke R, Arnold W, Oestreicher E (2003) Auditory nerve fibre responses to salicylate revisited. *Hear Res* **183**: 37–43.

Noreña A, Micheyl C, Chery-Croze S, Collet L (2002) Psychoacoustic characterization of the tinnitus spectrum: implications for the underlying mechanisms of tinnitus. *Audiol Neurootol* **7**: 358–69.

Noreña AJ, Eggermont JJ (2003) Changes in spontaneous neural activity immediately after an acoustic trauma: implications for neural correlates of tinnitus. *Hear Res* **183**: 137–53.

Noreña AJ, Eggermont JJ (2005) Enriched acoustic environment after noise trauma reduces hearing loss and prevents cortical map reorganization. *J Neurosci* **25**: 699–705.

Noreña AJ, Eggermont JJ (2006) Enriched acoustic environment after noise trauma abolishes neural signs of tinnitus. *Neuroreport* **17**: 559–63.

Ozimek E, Wicher A, Szyfter W, Szymiec E (2006) Distortion product otoacoustic emission (DPOAE) in tinnitus patients. *J Acoust Soc Am* **119**: 527–38.

Peng H, Derrick BE, Martinez JL Jr (2003) Identification of upregulated SCG10 mRNA expression associated with late-phase long-term potentiation in the rat hippocampal Schaffer-CA1 pathway in vivo. *J Neurosci* **23**: 6617–26.

Puel JL, Ruel J, Gervais d'Aldin C, Pujol R (1998) Excitotoxicity and repair of cochlear synapses after noise-trauma induced hearing loss. *Neuroreport* **9**: 2109–14.

Rauschecker JP (1999) Auditory cortical plasticity: a comparison with other sensory systems. *Trends Neurosci* **22**: 74–80.

Read HL, Winer JA, Schreiner CE (2001) Modular organization of intrinsic connections associated with spectral tuning in cat auditory cortex. *Proc Natl Acad Sci USA* **98**: 8042–7.

Robertson D, Paki B (2002) Role of L-type Ca^{2+} channels in transmitter release from mammalian inner hair cells. II. Single-neuron activity. *J Neurophysiol* **87**: 2734–40.

Schaette R, Kempter R (2006) Development of tinnitus-related neuronal hyperactivity through homeostatic plasticity after hearing loss: a computational model. *Eur J Neurosci* **23**: 3124–38.

Simpson JJ, Davies WE (2000) A review of evidence in support of a role for 5-HT in the perception of tinnitus. *Hear Res* **145**: 1–7.

Singer W, Gray CM (1995) Visual feature integration and the temporal correlation hypothesis. *Annu Rev Neurosci* **18**: 555–86.

Smits M, Kovacs S, de Ridder D, Peeters RR, van Hecke P, Sunaert S (2007) Lateralization of functional magnetic resonance imaging (fMRI) activation in the auditory pathway of patients with lateralized tinnitus. *Neuroradiology* **49**: 669–79.

Stypulkowski PH (1990) Mechanisms of salicylate ototoxicity. *Hear Res* **46**: 113–45.

Suneja SK, Potashner SJ, Benson CG (1998) Plastic changes in glycine and GABA release and uptake in adult brain stem auditory nuclei after unilateral middle ear ossicle. *Exper Neurol* **150**(2): 273–88.

Turner JG (2007) Behavioral measures of tinnitus in laboratory animals. *Progress Brain Res* **166**: 147–56.

Turner JG, Hughes LF, Caspary DM (2005) Affects of aging on receptive fields in rat primary auditory cortex layer V neurons. *J Neurophysiol* **94**: 2738–47.

Turrigiano GG (1999) Homeostatic plasticity in neuronal networks: the more things change, the more they stay the same. *Trends Neurosci* **22**: 221–7.

Valentine PA, Teskey GC, Eggermont JJ (2004) Kindling changes burst firing, neural synchrony and tonotopic organization of cat primary auditory cortex. *Cereb Cortex* **14**: 827–39.

Wallace MN, Kitzes LM, Jones EG (1991) Intrinsic inter- and intralaminar connections and their relationship to the tonotopic map in cat primary auditory cortex. *Exp Brain Res* **86**: 527–44.

Wang J, Ding D, Salvi RJ (2002) Functional reorganization in chinchilla inferior colliculus associated with chronic and acute cochlear damage. *Hear Res* **168**: 238–49.

Wang Z, Ruan Q, Wang D (2005) Different effects of intracochlear sensory and neuronal injury stimulation on expression of synaptic N-methyl-D-aspartate receptors in the auditory cortex of rats in vivo. *Acta Otolaryngol* **125**: 1145–51.

Weisz N, Wienbruch C, Dohrmann K, Elbert T (2005a) Neuromagnetic indicators of auditory cortical reorganization of tinnitus. *Brain* **128**: 2722–31.

Weisz N, Moratti S, Meinzer M, Dohrmann K, Elbert T (2005b) Tinnitus perception and distress is related to abnormal spontaneous brain activity as measured by magnetoencephalography. *PLoS Med* **2**: e153.

Weisz N, Müller S, Schlee W, Dohrmann K, Hartmann T, Elbert T (2007) The neural code of auditory phantom perception. *J Neurosci* **27**: 1479–84.

Yan J, Ehret G (2002) Corticofugal modulation of midbrain sound processing in the house mouse. *Eur J Neurosci* **16**: 119–28.

Yang G, Lobarinas E, Zhang L, *et al.* (2007) Salicylate induced tinnitus: behavioral measures and neural activity in auditory cortex of awake rats. *Hear Res* **226**: 244–53.

Zacharek MA, Kaltenbach JA, Mathog TA, Zhang J (2002) Effects of cochlear ablation on noise induced hyperactivity in the hamster dorsal cochlear nucleus: implications for the origin of noise induced tinnitus. *Hear Res* **172**: 137–43.

Zhang JS, Kaltenbach JA, Godfrey DA, Wang J (2006) Origin of hyperactivity in the hamster dorsal cochlear nucleus following intense sound exposure. *J Neurosci Res* **84**: 819–31.

Zhou J, Shore S (2006) Convergence of spinal trigeminal and cochlear nucleus projections in the inferior colliculus of the guinea pig. *J Comp Neurol* **495**: 100–12.

Chapter 22

Auditory prostheses for the brainstem and midbrain

Robert V. Shannon

22.1 Introduction

Cochlear implants (CIs) have been successful beyond our wildest speculation. In the 1970s few people would have predicted that deaf patients with CIs would be able to converse normally on the telephone or enjoy music. Yet telephone use is common and even expected from modern CIs (e.g., Spahr and Dorman, 2004; Krueger *et al.*, 2008), while music appreciation is uncommon but possible. We now know that we greatly underestimated the pattern recognition abilities of the brain and that speech can be recognized when it is represented at the auditory periphery by very coarse tonotopic patterns of activity changing slowly in time (Shannon *et al.*, 1995, 2004). Fine frequency tuning and temporal phase locking are not necessary for understanding speech in quiet listening conditions, but become increasingly important as the listening conditions become more difficult (Smith *et al.*, 2002; Shannon *et al.*, 2004). Efforts are now underway to improve the delivery of temporal and spectral fine structure to CIs (Lorenzi *et al.*, 2006; Koch *et al.*, 2007), to provide localization of sounds in space via bilateral CIs (Litovsky *et al.*, 2004), to combine electrical hearing and acoustic residual hearing (Gifford *et al.*, 2007), and to implant deaf infants below 1 year of age (Svirsky *et al*, 2000; Robbins *et al.*, 2004; Dettman *et al.*, 2007). However, some patients are not able to use CI technology, such as those who have damaged auditory nerves. If people with damaged auditory nerves are to benefit from implant technology the site of stimulation must go beyond the cochlea. In this chapter we discuss attempts to provide hearing by stimulating neural structures in the central auditory system beyond the cochlea: in the cochlear nucleus (CN) and inferior colliculus (IC).

In electrical stimulation of the CN and IC we need to consider the tonotopic organization and the specialization of neural circuitry when we design electrodes and stimulation strategies. The CN contains many different specialized cell types and a complex tonotopic structure. In spite of this, excellent speech recognition has been observed in some patients with an auditory brainstem implant (ABI) (Colletti and Shannon, 2005). Due to the tonotopic organization of the cochlea, CI electrodes are nicely arranged along the primary spectral axis of the cochlea, so that electrodes at the base elicit high pitch sensations and electrodes at the apex elicit low pitch sensations. However, central auditory nuclei often have complex and multiple tonotopic representations within the nucleus, so that matching the electrodes to the tonotopic dimension is not always possible. In the case of the ABI the presumed mismatch between the stimulation presented to the surface electrode array and the tonotopic dimension of the CN did not appear to adversely affect the effectiveness of the device, but that may not be true as we target auditory nuclei higher in the system. However, there is likely a point of diminishing returns as we stimulate more and more centrally. At some point the artificial electric activation will produce a pattern of neural activity that is inappropriate for further processing and will not result in useful hearing sensations. Electrical stimulation of the visual cortex has not been successful probably because the evoked sensations from each electrode are complex and the sensations from different electrode locations do not coalesce into a single perceptual object. It is possible that auditory cortex will present the same problems as a target for prosthetic stimulation, but it is not yet known.

22.2 Electrical stimulation of the brainstem

22.2.1 Auditory brainstem implant

Auditory brainstem implants (ABIs) were developed to provide auditory sensations to patients with neurofibromatosis type 2 (NF2) (Brackmann *et al.*, 1993). NF2 is a genetic disorder located on chromosome 22 that is characterized by bilateral vestibular schwannomas (VS) and other schwannomas at or near the myal/glial junction in the brain and along the spinal cord (Trofatter *et al.*, 1993). VS are slowly growing tumors, but are life threatening and so must be removed. VS removal usually severs the auditory nerve so that a CI is of no use. The original ABI was a single electrode placed into the CN and the electrode design evolved over the years to become a multichannel array (Fig. 22.1). The ABI electrode array is inserted into the lateral recess of the IVth ventricle following tumor removal (Brackmann *et al.*, 1993). ABI patients receive sound awareness, some environmental sound discrimination and identification, and a significant improvement in face-to-face communication when the ABI is combined with lip reading (Shannon *et al.*, 1993; Lenarz *et al.*, 2001; Nevison *et al.*, 2002; Otto *et al.*, 2002). However, out of more than 600 ABIs worldwide, no ABI patients with NF2 have been able to achieve the high level of speech recognition that is common with CIs. Only ABI patients with other pathologies have been able to achieve CI-like speech recognition.

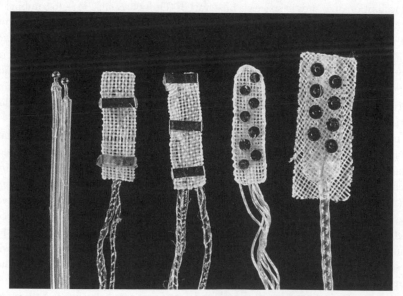

Fig. 22.1 Evolution of electrode designs for the surface array auditory brainstem implant. The initial patient in 1979 received a simple two-ball electrode. Subsequent patients received multi-electrode arrays on fabric backing inserted into the lateral recess of the IV ventricle. The fabric backing allows array fixation by encouraging fibrous ingrowth. (Copyright House Ear Institute, reproduced with permission.)

The CN has multiple tonotopic representations and none is arrayed along the surface in a manner that provides easy access from a surface electrode array. ABIs in patients typically produced a limited range of pitch sensations in the low pitch range and an absence of high pitch sensations presumably because high-pitch neurons are located deep inside the CN surface. Animal experiments showed that penetrating microelectrodes can provide low threshold levels, access to high-frequency neurons, and better tonotopic selectivity than surface electrodes (McCreery *et al.*, 1998).

22.2.2 Penetrating electrode ABI

A new type of ABI, the penetrating electrode ABI (PABI), was developed on the assumption that the limited performance in the NF2 ABI patients was due to the poor selectivity of the implant along the tonotopic dimension of the auditory system (compared to CIs). Thus, PABI results should be better than regular ABI results if ABI performance has been limited by tonotopic selectivity and the lack of high pitch activation. Patients fitted with PABIs achieved the goals of low stimulation thresholds, excellent tonotopic selectivity, and distinct pitch across electrodes, but have not demonstrated the expected high levels of open-set speech recognition (Otto *et al.*, 2008). In 2003 it appeared that the CN was already too high in the auditory system for effective prosthetic stimulation. NF2 patients with either surface or penetrating electrodes in the CN could not understand speech as well as CI listeners. However, a new development was taking place in Verona, Italy, that would change the future of ABIs: patients who did not have NF2 were implanted with the ABI and their performance was much better than that of NF2 ABI patients.

22.2.3 ABI in non-NF2 patients

The ABI was initially not offered to non-NF2 patients because it was thought that the risk–benefit ratio was not favorable. The average speech performance of NF2 patients with the ABI was poor compared to cochlear implantees – similar to results from older single-channel cochlear implantees. It was widely thought that the risks of a craniotomy and surgical approach to the brainstem were too great for voluntary surgery. In NF2 patients the surgery was performed primarily to remove life-threatening tumors; the additional risk of placing the ABI was minimal. To perform the surgery simply to obtain the apparently minimal auditory benefits of the ABI was not thought to be an acceptable trade-off.

However, Colletti felt that the risks of surgery to place an ABI were minimal and that it might be possible to obtain better results with an ABI in patients who did not have the tumors of NF2: patients who have lost cochlear nerve function due to other etiologies, including trauma and severe ossification of the cochlea and modiolus. Many of these non-tumor (NT) ABI users are capable of excellent speech understanding (Colletti *et al*, 2005; Colletti and Shannon, 2005) – similar to the high levels seen in CIs (Fig. 22.2). Figure 22.2 shows the percentage of patients whose performance on open set sentence recognition falls in each quintile. Four groups of patients are compared: 220 NF2 ABI patients from the House Ear Institute and Clinic, 10 PABI patients from Otto *et al.* (2008), 29 non-tumor (NT) patients from Colletti and Shannon (2005), and 30 CI patients from Spahr and Dorman (2004). Note that most of the NF2 ABI patients scored less than 20% correct on open set sentence recognition (most of these patients actually scored zero on this test). In contrast, the performance of NT ABI patients was evenly distributed from 0 to 100% correct, with approximately 50% of subjects scoring above 50% correct.

Because both NF2 and NT ABI patients use the same device, the same electrode placement, and the same speech processing strategy, the difference in patient outcomes appears to be due to the difference in etiology. It appears that the NF2 tumor growth and/or removal may damage neural

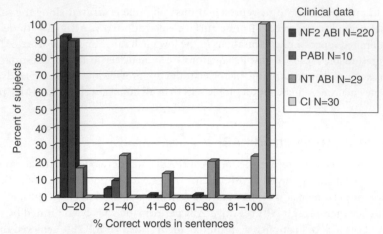

Fig. 22.2 Comparison of sentence recognition across implant devices and etiologies NF2 ABI, PABI, NT ABI, and CI. These sentences were presented in the auditory modality alone, i.e. without lip reading cues. The NF2 ABI results are updated from the results presented by Otto *et al.* (2002). PABI data are from Otto *et al.* (2008). NT ABI data are from Colletti and Shannon (2005). CI data are from Spahr and Dorman (2004).

elements in the CN that are essential for speech recognition. The results with NT ABI patients demonstrate that effective prosthetic stimulation is possible at the CN, despite the missing cochlea and auditory nerve and the highly unnatural neural activation patterns in the CN. This result has important implications for understanding the relative roles of the auditory periphery and the brain in hearing, as will be discussed later in greater detail.

22.2.4 **ABI in children**

Conditions that destroy the auditory nerve also occur in young children. Based on the experience with CIs in children, it appears that prosthetic devices applied in early childhood have an even greater chance of being successful due to early developmental plasticity. The early plasticity of the nervous system might allow young infants to better integrate the auditory patterns of neural activity from an ABI for speech recognition. However, it is probably important that children have sufficient neural survival in the CN to process the ABI activation. Conditions that produce abnormal development of the CN might not be suitable for an ABI. Anatomical and electrophysiological assessment tools are needed to determine whether or not an individual infant has a normally developed CN.

Of course the same critical periods for development apply equally to the CI and ABI. Studies have shown that CI performance is better when the device is implanted before 2 years of age (Svirsky *et al.*, 2000; Robbins *et al.*, 2004; Dettman *et al.*, 2007). Congenitally deaf children who receive the ABI prior to age 2 also would probably be more likely to learn to use the stimulation of the ABI for speech understanding. Children who were hearing at birth and then lost their auditory nerves due to ossification or trauma would also be more likely to gain benefit from the ABI for speech comprehension, because their brains are already experienced and trained with auditory stimulation patterns. As in CIs, congenitally deaf children who receive an ABI after the age of 5 would probably be less likely to develop speech understanding with the ABI alone.

Recently, ABIs have been used in children with cochlear malformation (Colletti *et al.*, 2005, 2009; Eisenberg *et al.*, 2008). Some of these children had hearing at birth and lost it due to meningitis or trauma. In some cases these children received a CI that provided no hearing sensations. Radiology subsequently showed the absence of an auditory nerve, explaining the failure of the CI. A few such children were implanted with an ABI and are now receiving auditory sensations. ABIs in children produce mixed results, with some children showing higher levels of auditory performance and learning than others (Colletti *et al.*, 2009). However, children of all etiologies fitted with ABIs do show improved auditory performance and improved cognitive development (Colletti and Zoccante, 2008).

Eisenberg *et al.* (2008) evaluated the performance of an ABI in a child with congenital cochlear malformation and cochlear nerve aplasia (Goldenhar syndrome). The child was implanted at age 3.5 years and was evaluated after 6 and 12 months of ABI experience. The child's performance with the ABI was comparable to that of a large cohort of congenitally deaf children implanted at a similar age with CIs. This result shows that the ABI can provide CI-like auditory development even in children with congenital absence of the auditory nerve. The different outcomes with ABIs in children appear to have a strong etiology component, but not enough cases are available at present to make definitive judgments of suitability of specific etiologies for the ABI.

22.2.5 Auditory midbrain implants and inferior colliculus implants

Two approaches have been used to deliver auditory stimulation to the IC in the midbrain: surface and penetrating electrodes. Colletti *et al.* (2007) reported useful auditory outcomes in a single patient with a surface electrode array on the IC, called the inferior colliculus implant (ICI). The surface electrode array was placed in a separate surgical procedure, gaining access to the IC via a supracerebellar-infratentorial approach. This patient was able to hear different pitch sensations on the different electrodes and had a full range of loudness on many electrodes. Threshold levels were low and showed changes in the first post-operative week, indicating that the electrode was in close proximity to the IC but moved slightly. The patient was able to integrate the sound from the device with lip reading to obtain an improvement in face to face communication. However, he was not able to recognize words and sentences only using the implant.

Lenarz and colleagues (Lim *et al.*, 2007, 2008) developed a penetrating electrode array for the IC and have implanted five patients as of June 2009. Only four of the five patients have been evaluated so far. The electrode array consisted of 20 contacts spaced along a single shaft. The electrode array had a stiffening rod in the center to aid penetration, which was then removed after electrode insertion. Electrodes were 0.126 mm^2 in surface area and were spaced 200 μm center-to-center. The entire array was 0.4 mm in diameter and 6 mm in length. Due to variations in anatomy and surgical landmarks three of the five implants were placed outside of the central nucleus of the IC. One of the first five patients had the array placed in the lateral lemniscus, two in the central nucleus of the IC, and two in the dorsal cortex of the IC. All patients received auditory sensations from most of the electrodes in the array, but the characteristics of their perception varied with the placement. The differences in the perceptual responses in the five patients give some insights into the functional differences in these locations. For example, the dorsal cortex of the IC produces perceptions that show dramatic adaptation, with a loud sensation fading to inaudibility after 10–20 s of continuous stimulation. The adaptation even occurs when the stimulation is modulated at a low rate (20 Hz). In contrast, adaptation was modest for the central nucleus of the IC and no adaptation was observed from stimulation of the lateral lemniscus. All other psychophysical measures were similar across the three stimulation sites.

All auditory midbrain implant (AMI) patients heard pitch changes across the electrodes, a full range of loudness as stimulus current was increased, and functional benefit in communication. The sound from the AMI allowed them to detect and discriminate environmental sounds, to recognize some distinctive sounds, and to improve communication over lip reading alone.

To date, no AMI patient has achieved significant open set speech recognition with electrical stimulation of the IC, but it is far too early to evaluate the ultimate success of these prostheses.

22.3 **Implications of prosthesis results for auditory processing**

With the wide variety of results from prostheses at different locations in the auditory system a picture emerges of the elements of pattern recognition in hearing. The excellent speech recognition that is common with CIs tells us that neither spectral nor temporal fine structure (TFS) is necessary. Once a brain is trained by 10-12 years of auditory experience, it is possible to understand speech when its acoustic representation has been reduced to four, octave-wide bands of noise, each modulated at temporal rates of less than 20 Hz (Shannon *et al.*, 1995). Such a signal is highly reduced in information relative to the full acoustic signal; it contains no harmonics, no formants, and no voice fundamental frequency. Yet it is highly intelligible. The tonotopic resolution in CIs has been measured to be considerably broader than comparable tuning curves measured in normal acoustic hearing (Nelson *et al.*, 2008). Furthermore, the signal processing for CIs removes TFS. Yet most CI listeners can converse on the telephone without difficulty.

Children less than 10–12 years of age cannot achieve the same level of speech understanding with degraded noise-band speech as adults (Eisenberg *et al.*, 2000). It appears that it takes the brain 12–15 years to fully develop complex pattern recognition to adult levels of fluency. Interestingly, this time scale roughly coincides with the time scale of myelination in the deep layers of auditory cortex (Moore and Guan, 2001). This suggests that experientially driven processes determine the connections in deep layers of cortex over more than a decade of learning. There are parallels to such a long time course in visual development as well: full maturation of object size constancy does not occur until 9–13 years of age.

One interesting question in the development of auditory pattern recognition is whether the unnatural patterns of activation provided by an auditory prosthesis are sufficient for learning in an infant who has not had experience with normal auditory input. In congenitally deaf children it appears that the coarse input from a CI is sufficient for the development of relatively normal speech recognition and even some limited development of musical production (Svirsky *et al.*, 2000; Robbins *et al.*, 2004; Dettman *et al.*, 2007). Thus, stimulation lacking spectral and TFS cues is sufficient for supporting the development of speech pattern recognition when applied to a cochlear implant.

There is some evidence that brainstem implants in congenitally deaf children can also provide sufficient cues for auditory development, but the extent of development with an ABI is not yet understood (Colletti *et al.*, 2005, 2009; Eisenberg *et al.*, 2008). ABI devices in NF2 adult patients have resulted in auditory benefit, but little open-set speech recognition (Otto *et al.*, 2002). Even the PABI device with penetrating microelectrodes has produced little open set speech recognition (Otto *et al.*, 2008). In contrast, excellent speech understanding has been demonstrated with the same, surface-electrode ABI device applied to patients without NF2 (Colletti and Shannon, 2005; Colletti *et al.* 2005). Let us examine the difference in outcomes between NF2 and non-tumor ABI patients. What differences could exist in perceptual capabilities and/or physiology that result in the dramatic difference in speech recognition shown in Fig. 22.2?

The only psychophysical ability that is correlated with speech recognition performance in ABIs is modulation detection (Colletti and Shannon, 2005), a correlation also observed in CI patients (Fu, 2002). Figure 22.3 shows a scatter plot of modulation detection and vowel recognition in 42 ABI patients. Open symbols show results from NF2 patients, while filled symbols show results from NT patients. The difference in scores between NF2 and NT ABI patients is significant for both modulation ($p < 0.001$) and for vowel recognition ($p < 0.005$). The correlation between the

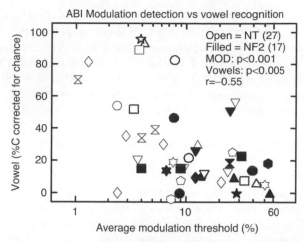

Fig. 22.3 Vowel recognition (%C indicates percent correct) plotted as a function of modulation detection score. The listener was presented with a single vowel and asked to select the presented item from a list of four possible vowels. Chance performance is 25% correct and the scores plotted are corrected for chance. The modulation detection scores represent the smallest amount of sinusoidal modulation detectable in a steady stimulus. The modulation frequency was 10 or 20 Hz and measures were collected from three to five stimulus levels that spanned the entire dynamic range, from very soft to very loud. *Open symbols* show results from ABI patients without tumors (NT) and *filled symbols* show results from ABI patients with NF2.

scores is modest ($r = -0.55$) but significant ($p < 0.01$). One interpretation of this correlation is that the neurons or pathways that support modulation detection are also important for speech recognition. In patients where modulation detection is impaired, speech recognition is also impaired. What neural pathways would support modulation and speech?

The limited performance of the ABI in NF2 patients appears to be due to something with regard to NF2: either the disease process itself, or negative sequellae of the tumor, or the tumor removal process. Some aspect of NF2 appears to damage a neural pathway that supports modulation detection and speech. The difference is probably not due to the disease process of NF2 because there are no known central manifestations of NF2; NF2 is primarily a disease of peripheral Schwann cells. The tumor growth typically occurs on the vestibular branch of the VIII nerve – it does not impact the CN directly. The presence of an NF2 tumor, even a very large tumor, does not necessarily damage the CN or disrupt hearing. Many NF2 cases exist where audiometrically normal hearing is present even with tumors exceeding 5 cm in diameter, a size at which there is considerable distortion of the brainstem. If the difference between ABI outcomes in NF2 and non-NF2 patients is not due to central manifestations of NF2, and is not due to tumor presence *per se*, then the most likely explanation is that tumor removal damages a critical portion of the CN.

Let us examine NF2 tumor removal surgery and its potential damage to the CN. NF2 VS are benign (non-metastatic) tumors that originate on the vestibular branch of the VIII nerve. These tumors can cause deafness even when they are quite small, if their point of origin is inside the internal auditory meatus. In such cases, they can cause deafness by pressure on the cochlear artery or by pressure directly on the VIII nerve itself. If, however, the tumor's point of origin is outside the meatus, the VS can grow into the cerebello-pontine angle without putting direct pressure on any auditory structure. In such cases, normal hearing can persist even with a large tumor. It is not common, but possible, that a 5- to 6-cm tumor can coexist with audiometrically normal hearing.

When the tumor diameter exceeds about 2 cm the tumor will contact the surface of the brainstem and start to distort the geometry of the brainstem. As the tumor grows it requires a blood supply and, as in most tumors, produces an angiogenesis factor at the surface that encourages capture of local blood supply to support the tumor. The primary blood supply to the CN derives from the posterior inferior cerebellar artery (PICA). The artery supplying the CN travels across the surface of the brainstem and then branches and descends into the CN. Thus, a tumor pressing against the surface of the brainstem could contact the vasculature that runs across the surface of the CN and compromise it.

During tumor removal surgery cautery is used to stop the bleeding. Since the vasculature is now shared between the tumor and the brainstem, this cautery may cause damage to the blood supply to the portions of the brainstem that are closest to the tumor and so most intimately interconnected in terms of vasculature. How much damage might such cautery produce? We know that most NF2 ABI patients can hear auditory sensations from electrical stimulation in the vicinity of the CN, so the damage is not so extensive that all auditory neurons are destroyed. Most NF2 ABI patients even hear different pitch sensations when different electrodes are stimulated, so some aspect of the tonotopic representation within the CN must be preserved. However, no NF2 ABI recipient has been able to achieve high levels of open set speech recognition. Thus, the putative damage to the CN from cautery during tumor removal must damage only a portion of the CN, but the portion that is damaged must be critical for speech recognition. In NT ABIs there is no tumor and so the surface vasculature is presumably intact.

Let us consider what region and cell type in the CN might be particularly susceptible to damage during surgery, thus resulting in deficits to speech recognition. In particular, consider the small cell cap (SCC) of the CN. The SCC is located on the surface of the CN, and while it is a relatively small structure in most mammals, it is greatly hypertrophied in humans (Moore and Osen, 1979; Moore, 1987) and porpoises. Because the SCC is on the lateral surface of the CN it is a structure that is most likely to be damaged by pressure from the tumor and trauma from the tumor removal. The SCC may be more susceptible to damage from cautery and vascular disruption during tumor removal because of its surface location.

Relatively little is known about the anatomical inputs and projections of the SCC and very little is known about its physiology. Liberman (1991) demonstrated that the SCC receives primarily the projections from the low-spontaneous rate (LSR) auditory neurons and that about half of the LSR neurons project only to the SCC. Goshal and Kim (1996) were able to measure response properties of neurons in the SCC. They have a large dynamic range, good response to modulated stimuli, and a sloping saturation, probably reflecting the properties of the primary auditory neurons with high thresholds and LSR. The SCC also receives some projections from the vestibular system, but their function is not clear. The projections from the SCC are not well documented, primarily because they are small fibers and difficult to maintain for recordings and injections. However, because they are small, they cannot maintain long axons and so probably project locally to within the CN.

Since the SCC is unusually large in humans and is in an anatomical location that would be susceptible to damage during tumor removal, we hypothesize that the SCC may be selectively damaged in NF2 patients, but not in patients who have lost their VIII nerve from other causes. Under this hypothesis, the presence or absence of the SCC leads to a major difference in outcomes with an ABI. If this hypothesis is correct it implies that the SCC is an essential part of the auditory pathway with respect to the processing of modulation and speech, and that the remaining auditory structures in the CN that are stimulated in NF2 patients are not sufficient to support speech understanding. It also suggests that speech pattern recognition is linked directly to specific cell types in the auditory periphery – as peripheral as the CN. Indeed, to the extent that the SCC is simply a relay structure for LSR neurons, speech pattern recognition may even be linked directly to a subset of primary auditory nerve fibers.

22.3.1 Separate processing streams for envelope and fine structure

Harmonic pitch and sound localization require fine-structure temporal information and probably fine spectral resolution as well, and may be served by a specialized independent processing pathway – the 'localization/pitch' pathway. One of the best-studied pathways in the auditory brainstem provides fine time structure information to the medial superior olive complex which allows localization of sound sources in space. In the auditory system such perceptual capability requires timing information in the order of tens of milliseconds, which necessitates its processing to be close to the periphery before the temporal information is smeared by the effect of intervening synapses. Several researchers and theorists have suggested that the medial superior olive with its specialization for encoding information about TFS may also play a role in harmonic pitch processing.

Implant results show that it is possible to recognize complex patterns of speech with only coarse spectral resolution and slowly changing temporal envelope information. This result suggests that central pattern recognition for speech, once trained, can resolve speech patterns with coarse information. Based on the difference in ABI outcomes in NF2 and non-NF2 patients we suggest that separate processing streams may originate as low as the brainstem splitting global pattern information from fine temporal and spectral structure information.

The processing of global spectral shape requires a different form of information and may reside in a separate physiological pathway as early as the CN. The cells of the SCC have a large dynamic range and so respond well to modulated stimuli over a wide amplitude range (Goshal and Kim, 1996). This large dynamic range is probably due to the fact that the low spontaneous rate auditory nerve fibers that project to the SCC have a higher threshold and so are active in an amplitude range where the peripheral cochlear amplifier is saturated (Liberman, 1991). Modulation detection over a wide range of amplitudes is a psychophysical capability that does correlate with speech recognition both in CIs (Fu, 2002) and in ABI (Colletti and Shannon, 2005; Fig. 22.3). Based on the difference in ABI outcomes between NF2 and NT patients, we propose that processing via the SCC may constitute a distinct and separate pathway of auditory processing.

Such separate processing pathways are well known in other sensory systems. In the processing of visual information it is now accepted that there are separate processing streams at the level of the visual cortex: termed the 'what' and'where' pathways (Borowsky et al., 2005). The 'what' pathway processes global pattern information that is necessary for object identification and is processed in the inferior ventral stream in the cortex, while the'where' pathway processes information that allows identification of the object motion and location in space and is processed in the superior dorsal stream in the cortex. Furthermore, recent physiological and behavioral studies have demonstrated two independent processing streams analogous to the'what' and'where' at the level of the auditory cortex: one for spectral pattern information and one for spatial localization and pitch (Kraus and Nicol, 2005; Lomber and Malhotra, 2008).

Let us consider two recent areas of research that support the separation of auditory processing into different streams: auditory chimeras and TFS cues for speech recognition.

22.3.2 Envelope cues vs temporal fine structure cues in speech recognition

The duality of TFS and envelope cues in perception has been the subject of several studies. In one experiment, temporal and spectral cues were put in conflict by the creation of auditory'chimeras'.'Chimeras' were created by combining the envelope of one sound with the fine structure of another using different numbers of spectral bands (Smith *et al.*, 2002). A wideband chimera is constructed by taking the TFS from one wideband signal and modulating it with the wideband envelope from a different signal. For such wideband signals the fine structure signal dominates the perception. This is because the wideband (single channel) envelope signal is not sufficient for speech recognition (van Tasell *et al.*, 1987; Shannon *et al.*, 1995). The wideband fine structure signal is refiltered by normal auditory filters which will reconstruct the multiband envelope signal from the fine structure signal (Ghitza, 2001). A different chimera can be constructed when the signal is filtered into 16 bands and then the fine structure and envelope signals are extracted from each band. The combination of the band-limited TFS of one sound and the band-limited envelope signal from another band has a different perceptual outcome compared to the wide band signal. In the multiband case the envelope signal dominates the perception. In this case a 16-band envelope signal is sufficient to convey clear speech intelligibility. The TFS signal from each band is now processed by one or two normal auditory filters, which is not enough to reconstitute the envelope signals of the original signal. This experiment demonstrated that envelope cues dominate perception; whether they are extracted explicitly as in the multiband case or reconstructed by the ear's own internal filters from the wideband temporal signal as in the wide-band case, it appears that, in quiet, envelope signals dominate over TFS cues in perception of speech.

In the presence of noise, however, TFS may be important. Qin and Oxenham (2003) measured speech recognition in fluctuating noise maskers for normal speech and for noise band vocoded speech. Noise vocoded speech represents speech using multiple bands of noise, each modulated by the envelope signal from that band of speech. Noise vocoded speech is typically intelligible with only four spectral bands when presented in quiet. Noise vocoded speech is more difficult to understand than unprocessed speech when presented in steady or fluctuating noise. In normal speech the signal to noise ratio at which 50% of the speech can be recognized is improved by almost 10 dB when the noise is fluctuating compared to steady noise. It is thought that this improvement is due to listeners being able to listen in the silent intervals of the fluctuating masker and synthesize the disjoint snippets of speech. However, when the speech was noise-band vocoded there was a clear deficit in recognition in both steady and fluctuating noise, even with 24 bands, a level of spectral resolution that results in an excellent representation of the spectral envelope. It appears that the loss of the TFS did not allow listeners sufficient harmonic pitch information to segregate the signal and maskers, even though the global spectral shape was providing excellent information about the speech signal.

Studies (Gilbert and Lorenzi, 2006; Lorenzi *et al.*, 2006) have demonstrated that at least part of the reason that hearing-impaired listeners have difficulty recognizing speech in noise is the loss of TFS. Some hearing-impaired listeners have difficulty in noise beyond what might be predicted from their degree of hearing loss. Psychophysical measures show that these listeners have a deficit in processing TFS information that may be independent from the loss of sensitivity and/or a broadened spectral resolution. Without good access to TFS it is difficult to derive the voicing fundamental frequency, a cue that helps formation of auditory objects and segregation of multiple sounds. Listeners with CIs have a similar deficit in accessing TFS information.

In summary, it appears that coarse envelope with no TFS is sufficient for speech understanding in quiet. However, TFS may be critical for music, harmonic pitch, and understanding speech in noise.

22.4 **Conclusions**

Clinical application of electrical stimulation to the auditory system has been more successful than was thought possible. At almost every stage of prosthesis development we have underestimated the potential benefit of the devices. For many years it was thought that CIs would never be able to allow normal conversation by telephone, but that is now a normal and expected outcome. It was thought that ABIs would never allow the same level of speech recognition as CIs, but many NT ABIs show comparable performance to CIs. Will AMIs allow open set speech recognition for NF2 patients or others with damage to the CN? It is still too early to know. Will children with cochlear nerve aplasia be able to learn to understand speech using the stimulation of an ABI? Early results suggest that this may be achievable for some etiologies. There are many questions still to be answered in the application of electrical stimulation to restore hearing. Properly controlled scientific and clinical studies are needed to 'push the envelope' of outcomes. Implant technology has been a great success story in otolaryngology and the ultimate limits of the technology are still not known. Clinical outcomes can feed back into auditory neuroscience to help us understand the functional consequences of damage to specific structures within the auditory pathway. The interplay between clinical outcomes and neuroscience will help to refine our knowledge of auditory processing pathways and to design improved prostheses in the future.

References

Borowsky R, Loehr J, Friesen CK, Kraushaar G, Kingstone A, Sarty G (2005) Modularity and intersection of "what", "where" and "how" processing of visual stimuli: a new method of FMRI localization. *Brain Topogr* 18(2): 67–75.

Brackmann DE, Hitselberger WE, Nelson RA, *et al.* (1993) Auditory brainstem implant. I: Issues in surgical implantation. *Otolaryngol Head Neck Surg* 108: 624–34.

Colletti L, Zoccante L (2008) Non-verbal cognitive abilities and auditory performance in children fitted with ABI: preliminary report. *Laryngoscope* 118(8): 1443–8.

Colletti V, Shannon RV (2005) Open set speech perception with auditory brainstem implant?. *Laryngoscope* 115: 1974–8.

Colletti V, Carner M, Miorelli V, Guida M, Colletti L, Fiorino F (2005) Auditory brainstem implant (ABI): new frontiers in adults and children. *Otolaryngol Head Neck Surg* 133(1): 126–38.

Colletti V, Shannon RV, Carner M, *et al.* (2007) The first successful case of hearing produced by electrical stimulation of the human midbrain. *Otol Neurotol* 28(1): 39–43.

Colletti L, Colletti V, Carner M, Veronese S, Shannon RV (2009) The development of auditory perception in children following auditory brainstem implantation. *Otol Neurotol* (in press).

Dettman L, Pinder D, Briggs R, Dowell R, Leigh J (2007) Communication development in children who receive the cochlear implant younger than 12 months: risks versus benefits. *Ear Hear* 28: 11S–18S.

Eisenberg L, Shannon RV, Martinez AS, Wygonski J, Boothroyd A (2000) Speech recognition with reduced spectral cues as a function of age. *J Acoust Soc Am* 107(5): 2704–10.

Eisenberg LS, Johnson KC, Martinez AS, *et al.* (2008) Comprehensive evaluation of a child with an auditory brainstem implant. *Otol Neurotol* 29(2): 251–7.

Fu Q-J (2002) Temporal processing and speech recognition in cochlear implant users. *Neuro Re* 13: 1635–9.

Ghitza O (2001) On the upper cutoff frequency of the auditory critical-band envelope detectors in the context of speech perception. *J Acoust Soc Am* 110: 1628–40.

Gifford RH, Dorman MF, McKarns SA, Spahr AJ (2007) Combined acoustic and contralateral acoustic hearing: word and sentence recognition with bimodal hearing. *J Speech Lang Hear Res* 50: 835–43.

Gilbert G, Lorenzi C (2006) The ability of listeners to use recovered envelope cues from speech fine structure. *J Acoust Soc Am* 119: 2438–44.

Goshal S, Kim DO (1996) Marginal shell of the anteroventral cochlear nucleus: intensity coding in single units of the unanesthetized, decerebrate cat. *Neurosci Lett* 205: 71–4.

Koch DB, Downing M, Osberger MJ, Litvak L (2007) Using current steering to increase spectral resolution in CII and HiRes 90K users. *Ear Hear* 28(2 Suppl): 38S–41S.

Kraus N, Nicol T (2005) Brainstem origins for cortical 'what' and 'where' pathways in the auditory system. *Trend Neurosci* 28: 176–81.

Krueger B, Joseph G, Rost U, Strauss-Schier A, Lenarz T, Buechner A (2008) Performance groups in adult cochlear implant users: speech perception results from 1984 until today. *Otol Neurotol* 29: 509–12.

Lenarz T, Moshrefi M, Matthies M, *et al.* (2001) Auditory brainstem implant: part I. Auditory performance and its evolution over time. *Otol Neurotol* **22**: 823–33.

Liberman MC (1991) Central projections of auditory nerve fibers of differing spontaneous rate. I. Anteroventral cochlear nucleus. *J Comp Neurol* **313**: 240–58.

Lim HH, Lenarz T, Joseph G, *et al.* (2007) Electrical stimulation of the midbrain for hearing restoration: Insight into the functional organization of the human central auditory system. *J Neurosci* **27**: 13541–51.

Lim HH, Lenarz T, Anderson DJ, Lenarz M (2008) The auditory midbrain implant: effects of electrode location. *Hear Res* **242**: 74–85.

Litovsky RY, Parkinson A, Arcaroli J, *et al.* (2004) Bilateral cochlear implants in adults and children. *Arch Otolaryngol Head Neck Surg.* **130**(5): 648–55.

Lomber SG, Malhotra S (2008) Double dissociation of 'what' and 'where' processing in auditory cortex. *Nat Neurosci* **11**(5): 609–16.

Lorenzi C, Gilbert G, Carn H, Garnier S, Moore BCJ (2006) Speech perception problems of the hearing impaired reflect inability to use temporal fine structure. *PNAS* **103**: 18866–9.

McCreery DG, Shannon RV, Moore JK, Chatterjee M, Agnew WF (1998) Accessing the tonotopic organization of the ventral cochlear nucleus by intranuclear microstimulation. *IEEE Trans Rehab Eng* **6**(4): 391–9.

Moore JK (1987) The human auditory brainstem: a comparative view. *Hear Res* **29**: 1–32.

Moore JK, Guan YL (2001) Cytoarchitectural and axonal maturation in human auditory cortex. *J Assoc Res Otolaryngol* **2**(4): 297–311.

Moore JK, Osen KK (1979) The cochlear nuclei in man. *Am J Anat* **154**: 393–417.

Nelson DA, Donaldson GS, Kreft H (2008) Forward-masked spatial tuning curves in cochlear implant users. *J Acoust Soc Am* **123**: 1522–43.

Nevison B, Laszig R, Sollmann WP, *et al.* (2002) Results from a European clinical investigation of the nucleus multichannel auditory brainstem implant. *Ear Hear* **23**: 170–83.

Otto SA, Brackmann DE, Hitselberger WE, Shannon RV, Kuchta J (2002) The multichannel auditory brainstem implant update: performance in 60 patients. *J Neurosurg* **96**: 1063–71.

Otto SR, Shannon RV, Brackmann DE, *et al.* (2008) Audiological outcomes with the penetrating electrode auditory brainstem implant. *Otol Neurotol* **29**: 1147–54.

Qin MK, Oxenham AJ (2003) Effects of simulated cochlear implant processing on speech reception in fluctuating maskers. *J Acoust Soc Am* **114**: 446–54.

Robbins KM, Koch DB, Osberger MJ, Zimmerman-Phillips S, Kishon-Rabin L (2004) The effect of age at cochlear implantation on auditory skill development in infants and toddlers. *Arch Otolaryngol Head Neck Surg* **130**: 570–74.

Shannon RV, Fayad J, Moore JK, *et al.* (1993) Auditory brainstem implant. II: Post-surgical issues and performance. *Otolaryngol Head Neck Surg* **108**: 635–43.

Shannon RV, Zeng F-G, Kamath V, Wygonski J, Ekelid M (1995) Speech recognition with primarily temporal cues. *Science* **270**: 303–4.

Shannon RV, Fu Q-J, Galvin J (2004) The number of spectral channels required for speech recognition depends on the difficulty of the listening situation. *Acta Oto-Laryngolog Suppl* **552**: 50–4.

Smith ZM, Delgutte B, Oxenham AJ (2002) Chimaeric sounds reveal dichotomies in auditory perception. *Nature* **416**: 87–90.

Spahr AJ, Dorman MF (2004) Performance of subjects fit with the advanced bionics CII and nucleus 3G cochlear implant devices. *Arch Otolaryngol HNS* **130**: 624–8.

Svirsky MA, Robbins AM, Kirk KI, Pisoni DB, Miyamoto RT (2000) Language development in profoundly deaf children with cochlear implants. *Psychol Sci* **11**(2): 153–8.

Trofatter JA, MacCollin MM, Rutter JL, *et al.* (1993) A novel moesin-, ezrin-, radixin-like gene is a candidate for the neurofibromatosis 2 tumor suppressor. *Cell* **72**: 791–800.

van Tasell DJ, Soli SD, Kirby VM, Widin GP (1987) Speech waveform envelope cues for consonant recognition. *J Acoust Soc Am* **82**: 1152–61.

Index